MX 0709132 X

KU-208-994

ESSENTIAL GENERAL SURGICAL OPERATIONS

W/d 25/3/2024

DEDICATION

To our families:
Peggy, Valentine, Jeremy and Louise (RMK)
and
Esther, Kitty, Harold and Jonah (MCW)

Commissioning Editor: **Laurence Hunter**
Development Editor: **Janice Urquhart**
Project Manager: **Emma Riley**
Text Design: **Charles Gray**
Cover Design: **Stewart Larking**
Illustrator: **Ian Ramsden**
Illustration Manager: **Gillian Richards**

ESSENTIAL GENERAL SURGICAL OPERATIONS

SECOND EDITION

EDITED BY

R. M. Kirk MS FRCS
Honorary Professor of Surgery, The Royal Free and University College Medical School, London, UK;
Honorary Consulting Surgeon, The Royal Free Hospital, London, UK

M. C. Winslet MS FRCS
Professor of Surgery and Head of Division of Surgery and Interventional Science, The Royal Free and University College Medical School, London, UK

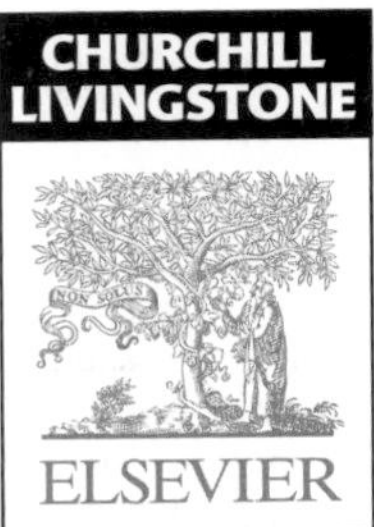

Edinburgh • London • New York • Oxford • Philadelphia • St Louis • Sydney • Toronto 2007

Site WH | MIDDLESEX UNIVERSITY LIBRARY
Accession No. 0709132
Class No. WO500 ESS
Special Collection ✓

CHURCHILL
LIVINGSTONE
An imprint of Elsevier Limited

© R. M. Kirk and M. C. Winslet 2001
© R. M. Kirk and M. C. Winslet 2007

The right of R. M. Kirk and M. C. Winslet to be identified as editors of this work has been asserted by them in accordance with the Copyright, Designs and Patents Act 1988

No part of this publication may be reproduced, stored in a retrieval system, or transmitted in any form or by any means, electronic, mechanical, photocopying, recording or otherwise, without the prior permission of the Publishers. Permissions may be sought directly from Elsevier's Health Sciences Rights Department, 1600 John F. Kennedy Boulevard, Suite 1800, Philadelphia, PA 19103-2899, USA: phone: (+1) 215 239 3804; fax: (+1) 215 239 3805; or, e-mail: healthpermissions@elsevier.com. You may also complete your request on-line via the Elsevier homepage (http://www.elsevier.com), by selecting 'Support and contact' and then 'Copyright and Permission'.

First edition 2001
Second edition 2007

ISBN: 978 0 443 10314 8

British Library Cataloguing in Publication Data
A catalogue record for this book is available from the British Library

Library of Congress Cataloging in Publication Data
A catalog record for this book is available from the Library of Congress

Note

Knowledge and best practice in this field are constantly changing. As new research and experience broaden our knowledge, changes in practice, treatment and drug therapy may become necessary or appropriate. Readers are advised to check the most current information provided (i) on procedures featured or (ii) by the manufacturer of each product to be administered, to verify the recommended dose or formula, the method and duration of administration, and contraindications. It is the responsibility of the practitioner, relying on their own experience and knowledge of the patient, to make diagnoses, to determine dosages and the best treatment for each individual patient, and to take all appropriate safety precautions. To the fullest extent of the law, neither the Publisher nor the Editors assume any liability for any injury and/or damage to persons or property arising out or related to any use of the material contained in this book.

The Publisher

ELSEVIER your source for books, journals and multimedia in the health sciences
www.elsevierhealth.com

Working together to grow libraries in developing countries
www.elsevier.com | www.bookaid.org | www.sabre.org
ELSEVIER BOOK AID International Sabre Foundation

The publisher's policy is to use **paper manufactured from sustainable forests**

Printed in China

Contents

CONTENTS

Preface

We have changed our priorities since the first edition in 2001 in response to the changes in training. Aspiring surgeons previously hoped to obtain junior posts in their selected specialty and join a stream of trainees who gained the trust of consultants, which was rewarded with delegation of increasing responsibility in well-recognized operative training procedures. As a result we concentrated on giving full coverage to procedures likely to be performed by trainees in each specialty.

In the past the common path to a surgical career was through general surgery. Aspiring surgeons honed their skills on minor general surgical procedures. Attachments now tend to be short and include a number of specialities; yours may bypass some or all of general surgery. In response to this we needed to widen the scope to provide information on frequently performed procedures within the generality of surgery. We hope that this will equip you, whatever your rotations, to understand the principles of a wide range of operations, to stimulate your interest, equip you to assist intelligently and inform you to provide the necessary peri-operative care. We have not neglected to give detailed accounts of those operations that may be delegated to you. Reinforce the descriptions by reviewing the relevant anatomy and you will be able to benefit from actively participating in interesting procedures. Many of the lessons you learn in one field are transferable to other areas.

In order to offer you the most comprehensive guidance possible we needed to make some difficult decisions to keep down the size and price. We reluctantly restricted some diagrams because you can compensate by reading the book alongside an anatomy text. This enabled us to mention some of the latest operative techniques while retaining the step by step guidance of operations which may be delegated to you.

This is a 'What to do' book. It assumes you have taken the trouble to study the basis of 'How to do it' in, for example, *Basic Surgical Techniques*. In order to keep the size of the book within limits we have omitted perioperative management; this is fully covered in *Clinical Surgery in General*. Both of these are also published by Elsevier.

We are well aware that you may not be fortunate enough to gain as much practical experience as you would like. Textbooks offer guidance but they cannot tell the whole story. You gain most from watching, assisting, and being assisted by, an experienced surgeon. You will be inspired and learn without effort, almost by 'osmosis'. A wonderful writer on acquiring skills wrote, 'By watching the master and emulating his efforts in the presence of his example, the apprentice unconsciously picks up the rules of the art, including those which are not explicitly known to the master himself.'* Make the most of your contacts with inspiring teachers and experts. Seize every offer to assist and perform practical procedures. Thomas Hardy, the novelist, stated, 'Experience is as to intensity, not as to duration.'

Many readers do not have English as a first language, and some who have been brought up with English accept new words without knowing their true meaning. We have given the origin of some unusual words in the hope of stimulating you to develop an interest in using words precisely. You may also enjoy the notes on some of your predecessors who have contributed to our advances in surgery.

Apology

We apologize to women surgeons and women in general if we occasionally use the male pronoun on its own. Constant repetition of, 'he and she', 'him and her', 'his and hers', and inappropriate use of plural pronouns can be irritating. There is no epicene third personal pronoun. 'Master' refers to someone possessing superior skills – 'Mistress,' has a very different connotation!

**Michael Polanyi, 1973, Personal Knowledge, Routledge & Kegan Paul, London, p. 53.*

Contributors

Hiroshi Akiyama MD FRCS(Eng) FACS
Senior Adviser, Toranomon Hospital, Tokyo, Japan

Shaun G. Appleton MS FRCS
Consultant Surgeon, Wycombe Hospital, High Wycombe, UK

Satyajit Bhattacharya MS MPhil FRCS
Consultant Surgeon, Royal London and St Bartholomew's Hospitals, London, UK

Michael D. Brough (Deceased)

Kevin G. Burnand MB BS FRCS MS
Professor of Surgery, Guy's, King's and St Thomas's Medical School, King's College London, London, UK

Peter Butler MD FRCSI FRCS FRCS(Plast)
Consultant Plastic Surgeon, Department of Plastic Surgery, Royal Free Hospital, London, UK

C. Richard G. Cohen MS FRCS
Consultant Surgeon, University College Hospitals, London, UK

Richard E. C. Collins MB BS FRCS(Eng) FRCS(Ed)
Consultant Surgeon, Kent and Canterbury Hospital, East Kent NHS Trust, UK

Frank W. Cross MS FRCS
Consultant Surgeon, Royal London Hospital, London, UK

Ara Darzi KBE HonFREng FMedSci MD FRCS FACS FRCS(I)
Professor of Surgery and Head of Division, Department of Surgical Oncology and Technology, Imperial College London, St Mary's Hospital, London, UK

Roy W. R. Farrell MA MB BAO BCL FRCSI FRCS
Consultant Otolaryngologist and Head and Neck Surgeon, Northwick Park Hospital, Harrow, UK

Chris Fowler BSc MA MS FRCP FRCS(Urol) FEBU
Professor of Surgical Education and Honorary Consultant Urologist, Barts and the London, Queen Mary's School of Medicine and Dentistry, University of London, London, UK

Nicholas Goddard MB BS FRCS
Consultant Orthopaedic Surgeon, The Royal Free Hospital, London, UK

Gareth Harper MA BM BChir FRCS(Orth)
Consultant Orthopaedic Surgeon, Queen Alexandra Hospital, Portsmouth, UK

Peter L. Harris MB ChB Md FRCS(Eng)
Consultant Vascular Surgeon and Director of Vascular Services, Regional Vascular Unit, Royal Liverpool University Hospital, Liverpool, UK

Michael Hobsley MA MB MChir PhD DSc FRCS
Emeritus Professor, Department of Surgery, University College London Medical School, London, UK

Jonathan D. Jagger MB BS FRCS DO FRCOphth
Consultant Ophthalmic Surgeon, Eye Department, The Royal Free Hospital, London, UK

Long R. Jiao MD FRCS(Eng)
Senior Lecturer, Honorary Consultant Surgeon, Department of Hepatopancreobiliary Surgery, Hammersmith Hospital Campus, Division of Surgery, Anaesthesia and Intensive Care, Imperial College School of Medicine, London, UK

Islam Junaid MB BS FRCS(Ed) FRCS(Urol)
Consultant Urological and Transplant Surgeon, Barts and The London NHS Trust, London, UK

Ajay K. Kakkar MB BS BSc PhD FRCS
Professor and Head, Centre for Surgical Science, Barts and The London, Queen Mary's School of Medicine and Dentistry, University of London; Consultant Surgeon, St Bartholomew's and Royal London Hospitals; Director Designate, Thrombosis Research Institute, London, UK

Robin R. Kanagasabay MB BS BSc FRCS(CTh) MRCP
Consultant Cardiothoracic Surgeon, Department of Cardiothoracic Surgery, St George's Healthcare NHS Trust, London, UK

R. M. Kirk MS FRCS
Honorary Professor of Surgery, The Royal Free and University College Medical School, London, UK; Honorary Consulting Surgeon, The Royal Free Hospital, London, UK

Iain M. Laws TD MB ChB FDSRCS
Emeritus Consultant, Maxillofacial Surgeon, The Royal Free Hospital, London, UK

Roger J. Leicester OBE MB FRCS(Edin & Eng)
Consultant Colorectal Surgeon, St George's Hospital, London; Endoscopy Tutor, Raven Department of Education, Royal College of Surgeons of England, London, UK

Robert Mason BSc MB ChB ChM MD FRCS(Eng) FRCS(Ed)
Consultant Upper GI Surgeon and Deputy Medical Director, Guy's and St Thomas's Hospitals, London, UK

R. S. Maurice-Williams MA MB BChir FRCP FRCS
Consultant Neurosurgeon, Neurosurgical Unit, The Royal Free Hospital, London, UK

Bridget Mulholland MD FRCOphth
Consultant Ophthalmologist, The Norfolk and Norwich University Hospital, Norfolk; The James Paget University Hospitals, Great Yarmouth, UK

Stephen J. Nixon MB ChB BSc FRCS FRCP
Consultant Surgeon, Royal Infirmary, Edinburgh, UK

P. A. Paraskeva PhD FRCS(GenSurg)
Department of Biosurgery and Surgical Oncology, Imperial College London, and St Mary's Hospital, London, UK

Arthanari Rajasekar MB BS MD(GenSurg) FRCS(Eng) FRCS(Ire)
Consultant Gastrointestinal and Laparoscopic Surgeon, Department of Gastroenterology and Endoscopic Surgery, Sri Gokulam Hospital, Salem, Tamilnadu, India

John A. Rennie MS FRCS
Consultant Surgeon, King's College Hospital, London, UK

Gavin S. M. Robertson MB ChB MD FRCS
Consultant Surgeon, Department of Surgery, Leicester Royal Infirmary, Leicester, UK

T. Rockall MD FRCS
Consultant Surgeon, Minimal Access Therapy Training Unit, Royal Surrey County Hospital, Guildford, UK

Keith Rolles MA MS FRCS
Consultant Surgeon, The Royal Free Hospital, London, UK

James M. Ryan MCh FRCS DMCC
Leonard Cheshire Professor of Conflict Recovery, University College London; International Professor of Surgery, USUHS, Bethesda, Maryland, USA

Richard Sainsbury MB BS MD FRCS
Reader in Surgery and Honorary Consultant Surgeon, Rogal Free and University College Medical School, University College London, London, UK

Marcus E. Setchell CVO MB BChir FRCS(Eng) FRCOG
Consultant Obstetrician and Gynaecologist, Whittington Hospital, London; Honorary Consultant Gynaecologist, King Edward VII Hospital, London, UK

Arjun Shankar MD FRCS
Consultant Surgeon, University College Hospitals, London, UK

Robert S. Simons QHP(C) MB ChB FRCA FANZCA
Consultant Anaesthetist, The Royal Free Hospital, London, UK

Lewis Spitz MB ChB PhD MD FRCS(Edin) FRCS(Eng) FRCPCH FAAP
Emeritus Nuffield Professor of Paediatric Surgery, Institute of Child Health, University College London; Consultant Paediatric Surgeon, Great Ormond Street Hospital for Children NHS Trust, London, UK

Michael P. Stearns MB Bs BDS FRCS
Consultant Otolaryngologist/Head and Neck Surgeon, The Royal Free Hospital, London, UK

Ian D. Sugarman MB ChB FRCS(Ed) FRCS(Paed)
Consultant Paediatric Surgeon, Leeds General Infirmary, Leeds, UK

Justin Tan MB BS MRCS
Academic Department of Surgery, St Thomas's Hospital, London, UK

Jeremy N. Thompson MA MB MChir FRCS
Consultant Surgeon, Chelsea and Westminster and Royal Marsden Hospitals, London, UK

Tom Treasure MD MS FRCS FRCP
Consultant Thoracic Surgeon, Guy's and St Thomas's Hospital, London; Professor of Cardiothoracic Surgery, Department of Cardiothoracic Surgery, University of London, London, UK

Matthew G. Tutton BSc MRCS
Specialist Registrar in General Surgery, London Deanery, London, UK

Harushi Udagawa MD DMSc FACS
Head of Gastroenterological Surgery, Toranomon Hospital, Tokyo, Japan

Carolynne Jane Vaizey MD FRCS(Gen) FCS(SA)
Consultant Surgeon, St Mark's Hospital, London, UK

David F. L. Watkin MChir FRCS
Retired Consultant Surgeon, Leicester Royal Infirmary, Leicester, UK

James M. Wellwood MA MChir(Cantab) FRCS(Eng)
Consultant Surgeon and Honorary Senior Lecturer, Whipps Cross Hospital, London, UK

Douglas E. Whitelaw MB ChB FRCS(Ed) FRCS(GenSurg)
Consultant Surgeon, Luton and Dunstable Hospital, Luton, UK

R. C. N. Williamson MS FRCS MChir FRCS PhD
Consultant Surgeon, Hammersmith Hospital, London; Professor of Surgery, Imperial College, London; Dean, Royal Society of Medicine, London, UK

Marc C. Winslet MS FRCS
Professor of Surgery and Head of Division of Surgery and Interventional Science, The Royal Free and University College Medical School, London, UK

Acknowledgements

Thank you to all of you who have helped to produce this book: the illustrator Ian Ramsden, copyeditor Laila Grieg-Gran, proofreaders Alison Breewood, Ian Ross and Sandra Slater, and the indexer, Lynda Swindells.

1

Choose well, cut well, get well

R. M. Kirk

CONTENTS

INTRODUCTION

'Choose well, cut well, get well' is a succinct American aphorism summing up the requirements for successful surgery. As in so many complex procedures, the whole is dependent upon every single step. The adage 'Complications are made in the operating room' is not altogether true. Although an incompetently performed operation is likely to bring disaster, it is equally dangerous to perform a skilful but inappropriate procedure on an ill-prepared patient and fail to monitor recovery. The American surgeon Frank Spencer has stated that good surgery is about 20–25% manual dexterity and 70–75% decision-making.[1]

It is worrying that close contact between master and apprentice has diminished, reducing valuable teaching by example, so that not only explicit knowledge but also tacit wisdom and attitudes that cannot be put into words[2] have been eroded in surgical training[3] in favour of 'modular' teaching. Module (Latin *modulus*, diminutive of *modus* = measure) has the connotation of teaching, by defined units, a series of competences each of which can be tested. At the end of the course the sum of the competences should represent all that the pupil requires. This is an unjustifiable assumption; it is of great importance how the aptitudes are applied. There is a danger that the important whole is delegated to secondary importance.[4] As the Gestalt psychologists emphasized at the beginning of the 20th century, the whole is greater than the sum of its parts. We are adjured to apply evidence-based management of patients, but the changes in surgical training are arbitrary – no evidence is presented that overall clinical care of patients is improved by compartmentalizing surgical training. There is a multiplicity of interacting and changing factors at work that affect surgical outcomes.

In the past, the decisions and actions made by physicians and surgeons were rarely questioned. Vogue and idiosyncratic treatments and operations were performed without discussion. The Guy's Hospital surgeon Sir William Withey Gull (1816–1890) stated, 'Make haste and use the new remedies before they lose their effectiveness'.

Public expectations, which were previously low, have risen, driving the medical profession towards greater intra-professional surveillance, more evidence-based treatments, with review of outcomes. There is corresponding pressure to identify and deal with those who do not maintain acceptable standards. Inevitably, outcome data for individual surgeons is increasingly collected. Because a surgical operation is a specific event in management, it is too easily, and uncritically, used to compare results between surgeons. We shall need to pay as much attention to the outcome in those patients we decide not to submit to operation, especially since there is now a choice in many traditional surgical fields between effective drugs and treatment using endoscopic and interventional radiological methods.

CHOOSE WELL

Decide

The existence of double-blind, controlled clinical trials is well known. Our patients reasonably expect us to choose the correct management for their surgical conditions. Of the treatment methods available, surely, they will say, it is possible, after testing them, to conclude that one is better than the others. Ideally, there should be but one variable, the treatment. Unfortunately, biological variability is so great that very often a conclusive answer cannot be given. The physical and psychological condition of patients and the extent and virulence of diseases make it difficult or impossible to study matched groups of people with matched disease severity. As new methods become available, conflicting evidence emerges about their effectiveness and safety compared with existing methods.

Our selection of facts from the available evidence varies as individuals and between surgeons. From the accumulated information, one investigator may be influenced to follow one path, whereas another may direct the focus to other evidence. In reaching a decision about a particular patient, not all pieces of evidence are of equal value. Some features are common to many conditions, but we need to be influenced more by those that are discriminant (Latin *discrimen* = that which separates).

KEY POINTS Assessing evidence, decisions and priorities

- When collecting or assessing evidence on which to make a decision, there is a tendency to prefer numerically (digitally) expressed indicators over analogue (continuously variable) evidence. This is natural, because numbers can be compared easily. However, ensure that what is chosen to be measured is valid, and not selected merely because it can be assigned numbers.
- If the results of your investigations conflict with your carefully and confidently obtained clinical findings, trust your clinical judgement.
- At intervals review the order of your priorities. They do not remain static.
- Be flexible. Anticipate, recognize and react to changed circumstances.
- If you are about to make a heterodox (Greek *heteros* = other + *doxa* = opinion; different from the generally accepted one) decision, ask yourself, 'If my selected course of management fails, can I justify my actions to the patient, to my peers and, most importantly, to myself?'

We tend to favour evidence that fits our recent experience, perhaps of a run of successes or disasters, to change our viewpoint and our existing beliefs. A postal questionnaire to surgeons revealed, as one would expect, that those with a declared interest in laparoscopic surgery were more likely to advise their patients to have a laparoscopic hernia repair and to select it for themselves, than those without a declared interest.[5]

In some cases we may not have a diagnosis but a clinical feature alone that demands action on our part. This is particularly true for some emergencies, when the exact cause of a life-threatening haemorrhage, cardiorespiratory failure, peritonitis or pyrexia typical of sepsis may not be clear, but urgent treatment is necessary.

We cannot concentrate on a single patient in circumstances where many people are ill. This is particularly true in wartime or a civilian disaster. In such cases we must make urgent, sometimes agonizing, decisions. This process of triage (Old French: to pick, select) involves choosing to treat first those whose lives can be saved by quick action, deferring treatment of those with multiple or peripheral injuries. Possible loss of a limb or a special sense is less urgent than cases whose very survival depends on quick, effective action: 'Life comes before limb'.

Even in elective circumstances we need to make decisions with incomplete information. We never have all the necessary facts available about the physical and mental state of our patient but make the best guess, based on our general knowledge, the results of appropriately selected investigations, and often by intuition.

Some surgeons get better results than others, although there is no objectively assessable difference in their competence from the average. Possibly they analyse their results more critically than others, make better judgements, set higher than average standards. The higher ratio of accurate decisions may be based on tacit knowledge, i.e. knowledge that cannot be explicitly stated or objectively identified. They are sometimes referred to as 'lucky surgeons'. Success in individual cases does not necessarily indicate good judgement; a robust patient may improve in spite of inappropriate treatment. Conversely, a susceptible patient may deteriorate despite the best treatment.

When seeking a solution to a difficult but not urgent problem, take the opportunity to set it aside while you do something else. In some cases you may leave it overnight. There is mounting evidence that the answer to a problem formulates during sleep.[6] It is remarkable how solutions often appear spontaneously, sometimes as a result of viewing the situation from a fresh point of view. It is also valuable to re-examine, after an interval, the patient who presents with, for example, an acute abdomen, since the physical signs can change rapidly.

If you reach a decision, regard it as only provisional. Since it is based on incomplete knowledge, you may discover further facts, or the observed effects of your management may suggest that you review and revise the course of action. Too often, initially good management fails because it is inexorably pursued when the circumstances change. Your initial plan is comparable with the *strategy* of a general before battle, but he may need to alter his *tactics* as the battle develops.

Attempts to rationalize decisions have resulted in the development of *algorithms*, or standard, step-by-step actions, and *protocols*, which provide a standard approach leading to an expected optimum outcome. Especially in the USA, pressure from managed care organizations and 'stakeholders' (insurers and those who pay the bills) has resulted in *guidelines* and *clinical pathways*, although not all of them have been verified.[7] Such methods have been worked out and evaluated by experts in the particular fields where they can be applied. They do not necessarily fit every circumstance but provide a routine approach that aims to give the best results in most cases. Such methods need to be re-evaluated from time to time as views change with improvements in diagnosis and therapeutics, and in the light of follow-up. *Decision analysis*, another aid in evaluating the best course of action, is discussed later.

Remember that all these procedural guides are made to give the best results in the majority of circumstances. They do not fit every situation. For example, when treating major abdominal injuries it is usually possible to stabilize the patient's condition and carry out relevant diagnostic tests. At laparotomy when indicated, you would stop bleeding, explore the whole abdomen, repair all damage and close up. However, you cannot deliberately follow this routine if the patient is bleeding calamitously. You need to recognize that controlling the bleeding is paramount. It may be necessary to pack the abdomen, close it and defer any further action until you have stabilized the patient (see Ch. 3, 'Damage-control laparotomy').

Do not be too proud to take advice. The very action of arranging and presenting the problem to another person often clarifies it.

When you have reached a decision, you must discuss it with the patient, who has the right to participate. However much we try to offer an objective judgement, it is inevitable that the presentation to our patients is biased. Our decision is the one in which we believe, and inevitably we weight the evidence towards our selected management. There is nothing dishonest about this. Indeed, it would be cowardly not to give positive advice. We have access to the available facts and have to weigh them, reach a decision and place that decision before the patient. It is our professional duty to take responsibility for our decisions and irresolute to place the whole burden on to the patient. This does not, of course, excuse us if we ignore or override the patient's wishes. Patients faced with treatment decisions look at different criteria from us, such as quality of life, maintenance of independence and dignity; our anxieties revolve more closely around survival.[8,9] Investigations, protocols, guidelines, risk and decision analyses are useful but based on generalizations.[10] For individual cases, the decision of an experienced clinician must be paramount.[11]

Decision analysis (Fig. 1.1) offers a means of weighing all the factors and possible outcomes. In most cases the probable outcome of operation can be estimated from a study of the relevant literature. However, the outcome of with-

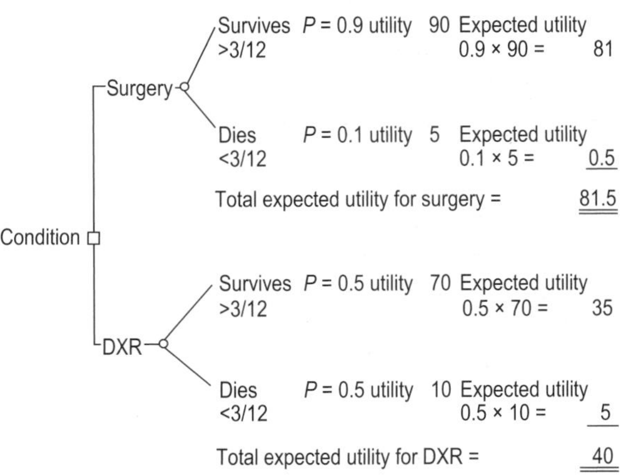

Fig. 1.1 Decision analysis, taking only short-term survival into account. The probability (*P*) of each outcome following surgery or deep X-ray therapy (DXR) is calculated from published results and local experience. The utility of each outcome is given a value between 0 (worst) and 100 (best). The expected utility is the product of probability and utility for each outcome. The sum of the expected utilities for each decision is compared with those of the other decisions. The highest scoring decision offers the best outcome. The square node is a 'decision node'; the circular nodes are 'chance nodes'.

holding operation in circumstances where it is routinely offered is often not known and must be estimated from reports written before surgery was possible, or from the records of patients who have refused operation. Added into the equation are the value judgements placed by you and the patient on the sequelae of surgical versus conservative management, and the likelihood of benefit from different operations. These subjective values are termed *utilities*. The possibility of curing a threatening condition by major operation has to be placed against the mortality and morbidity associated with it. If the condition is likely to be fatal, life expectation has to be balanced against the quality of life. There are a number of terms used in assessing this. One such is quality-adjusted life-year (QALY) expectancy. One year of life in perfect health is 1 QALY; a lower figure is allocated for a portion of a year in perfect health or a full year spent with a disability. Also added in are the economic implications: the *cost–benefit* analysis. Decision analyses have been published for a number of common conditions.

The main value of such analyses is in bringing into focus all the possibilities. In the distant past, surgery was often carried out as the last resort. As new methods of management become available, as the effects of various treatments become known, and as the knowledge and desire of patients to participate in the decision-making process increase, so we need to consider and evaluate all the choices.

REFERENCES

1. Spencer FC 1979 Competence and compassion: two qualities of surgical excellence. Bulletin of the American College of Surgeons 64:15–22
2. Polanyi M 1958 Personal knowledge. Routledge & Kegan Paul, London
3. Kirk RM 1998 Surgical excellence: threats and opportunities. Annals of the Royal College of Surgeons of England 80(6 Suppl):256–259
4. Kirk RM 2006 Surgical skills and lessons from other vocations; a personal view. Annals of the Royal College of Surgeons of England 88(2):95–98
5. Williams N, Scott A 1999 Conventional or laparoscopic inguinal hernia repair? The surgeon's choice. Annals of the Royal College of Surgeons of England 81:56–57
6. Nelson L 2004 While you were sleeping. Nature 430:962–964
7. Weiland DE 1997 Why use clinical pathways rather than practice guidelines? American Journal of Surgery 174:592–595
8. Mazur DJ, Hickam DH 1996 Five-year survival curves: how much data are enough for patient-physician decision making in general surgery? European Journal of Surgery 162:101–104
9. Newton-Howes PA, Bedford ND, Dobbs BR et al 1998 Informed consent: what do patients want to know? New Zealand Medical Journal 111:340–342
10. Kirk RM, Cox K 2004 Decision making. In: Kirk RM, Ribbans WJ (eds) Clinical surgery in general, 4th edn. Churchill Livingstone, Edinburgh, pp 144–151
11. Jewell ER, Persson AV 1985 Pre-operative evaluation of the high risk patient. Surgical Clinics of North America 65:3–19

CUT WELL

Routines

Sterile techniques in the operating theatre have been worked out over many years. Most, but not all, have been subjected to scientific evaluation. Although experienced people carry out the correct procedures instinctively, many of us acquire bad habits that go uncorrected. Accept the need to follow strict routines and so be free to concentrate on other aspects of the operation. Question the routines

KEY POINTS Achieving success

- If operation is indicated, should you perform it? Except in an emergency, avoid carrying out operations that can be better performed by someone else who is available.
- A major operation is merely a series of small operations, but a successful outcome depends upon each step being accomplished perfectly. Do not rush! Hurried movements result in mistakes and the need to repeat actions. Hand speed does not equate with operative speed. Deliberate, accurate movements are faster than rapid, 'flashy' actions that need to be undone or repeated.[1]
- In an emergency, you may often overcome a dangerous situation, not by rapid action but by intelligently deferring in essential routine procedures.
- **Concentrate on getting everything right first time.**

of fine absorbable synthetic material that does not require attendance by the patient for removal. Alternatively, use adhesive strips. The newer fibrin tissue adhesives may come into common use.

4 Employ delayed primary closure selectively in traumatized, contaminated, doubtfully viable wounds and those presenting after a delay. Do not close wounds if there is any possibility of increased tension, liable to produce local compartment syndrome.

5 Occasionally the wound needs to be packed because of bleeding that cannot be controlled by any other method. It can occur as a result of an uncorrected or uncorrectable bleeding diathesis, from a localized cause such as a vascular tumour that cannot be removed, or following trauma.

6 An oedematous wound, or one from which superficial tissue is lost, as following trauma or ablative surgery, may be better treated by delayed primary closure after swelling has subsided. After ensuring that the remaining tissues are viable, clean and dry, apply a single layer of non-adherent net, over which apply gauze to seal off the wound.

7 Achieve primary closure of defects using grafts or flaps, for example when bone is exposed or after repairing nerves or blood vessels (see Ch. 39).

DRESSINGS

1 Make sure you know why you are applying dressings and what function they will serve. They may merely protect the wound from damage, prevent the patient from inspecting it or picking at it, protect it from becoming infected or spreading infection elsewhere, soak up exudate, compress the wound to reduce or prevent swelling and act as a supporting corset to reduce tension.

2 Perfectly closed clean minor wounds require no dressing, since they seal within a few hours. Apply a strip of adhesive tape or a varnish if it is necessary to protect the area. If you expect oozing or exudation, apply sufficient sterile gauze to absorb it without 'strike through', ensuring that the gauze is changed before the exudate soaks through and forms a moist pathway for organisms to track down to the wound. If you wish to apply compression, ensure that this is evenly distributed. First apply gauze to absorb any exudate, then evenly laid cotton wool. Do not use the cotton wool as an extra absorbent as it will form a hard, useless cake. Alternatively, use sponge or an inflatable air cushion.

3 It is generally agreed that wounds should not be allowed to dry out. Particularly for wounds associated with burns, cream containing 1% silver sulfadiazine (Flamazine), is often applied. If you intend leaving the wound open, it is usual to apply a hydrophilic dressing. This will absorb any exudate but should not occlude the wound. Alternatively, apply a single layer of non-adherent net (but not tulle gras which has petroleum jelly that makes the wound soggy), followed by a bulky, absorbent layer of sterile gauze. Some surgeons pack cavities with gauze soaked in flavine emulsion. Do not pack or plug a deep wound as this will seal it from the air. In conflict situations, if all dead and ischaemic tissue and slough and foreign material has been removed and the wound appears clean and healthy, it is often left undisturbed until it is re-dressed 4–5 days later in the operating theatre. Although such wounds usually smell, they can be safely left, provided the patient is well and does not develop signs of sepsis. Of course the dressings must be taken down in the operating theatre if the patient shows features of pain and developing sepsis. In peacetime circumstances and if further removal of dead tissue will probably be required, be prepared to inspect the wounds more frequently.

4 Cavities can also be filled with polymerized foam formed within the cavity. This can be removed for wound cleaning, then washed and reapplied on some exposed areas, as after laying open a pilonidal sinus.

5 To hold dressings in place and exert compression, apply if possible an encircling bandage such as crepe bandage. If you use this method on limbs, always encase the limb with bandage from the extremity up to the site of the wound to avoid producing a garter effect, which would ensue if the bandage were applied only proximally, thus causing venous congestion and distal swelling. Always leave the tips of fingers and toes visible and inspect them regularly to ensure that they are not rendered ischaemic. For the abdomen, many-tailed bandages have been replaced by disposable elastic corsets. Adhesive elastic strips may be applied across the wound under slight tension but they tend to cause excoriation. However, when a wound needs frequent changes of dressing, adhesive strips may be placed on each side of

the wound and can be laced together over the dressings to retain them.

REFERENCES

1. Kirk RM 1996 Teaching the craft of operative surgery. Annals of the Royal College of Surgeons of England 78 (1 Suppl):25–28
2. Kording KP, Wolpert DM 2004 Bayesian integration in sensorimotor learning. Nature 427:244–247
3. Hopf H 2003 Development of subcutaneous wound oxygen measurement in humans: contributions of Thomas K Hunt. Wound Repair and Regeneration 11:424–430
4. Greif R, Akca O, Horn E-P et al 2000 Supplemental perioperative oxygen to reduce the incidence of surgical-wound infection. New England Journal of Medicine 342:161–167

GET WELL

It is not sufficient to carry out the correct procedure perfectly. However well the operation has been performed, the patient has undergone a physiological and psychological disturbance. Aim to help the patient achieve maximum functional recovery and satisfaction as soon as possible. The more ill the patient before operation, the bigger the operation, the greater the risk of short- and long-term complications. Following a general anaesthetic, the anaesthetist supervises the general care of patients until they have safely recovered and are in a stable condition (see Ch. 2); the recovery room nurses observe the patient and call for assistance as necessary. Give clear oral and written instructions about the procedure, the likely sequelae and any special observations or actions you require. The conscious, stable patient is returned to the ward on instructions from the anaesthetist. The pharyngeal airway is removed before the patient leaves the recovery room. Transfer ill, unstable patients to the intensive care unit.

Always make a full record as soon as possible of the operative findings, giving details of the procedure and any special points such as the insertion of drains. In complicated cases, ensure that drains are labelled; in addition, provide a sketch of the incisions and of attached drains, cannulas or other apparatus, with clear instructions about the management of each one.

Following a major operation, or one carried out on a poor-risk patient, inform the relatives and the general practitioner as soon as convenient, personally or by telephone. It is usually best to defer passing on the full impact of distressing news to relatives until you can speak under less stressful circumstances.

Recovery phase

Regard the patient who has just been submitted to an operation in the same light as one brought into the hospital following an acute illness or trauma.

Monitor

1 Airway, breathing and circulation (ABC) are vital functions to observe during the recovery from anaesthesia. Frequently check the consciousness level of the patient by noting the response to stimuli such as calling the name. In case of doubt, note pupillary and other reflexes and peripheral tone.

2 Do not have a fixed attitude to the amount of pain the patient is likely to suffer. Be willing to administer small, repeated doses of analgesics if the patient recovering consciousness is in pain.[1] Restlessness may have causes other than wound pain. Check that the bladder is not overfull, that the patient is lying comfortably and is not pressed upon by any sharp or hard apparatus.

3 In appropriate circumstances check the wound and drains. If blood emerges from an abdominal or chest drain it may be because intra-abdominal or intrathoracic tension has increased as the patient strains. It may also signify that straining has dislodged a ligature. If you suspect that severe bleeding has restarted, do not hesitate to return the patient to the operating theatre.

4 As soon as the patient is responsive, offer information as reassuring as possible about the operation and the present situation. Encourage the wakened patient to breathe deeply, cough and exercise the legs, within the limits posed by the procedure. Moisten the patient's lips or give a mouth wash.

5 Check aspects particular to the patient or the operation. For example, monitor the electrocardiogram (ECG) in patients with cardiac disease, the central nervous system following neurosurgical procedures, the urinary output if renal function is impaired, and the blood sugar in diabetics.

Intermediate phase

1 Transfer to the ward can be unsettling and uncomfortable. Carefully check airway, breathing, circulation,

temperature and other appropriate measurements and record them as a baseline. As the patient recovers, progressively reduce the frequency of monitoring until it is stopped.

2 Maintain adequate analgesia. Pain is reduced if you carried out a field block or instilled long-acting local anaesthetic such as bupivacaine into the wound before closing. The anaesthetist may have inserted an epidural catheter for the instillation of local anaesthetics or opiates. Intramuscular opiates may be titrated, or analgesics may be controlled by the patient. Ensure that the patient's discomfort and pain are reduced to a minimum. Anxiety about respiratory depression or fixed ideas on how much analgesic is needed often lead to inadequate control of pain.

3 Mobilize the patient as quickly as possible, giving breathing and coughing exercises to prevent pulmonary collapse. Encourage leg and foot movement to reduce venous stasis, and frequent changes of posture to prevent pressure sores, and allow drainage of the lung bases. Depending upon the operation, aim to have the patient ambulant as soon as possible. In recent years the length of time patients stay in bed after almost all operations has been drastically reduced.

4 Maintain fluid, electrolyte and acid–base balance,[2] especially in patients who were out of balance before operation, those who must have parenteral intake following, for example, gastrointestinal surgery, and those with renal failure. Following gastrointestinal surgery, aspiration of the digestive tract is usually needed. Check the volume and character of the aspirate.

5 Frequently check the wound and the function of the system subjected to operation. Check the discharge from drains. Remove most wound drains after 24–48 hours unless they are draining profusely. Chest drains are also removed after 1 or 2 days unless they are draining profusely or if there is a pulmonary leak as evidenced by persistent bubbling through the underwater seal.

6 Insulin-dependent diabetes is usually treated throughout the operation with an infusion of 10% dextrose containing 20 mmol potassium chloride and 300 units of insulin. Approximately 100 ml an hour is given, with frequent checks on blood glucose. It is usually possible to return progressively to the preoperative regime within 2–3 days. Some non-insulin-dependent diabetics need to be given soluble insulin over the operative period but should soon be able to return to their diet or oral islet-cell-stimulant drugs.

7 Long-term drugs often need to be given in a modified form over the perioperative period,[3] and the drugs are restored as the patient recovers. Those on steroid drugs need to have hydrocortisone over the operative period and this is continued, usually in a dose of 100 mg hydrocortisone intravenously by slow infusion every 6 hours, with progressive diminution of the dose so that the preoperative maintenance dose can be restored after 3–5 days. Ensure that there is adequate fluid and salt replacement and urinary output, and monitor the serum electrolytes and blood glucose. Patients with renal failure taking fludrocortisone should have it restarted, preferably within 3–5 days. Patients with prosthetic heart valves who take long-term warfarin will have been given heparin over the operative period, usually as a slow intravenous infusion, controlled by maintaining the activated partial thromboplastin time (APTT) at 1.5–2.5 times normal. After operation, restart warfarin to overlap the heparin; now also check the international normalized ratio (INR). Antidepressant, anxiolytic, anticonvulsant and antiparkinsonian drugs need to be restored. Drugs of abuse, including alcohol and opiates, must also be restored or alternative treatment given.

8 Most patients develop a mild pyrexia during the first 24 hours after operation. If it remains, there may be a known reason, but, if not, thoroughly investigate the cause.[4] A swinging pyrexia denotes sepsis and this is most likely to be at the site of operation. Interpret the pyrexia in association with other features, such as the general condition of the patient and any associated circulatory disorder. If you cannot discover the cause, routinely check the possibilities:

- Remember that patients may develop upper respiratory infection, including tonsillitis and ear infections, incidentally. Consider these, especially in young children. Clinical examination, chest X-ray and sputum culture may suggest pulmonary collapse, pneumonia or pulmonary embolus. Improvement following inhalations and physiotherapy may confirm a pulmonary cause.

- Apart from the presence of unilateral leg oedema, clinical detection of deep vein thrombosis is unreliable. Clinical evidence of pulmonary embolus may be supported by chest X-ray and ECG.

- Examine the cardiovascular system for features of myocardial infarction and check the ECG and cardiac enzymes.
- Examine the wound and, in the case of abdominal surgery, carefully examine the abdomen and perform a rectal examination. Plain X-ray of the abdomen may reveal air or fluid levels under the diaphragm, dilatation of small and large bowel suggesting adynamic ileus, and thickening of the interfaces between bowel segments, so-called 'layering', which is indicative of peritonitis. Order a white blood cell count.
- Send a midstream urine (MSU) specimen for microscopy and culture.
- Examine intravenous injection and infusion sites for phlebitis.

9 Look at the whole skin surface to exclude raw areas, including pressure sores.

10 Has the patient an artificial cardiac valve? You knew this before operation and should have given the patient prophylactic antibiotics. Nevertheless, order a blood culture. You may still be uncertain. If you have already sent blood for culture that was unrevealing, send another one: a single specimen may not culture organisms successfully. Re-examine the patient after an interval.

11 If you initiate non-specific supportive treatment and the patient improves, do not assume that the problem is solved. Remain vigilant and anticipate possible deterioration (Fig. 1.2). Consider what is the likely cause in this patient after the operation that was carried out. Do not order a battery of investigations in the hope that 'something will turn up'. First call in a senior, experienced colleague to examine the patient.

Day case

1 The monitoring of recovery from a general anaesthetic must be as thorough as that of an inpatient. Sedation with benzodiazepines and administration of analgesics may depress respiration, so have this monitored for 2 hours.

2 The normal assessment of recovery has to be compressed into a shorter period, but ensure that the cardiovascular and respiratory functions are normal before discharge.

3 Check the wound.

4 Fully inform the patient of the procedure, the likely sequelae, danger signs and what to do about them. It is wise to give written instructions for later reference.

5 If a follow-up appointment is to be given, arrange it now.

6 Ensure that those who have had a general anaesthetic or sedation are accompanied home.

7 Record the findings and procedure immediately. Because a similar series of day cases are often arranged, it is easy to confuse the details if they are not recorded individually, between procedures.

Audit

- Remarkable changes have occurred during the last 10 years, and especially during the last 5 years, from changes in public expectation and from media coverage of the complications that developed following the general adoption of minimal access techniques, often by surgeons with minimal training. However, the investigation in 1998 of the results of paediatric cardiac surgery in Bristol brought matters to a head.
- We should all ensure our results are open to scrutiny – not, as formerly, just to our own consciences, but also to our patients and peers.
- Although mortality and morbidity conferences and audit meetings are as yet fairly crude, efforts are being made to grade the severity of acute conditions, such as the modified acute physiology and chronic health evaluation (APACHE II)[5] combination of clinical and laboratory findings. Surgical outcome can be assessed using POSSUM (Physiological and Operative Severity Score for Enumeration of Mortality and Morbidity),[6,7] and this has been used with a modification for the evaluation of vascular surgical operations – the Portsmouth predictor equation.[8] Undoubtedly, these methods will be refined so that reliable comparisons will be possible between the likely outcomes following available operations and also of non-operative management.

Follow-up

You follow up patients to ensure that they recover without complications, to reassure them, to give further treatment,

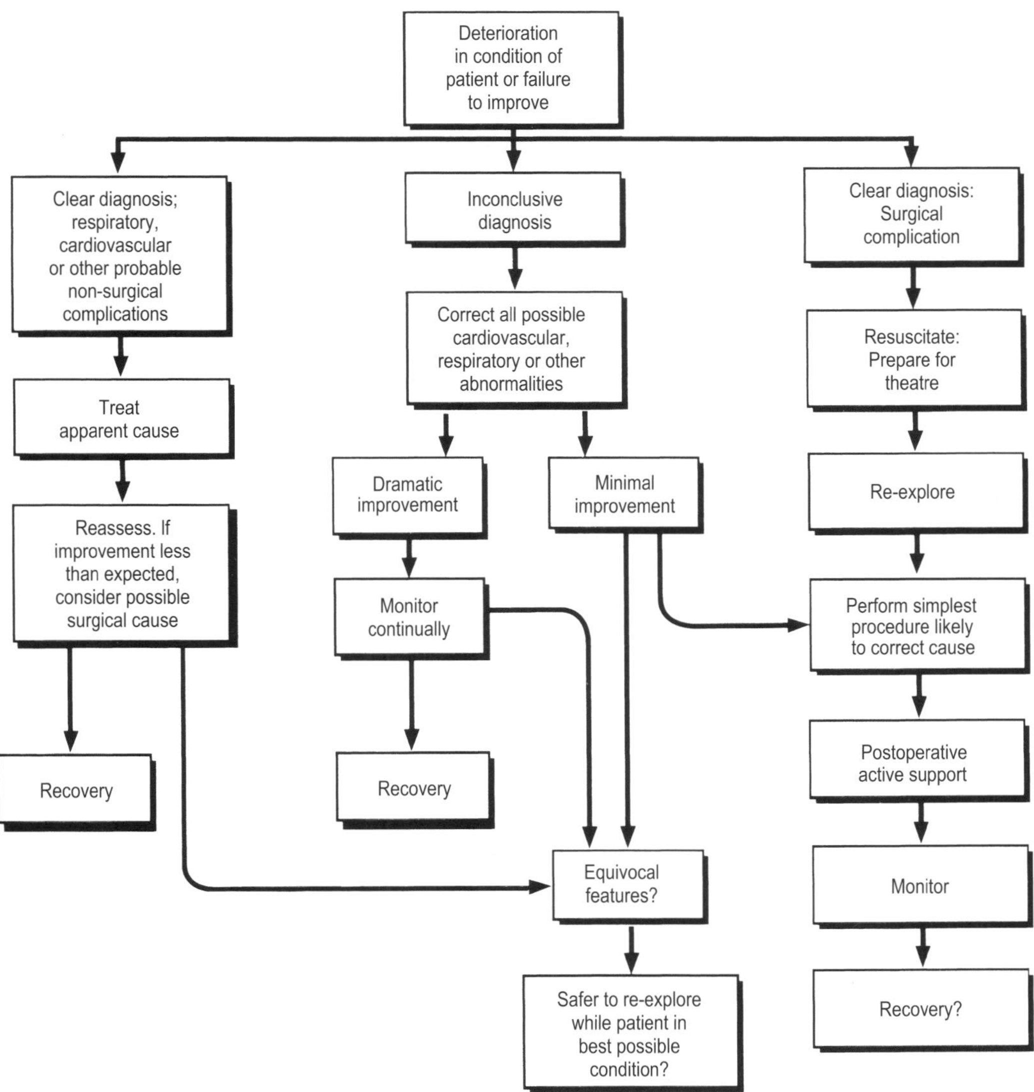

Fig. 1.2 Scheme for management of a patient who develops a complication or fails to recover satisfactorily following an operation. (Adapted with permission from Kirk RM 1990 Reoperation for early intra-abdominal complications following abdominal and abdominothoracic operations. Hospital Update 16:303–310.)

to assess your own results for comparison with published figures and to detect long-term sequelae.

Make sure that you know why each patient is returning to your clinic. If patients attend unnecessarily, the clinic becomes overfilled and those who need attention are deprived of it. Sometimes attendance at the clinic can be averted by allowing patients to write in or telephone when they have a problem or at fixed intervals.

REFERENCES

1. Sodhi V, Fernando R 2004 Management of post-operative pain. In: Kirk RM, Ribbans WJ (eds) Clinical surgery in

general, 4th edn. Churchill Livingstone, Edinburgh, pp 357–369

2. Aveling W, Hamilton MA 2004 Fluid, electrolyte and acid-base balance. In: Kirk RM, Ribbans WJ (eds) Clinical surgery in general, 4th edn. Churchill Livingstone, Edinburgh, pp 107–124
3. Tate JJT 2004 Post-operative care. In: Kirk RM, Ribbans WJ (eds) Clinical surgery in general, 4th edn. Churchill Livingstone, Edinburgh, pp 349–356
4. Smith JAR 2004 Complications: prevention and management. In: Kirk RM, Ribbans WJ (eds) Clinical surgery in general, 4th edn. Churchill Livingstone, Edinburgh, pp 373–387
5. Goldhill DR, Sumner A 1998 APACHE II, data accuracy and outcome prediction. Anaesthesia 53:937–943
6. Copeland GP, Jones D, Walters M 1991 POSSUM: a scoring system for surgical audit. British Journal of Surgery 78:355–360
7. Jones HJS, de Cossart L 1999 Risk scoring in surgical patients. British Journal of Surgery 86:149–157
8. Midwinter MJ, Tytherleigh M, Ashley S 1999 Estimation of mortality and morbidity risk in vascular surgery using POSSUM and the Portsmouth predictor equation. British Journal of Surgery 86:471–474

FURTHER READING

Birkmeyer JD, Welch HG 1997 A reader's guide to surgical decision making. Journal of the American College of Surgeons 184:589–595

Bunker JP, Barnes BA, Mosteller F 1977 Costs, risks, and benefits of surgery. Oxford University Press, Oxford

Finlayson SRG, Birkmeyer JD 1998 Cost effectiveness analysis in surgery. Surgery 123:151–156

Kirk RM 2002 Basic surgical techniques, 5th edn. Churchill Livingstone, Edinburgh

UK Health Departments 2000 Hepatitis B infected health care workers. HSC 2000/020. Department of Health, London

2

Anaesthesia-related techniques

R. S. Simons

CONTENTS

INTRODUCTION

The topics in this chapter are confined to the practical skill-mix listed above. To obtain a wider understanding of the anaesthetist's contribution to surgical patients, read the relevant chapters in the companion volume: Kirk RM, Ribbans WJ (eds) 2004 Clinical surgery in general, 4th edn. Churchill Livingstone, Edinburgh (an RCS course manual). These skills, applicable to anaesthetists and surgeon alike, include the ability to:

1. Evaluate co-morbidities that the patient may have, typically but not exclusively involving cardiovascular, renal, respiratory and metabolic systems.
2. Assess preoperative investigations (including blood transfusion requirements) required for surgery in conjunction with the patient's age, co-morbidity and extent of intended surgery.
3. Demonstrate proficiency in the ABC (airway, breathing, circulation) of resuscitation.
4. Confidently undertake peripheral and central venous access and restore acute and chronic fluid losses.
5. Use local anaesthetic techniques to supplant or augment general anaesthesia, including its use in postoperative analgesia.
6. Provide effective postoperative pain relief.
7. Utilize intensive therapy facilities in a coordinated and efficient manner.

RESPIRATORY SUPPORT

To maintain the heart and the brain,
Give oxygen now and again.
Not now and again, but NOW, AND AGAIN, AND AGAIN, AND AGAIN, AND AGAIN.
(Adapted from a well-known limerick.)

All doctors in clinical practice, regardless of speciality, should receive training and certification in cardiopulmonary resuscitation (CPR) to the level of basic life support (BLS). You should also attend an advanced trauma life support (ATLS) course. Advanced cardiac life support (ALS) requirements are just as simple to learn and perform (see Further reading).

▶ KEY POINT Get oxygen to the brain

- Anoxia damages all organs eventually, but failure of oxygen supply can damage the brain within 3–4 minutes. It is vital that you ensure a patent airway, satisfactory exchange of gases and adequate circulation.

OXYGEN THERAPY

Appraise

Oxygen is vital for metabolism. In the presence of ineffective ventilation, impaired pulmonary gas transfer or low output states, high inspired concentrations may be required to restore a deficient cellular oxygen supply to normal.

Give oxygen for all hypoxic states if ventilation, oxygen transfer, or circulation is impaired, for intracranial, spinal and chest injuries, postoperatively, especially when ventilation is surgically affected or pulmonary disease coexists, for shock of all types and for hypermetabolic states such as shivering and hyperthermia.

Action

1 A clear airway is essential. Partial or broken dentures, food and foreign debris, blood (active bleeding or clots) and vomited or regurgitated stomach contents represent additional sources of airway obstruction or which may be inhaled into the lungs. Altered consciousness (intracranial damage, drug overdose and profound shock) may compromise the airway by obstruction in the oro- or laryngopharynx. In the supine patient this is typically caused by the tongue falling back against the posterior pharyngeal wall. In emergencies such as shock, post-arrest and multiple trauma, a high inspired oxygen concentration of 80–95% is desirable. In self-ventilating patients this is best achieved by the use of a 'trauma' or 'non-rebreathing oxygen mask' which has a plastic oxygen reservoir bag incorporating a non-rebreathing valve. Use high oxygen flow rates of 12–15 litres/min.

2 In patients with impaired consciousness, remove any dentures and clear the pharynx and mouth of any gross contamination from blood, gastric contents or foreign material. Have available at all times Magill forceps and suction equipment with a semirigid Yankauer handpiece already attached.

3 Following trauma be suspicious of cervical spine injury. Conduct manoeuvres to ensure airway patency with the head centrally aligned. Do not allow the head and neck to be flexed or extended. Stabilize the head with a firm cervical collar, supports or straps, to prevent axial rotation of the spine.

4 Assess whether simple airway adjuncts, such as the Guedel oropharyngeal airway or soft curved nasopharyngeal tube, will secure patency. Insert a Guedel airway 'upside down' under the upper teeth, then rotate it downwards behind the tongue. After insertion, continue to support the jaw by jaw lift or jaw thrust. Lubricate a nasopharyngeal airway and insert it into the nose parallel to the hard palate to lie behind the soft palate and tongue. Put a safety pin through the tube to ensure it cannot migrate into the nose.

5 If ventilation is adequate, nurse the patient in the lateral or semiprone recovery position with head dependent to avoid regurgitation and aspiration into the trachea. This posture may be impracticable while you examine, resuscitate or treat the patient, or if spinal trauma is present or suspected. If necessary, reverse the effect of opioid or benzodiazepine drugs with their respective specific antagonists: 0.2–0.4 mg naloxone or 0.3–0.6 mg flumazenil given intravenously.

6 If spontaneous ventilation is inadequate despite the insertion of an oropharyngeal airway, apply the mask (adult sizes 4–6) of a self-inflating bag-mask resuscitator to the nose and mouth (Fig. 2.1). Hold it securely on the face with one hand while lifting the jaw upwards and forwards, with the airway still in place, and create a tight seal. Try to achieve tidal volumes of 500–800 ml at a rate of 10–15 /min. Common problems encountered are an obstructed airway or failure to obtain an adequate seal. If the former is the case, elevate the jaw further and extend the head, provided you do not

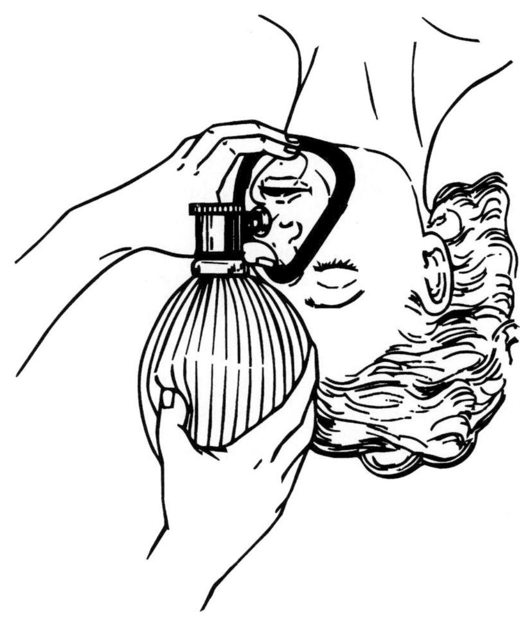

Fig. 2.1 Resuscitation with a bag–valve mask (single-handed).

suspect cervical spine injury. If mask seal is a problem, reapply the mask more evenly or ask an assistant to squeeze the bag while you use both hands to hold it firmly in position. Add oxygen to the bag at 8–10 litres/min to increase the inspired oxygen concentration to 40–60%. Where possible, add a reservoir bag to the resuscitation device. This increases the inspired oxygen level to 80–90%.

7 If you cannot achieve any chest movement, consider the possibility of a foreign body obstructing the hypopharynx, larynx or trachea. Attempt the Heimlich manoeuvre if appropriate and/or use a laryngoscope and Magill forceps to remove the offending foreign body if you can see it at laryngoscopy. If this fails or if severe maxillofacial trauma prevents effective ventilation by conventional methods, prepare for cricothyrotomy as an emergency procedure.

8 *Cricothyrotomy.* Make an incision horizontally in the cricothyroid membrane and insert a suitable hollow device through the membrane into the trachea, below the level of the vocal cords. A 5-mm (internal diameter, ID) tube may be adequate for resuscitation purposes, but presents a high resistance to both inspiratory and expiratory flow. Increased resistance with spontaneous ventilation may induce pulmonary oedema from any forceful negative intrathoracic efforts the patient may attempt. Therefore prefer a 6–7-mm tube if possible and convert it to a formal tracheostomy as soon as practicable. Do not attempt tracheostomy as a primary emergency procedure since it is difficult to perform under emergency conditions in inadequate surroundings on hypoxic patients.

9 Regurgitation with pulmonary aspiration is not uncommon in semiconscious patients and usually develops insidiously. It more commonly occurs in the presence of a full stomach, ileus, pregnancy, hiatal hernia, maxillofacial trauma or muscle relaxants, and may be compounded by air blown into the stomach during mask ventilation. Use cricoid pressure – the Sellick manoeuvre – during resuscitation and intubation to avoid or minimize this risk. Have an assistant press firmly with three fingers straddling the cricoid ring to compress the oesophagus between the cricoid ring and the body of the sixth cervical vertebra.

10 Vomiting, unlike regurgitation, is an active process and usually occurs at lighter levels of unconsciousness. If you observe prodromal (Greek *pro* = before + *dromos* = a run: forerunner) retching or vomiting, release cricoid pressure to avoid gastric rupture. Turn the patient quickly into the recovery position with head dependent if possible.

11 The hazard of pulmonary aspiration is accentuated if the aspirate has a pH of less than 3, when the risk of a chemical pneumonitis from acid aspiration (Mendelson's syndrome) is considerable. If you suspect pulmonary contamination, immediately intubate the patient (see below) to secure airway isolation and if possible set aside a suction trap specimen from the lungs or pharynx to measure the acidity of the aspirate with wide-range pH paper (not litmus). Immediately lavage the lungs several times with aliquots of 20–50 ml of saline, using 100% oxygen, large tidal volumes and tracheal suction. The procedure may well avert a full-blown aspiration syndrome, which can develop within 2–4 hours and resemble acute adult respiratory distress syndrome (ARDS). Give broad-spectrum antibiotic therapy. Intravenous steroids and tracheal bicarbonate instillation are of doubtful benefit. Involve anaesthetists or intensivists in the further care of such patients as soon as possible.

TRACHEAL INTUBATION

1 Achieve competence in tracheal intubation by practising on an intubation training simulator and under supervision by anaesthetists during induction of anaesthesia for routine surgery. It is a useful skill to have when faced with airway emergencies in or out of hospital. Always have functioning suction equipment available for unconscious patients.

2 Patients tolerate tracheal intubation only at deep levels of unconsciousness, typically associated with general anaesthesia or 'coma'. Intubation ensures the patency of the upper airway, avoiding obstruction from haemorrhage or swelling, and prevents entry of blood, gastric contents, secretions and other foreign matter into the tracheobronchial tree. It is the most effective form of airway isolation when undertaking positive pressure ventilation.

3 When deciding whether an unconscious patient requires tracheal intubation in order to safeguard the airway, be guided by the state of the laryngeal reflexes and the degree of muscle tone. If these are such that intubation is unlikely to be tolerated without great difficulty or

sedation, then abandon intubation and use an oral or nasal pharyngeal airway instead.

4 *Laryngoscope*. The Macintosh-pattern curved laryngoscope blade is still the most popular and the easiest to learn to use. The standard adult size 3 Macintosh blade is suitable for most patients over 5 years of age, although a size 4 may be required for large males. Check that the laryngoscope bulb and blade are well secured.

5 *Endotracheal tube*. These slightly curved plastic tubes have an ID range of 2.5–10.0 mm in 0.5-mm increments. They are presented as disposable, prepacked items complete with one bevelled end (cuffed above 6.0 mm) and a 15-mm plastic connector lightly inserted into the other end. The tube is stamped with the internal diameter in millimetres near the bevel and the length is often marked in centimetres at the connector end, which requires cutting to length before use. Use 7.0–8.0 mm ID for adult females and 8.0–9.0 mm for adult males. Use cuffed tubes for patients over 7–8 years, uncuffed below that age. A convenient guide to tube diameter can be based on the tip of the patient's little finger; this is a good measure of overall tube size as it closely matches the size of the cricoid ring.

For children, ID (mm) = [(age in years)/4] + 4.5. Length for adults ranges from 22 cm for females to 24 cm for males. For nasal intubation add 2–4 cm. As a convenient guide to length, hold the tube alongside the patient's face, allowing for the curvature in the mouth and measure the distance from lips to cricoid ring; add an allowance for the portion outside the mouth and a safe length in the trachea. For children, length (cm) = [(age in years)/2] + 12.

6 *Connections* (Fig. 2.2). Having cut the tube to the recommended length, fit the tapered tube connector tightly into the cut end. The 15-mm end connector is a standard fit for use with a catheter mount to adapt it to a resuscitation device, anaesthetic circuit or ventilator. It also fits directly to a self-inflating bag–valve resuscitator if the catheter mount is not available. Test the cuff of the tube with a few millilitres of air from a 10-ml syringe. Deflate it and apply water-miscible lubricant over the cuffed portion of the tube. Have ready a curved malleable metal stylet or a long gum-elastic bougie to assist in case the intubation is difficult. Test the good working order of the suction equipment. Have available Yankauer semirigid handpieces in addition to a range of plastic suction catheters.

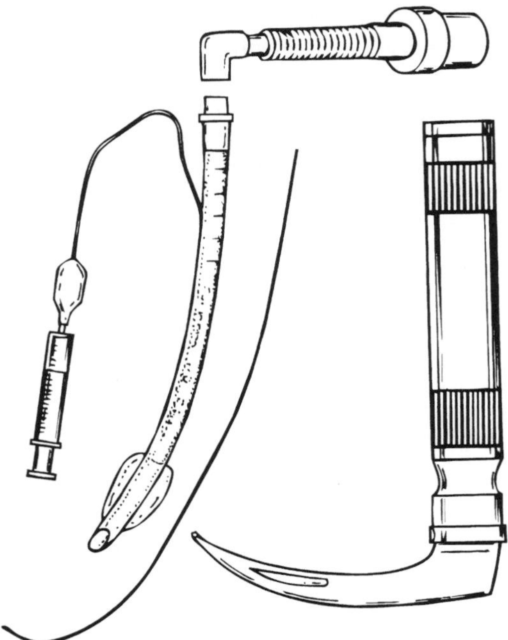

Fig. 2.2 Tracheal intubation equipment: cuffed endotracheal tube with inflation syringe, catheter mount, gum-elastic bougie and laryngoscope.

7 Correctly position the patient. Moderately flex the cervical spine by raising the head on one pillow, and then extend the head at the atlanto-occipital joint, as when 'sniffing the morning air'. Inspect the mouth. Remove any dentures and look for loose teeth, crowns or bridges, especially in the upper incisor area, to avoid damaging or dislodging them during intubation.

Action

1 Hold the laryngoscope handle vertical in your left hand with the blade downward and the light shining towards the patient's feet. Open the mouth by gently extending the head with the right hand. Maximum opening can be obtained by placing your right index finger along the line of the upper right premolars and molars, and further extending the head. Avoid damage to the incisors. With the head extended, insert the blade into the right side of the mouth in an arc over the tongue, directing the blade tip towards the uvula. The laryngoscope blade holds the bulk of the tongue out of the way to the

left and allows you a clear view down the right side of the mouth. Continue advancing the blade in a gentle curve along the back of the tongue until you see the epiglottis. Then pass the blade anterior to the epiglottis, between it and the base of the tongue, and lodge the tip firmly in the vallecula. The vocal cords may be visible now but it is usually necessary to lift the tongue and jaw together vertically to adequately visualize the glottis. Do not lever on the upper teeth or gums. This causes damage and does not improve the view.

2 If you cannot see the epiglottis, either the laryngoscope blade is not in the midline or it may have passed over the epiglottis into the laryngopharynx. Withdraw the blade to about two-thirds along the tongue and re-advance it.

3 When you see the glottis, hold the tracheal tube near its connector in the right hand, concavity forward, and pass it via the right side of the mouth, so that the tip comes into the midline immediately above the laryngeal opening. Insert the bevel between the vocal cords and slide the tube onwards through the larynx so that the cuff lies below the level of the vocal cords. Hold the tube firmly while gently withdrawing the laryngoscope.

4 To check that the tube is in the correct position, press firmly on the subject's chest. A puff of air emerging from the tube gives some reassurance that it has entered the trachea rather than the oesophagus. Connect it to a ventilating device such as a self-inflating bag or anaesthetic circuit, and apply positive pressure to ventilate the patient's lungs. If you use a cuffed tube, slowly inflate the cuff with an air-filled 10-ml syringe until audible leakage ceases during inspiration; this is typically 3–7 ml. Check for reasonable tension in the pilot cuff. Remove the syringe from the self-sealing Luer-lock valves of the pilot tube.

5 Uniform expansion of the chest indicates correct placement. Confirm correct placement by auscultation with a stethoscope while ventilating the lungs. Also auscultate the epigastrium to ensure the tube was not inadvertently placed in the oesophagus. If one side of the chest expands more than the other then the tube may have passed too far into a main bronchus, usually the right. Deflate the cuff and withdraw the tube until chest expansion is uniform. Re-inflate the cuff. Exclude less frequent causes of unilateral chest expansion such as pneumo- or haemothorax.

6 Secure the tube to the patient's face with strapping or by means of a loop of tape or bandage around the neck, having first knotted it securely around the tube. Avoid constricting the jugular or facial veins by tying too tightly.

? DIFFICULTY

A common difficulty during intubation is an inability to lift the jaw sufficiently forward to expose the glottis fully, or to persuade the tube to follow the curve behind the epiglottis. Bend the tube to increase its curvature and try again. A further option is to pass a lubricated malleable metal stylet into the tube to within 1 cm of the tip, and angulate the tube more sharply. Alternatively, pass a long gum-elastic bougie through the tube so that it protrudes for a few centimetres and angulate the end of this to aid laryngeal entry. In difficult cases, first insert the gum-elastic bougie into the trachea alone and then railroad the tracheal tube over the bougie into the trachea.

Alternative

The laryngeal mask airway (LMA) is very popular with anaesthetists (Fig. 2.3). It has a curved tube with a hollow, soft rubber spoon at one end bearing an inflatable rim. The device is inserted via the mouth into the laryngopharynx, concavity forward, and the cuff is inflated to 'seal' the rim against the laryngeal inlet, so maintaining patency and providing a degree of airway isolation. It is tolerated at lighter levels of consciousness than a standard tracheal tube and may allow positive pressure ventilation, although some leakage is likely. Its ability to isolate the trachea reliably against aspiration cannot be guaranteed, but with practice it is easy to use and is likely to prove a useful adjunct in situations where conventional intubation would be impracticable.

Recent modifications of the device include an intubating LMA and a further device which allows decompression and suction of gastric contents via a venting tube.

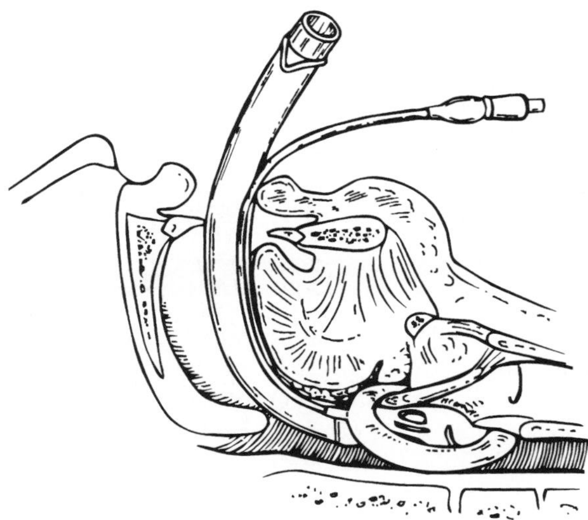

Fig. 2.3 Laryngeal mask airway.

ARTIFICIAL VENTILATION

1 Institute IPPV (intermittent positive pressure ventilation) without delay whenever spontaneous breathing is inadequate to provide effective gas exchange. Room air contains 21% oxygen, and the immediate application of 35–60% oxygen via an oxygen mask is a useful emergency measure to compensate for the hypoxia associated with impaired ventilation while preparing for intubation and ventilation. If breathing is totally absent, immediately institute artificial ventilation.

2 In lay emergency situations, start expired air resuscitation using mouth-to-mouth, mouth-to-nose or mouth-to-airway adjuncts, using the 16% oxygen available in expired air. Mouth-to-mouth ventilation may be hazardous in the presence of oral trauma, and resuscitation equipment for health-care professionals should include self-inflating resuscitation bags with oxygen reservoirs in addition to a range of airway adjuncts: Guedel oropharyngeal airways and soft rubber or plastic nasopharyngeal tubes.

3 Ensure airway patency and ventilate the patient with a bag–mask device. As soon as possible add oxygen from a pipeline or portable cylinder to the inlet valve of the resuscitation bag. At oxygen flows of 6–10 litres/min the inspired oxygen level can be increased from 35% to 80% by adding an oxygen reservoir bag to the self-inflating resuscitator. When using portable oxygen cylinders ensure you have adequate reserves for unexpected delays, especially during transport.

4 Isolate the trachea by passing a tracheal tube or similar device and continue bag–mask ventilation until the patient is connected to a functioning ventilator. Semi-conscious patients may need sedation to tolerate airway isolation and IPPV (see below).

▶ **KEY POINT Ventilation**

- **Underventilation is harmful, overventilation rarely so.**

5 Aim for a minute volume of 6–8 litres/min in an adult by ventilating at a rate of 10–15 breaths/min with tidal volumes of 500–800 ml. Commence ventilation with 60% inspired oxygen. Inflate the lungs over 1–1.5 seconds and allow 2–2.5 seconds for expiration to occur passively. The expiratory pause is necessary as IPPV raises intrathoracic pressure and impairs venous return.

6 Seek the assistance of anaesthetists and/or intensivists to provide continuing care. Adjust oxygen flow to maintain pulse oximeter saturation readings in excess of 94%, equivalent to arterial oxygen tensions of 11.5–14 kPa (87–105 mmHg). Maintain ventilation to achieve end-tidal carbon dioxide readings or arterial carbon dioxide gases range of 4.0–5.5% (kPa), equivalent to 30–42 mmHg.

7 *Secretions*. Tracheobronchial toilet is necessary during artificial ventilation. Sterility is important. Select sterile disposable catheters with a rounded tip and having several side holes in preference to those with a single end aperture. The latter are traumatic, stick to the tracheal wall and are difficult to advance. Choose a suction catheter that is less than half the tracheal tube diameter (12–14F in adults) and use it once only. Insert the catheter using sterile gloves or forceps and apply suction intermittently during its withdrawal, avoiding prolonged suction as this causes hypoxia. Collect a sputum-trap specimen for culture initially. A saline nebulizer or repeated saline instillation of 5–10 ml may be useful when secretions are tenacious.

PERIPHERAL VENOUS ACCESS

A high-capacity, trouble-free intravenous infusion necessitates one or two large cannulas (16–14FG) in large veins. Prepare carefully and do not rush. For the standard percutaneous technique have ready an infusion stand bearing the container of the chosen fluid attached to an intravenous fluid administration set primed to remove air, a venous tourniquet (elasticated Velcro band, etc.), swabs, infusion needle–cannula assembly, a 2-ml syringe containing 0.5 ml of 1% plain lidocaine with attached 25SWG needle for infiltration of local anaesthesia, scalpel blade, good light source and adhesive strapping.

Action

1. Explain what is to be done, reassure the patient, select a suitable vein, apply a tourniquet to distend the vein and clean the skin. Inject a small quantity of local anaesthetic to raise a weal, wait 3–5 minutes and insert the needle through the weal, if necessary after making a small skin incision.
2. Insert the needle, bevel upwards, at a shallow angle in the long axis of the vein to enter it, confirming the flowback of blood into the chamber and advance it. If the needle carries a cannula, advance this, then withdraw the needle.
3. Remove the venous tourniquet, attach the infusion set and secure the needle or cannula and adjacent tubing.

CENTRAL VENOUS ACCESS

Central venous cannulas or catheters, available as single or multichannel devices of up to four channels (mixed 20–14G size), provide a route for the infusion of fluids, especially veno-irritant medications (e.g. potassium chloride, 50% dextrose, parenteral nutrition) and regulated infusions of inotropes and vasoactive drugs. The resistance in these catheters rather mitigates against their use for rapid intravenous infusion except when large-bore (12G or larger) catheters are used.

Central venous access can be gained through the internal jugular, subclavian or femoral veins. Vascular dialysis catheters and tunnelled cuffed Hickman lines can also be inserted through these sites, as can balloon-tipped, flow-directed pulmonary artery (wedge) catheters capable of monitoring mixed venous oxygen saturation, thermal cardiac output and pulmonary capillary wedge pressures (PCWP). Access is via the internal jugular or subclavian vein or femoral vein using a percutaneous cannula.

LOCAL ANAESTHESIA

Operative procedures under local anaesthesia are regularly undertaken in hospitals, clinics and surgeries. Local anaesthetic techniques are particularly well suited for minor operations such as removal of small non-infected superficial lesions and minor surgery of the hands. It may be useful when general anaesthesia is not readily available or is impracticable (e.g. recent ingestion of food). Local anaesthesia is inexpensive as it does not require the specialized staff and facilities that general anaesthesia demands, is relatively safe, causes less systemic upset than general anaesthesia and enables patients to be discharged soon after surgery.

More extensive procedures involving large field blocks may not be as safe as general anaesthesia due to the toxic effect associated with the large volume of local anaesthetic required. Moreover, local anaesthesia does not necessarily block the physiological disturbances such as bradycardia and vomiting which arise from autonomic reflexes during some surgical procedures.

Local anaesthetic drugs can be administered in various ways according to the required area of analgesia:

Topical anaesthesia: application of local anaesthetics to the mucous membranes of the conjunctival sac, mouth, nose, tracheobronchial tree and urethra.

Local infiltration: direct injection of the anaesthetic into the operative site.

Field block: injection of local anaesthetic around the operative site so as to create an analgesic zone.

Individual peripheral nerve blocks: e.g. ulnar, pudendal, femoral, common peroneal, etc. The extent of the block varies according to the cutaneous distribution the nerve supplies.

Regional block: injection of local anaesthetic around the individual nerves or nerve trunks supplying the region to be operated upon. Where nerves are grouped together as plexuses then several nerves can be blocked at the same time. The brachial plexus is the best known, but the lumbosacral plexus block is occasionally used. The large volumes required for these blocks approach toxic levels.

Spinal anaesthesia: insertion of local anaesthetic drugs directly into the subarachnoid space in small volumes (1.5–3 ml) produces effective sensory and motor block as the nerve roots in this space have negligible covering; low-pressure headache due to cerebrospinal fluid leak is not uncommon following this technique.

Extradural block: injection of local anaesthetic into the epidural or caudal space; these blocks require 4–10 times the volumes used in subarachnoid block because of local diffusion and the presence of dural and myelin covering of the nerve roots. Combined spinal–epidural techniques, pioneered for obstetric anaesthesia, are increasingly popular for their ability to provide effective intraoperative analgesia combined with good postoperative pain relief.

Regional intravenous anaesthesia: injection of a large volume of dilute local anaesthetic into the veins of a previously exsanguinated limb.

Agents

Various local anaesthetic drugs are available, of which amino amide derivatives are the most commonly used. Most drugs are marketed in the form of their water-soluble salts, usually the hydrochloride. Before they can act in the body they must dissociate to liberate the free base. Dissociation is inhibited in an acid medium, which explains why analgesia may be unpredictable when local anaesthetics are injected into inflamed tissues.

▶ KEY POINTS Caution when administering local anaesthesia

- Never perform any but the most trivial of blocks single-handed. Serious cardiovascular and neurological consequences can develop suddenly if local anaesthetics are inadvertently injected into the wrong place, while other side-effects or complications may develop some time after the local anaesthetic has been injected. It is desirable to have another competent person who is capable of recognizing and dealing with unexpected problems attending the patient. This is particularly important if the patient is unwell, if concurrent sedation is being administered or if equipment such as a tourniquet is in use. At times another doctor (e.g. an anaesthetist) may be responsible for the patient's care during surgery. Otherwise you are accountable for your patient's safety. You cannot properly observe the patient or treat untoward reactions if you are a single-handed operator–anaesthetist engrossed in the surgery you are performing.
- Do not use local anaesthetic techniques until you are well versed in the relevant aspects of resuscitation. The morbidity and mortality associated with local anaesthesia relate more to the ability of the surgeon to deal rapidly and effectively with unexpected side-effects than to surgical ability.
- Do not attempt to block the ulnar nerve at the elbow or the common peroneal nerve in the leg in unconscious patients. There is a high risk of causing intraneural injury.

The duration of action of some local anaesthetics having a low tissue affinity is increased if they are combined with a vasoconstrictor such as adrenaline (epinephrine). This will also reduce the systemic absorption and toxicity of these agents. For infiltration, concentrations of 1 in 250000 of adrenaline (epinephrine) may be used by the addition of 1 mg (1 ml of adrenaline tartrate 1/1000) to 250 ml of local anaesthetic solution. There is no advantage in using higher concentrations than this. The total amount of adrenaline (epinephrine) injected should not exceed 0.5 mg. Adrenaline (epinephrine) may cause tachycardia and hypertension and should be used with caution in patients with cardiovascular disease and those taking cardiac medication (e.g. beta-blockers). Less toxic vasoconstrictors (e.g. felypressin) are available. Injection of vasoconstrictors is absolutely contraindicated in areas supplied by end arteries (e.g. the fingers, toes and penis) as prolonged ischaemia here may lead to tissue necrosis.

The most commonly used agents include:

Lidocaine. This is the most widely used local anaesthetic. It is stable, only moderately toxic, produces no vasodilation and has an onset of action within a few minutes and a duration of action of 60–90 minutes. It is used in concentrations of 4% for topical anaesthesia and concentrations of 0.5–2% for infiltration and nerve blocks. The maximum safe dose is 3 mg/kg body weight when used without adrenaline and 7 mg/kg with adrenaline.

Prilocaine. Chemically related to lidocaine, prilocaine is less toxic but also less potent. Duration of action is less affected by adrenaline (epinephrine) than lidocaine is. Prilocaine is used as a 4% solution for topical anaesthesia and in concentrations of 1–3% for nerve blocks. The maximum safe dose is 10 mg/kg. Excessive doses of prilocaine produce methaemoglobinaemia, which may manifest as apparent cyanosis. Hypoxaemia results if more than 15 mg/kg of the agent is administered. Treatment involves the administration of 1% methylthioninium chloride (methylene blue), 1–2 mg/kg.

Bupivacaine. This agent is two to three times as toxic as lidocaine but about four times more potent. It is used in concentrations of 0.25–0.5% and has a maximum safe dose of 2 mg/kg. It is extensively bound in the tissues and hence has the advantage of a long duration of action (3–12 hours). It has a delayed onset compared to lidocaine, although this may be overcome by mixing bupivacaine and lidocaine together (see Methods below).

Toxicity

All local anaesthetics exert toxic effects when given in large doses, and inadvertent intravascular injection, even in small doses, can cause central nervous and cardiovascular disturbances resulting in restlessness, convulsions, hypotension, bradycardia and, in extreme cases, respiratory and cardiac arrest.

Management of these toxic effects includes the use of intravenous sedatives with anticonvulsant properties (benzodiazepines or thiopental), oxygen, intravenous fluids and pressor agents (ephedrine or metaraminol). In extreme circumstances tracheal intubation and artificial ventilation may be necessary. The importance of securing intravenous access before local anaesthesia is commenced is obvious.

The conduct of thoracic or lumbar spinal and epidural anaesthesia involves blockade of the T1–L1 sympathetic outflow tracts. This results in vasodilation below the block with compensatory vasoconstriction above this level. If the block reaches above T10, hypotension is likely. Compensatory tachycardia may not occur, especially if a high block affects the T1–T4 outflow or the patient is on beta-blockers or has a pacemaker. For this reason good venous access is important; a preload infusion of 300–500 ml of crystalloid is recommended before such blocks are commenced. Administer a small subcutaneous or intravenous dose of a vaso- and venoconstrictor such as ephedrine or metaraminol before or during the procedure to protect against hypotension.

The risk of hypotension is particularly high when pre-existing hypovolaemia is present, during supine hypotension syndrome of pregnancy or when unexpected subarachnoid (spinal) anaesthesia occurs. This latter hazard may arise when an epidural technique is complicated by dural puncture or where an existing epidural catheter perforates the subarachnoid space. Partial or extensive spinal anaesthesia may also occur from misplaced spinal injection during the conduct of pre- or paravertebral blocks. Profound hypotension, unconsciousness and respiratory paralysis can occur. Emergency management involves oxygenation, intubation, ventilation, intravenous infusion and pharmacological support of the cardiovascular system.

Prepare

1 Check that resuscitation equipment is present and in working order and that competent assistance is available if needed urgently. The minimum equipment required is a self-inflating bag with mask and airways, an oxygen cylinder capable of delivering 8–10 litres/min via oxygen mask and resuscitation bag, sedatives to deal with convulsions, intravenous fluids and vasopressors for sudden circulatory failure. Ensure that a quiet environment will be maintained for the duration of surgery. Quiet music may be beneficial but keep casual conversation to a minimum. Explain to the patient what surgery you are proposing to perform under local anaesthesia, check that the correct site (and side) is being operated on and obtain written consent. Explain the sequence of the events that are going to take place, including the initial preparation of the area, the injection of local anaesthetic and the subsequent surgery. Reassure the patient that the pain from any injection will be temporary and that during surgery there should be no pain, although the sense of touch may remain.

2 Enquire particularly about current therapy, allergies, cardiorespiratory and neurological disease. Check the pulse rate, rhythm and blood pressure. If you suspect myocardial disease have the pulse, blood pressure and

ECG monitored throughout the procedure. Study the landmarks of the area carefully before proceeding. Place a catheter in a vein well away from the operative site in case resuscitation is required. Choose local anaesthetic drugs with attention to the likely volume required: 0.5% or 1% lidocaine or prilocaine without adrenaline (epinephrine) is suitable for most infiltrations or nerve blocks, respectively. Calculate the maximum safe dose based on the patient's measured weight. In a 70-kg adult the maximum dose of plain lidocaine is 210 mg (3 mg/kg). As 1% lidocaine contains 10 mg/ml, the maximum safe volume is 21 ml. If larger volumes are required, either reduce these concentrations, add adrenaline (epinephrine) or perform part of the block 15–20 minutes later.

Action

1 Exercise full sterile precautions. Wash hands and arms thoroughly before donning gown and gloves. Prepare the skin with 2% iodine in spirit or 0.5% chlorhexidine in 70% alcohol and cover with suitable drapes. Maintain a sterile environment throughout the procedure. Use fine 25SWG needles for initial intradermal injection of local anaesthesia and 22–23SWG needles for infiltration.

2 When performing local infiltration, inject as the needle is being moved. When injecting round specific nerves this is less practicable. Check by aspiration before injecting to minimize the likelihood of intravascular injection. Constantly anticipate untoward reactions such as drowsiness and slurring of speech which are early signs of central nervous system toxicity. If they appear stop injecting local anaesthetic and be prepared to initiate urgent treatment.

3 Wait 10–15 minutes after injection for the local anaesthetic to take full effect. Be careful when testing whether a block is working that the patient does not confuse the sensation of pain with that of touch. Warn the patient that there may be some discomfort when the effects of the block begin to wear off.

4 According to the clinical practice and your confidence, use the following procedures. Unless otherwise indicated, use the concentrations of local anaesthetics shown in Table 2.1.

5 Lidocaine and bupivacaine can be mixed to combine the rapid onset of the former with the longer action of the latter. For infiltration anaesthesia, equal volumes of 1% lidocaine (with or without adrenaline (epinephrine)) and 0.5% bupivacaine may be used, providing the combined dose of drugs does not exceed their cumulative toxic level. Amongst anaesthetists, 2% lidocaine and 0.75% bupivacaine have some popularity for use in epidurals to ensure profound sensory and motor block, but such concentrations should not be used routinely.

TABLE 2.1 Use of local anaesthetics

Method	Anaesthetic
Infiltration	0.5% lidocaine, 0.25% bupivacaine
Nerve blocks	1% lidocaine, 1% prilocaine or 0.5% bupivacaine
Epidural	1.5% lidocaine, 0.5% bupivacaine
Spinal	0.5% heavy bupivacaine

Infiltration anaesthesia

Infiltration anaesthesia provides good operating conditions for the removal of small superficial lesions, such as sebaceous cysts and lipomata. Do not use infiltration anaesthesia in infected sites because of the risk of spreading infection and because adequate sensory block is unlikely to be achieved. Follow the general advice on equipment and actions detailed above. 0.5% lidocaine is generally recommended, avoiding adrenaline (epinephrine) where blood supply may be tenuous. Raise a small skin bleb close to the lesion then infiltrate through this bleb, attempting to place the local anaesthetic so that it spreads along tissue planes and the lesion 'floats' in an anaesthetized area.

Allow an adequate time for the anaesthetic to take effect before commencing surgery.

Digital nerve block

Digital nerve block to the fingers and toes passes along the anterolateral line of the phalanx. A digital tourniquet may be used but never use adrenaline (epinephrine).

Raise a skin bleb over the dorsum of the proximal phalanx using 1 ml of 1% plain lidocaine. Pass a 23SWG needle through this to deposit about 1–2 ml of the agent on either side of the phalanx. Inject the agent close to the web space to avoid undue distension of the tissues. Unlike infiltration analgesia, nerve blocks may require up to 20 minutes to have an effect.

Lower limb nerve blocks

Lower limb nerve blocks involve several major nerves of the thigh and leg, which are technically more difficult to block than those of the upper limb and require large doses of local anaesthetic agent. Surgeons interested in these blocks should consult the texts quoted at the end of the chapter.

Thoracic and lumbar epidurals, and spinal anaesthesia

Thoracic and lumbar epidurals, and spinal anaesthesia require expert techniques. Never perform these single-handed. Learn them under guidance.

INTRAVENOUS REGIONAL ANAESTHESIA

The technique is known as Bier's block, having been initially described in 1908 and revised by McHolmes in 1967. A dilute solution of local anaesthetic is injected into the venous system of a limb that has been exsanguinated and is kept isolated from the rest of the circulation. The anaesthetic exerts its action by diffusing from the vascular system into the tissues and thus affecting the terminal branches of sensory nerves. This is a very useful but potentially dangerous block.

POSTOPERATIVE ANALGESIA

A review on pain after surgery by the Royal College of Surgeons of England identified that many doctors considered postoperative pain to be an inevitable consequence of surgery and failed to control it adequately. In many countries, in-hospital 'acute pain teams' are responsible for the management of postoperative pain and these are now becoming increasingly common in UK practice.

The financial implications of instituting such a system are considerable, but improvements in pain control and earlier mobilization can be made within the financial constrains of health service practice.

You have an important commitment to minimize postoperative pain and provide leadership to the surgical team (junior staff, anaesthetists, nurses, physiotherapists, etc.) in the way pain control is monitored and managed.

Appraise

Failure to relieve pain adequately may have significant repercussions. Pain (real or feared) impairs mobility, and circulation to skin and muscles is reduced. As a consequence, healing is slow and pressure sores may develop with frightening rapidity. The risk of thromboembolic disease is significantly increased in immobile patients. Pain is frequently associated with hypertension and tachycardia, which may exacerbate myocardial ischaemia in susceptible individuals. After abdominal and thoracic surgery, pain will limit respiratory function with attendant risk of hypoxia and chest infection. The return of normal gut motility and absorption may be delayed, resulting in dehydration and the need for extended intravenous therapy. Even after straightforward musculoskeletal operations, pain profoundly limits activity and full function may be delayed for weeks. In financial terms alone, unrelieved pain delays healing, prolongs hospital stay and retards the patient's return to taxpayer status.

Analgesia can be achieved using many agents, administered by a variety of routes. Read the chapter on management of postoperative pain in the companion manual to this book (Kirk RM, Ribbans WJ (eds) 2004 Clinical surgery in general, 4th edn. Churchill Livingstone, Edinburgh, pp 357–369; an RCS course manual) to familiarize yourself with the various classes of analgesics available and their methods of delivery.

The use of microprocessor-controlled devices for continuous or intermittent intravenous or epidural infusions provides a more consistent pattern of pain relief. Increasingly popular are the more complex devices which permit patient-controlled analgesia (PCA), thereby enabling patients to retain some independent control of their pain. However, these sophisticated techniques do require a good understanding of the pharmacology of the drugs being administered and the complications that may ensue. Regular surveillance during their use must include frequent clinical observation and documentation of the patient's vital signs.

FURTHER READING

American College of Surgeons Committee on Trauma 1997 Advanced trauma life support for doctors. American College of Surgeons, Chicago, IL

Colquhoun MC, Handley AJ, Evans TR (eds) 2003 ABC of resuscitation, 5th edn. BMJ Books, London

Commission on the Provision of Surgical Services 1990 Report of the working party on pain after surgery. Royal College of Surgeons of England/College of Anaesthetists, London

Kirk RM, Ribbans WJ (eds) 2004 Clinical surgery in general, 4th edn. Churchill Livingstone, Edinburgh

Skinner D, Driscoll P (eds) 1999 ABC of major trauma, 3rd edn. BMJ Books, London

3

The severely injured patient

F. W. Cross, J. M. Ryan

CONTENTS

INTRODUCTION

We offer advice on appraising seriously injured patients, including definitive management. Initial management and resuscitation are described elsewhere in this textbook.

However, be aware that your approach to an injured patient is different from that adopted with other surgical illness, in that potentially life-threatening injuries involving the airway, breathing and circulation (ABC) must be corrected as they are diagnosed. You must largely abandon the usual algorithm of taking a detailed history followed by making a detailed clinical examination. For example, damage-control laparotomy as a resuscitative procedure, when the patient fails to respond to transfusion, is now well described. It is occasionally required almost as an initial procedure, leaving other injuries to be dealt with later.

SURGICAL MANAGEMENT

You should, if necessary, be able to carry out life-saving operations on most parts of the body. One test of your judgement is knowing how to modify a standard operation to meet the prevailing requirements. This includes knowing how and when to 'cut corners' safely. The ability to explore a wound successfully is a good test of basic surgical understanding and tissue craft. It is the last stage in diagnosis and at the same time it is the first stage in treating a wound.

In this chapter, we assume that the patient has been fully assessed and resuscitated and you have made a decision to operate. Early management of chest and abdominal wounds, and complex superficial lacerations, falls to general surgeons. The management of trauma is truly general surgery. The surgical management of the multiply injured should involve multiple surgical specialists working together. In many countries, specialist trauma surgeons trained in general surgery, neurosurgery and orthopaedics undertake the definitive management of these patients from admission to discharge. This chapter deals with basic procedures in the head and neck, chest, abdomen and pelvis, whether sustained in civilian or military circumstances.

SOFT TISSUE WOUNDS: GENERAL PRINCIPLES

Exploration of wounds can be a hazardous procedure, especially in the neck. In some situations, if exploration is indicated, you should decide to make a generous incision and achieve control of the major vascular structures as part of the exploration rather than provoke haemorrhage by disturbing the wound with fingers or instruments.

We describe the principles of wound exploration in general terms, which can be applied to most superficial areas of the body including scalp, face, extremities and superficial wounds of the trunk and perineal area. We give specific instructions for particular problems later in the chapter or elsewhere in the book where appropriate.

Learn as much as you can before operation. In particular, examine for potential nerve injury. When there is a penetrating missile injury obtain preliminary biplanar X-rays. They are invaluable, revealing retained missile fragments and providing clues to the missile track. In the abdomen, probing the wound is useless as a means of determining whether or not it enters the peritoneal cavity; the layers move across creating a series of baffles in a different relationship from that at the time of injury. Make sure the anaesthetist is prepared for a prolonged procedure.

Manage soft tissue wounds as a formal procedure consisting of clearly defined stages. This is the part most frequently neglected by those with limited or no experience of trauma and war wound surgery. The entry and exit wounds of missile injuries give little indication of the damage that may have occurred to deeper structures. The extent of injury can be detected only by full wound exploration. After exploring limb wounds, carry out thorough wound excision. With very few exceptions, you should leave the wound open. Perform delayed primary closure after 4–7 days.

Prepare

Prepare the wounded area and a large enough surrounding area to allow for a necessary but unplanned extension of the skin incision. If possible photograph the injured area or make a sketch; this is particularly useful to pass on to the receiving doctor if you need to transfer the patient. Clean the skin thoroughly with an antiseptic solution of your choice. Retain pressure dressings over bleeding wounds until the last minute. Wounds are usually already contaminated and such dressings rarely contribute to further overall contamination.

Access

1 Identify the extent of visible damage. Knowledge of the force and mechanism of injury and the position of the patient at the time provides added information on the likely extent of the damage.

2 Arrange for adequate assistance, retraction and lighting in order to make a firm assessment.

3 You usually need to enlarge the wound in order to obtain adequate access to damaged structures. Further enlargement may be necessary later during definitive repair.

4 Digital exploration may indicate the direction of the wound but cannot reliably reveal its depth or eventual extent. The most direct way of doing this is usually to incise tissue immediately overlying the track. Bear in mind the site and extent of the resulting wound, particularly if it needs to be extended as part of the definitive procedure, or if it crosses major skin creases. However, cosmesis (the future appearance) is not of primary concern during life-saving surgery. Whenever possible, incise in the long axis of a limb. In some circumstances you may need to make counter-incisions.

Assess

You need good lighting, intelligent retraction, a knowledge of local anatomy and the possible distortions to perform safely. Look carefully into the existing wound and identify its extent, if possible without initial dissection. The presence of blood indicates the site of tissue injury. Follow it by retracting the tissues and observing. Do not initially carry out any dissection because it destroys the natural tissue relationships, so defer it as long as necessary. Explore the wound in layers. Follow any puncture wound through the layers, opening each in turn until you can detect no further penetration. Remember that the tissues may no longer be in the same relationship that they were at the time of the injury, and a penetrating wound may seem to take a different course from that expected. The tissue layers form a series of baffles, as in the abdomen, mentioned above.

Identify neurovascular bundles in the wound track and note any damage, but you need not dissect out nerves. The majority of nerve injuries are neurapraxias [Greek *neuron* (= nerve) + *a* (= not) + *prassein* (= to do)], described by H. J. Seddon as temporary paralysis without degeneration, and recover spontaneously. If a nerve appears to be injured, requiring later exploration, mark its position with a non-absorbable suture. Record in the operation notes the nature and extent of any nerve injury that you detect.

Action

1 Arrest haemorrhage, temporarily compressing the bleeding point with swabs, controlling major vessels proximally and distally with slings or with arterial clamps. Do not apply haemostatic arterial clamps indiscriminately but capture and ligate small bleeding vessels under vision as you encounter them. Do not attempt to explore or repair wounds in the presence of bleeding. It is futile and dangerous.

2 Once you have done this, start by cleaning the wound. Irrigate it with copious quantities of saline followed by aqueous antiseptic. This removes most superficial foreign material and improves visualization. Remove deeper contaminants as the exploration progresses.

3 Radio-opaque objects localized with preoperative films may still be difficult to find; employ intraoperative

screening if it is available. Most glass is radio-opaque. Make sure you can identify the layer of tissue in which the object lies, otherwise you are not likely to localize it at all. Approach long narrow objects such as glass slivers or needles from the side rather than end-on, since they seldom leave discernible tracks. It is not necessary to remove every piece of metal or glass visible on a radiograph. Use your clinical judgement; for example, you may leave a small piece of smooth-edged windscreen glass in the face, but vegetable material or slivers of wood are potent sources of chronic infection.

KEY POINT Criteria for muscle excision

- Identify and rigorously excise dead muscle, which is pale, non-contractile, mushy and does not bleed when incised.

4 Inspect for tendon damage. Tendon repair need not be performed initially. Trim tattered ends and mark them with a non-absorbable suture as for nerves (see above).

5 Now repair any major vessel damage that you had previously noted. Trim damaged vessel ends and carry out a primary anastomosis wherever possible. Avoid tension; if necessary, mobilize the vessel proximally and distally. It is possible to achieve considerable length by simple mobilization. If this does not work, interpose a graft. If possible use reversed vein because of problems with infection. You may be forced to use a synthetic graft; in this case put antibiotic powder directly into the wound at the end of the operation and cover the repair with healthy muscle. Always repair interrupted major veins at the same time as arteries. Use a plastic shunt to restore the circulation if immediate repair is not possible (see below). Shunt both the damaged artery and vein if possible since venous engorgement of a limb may compromise its viability. For precise details of vascular repair see Chapter 32.

6 Pay particular attention to comminuted bony injuries. Clean contaminated bone but do not remove it if it is still attached to viable periosteum or healthy muscle. Discard small detached bony fragments, which contribute to postoperative wound infection. Carry out orthopaedic fixation after completing vascular repair. In the event of major long bone fractures, allow for the presence of shortening that will be corrected at orthopaedic repair, particularly when you need to repair blood vessels.

7 Identify injuries to joints and clean them rigorously. Cover exposed cartilage with at least one layer of healthy tissue, ideally with synovium.

8 Make sure that all dead tissue has been removed, that an open wound is open enough to drain and that haemostasis is secure.

9 Irrigate the wound again at the end of the repair procedure. Secure haemostasis before closing a clean wound or dressing an open contaminated wound with lightly fluffed gauze to allow free drainage, avoiding constriction.

KEY POINT Delayed primary closure

- Always leave contaminated wounds open including the fascia, since damaged muscle deep to fascial layers inevitably swells, potentially causing compartment syndrome.

Closure

1 Do not close a wound unless you are sure it is recent, clean and healthy. Use delayed primary closure if in doubt. Approximate tissue loosely during closure, never under tension, and in its natural layers. It is seldom necessary to repair muscle, but approximate subcutaneous tissue with absorbable sutures, preferably interrupted, to reduce the risk of tissue fluid collecting in dead spaces.

2 Close the skin with interrupted non-absorbable sutures, trimming the edges where required to reduce bevelling.

3 Consider using primary split-skin grafting in addition to suturing at delayed primary closure, particularly when there has been tissue loss.

4 Always check distal limb viability before leaving the operating theatre, particularly in the presence of constrictive dressings.

Postoperative

1 Immobilize the injured soft tissue with cotton wool, conforming bandages and, if necessary, a splint, even in the absence of bony injury. Keep the limb or other wounded part immobilized as far as possible. Watch for the signs of sepsis outlined below.

2 Watch for signs of postoperative limb ischaemia or overt haemorrhage.

3 Continue the antibiotic cover started preoperatively.

KEY POINT Signs of sepsis

- Increasing pain, increasing temperature, soiling of dressings and an offensive smell.

SPECIFIC SOFT TISSUE SITES

NECK

Blunt injury to the neck rarely requires operative intervention. The cervical collar provides first-aid immobilization. Institute skull traction to decompress the spinal canal if there are neurological signs. If this fails, neurosurgical intervention is needed to decompress it directly. Treat partial section of the cervical spinal cord by early operative decompression and fixation to reduce the amount of residual disability, but this is controversial and it is not indicated for complete section. Seek an urgent neurosurgical referral.

Do not explore penetrating wounds that remain superficial to the platysma muscle. If the wound goes deeper, explore it if there is brisk bleeding, an expanding haematoma, haemoptysis or haematemesis, neurological injury, surgical emphysema or an obvious air leak. Do not explore the neck if there is a pneumothorax in the absence of any of these signs. If none of these is present and arteriography and X-ray examination of the pharynx as the patient swallows thin barium are negative, then it is safe to observe the patient. Oesophagoscopy and bronchoscopy are often advised but seldom helpful; in any case, any visible lesion is likely to produce one of the above features.

Whilst knife wounds and handgun injuries to the neck may be handled conservatively in the absence of major damage, high-energy-transfer missile wounds often cause extensive disruption and almost always require emergency exploration for the arrest of major haemorrhage.

Action

1 Explore the neck through one of the standard vascular access incisions, either along the clavicle or the anterior border of the sternocleidomastoid muscle, so that you can control the carotid and subclavian vessels if there is sudden bleeding. Be prepared to remove the middle third of the clavicle with a Gigli or air-driven saw to gain better access. You may need to expose injuries to the roots of the great vessels by splitting the sternum with a saw in the midline and progressively opening the cut edges with a self-retaining retractor (Fig. 3.1).

2 Haemorrhage from one or other of the major vessels can normally be controlled by simple oversewing, but if the main arteries are contused use a vein patch; alternatively replace a short section with an artificial graft. Always repair the common or internal carotid unless it is actually clotted; in that case there is a risk of embolus to the brain if you disturb the clot. You may safely ligate the external carotid. Haemorrhage from the vertebral artery is usually more difficult to deal with, through a prevertebral approach. Repair the internal jugular veins

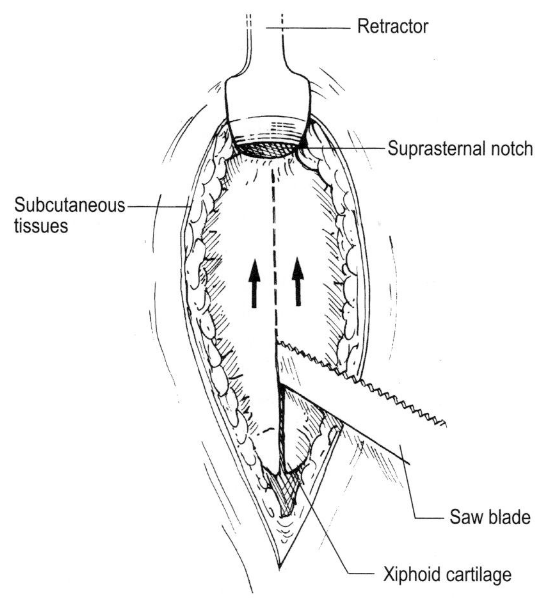

Fig. 3.1 The midline sternotomy for access to all chambers of the heart, the pulmonary vessels and the arch of the aorta. You may use a Gigli saw if you do not have a powered sternal saw available.

whenever possible but you may safely ligate all the other neck veins. Head-down tilt reduces risk of air embolus to the heart but increases bleeding. Try to clamp the vessel on either side of the damage before attempting repair.

3 You can normally repair the trachea using a single layer of absorbable material over the endotracheal tube. Defects need to be patched. Repair the injured pharynx in two layers and drain the wound.

> **? DIFFICULTY**
>
> On occasion you explore a neck wound because of severe haemorrhage and cannot identify any vascular injury, so explore the wound to its fullest extent. If you miss a vascular injury and bleeding, the patient is in severe danger.

SURGICAL AIRWAY

If the airway is obstructed and it is not possible to perform either an orotracheal or nasotracheal intubation you need to create a surgical airway. The commonest indication is severe faciomaxillary injury.

Action

1 Cricothyroidotomy is a relatively safe and bloodless method of securing an airway. It is not recommended in children under 12 years of age because the cricoid cartilage is the sole support for the trachea at this level. Instead employ jet insufflation. Insert a 14G intravenous cannula percutaneously through the cricothyroid membrane and connect this to an intermittent oxygen insufflator, a simple oxygen tube with a Y connector cut into it in series such that oxygen passes through the cannula only when the Y connector is digitally occluded. This procedure leads to a certain amount of carbon dioxide retention so use it for no more than 40 minutes. This buys the time to arrange either an expert intubation or a formal tracheostomy. There is no need for special positioning of the patient since the cricothyroid membrane is easily accessible.

2 Check the balloon on the cricothyroidotomy tube before starting. Remove any cervical collar. Have an assistant support the neck rigorously between hands or bent knees. A rigid cervical support collar is normally fenestrated and can be replaced after the procedure, passing the airway tube through the fenestration. Identify the cricothyroid membrane between the thyroid and cricoid cartilages and make a 3-cm transverse incision in the skin down onto it. Divide the cricothyroid membrane and enlarge the resulting hole in the trachea with a tracheal dilator or artery forceps. Insert a suitable-sized cuffed adult tracheostomy tube or a purpose-made cricothyroidotomy tube if one is available. Replace the rigid cervical collar.

> **? DIFFICULTY**
>
> 1. Keep the cricothyroidotomy incision small, no wider than a stab incision with a large blade – a larger incision risks damaging the anterior jugular vein and brisk venous haemorrhage. You can stop it by pressing on it but prefer to identify, clamp and ligate the cut end after you have safely secured the cricothyroidotomy tube. Remember that airway is more urgent than bleeding and, if this mishap occurs, ignore bleeding until the tube is secure in the trachea.
> 2. Regard tracheostomy as an elective technique, best performed in an anaesthetized, intubated patient. It is a requirement in children. The only real emergency indication in an adult is for penetrating laryngeal trauma with associated damage in the cricothyroid. The technique is described in Chapter 49. When there is an open defect in the trachea, the tracheostomy tube can often be placed in the trachea directly through the wound.

CHEST

Chest wounds, whether blunt or penetrating, range between trivial and fatal. In war, chest injury is common with a high immediate mortality, usually from mediastinal disruption, open pneumothorax or massive haemothorax. In blunt injury, haemothorax and pneumothorax often accompany falls or other deceleration injuries.

THORACOCENTESIS

Emergency intervention in chest trauma is largely confined to thoracocentesis for tension pneumothorax, haemothorax or a combination of the two. You should be able to insert an intercostal tube drain gently and painlessly after injecting plenty of local anaesthetic; allow 5 minutes for the anaesthetic to work, unless it is urgent.

Prepare

Unless it is impossible in an unconscious patient with multiple injuries, insert the drain with the patient sitting upright. Emergency thoracocentesis is occasionally required for tension pneumothorax, but there is usually time to prepare the patient and use an aseptic technique. Use at least a 32G fenestrated (with a side window) chest drain. Place the incision in the anterior axillary line, just above the nipple line to avoid diaphragmatic or, particularly on the right, hepatic injury. This leads you to the fifth or sixth intercostal space, which is relatively free of complications. Prepare the chest with antiseptic solution. Inject at least 15 ml of 1% lidocaine, preferably with adrenaline (epinephrine) 1:200000, into the skin and deeply and widely into the intercostal muscle.

Action

1 Make a 1-cm transverse incision in the skin and deepen it into the muscle just above the upper border of the rib or you may damage the intercostal vessels. Insert two heavy nylon stitches, one as a mattress suture across the hole (not a purse-string) for closing the hole later, and the other to the side of the incision to secure the drain. Separate the intercostal muscles using scissors or artery forceps, and puncture the parietal pleura. If possible, sweep a finger around the inside of the hole to exclude or separate lung adhesions. If there is a tension pneumothorax there is a brisk gush of air at this point. Select a fenestrated trocar drain, remove the trocar completely, and place the drain gently in the pleural cavity about 6 cm deeper than the most proximal fenestration, using an artery forceps to stiffen the tip. There is no need to introduce the drain to the hilt; expansion of the lung forces both air and blood into its lumen, whatever its position. Under no circumstances use the pointed trocar to force the drain through the intercostal muscle. Connect the drain to a flutter valve or to an underwater seal drain if available (see Ch. 36). Secure it with the previously placed suture and apply a light dressing; do not use strips of adhesive plaster.

2 Insertion of the drain through a high interspace in the anterior axillary line is dangerous because of the proximity of hilar structures and the mediastinum. Avoid the mid-axillary line because of the slight but significant risk of injuring an accessory mammary artery which passes down the inside of the chest wall in the mid-axillary position.

Postoperative

Underwater sealed thoracocentesis drains may bubble for days without problems, but persistent drainage of blood is more serious. Carry out thoracotomy if there is immediate drainage of more than 1 litre of blood, or persistent drainage of more than 250 ml/hour.

PERICARDIOCENTESIS

This is occasionally beneficial when managing pericardial tamponade. It is recommended in the Advanced Trauma Life Support (ATLS) core curriculum as an emergency procedure for inexperienced doctors working alone. If emergency pericardocentesis is required for life-threatening tamponade, first call for cardiac surgical assistance since emergency thoracotomy will almost certainly be required.

Prepare

Prepare the skin with antiseptic solution and identify the xiphoid process. Place electrocardiographic (ECG) chest electrodes; if you touch the myocardium with the needle during this procedure you often see ectopic contraction waves on the monitor.

Introduce a wide-bore needle to the left of the xiphoid process, pointing towards the tip of the left scapula. Aspirate, using a syringe, as you advance the needle. If you obtain blood, attach a three-way tap and 50-ml syringe, to remove larger quantities. Watch the ECG monitor for ectopic activity. The blood is almost always clotted and often impossible to remove sufficiently to relieve the tamponade. Aspiration of blood is not a definitive treatment and the condition will recur, in which case perform immediate thoracotomy (see Ch. 36).

THORACOTOMY

Appraise

Emergency thoracotomy is rarely needed. It is usually indicated for intractable intrathoracic bleeding, as diagnosed by persistent bleeding into the chest drain. Formal thoracotomy is demanded if there is initial blood loss of more than 1 litre, continued loss of more than 250 ml/hour, cardiac tamponade, other mediastinal injuries, persistent air leak and retained foreign bodies >1.5 cm in diameter. Reserve 'emergency room thoracotomy' for penetrating cardiac wounds in which you perceive that tamponade, or brisk exsanguination through the entry wound, are immediate threats to life. It is indicated only when the vital signs are present on arrival in the emergency room, but are lost despite immediate resuscitative measures. If you can maintain cardiac output, immediately transfer the patient to the operating theatre. Do not carry out this procedure following blunt trauma to the mediastinum or aorta since the damage is nearly always diffuse.

The outcome is far better following penetrating trauma than after blunt trauma. Stab wounds usually produce single small lacerations that can be repaired relatively easily. Blunt trauma often causes widespread contusion and laceration which are more difficult to repair.

When possible, plan an urgent procedure in the operating theatre. The commonest causes of such bleeding after both blunt or penetrating trauma are damage to the intercostal vessels or lung parenchyma caused either by rib fracture or by direct rupture.

Mediastinal trauma is less often a cause of bleeding, but when it is, it is much more serious. Lung resection is seldom required in trauma cases; when it is, try to avoid pneumonectomy which carries a high mortality, even in previously fit individuals.

Prepare

Give an anaesthetic if the patient is conscious. The procedure is facilitated if there is sufficient time and the anaesthetist is able to insert a double-lumen tube in order to collapse one lung completely. This is not likely to be feasible during a conflict. Apply antiseptic skin preparation since this takes a few seconds only.

Access and assess

Thoracotomy is described in Chapter 36. Approach cardiac injury through a left anterior approach (Fig. 3.2), or if less urgent, a posterolateral incision, which gives access to lungs and pleura and mediastinum; midline sternotomy gives the best access to mediastinal structures (Fig. 3.1). There is seldom time to carry out high-resolution computed tomography (CT) even when it is available. If laparotomy is also needed, use a midline sternotomy but if there is penetrating abdominal injury, keep the laparotomy separate from the thoracotomy to avoid possible faecal contamination of the chest. For posterolateral thoracotomy incise the intercostal muscles, expose the chest cavity, insert a rib spreader and examine the thoracic cavity. Evacuate any clot, keep the operative field clear with retraction and suction. Have the lung collapsed if a double-lumen tube is in place or have it gently retracted. Examine the chest wall for injury to the intercostal or internal thoracic (mammary) arteries, and

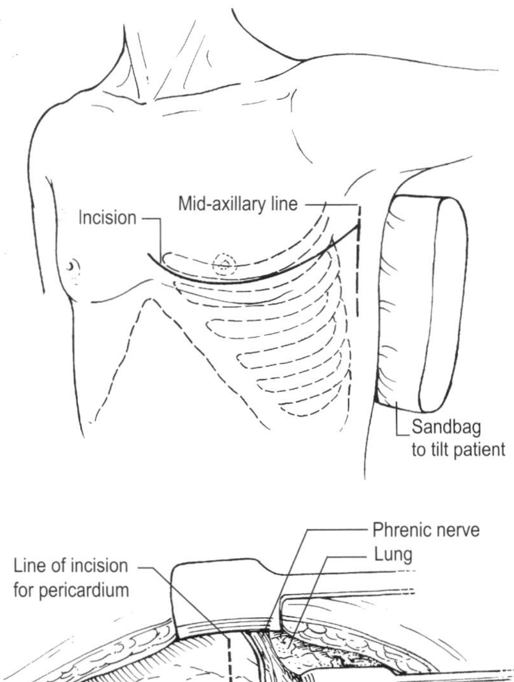

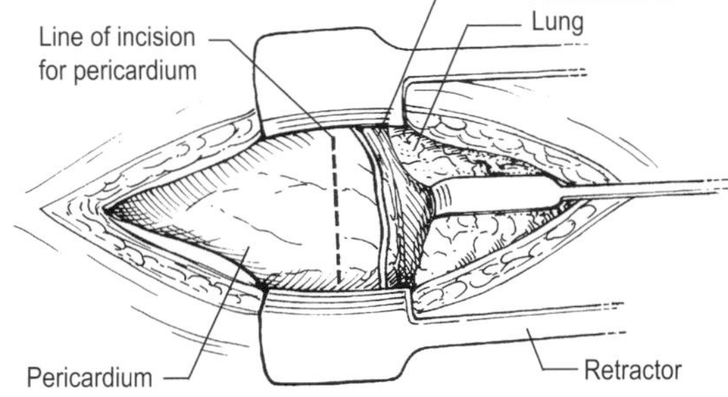

Fig. 3.2 Left anterior thoracotomy, which provides access especially to the left ventricle and pulmonary conus. Avoid the phrenic nerve.

the lung surfaces for lacerations, which may bleed profusely, and finally the aorta and lung root vessels.

If necessary lengthen the thoracotomy wound across the sternum to the contralateral side to access the other lung because of bleeding or air leak – the 'clamshell' incision (Fig. 3.3). For access to the heart, incise the pericardium, sparing the phrenic nerve, to evacuate the pericardial clot and gently deliver the heart. Excessive traction stops the circulation.

Action

1 First control bleeding from thoracic wall vessels unless there is massive exsanguination from the pulmonary vessels or aorta; control major bleeding by direct pressure. Encircle the intercostal bundle or other vessel with a suture to ligate it, avoiding, if possible, the intercostal nerve to prevent postoperative pain. Compress or oversew minor and moderate lung tears; bleeding often stops and tears seal spontaneously when the lung is deflated. Control a more extensive tear from a penetrating missile injury by applying clamps on either side of the tear; divide the tissue between them and oversew the bleeding vessels in the exposed wound track. If major hilar vessels are bleeding, consider lobectomy or pneumonectomy (see Ch. 36) if expert help is available.

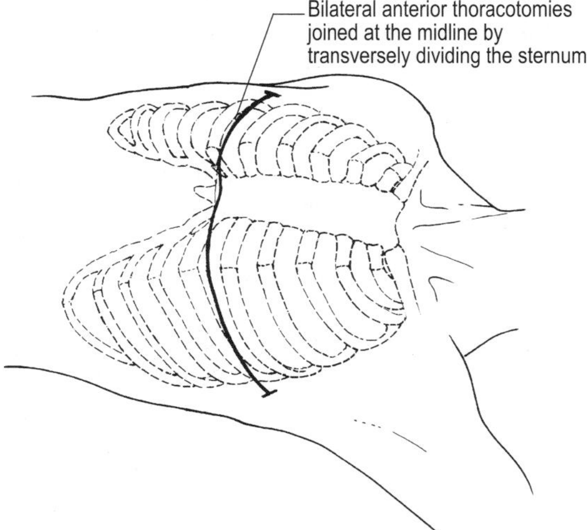

Fig. 3.3 The clamshell incision for access to both thoracic cavities and the mediastinum. The internal mammary (internal thoracic) arteries on both sides need to be cut. Secure both ends of each.

Pulmonary artery tears often extend into the left atrium and the mortality is extremely high.

2 Aortic tears or penetrating wounds are difficult to control but may seal spontaneously if the blood pressure falls. Oversew the tear with interrupted, non-absorbable sutures mounted on a round-bodied needle. Control small tears by applying a side clamp such as Brock's or Satinsky's. Cross-clamp above and below large tears before repairing them or resecting and interposing a tube graft. The superior vena cava (SVC) tends to shred when stitched so ask for expert help. In an emergency or when the thoracic wound is contaminated, oversew the cut ends of the cava.

3 Place deep sutures in injured myocardium with a large curved round-bodied needle, identifying and avoiding the coronary arteries (see also Ch. 36). Temporarily control bleeding from a penetrating ventricular wound by inserting a collapsed Foley catheter into the ventricle, inflating the balloon and pulling it against the inner edges of the defect, held there with a stitch ligature into the ventricular muscle (Fig. 3.4). Injured right atrium is thin-walled and floppy, so insert full-thickness continuous sutures to appose the wound edges. Occasionally a penetrating cardiac injury results in a large tear in one of the cardiac chambers. Urgently call for expert help. A damaged coronary artery bleeds briskly, requiring expert repair using magnification.

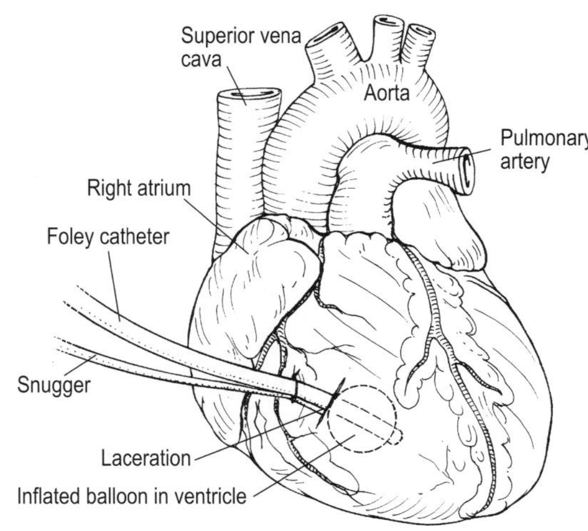

Fig. 3.4 A method for achieving temporary haemostasis in penetrating cardiac trauma, using a Foley catheter.

4 Do not close the chest until you have ensured that all major bleeding has been controlled and that the continuity of all damaged structures has been restored. Close the chest as for elective procedures and use wide-bore larger than 32G fenestrated chest drains. If the wound is contaminated or infected, leave the skin and subcutaneous layers open but not, of course, the chest cavity. Secure the drains with strong, tight no. 1, nylon stitches to avoid the disaster of them being inadvertently pulled out during transport. Never clamp drains prior to evacuation by air or road; this can lead to an unrecognized tension pneumothorax and death.

Postoperative

Ensure that the patient is carefully monitored, preferably in a critical care unit. This may be possible even during war and conflict, with robust, field-tested, modern monitoring devices. Probably the most useful device is the pulse oximeter. If the patient cannot maintain an adequate oxygen saturation despite oxygen therapy, you may need to order vigorous physiotherapy or even assisted ventilation. Always carry out a full, thorough re-examination to exclude a simple correctable cause such as a pneumothorax or haemothorax. If you fail to detect and deal with the cause, you risk allowing progressive lung infection with atelectasis possibly proceeding to an acute lung injury syndrome such as adult respiratory distress syndrome (ARDS).

Complications

These include bleeding, infection, continuing air leak and cardiac dysrhythmias. Persistent profuse bleeding of more than 250 ml/hour is a problem but postoperative bleeding tends to diminish and stop with time and possible transfusion. Reopen the chest only if the patient becomes shocked despite adequate resuscitation. Infection of the thoracotomy incision or of sustained entry and exit wounds is common, particularly if resources are constrained. Follow first principles, including reopening the wound, draining pus and giving appropriate antibiotics. Intrathoracic infection usually presents later as an empyema.

Continuing air leak is common following lung parenchymal injury. Provided the lung is fully expanded it stops spontaneously over 24–48 hours. Continuing leaks may result from previously unrecognized bronchial or even tracheal injury; suspect it if the lung fails to expand despite the presence of two large drains and suction. If possible evacuate the patient to a specialist centre.

The commonest cardiac dysrhythmia following chest injury is atrial fibrillation, usually associated with shunting and hypoxia. Ventricular ectopic beats are associated with post-traumatic myocardial ischaemia. Remember, older patients may already have an underlying cardiac problem.

TRACHEAL INJURIES

Appraise

Injury to the trachea in the neck is open or closed. Open injury is obvious. Closed injury may lead to surgical emphysema in the neck with characteristic crepitus. The trachea is rarely injured in isolation from a penetrating injury. Always investigate the oesophagus (see below). The diagnosis is more difficult following blunt trauma but you must carry out an exploration, if possible preceded by endoscopy.

Injury to the trachea and main bronchi in the chest is unusual but leads to a massive air leak. On examination you find only a tension pneumothorax but when you insert a chest drain there is a persistent air leak. If the lung does not re-expand after drainage, suspect a major airway injury, so insert a second chest drain and apply suction to both of them.

Prepare

Secure the airway. Because of the likelihood of damage to other structures including the thyroid and major vessels, seek expert help before embarking on a major exploration and repair.

Access

Injuries in the neck are dealt with locally. Otherwise carry out a posterolateral thoracotomy.

Assess and action

These two sections are dealt with together because the extent of injury will determine your technique.

1 Oversew closed injuries to the trachea in the neck, using interrupted absorbable sutures.

2 Open injuries such as those associated with high-energy transfer missiles may be associated with extensive tissue loss, precluding direct primary repair. You may be able only to insert an endotracheal tube into the disrupted trachea, thus securing the airway and closing the leak at the same time. Seek help from an expert.

3 In the chest, oversew a simple tear of the trachea or main bronchus using interrupted non-absorbable sutures. This requires expertise; the consequences of a bronchopleural fistula are lethal. More extensive injury involves the blood vessels, again demanding expert help if available.

4 Hilar near-avulsion probably requires pneumonectomy. You are unlikely to encounter this in the operating theatre since it is usually rapidly fatal.

OESOPHAGEAL INJURY

Appraise

This is usually occult. Clinically, you detect subcutaneous surgical empyema in the supraclavicular fossae. Chest X-ray may demonstrate air in the mediastinum. Oesophageal injury is normally associated with other mediastinal injuries, whether blunt or penetrating. Order a Gastrografin swallow X-ray to confirm the diagnosis.

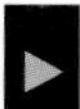

KEY POINT Do not miss oesophageal rupture

- A missed rupture carries the gravest of prognoses.

Prepare

Prepare the patient for a left posterolateral thoracotomy, possibly with a separate neck access incision or a thoracoabdominal extension. Covering antibiotics are essential.

Access

Most of the intrathoracic oesophagus can be reached through the posterolateral incision. Look out for and protect the phrenic nerve crossing the pericardium, and also the descending thoracic aorta, which is also vulnerable.

Assess

A fresh injury is relatively clean and easy to repair. If there is any delay at all, anticipate mediastinitis with pleural cavity contamination.

Action

1 Dissect the oesophagus free from surrounding structures and introduce slings above and below the site of injury. Repair a fresh injury by approximating the mucosa with interrupted absorbable sutures. This is the most important layer; a second muscular suture adds security to the repair. Drain the injury site and close the chest in the usual way.

2 A contaminated ruptured oesophagus is irreparable. It has the consistency of wet blotting paper. Manage it by draining and isolating it.

3 Drain the site and insert a tube gastrostomy into the stomach.

4 Through an incision through the sternomastoid in the neck, carry out an open formal pharyngostomy, suturing mucosa to skin. This acts as a diversion to keep the saliva out of the mediastinum.

Checklist, closure and postoperative care

These are the same as for thoracotomy.

ABDOMEN

LAPAROTOMY

Have you examined the back? Fail to look, fail to diagnose. Having done so, conducting a laparotomy for trauma follows standard guidelines which apply irrespective of whether this is a blunt or penetrating injury. Some techniques vary depending on the locally available resources.

KEY POINTS Laparotomy is indicated:

- When there is unequivocal clinical evidence of peritonitis.
- When the patient is difficult to resuscitate, requiring continuing intravenous fluids, and bleeding has been excluded in other areas.
- When air is present under the diaphragm or there is evidence of diaphragmatic rupture on the erect chest X-ray.
- When there is a positive diagnostic peritoneal lavage or a CT scan reveals the presence of blood and ruptured solid viscera.
- When there is a penetrating or perforating missile wound in a resource-constrained environment.

If an unconscious patient is stable, take advantage of available diagnostic aids. CT scan of the abdomen with contrast injection is the best single test, especially when the patient is undergoing a CT scan of the head – but insufficient blood may not yet have accumulated to show unequivocally on an abdominal CT scan performed very soon following injury. Constantly reappraise the patient's clinical condition. If CT is not available, ultrasound may be useful. If this is also not available, employ diagnostic peritoneal lavage, which remains a reliable tool (Ch. 7). If the patient is not stable, proceed to resuscitative laparotomy without delay. The laparotomy is being carried out because the patient has either shown signs of peritonitis or haemorrhage into the peritoneal cavity, or because a diagnostic test has given a positive result.

Penetrating wounds may initially present with few clinical signs but there is always a danger of the patient's condition suddenly deteriorating. Blunt injury giving rise to visceral damage normally leaves tell-tale signs on the abdominal wall such as bruising, abrasion, tyre marks, or seatbelt tattooing.

KEY POINT Exploration of penetrating wounds

- Conventional advice is that all penetrating abdominal wounds should be explored, but this is not necessary provided that:
  - The patient is absolutely stable, with no signs of intra-abdominal injury or shock.
  - You reassess the patient at frequent intervals, every 2 hours if necessary.
  - At the first sign of deterioration such as increasing pulse rate, falling blood pressure or increasing abdominal tenderness, you carry out a laparotomy. Treat such an event not as a failure but as a natural resolution of the equivocal physical signs.

Prepare

1 If the patient has not been given prophylactic antibiotics, give an initial intravenous loading dose of a versatile appropriate antibiotic now. Pass a nasogastric tube into the stomach and a urinary catheter into the bladder. There is always time to prepare and drape the abdomen properly before laparotomy.

2 Make sure that rapid transfusion of blood or fluids can be started as soon as the abdomen is opened. The abdominal wall often tamponades bleeding and this is released when the abdomen is opened.

3 Warn the theatre staff to have available necessary equipment such as two powerful suckers, adequate numbers of large packs, and vascular instruments if massive bleeding is likely.

4 Cover as much of the patient as possible with heat-reflective blankets to prevent hypothermia. A warm-air blanket is most useful if available. Bleeding patients cool off rapidly even in hot climates.

Access and assess

1 Explore the abdomen through a midline incision which can be extended in both directions, even into a median sternotomy if necessary.

2 Examine all viscera, explore the lesser sac, identify all sources of bleeding and explore all stab wounds to their fullest extent (Ch. 7).

Action

1 Your first priority is to control haemorrhage. Major intraperitoneal bleeding can be a daunting prospect. Have available two suckers and a number of large packs. As soon as the peritoneum has been opened try to identify the general area from which the bleeding is coming and clear away as much clot and free blood as possible to identify the specific source.

2 Treat life-threatening exsanguination from abdominal bleeding by opening the left chest and cross-clamping the aorta. You may leave the clamp in place for a maximum of 45 minutes while seeking and controlling it. Following penetrating trauma explore expanding retroperitoneal haematomas to exclude major vessel injury. In blunt trauma, especially that associated with pelvic fractures, leave haematomas alone as exploration may lead to uncontrollable venous haemorrhage. Control bleeding from major abdominal vessels with pressure whilst dissecting around the wound to achieve control above and below the leak, then repair the vessel with polypropylene sutures. You require expert assistance to repair major damage to aorta and vena cava. Oversew smaller bleeding mesenteric vessels. Always

examine distal bowel afterwards and resect it if you doubt its viability.

3 Repair damaged hollow viscera next, thereby limiting contamination of the peritoneum. Examine both surfaces of the stomach. Oversew tears or penetrating injuries. Watch for doubtful viability of the greater curve if there is a longitudinal tear parallel to it and resect it in case of doubt.

4 Explore the area of the duodenum if there is local retroperitoneal haemorrhage or biliary discoloration; mobilize it by Kocher's manoeuvre to examine its posterior surface. If possible repair rather than resect it. Most duodenal tears can be repaired primarily or patched with a loop of jejunum. Perform a diversionary gastrojejunostomy and place a T-tube in the common bile duct in addition to the repair if there is extensive duodenal damage. Make sure that you adequately drain the area afterwards. Resect the duodenum only if there is severe tissue loss and major concurrent pancreatic trauma, but the morbidity is formidable.

5 Small bowel injuries are easier to deal with than those of the duodenum. It is not uncommon for a single stab wound to traverse several loops of small bowel. Carefully oversew all penetrating wounds or tears with absorbable sutures in a single interrupted layer. Resect only if there are many tears in a short length of bowel, or if the viability is in doubt.

6 Large bowel injury is more likely to require resection. Prefer to oversew a small penetrating wound less than 6 hours old, particularly on the right side of the colon. Perform right hemicolectomy or left hemicolectomy if there is gross contamination, with primary anastomosis but on the left side protect this with a proximal colostomy. If there is established, generalized faecal peritonitis from the distal colon, choose the safer Hartmann's procedure (Ch. 7). If you are inexperienced, call for advice from a senior colleague.

7 Hepatic tears are often mild and may have stopped bleeding by the time you perform the laparotomy (Ch. 25). Suture major tears using a liver needle, taking care to prevent the needle from moving laterally in the parenchyma and so making the tear worse. If there is substantial haemorrhage from the liver use the manoeuvre described in 1908 by the Glaswegian surgeon J. Hogarth Pringle (1863–1941). Place a non-crushing clamp across the portal triad, with one blade through the foramen of Winslow into the lesser sac. This compresses the hepatic artery and portal vein while you assess and repair the liver damage. If bleeding continues after clamping, it is from the hepatic veins or inferior vena cava (IVC). Do not leave the clamp in place for more than 20 minutes. Major hepatic injury may demand lobectomy. Damage to the retrohepatic IVC can be difficult to reach in order to control problems. You may need to control the IVC in the chest through a midline sternotomy, then insert a bypass tube from the right atrium to the infrarenal cava, isolating the hepatic veins and retrohepatic cava for repair. Summon expert help. Survival rates from this injury are extremely disappointing. Pack otherwise uncontrollable haemorrhage and reoperate at 24 hours to remove the packs and reassess the position. Repack if the bleeding restarts. Conservative management of hepatic trauma may be effective in up to 20% of cases.

8 Splenectomy is the safest management of ruptured spleen. Sweep your hand between the diaphragm and the spleen to break down any adhesions and deliver the spleen forwards into the wound. Clamp and divide the gastrosplenic and lienorenal ligaments, avoiding the tail of the pancreas. Resect the spleen and double-tie the pedicles with strong absorbable ligatures. Oozing from disrupted adhesions usually stops after packing; if not, use diathermy current coagulation. Splenic salvage surgery involves applying haemostatic agents to the injury such as microfibrillar collagen or Vicryl mesh bags, together with diathermy coagulation and oversewing the defect (Ch. 26). Conservative management suffices in up to a quarter of patients. Favour it in children who are haemodynamically stable since they are more likely than adults to develop overwhelming post-splenectomy infections. Institute active conservative management (Ch. 26). Do not forget to arrange for immunization against pneumococcus and long-term antibiotics if the spleen does have to be resected.

9 Avoid operating for blunt renal trauma unless there is intractable parenchymal bleeding, signified by gross haemodynamically significant haematuria for more than 24 hours, or a urinary leak, or an expanding perirenal haematoma discovered at laparotomy. It is less often possible to manage penetrating trauma conservatively, but intravenous urography (IVU) and CT are helpful in excluding blood or urine leaks. The IVU demonstrates whether both kidneys are functioning if you need to consider nephrectomy. Always approach the damaged kidney through a midline laparotomy

since other viscera may be damaged which cannot be dealt with through a loin incision. Oversew contused or penetrated bleeding areas with deep liver sutures. Conserve as much kidney as possible, bearing in mind the end artery anatomy of this organ. Repair injured ureters and bladder primarily, using absorbable sutures. Insert a single layer to the ureter over a double 'J' stent. Insert a double layer into the bladder, over a suprapubic catheter. Urethral repair is described in Chapter 45.

10 If pancreatic injury is slight and the ducts are intact, stop all bleeding. Do not try to repair the injury but leave a drain down to the injured part. Treat distal injuries involving the duct by distal resection. Repair an injured duct of the head of the pancreas or unite it to a jejunal loop (Ch. 24), and call for experienced assistance.

11 If there is retroperitoneal bleeding achieve access to the IVC in the right abdomen by dividing the congenital adhesions in the right paracolic gutter and sweep the entire right colon and duodenum to the left. Now control the cava proximally and distally. Injuries to the retrohepatic cava high up at the level of the hepatic veins are nearly always fatal; they may require the insertion of an excluding shunt within the cava (see Ch. 25). Expose injuries to the aorta in a manner similar to exposing the IVC. Divide the congenital adhesions in the left paracolic gutter and swing the entire left colon, including if necessary the spleen and left kidney, to the right. In this way you can expose, control and deal with injuries to the suprarenal and coeliac levels of the aorta.

Checklist

Check that you have secured haemostasis. Is the peritoneal cavity well washed out, even in cases of recent injury, before you close the abdomen? Also confirm that all the viscera are viable once they have been returned to the abdomen. Make sure they are not under tension. Check that you have placed adequate drains and that they are properly placed and secured to the abdominal wall. Are stoma bags correctly placed, and stomas covered with dressings to avoid wound contamination?

Closure

Close the laparotomy wound using a mass closure technique, usually with a single layer looped no. 1 nylon thread. You may leave open a grossly contaminated abdomen or one with major retroperitoneal oedema. Cover the wound with wet gauze swabs. Alternatively and probably appropriately, apply a Bogota bag. Open up an intravenous fluid bag, shape it, apply the inner sterile surface over the wound and loosely suture it to the skin edges with a continuous nylon suture. It is a crude but highly effective technique, allowing continuous inspection of abdominal contents and their drainage, and it is particularly useful if you are worried concerning abdominal compartment syndrome or bowel viability (see Ch. 7). It is particularly appropriate when resources are constrained. Leave open associated missile entrance and exit wounds in the abdominal wall. Excise them and leave them for delayed primary closure.

Postoperative

Major abdominal surgery may lead to surprisingly few postoperative problems provided you have prepared adequately but this is seldom possible in trauma patients, so the immediate postoperative management is crucial. This requires a critical care environment. Following a resuscitative 'damage-control' laparotomy you nearly always need to carry out a subsequent 'second-look' laparotomy to check tissue viability and to search for, and correct, injuries missed during resuscitation.

Complications

The most important postoperative complication is bleeding. It demands re-laparotomy and control may be simple or extremely difficult with few in between. Avoid bleeding from clotting deficiency to some certain extent by giving 1 unit of fresh frozen plasma to every 4 units of transfused stored blood, and calcium gluconate injections to reverse the ethylenediamine tetra-acetic acid (EDTA) in the blood. Give platelets once the total transfused volume exceeds 10 units, even if the platelet count appears relatively normal, since many of these platelets are non-functional. A low body temperature wrecks the clotting system completely, so keep the patient warm.

Sepsis is a potent cause of collapse after 48–72 hours. Immediate postoperative pyrexia is nearly always respiratory; actively treat the patient with physiotherapy and appropriate antibiotics, and with suction if the patient is on a ventilator. Progressive abdominal sepsis is relentless in its course and leads to multisystem failure including renal, respiratory and hepatic collapse unless you deal with it surgically by drainage. Do not ignore progressive abdominal sepsis; urgently re-explore the abdomen to determine the cause and deal with it.

Anastomotic leaks are more likely following trauma surgery than after elective operations, so institute judicious drainage at the initial procedure to provide early warning of a leak. Treat such leaks conservatively. Low-output fistulae usually respond to a few days without oral feeding and instituting nasogastric aspiration. High-output fistulae demand parenteral nutrition, somatostatin or a similar agent and a critical care environment if possible. Management of multi-organ failure is complex, requiring expert care and back-up.

DAMAGE-CONTROL LAPAROTOMY

This term describes laparotomy to control massive haemorrhage following abdominal injury. The technique differs little from that described previously. Studies in the USA in the 1980s showed deaths occur at the scene following multiple handgun injuries, the great majority associated with vascular damage and bleeding, although some died later from sepsis and multi-organ failure. The risks are highest with high-energy injury, penetrating injury and multi-organ injury.

Standardized treatment was developed but, following devastating trauma to the torso, mortality remains high from exsanguination. Exsanguination and resulting hypoperfusion reduces tissue oxygenation, with consequent anaerobic metabolism, causing a build-up of lactic acid and acidosis. Hypothermia develops at the site of injury, during transfer and on exposure of the body cavities at operation. Coagulopathy develops as a result of the exsanguinations, trauma, acidosis, and also from the effects of the hypothermia on the temperature-sensitive clotting cascade. These three factors combine to increase mortality and demand damage control.

Transfer the patient to operating theatre as quickly as possible. Open the abdomen through a generous midline incision. If you need to enter the chest, employ a 'clamshell' incision (Fig. 3.3). The laparotomy proceeds in three parts. Rotondo[1,2] suggests that a survival rate approaching 60% can be achieved. The initial laparotomy is intended to control damage which can be controlled and pack damage which cannot. Secondly there is an intensive care phase, aimed at correcting the metabolic acidosis, haemoglobin and blood clotting. The third phase is a return to theatre, with definitive repair of packed injuries at a second-look laparotomy. Never forget why you are operating: to save life. Life lost is irrecoverable; sepsis or organ failure may be recoverable.

REFERENCES

1. Rotondo MF, Zonies DH 1997 The damage control sequence and underlying logic. Surgical Clinics of North America 4:761–777
2. Rotondo M, Schwab CW, McGonigal D et al 1993 Damage control: an approach for improved survival in exsanguinating penetrating abdominal injury. Journal of Trauma 35:373–383

FURTHER READING

American College of Surgeons 1989 Advanced trauma life support course for physicians. American College of Surgeons, Chicago

Shapiro MB, Jenkins DH, Schwab CW 2000 Damage control: collective review. Journal of Trauma 49:969–978

Skinner D, Driscoll P, Earlam R J (eds) 1991 ABC of major trauma. BMJ Books, London

4

Minor soft tissue injuries

R. M. Kirk, M. C. Winslet

Appraise

1 Minor injuries are differentiated from severe injuries only by their extent and usual singularity. This allows you to focus on the local injury, usually without the need to concentrate on the patient's general condition, or identify which of several problems takes precedence. However, do not misinterpret 'minor'. Damaged tissue is susceptible to complications irrespective of its extent. You may discover that a small injury is very serious and the patient is severely injured (Ch. 3).

2 Do not, therefore, concentrate on the local lesion to the exclusion of considering other possible injuries, or a disability including epilepsy and diabetes making the patient susceptible, or physical or mental failure to guard against sustaining the injury, an undeclared malicious injury, and occasionally, a self-inflicted injury. Identify coexisting medical conditions, and medication, both prescribed and proscribed drugs, and excessive alcohol.

KEY POINTS 'Minor' does not excuse complacency

- Minor often means single, local – but the injuries may be severe and dangerous.
- Many 'minor' injuries prove to be of major consequence.
- Examine and manage them as potentially serious.
- Respond to unexpected findings.

3 While you are appraising the injury first stop any bleeding. Do this by applying pressure over the site. Do not rush to apply clamps, since the bleeding vessel may be important and needs to be repaired. If there is a delay it may be convenient to place a pad over a wound in an extremity, position a blood-pressure cuff over this, and slowly inflate the cuff until it controls the bleeding; thereafter monitor the distal pulses and the colour of the extremities. After 5–10 minutes, deflate the cuff and watch to see if the bleeding is controlled.

4 You can now quietly establish a relationship with the patient, who is likely to be apprehensive, may be volatile, and is easily panicked by feverish activity. Try not to rush this encounter because you need to assess the patient's general condition and state of mind, and the possibility of a so far undisclosed background of illness, drugs, or assault. You discover this information only by gaining the patient's trust.

5 If the patient is accompanied, or brought in by ambulance, obtain as much relevant information as possible. From the patient's history decide the interval since injury, the mechanism, the likely degree of contamination, and the likely viability of the tissues.

6 If the patient trusts you it is possible to examine the wound visually and by palpation, to determine its type and severity. As thoroughly as you can, determine the extent of the injury. Decide if the area is sensitive. Are the major vessels intact, and motor and sensory functions normal? Are there likely to be foreign bodies or contaminating particles? Is there previously unsuspected bone or joint injury? Is the appearance of the wound compatible with the patient's and any witnesses' accounts of when and how the injury was sustained? Exclude other injuries and assess possible co-morbidity.

7 Wounds may be classified as contusions (Latin *tundere* = to bruise), haematomas (Greek-*oma* = suffix indicating tumour thus a collection of blood rather than a diffuse bruise), abrasions (Latin *ab* = from + *radere* = scrape), incisions (Latin *in* = into + *caedere* = to cut), punctures (Latin *pungere* = to prick), penetrations – both low velocity and high velocity, or lacerations (Latin *lacerare* = to tear). There are also particular injuries such

as bites, pressure sores, degloving injuries, hydraulic injection of fluids, and implantation of foreign bodies.

8 The site of the wound has important consequences. If it is on the scalp the blood supply is generous and it will heal well. If it is on the face the blood supply is also rich but it is important to ensure that you achieve the best cosmetic result. Injuries to or near the eyes demand specialized care as do injuries to the ears and nose. Hand injuries demand the greatest attention because of their sensory and functional capabilities and also their appearance. Wounds in certain sites are notorious for poor healing, notably injuries over the shins which often raise traumatized skin flaps over the bone that frequently fail to survive.

9 A common and challenging injury is a splinter – usually in the hand or foot, often of wood including thorns, glass, and among butchers, spicules of bone. Retained organic splinters frequently turn septic. Metal and most glass fragments are radio-opaque, especially to mammography strength X-rays. Take X-rays in two planes at right angles to each other and be willing to attach a metal marker such as a paper clip over the site of the foreign body to guide you when you remove it. Ultrasound scans are sometimes helpful in identifying radiolucent materials.

10 Bites are notoriously liable to infection, the most contaminating often being human bites. Dog and cat bites may also transmit infection. In all cases take care to follow the principles of wound injuries. Give systemic antibiotics, and in the case of animal bites ensure that the patient is immunized against tetanus. Bites from rabid dogs and snake bites require specialist treatment.

11 If possible photograph the injury before you disturb it. If there is possible bony injury or radio-opaque foreign body, should you obtain bi-planar X-rays?

12 Carefully, accurately and fully record your findings.

▶ KEY POINTS Possible implications

- Many wounds that you see have legal and insurance implications.
- Take a photograph or make a sketch for future reference.
- Consider if you should ask for senior advice.
- Are there any further tests or investigations that might be demanded?

13 Consider the likelihood of tetanus developing. Remember that the size of the wound does not determine the risk. High-risk circumstances include those sustained in agricultural surroundings, punctured, frostbitten, crushed and avulsed wounds, old neglected wounds, those with embedded foreign bodies, missile wounds and burns. Elderly, pregnant and drug-addicted patients are at high risk. Is the patient actively immunized?

14 Is there a possibility of necrotizing fasciitis? (See Chs 2, 42.) It may complicate an apparently trivial injury, especially in the presence of co-morbidity such as diabetes, immunosuppression or drug abuse. Common sites include the limbs and perineum.

15 Although gas gangrene is rare, be aware of the possibility. The organism is usually *Clostridium perfringens (welchii)* and this is a normal commensal of the gastrointestinal and female genital tracts, so suspect the possibility if the minor injury is sited close to these tracts. It usually complicates trauma. Suspect it if there is obvious swelling, skin discoloration and crepitus.

Prepare

1 Maintain control of bleeding.

2 Discuss the management and risks with the patient and obtain informed consent for the proposed treatment.

3 For routine non-contaminated wounds do not prescribe antibiotics but if there is any doubt, and especially if the patient has a hip or cardiac prosthesis, diabetes, peripheral vascular disease or is prone to endocarditis, give a versatile systemic antibiotic.

4 For clean, recent wounds in a fully immunized patient, you need not give a further tetanus booster. You may be in doubt about full immunization in which case give a deep subcutaneous or intramuscular dose of absorbed diphtheria [low dose], tetanus vaccine. The wound may be more than 6 hours old, punctured, devitalized, with foreign bodies, likely to be contaminated with manure, and in an immuno-compromised patient or one in whom you are uncertain about the immunization status. Primarily concentrate on cleaning the wound and removing devitalized or foreign material to leave it clean and healthy. Give an antibiotic such as benzylpenicillin or metronidazole. Give a tetanus booster now, to start or continue full immunization, and through a different site, give an intramuscular injection of tetanus immunoglobulin.

5 Is there any risk of gas gangrene? Start a course of prophylactic, systemic penicillin if you have any doubt. Remember, though, that the best prophylaxis is adequate surgery.

KEY POINTS Tetanus and gas gangrene protection

- The best protection is not with injections but with wound care.
- Make sure the wound toilet is meticulous.

6 Clean the surrounding skin and apply a water-based antiseptic but do not allow this to enter the wound. In a limb extend the cleansing and antiseptic distally because you may need to inspect or operate on a distal area. Similarly, consider possible extensions of exploration of the trunk or head and neck.

Anaesthesia

1 What method of anaesthesia do you need? Except for the simplest, cleanest uncomplicated wound you need some sort of anaesthesia to explore and treat the wound properly. Remember that someone who has sustained an injury is already anxious. If you handle the wound roughly you will lose the cooperation of the patient.

2 Is it possible to carry out an examination and simple treatment using some form of local anaesthesia (Ch. 3)? You cannot thoroughly explore the wound if it is painful. Irrigate a simple wound with 1% lidocaine. Alternatively, soak a swab with 5 ml local anaesthetic and pack it in the wound for 10–15 minutes.

3 Do not underestimate the painfulness of splinter removal, especially in a young child. It is sometimes valuable to soak the area in warm water for 15–30 minutes to macerate the skin. If the splinter is in a finger or toe, especially if it is deep, beneath the nail, be willing to produce a digital block. Inject lidocaine from the dorsum of the root of the finger or toe to anaesthetize the dorsal and palmar or plantar nerves on each side of the proximal phalanx. Inject local anaesthetic at the level of the web space to avoid raising tissue tension in the digit (Fig. 4.1).

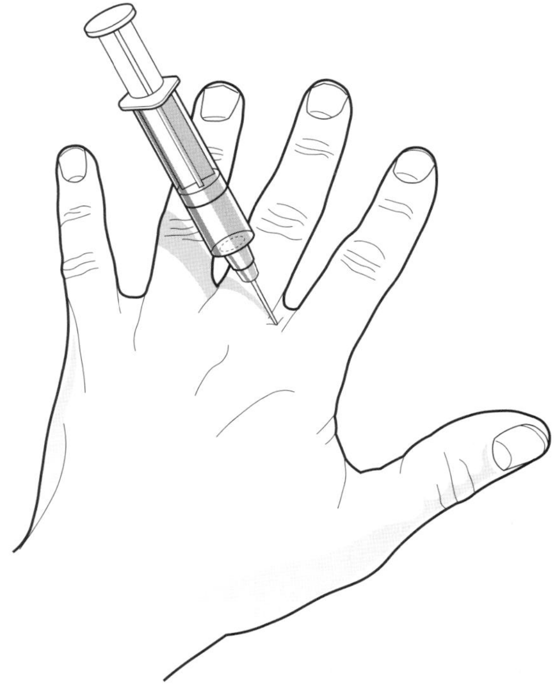

Fig 4.1 Never increase tissue tension when injecting local anaesthesia before incising an abscess, particularly for an infected finger. It is often referred to as 'ring block', suggesting the raising of a circular swelling, but this would compress the digital vessels. Inject at the level of the interdigital web where there is plenty of space.

4 You can obtain a more certain effect by infiltrating the tissues within the wound with lidocaine, inserting the needle subcutaneously from within the wound, avoiding puncturing the intact skin. Remember that the maximum dosage is 50 mg/hour for a 70-kg man. In each case leave sufficient time for the local anaesthetic to take effect, at least 5, and preferably 20 minutes.

5 If there is oozing you may add 1:2000 adrenaline (epinephrine) to lidocaine provided there is no area already ischaemic and no possibility of distal ischaemia in an extremity.

6 You may need to use regional or general anaesthesia in some cases (see Ch. 2).

Action

1 Have all the necessary clothing and dressings removed.

2 Under sterile conditions carefully inspect the wound and the surroundings. If you apply a skin sterilizing agent such as povidone-iodine, keep it from entering the wound.

3 Meticulously obtain haemostasis in order to see the whole wound. Remove all clot, since this signals a cut vessel that could re-bleed and may need to be suture-ligated using a fine absorbable synthetic stitch.

4 Look for colour changes, obvious contamination, and exposure of, for example, bone, joint, vessels, tendons and nerves.

5 Pick out foreign material such as clothing, grit, vegetable matter, and wash out dirt using plenty of sterile saline – although clean tap water appears to be just as safe. If there is ingrained dirt use a jet from a capacious syringe, through a medium-sized needle, rather than scrubbing the tissues, although gentle scrubbing with a soft brush is often used when dealing with extensive, ingrained wounds.

6 Splinter removal may be easy if you can grasp a protruding piece with fine forceps and draw it out completely in the line along which it entered. Very often this is not possible. Occasionally you can gently dilate the entry puncture wound with very fine pointed forceps, sufficiently to grasp the buried end. If not, be willing to create an access track by making an incision down to the splinter in the line of its entry. Use this method to remove a retained portion of a broken splinter. You may succeed in grasping the end of a subungual splinter by cutting a 'V' in the distal end of the nail after carefully anaesthetizing the area (Fig. 4.2). Soft splinters of, for example rotten wood, may require to be 'de-roofed' along the whole length of the splinter by incising the overlying skin or nail in the line of the splinter. Use your discretion when faced with an inert splinter or other deeply embedded foreign body, such as a broken needle, in an area at risk of damage such as the palm of the hand. Call for assistance or guidance, or defer exploration, allowing an experienced colleague to decide whether or not to leave the wound unexplored.

7 Excise all dead, crushed, avulsed, shredded, heavily contaminated tissue, using discretion. Be sparing with skin, and especially specialized skin on, for example, the fingers, hands and face. If the wound is dirty but the skin is healthy, merely pare a minimum from the skin edges.

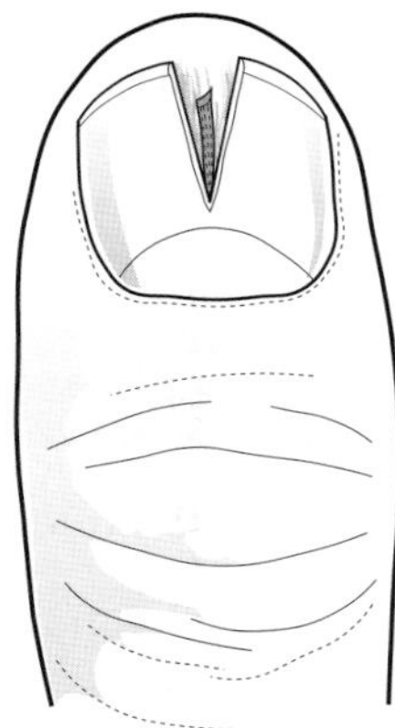

Fig. 4.2 Be willing to cut a 'V' out of the nail to remove a splinter safely and completely.

8 Boldly excise damaged or contaminated subcutaneous tissue and fat. Retained damaged, dead muscle is particularly dangerous; unless it is obviously pink and healthy, pinch up small pieces with dissecting forceps. If it contracts, release it; if it does not, snip it off; does the cut surface bleed? Continue until you reach healthy contractile muscle which bleeds from the cut surface.

9 Explore the whole of a dirty wound. Be willing to incise the skin to reach all the damaged area but do not open up fresh healthy tissues to pursue metal fragments. If there is tight fascia, incise it in the line of the skin incision.

10 However small the wound, it may prove to be heavily contaminated, to have foreign material, embedded organisms and bone or joint injuries. Meticulously remove all clot, since this signals a cut vessel that could re-bleed and may need to be suture-ligated using a fine absorbable synthetic stitch. In the presence of heavy contamination it may be unwise to attempt to repair fractures, or tendons and nerves. Mark the cut ends of nerves with black silk stitches placed through the adventitia. Cover the repair with healthy tissue.

11 Do not put any antiseptic in the wound. It damages previously viable tissues as much as bacteria.

12 Save pieces of tissue for staining and culture.

Check

1 Have you looked everywhere to exclude dead or diseased tissue?

2 Is there any persistent bleeding?

3 Have you washed away or picked out all the contaminating material?

4 Is there any potential tension from oedema?

Immediate primary closure?

1 Many simple wounds can be closed immediately provided there is no remaining devitalized tissue, no foreign material and no contamination. The earlier you see and treat the wound following injury the more likely that it is safe to close it immediately. A lapse of 6 hours is often quoted as a limit but the risk depends on many factors including the site, the amount of associated trauma, the likelihood of contamination and the type of organisms.

2 Primary wound closure implies immediate covering of the wound with skin. This may be by re-apposing clean wound edges if there is no skin loss, especially in areas with a rich blood supply such as the face and scalp. If this is a simple, clean, dry, uncontaminated wound, make the most careful apposition provided you can achieve it without tension.

3 The face, scalp and neck have such a rich blood supply that many wounds heal well even thought there may be some contamination and minimal crushing.

4 In some cases when the wound is contaminated with anaerobic organisms it may still be closed provided the patient is given prophylaxis against the organisms, perhaps with metronidazole.

5 Do not attempt immediate suturing of a traumatized skin flap on an area such as the shin, especially if the base is sited distally. Stop the bleeding, clean the wound carefully, elevate the part overnight if possible, to allow the swelling to settle and examine it next day. As a rule avoid stitches; prefer to replace a flap that is likely to survive, and after carefully drying the skin, apply adhesive tape to hold it in place (Fig. 4.3).

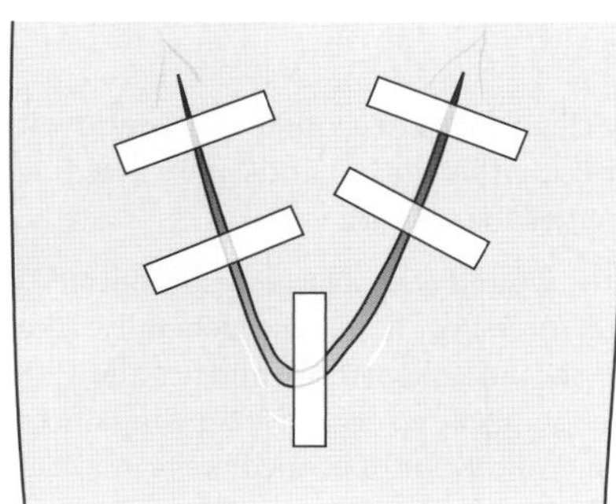

Fig. 4.3 Taping down a raised, traumatized skin flap in an area of doubtful viability.

> **KEY POINTS Inappropriate wound closure is disastrous**
>
> - Do not close if the wound is not recent, is dirty, crushed, neglected or is contaminated.
> - Do not close if the wound was sustained by human or animal bites.
> - Do not close if the vascular supply is uncertain.
> - Do not close if there are signs of inflammation or oedema.
> - Do not close if doing so will create tension.

Delayed primary closure

1 Tissues in open wounds are exposed to atmospheric oxygen; in closed wounds it may fall as low as 5–10 mmHg especially if it is cold or there is hypovolaemia (Ch. 1). Anaerobic organisms in particular flourish and wounds deprived of oxygen have a diminished defence against infections and also heal less well than those that are well oxygenated.

2 If the wound is recent, clean, healthy, viable, and uncontaminated but would produce tension from oedema, closure is likely to increase the tension, compress the blood vessels and exacerbate the anoxia. Delayed primary closure is the safest choice in case of doubt. If the wound is left open, blood flow and tissue nutrition are improved. Bacterial studies demonstrate a reduction in anaerobic organisms in the wound during

the delay period, in contaminated wounds, so defer closure.

3 Widely clean the skin around the wound with a detergent, followed by a mild antiseptic, avoiding allowing any to enter the wound.

4 Cover the wound with a large absorbent sterile pad or a hydrogel dressing. It is now generally accepted that wounds should be kept moist and not allowed to dry. Do not, though, apply an occlusive dressing since this reproduces the conditions of immediate primary closure. Do not, either, plug the wound with a large pack which occludes it. If you delayed closure because of oedema or potential swelling, elevate the part if possible.

5 Delayed primary closure is sometimes underused because there is a sense of failure; do not allow this to cloud your sense of the need for delay. Over-optimistic closure is much more of a failure. Delay may be resisted because of the apparent need for a second operation to close the wound; this is not necessarily so. You can insert sutures for closure at the initial operation and leave them untied; when the wound is healthy, tie the stitches, adding, if necessary, adherent strips between the stitches to perfect the closure.

6 It has been shown that following adequate excision of all devitalized tissue, removal of foreign material and thorough washing of the wound, it is safe to dress the wound and leave it undisturbed for several days even though it smells, provided that the patient is well, with no systemic signs of sepsis. It is difficult to resist inspecting the wound at intervals under sterile conditions, being prepared to excise devitalized tissue and take swabs and tissue samples for culture. Although objective tests are sometimes applied, you should take advice from an experienced surgeon before closing the wound. A small amount of serous discharge and fibrinous exudate is no bar to closure provided the tissues appear healthy. Be willing to repeat the inspection until you are satisfied that the wound can be closed safely, often within 3–7 days

Secondary closure

1 This is variously defined as closure delayed until granulation tissue has formed, or healing occurring spontaneously. It is infrequently used on acute injuries but you may see the wound for the first time that has resulted from an injury sustained several days or weeks ago.

2 Primary closure may not have been attempted or it may have been attempted and failed, perhaps from infection, ischaemia, subsequent trauma, nutritional deficiency or lack of viable tissue.

3 It has been known for many years that abdominal wound dehiscence and resuture almost invariably heals.

4 If you control infection, excise non-viable tissue and remove foreign material, the base fills with granulation tissue – capillary loops and fibroblasts, some of which are myofibroblasts. The myofibroblasts attach themselves and act like muscle fibres, causing wound *contraction*. Fibroblasts lay down collagen which contracts as it matures, drawing in the edges as wound *contracture*. If this process continues, drawing in surrounding tissues and skin, it results in ugly scarring and restriction of movement. In consequence, the earlier that you can overcome infection, and create a healthy, viable base, the earlier you can close the wound using free grafts or flaps (see Ch. 42).

Dressings and support

1 Make sure you know what dressings you are applying and your purpose in applying them. Closed wounds may require nothing, a simple plastic spray, an adherent tape cover or a protective pad held with an elastic adhesive strip or bandage.

2 If you expect any exudation, apply adequate absorptive dressings to avoid creating a moist track from wound to the surface which would allow microorganisms to reach the wound from the surface.

3 It is now accepted that open wounds should be kept moist. It is not yet sufficiently realized that open wounds should not be occluded from atmospheric oxygen. Especially if compression is applied, the blood flow through the local vessels is diminished. Different wound dressings are claimed to offer certain advantages. Among dressings in direct contact with open wounds, tulle gras – net impregnated with soft paraffin – has been traditionally used but is claimed to make the tissues soggy. Other non-stick dressings include soft silicone such as Mepitel®. Alginate Dressing BP 1993, type C (Kaltostat®) is valuable if there is likely to be moderate exudation, and polyurethane foams are highly absorbable; hydrogel dressings keep clean wounds moist, hydrocolloids are also claimed to facilitate autolysis – self-digestion of dead tissues.

5

Removal of superficial lumps

R. M. Kirk, M. C. Winslet

Appraise

1 Many lumps are discussed in other chapters devoted to individual organs and tissues, such as the breast (Ch. 28). However, some lumps are not specifically described. You often know or suspect the diagnosis from clinical examination. Tests may be helpful, including fine-needle aspiration cytology (FNAC) or Tru-Cut biopsy. Other lumps are determinable only by removing them and subjecting them to histological and other investigations.

KEY POINTS Single or multiple?

- Consider the possibility that the single lump that you have identified is part of a widespread condition.
- Explain this to the patient and carry out a thorough, complete examination.

2 If the lump could be malignant, decide the possible routes of spread: continuity, contiguity (Latin *con* = wholly + *tangere* = to touch; adjoining), lymphatic, vascular and, in the case of tumours lying in, or invading, serous spaces, by intracavity spread. In planning your access to such a lump bear in mind the possibility of a subsequent wide excision and try to ensure that your biopsy incision does not extend beyond the boundaries of an en bloc excision. Although the cosmetic result remains important, your first priority is safe and complete removal. If you intend to remove a biopsy specimen, plan your incision to lie within the confines of a wider radical excision if necessary.

KEY POINTS Anatomy

- Before attempting to remove a lump from an unfamiliar site, revise the anatomy – not just in relation to the surface but also in depth.
- Remember that the anatomy is often altered by disease processes.
- Always treat a lump near the parotid gland as parotid; ignore this advice at the patient's peril – it nearly always is!

Prepare

1 Obtain informed consent. If you are unsure about the nature of the lump discuss all the likely possibilities with the patient and therefore your likely course of action – and the possible consequences.

2 Mark the lump whenever possible. The position of the patient in which you examined the lump may be different from the position of the patient during the operation – and this may change the relationship of the lump to the surface.

3 Pre-plan how to place the patient and the part to be operated upon. Often, by positioning the patient or the part, you can elevate the site of operation, avoiding venous congestion and reducing bleeding. For example, a lesion on the head is easier to access if the patient lies slightly head up, emptying the veins, reducing congestion and bleeding, often termed 'reverse Trendelenburg' to distinguish it from the head down, legs up position in which the Leipzig surgeon Friedrich Trendelenburg (1844–1924) placed his patients to operate upon varicose veins.

4 If any X-rays or other images are available, have them on the screen so you can refer to them.

5 Make sure you have all the equipment and instruments you require. In the case of suspected or known malignancy make sure you have discussed with the pathologist how to preserve and present the specimen – it may need to be sent immediately in saline, or simply placed in formalin – but it may need to be split up and parts placed in different media. Before you start, make sure that the correct, labelled receptacles are to hand, the forms filled out and that a trustworthy person will deal appropriately with the specimen.

6 Study the skin creases and tension lines; they usually encircle joints rather than cross them. Although the primary consideration is the safe and effective removal of the lump, if you can do so through an incision along the lines of tissue tension, the resulting scar is fine with minimal distortion of the skin.

7 If you intend to shave the skin over the lump do so at the last possible moment. When you use local anaesthesia, clean and gently shave the skin while the anaesthetic takes effect.

8 If you are operating under local anaesthesia on a lump such as a simple cyst that you are confident is benign, inject dilute local anaesthetic around it, not into it. The oedema helps delineate and separate the surrounding tissues. If there is no infection or fear of causing ischaemia, you may incorporate adrenaline (epinephrine), 1:200000, with the local anaesthetic; this produces vasoconstriction and reduces bleeding. Start with the finest needle and raise an intracutaneous bleb a short distance, such as 1 cm, from the lump, in sensitive areas around the face, palmar skin of the hand or foot, or the nipple, or in the presence of inflammation. After 5–10 minutes, insert a longer needle through the bleb and gently advance it towards and over the lump, injecting as you proceed. If the lump is subcutaneous, inject around and beneath it. If it is a cyst, such as a sebaceous cyst, inject cautiously over the crown or you will puncture it where it connects with the blocked duct. Slightly angle your injection to each side of the skin attachment.

9 Apply antiseptic with a forceps-held swab onto the lesion and then swab round it in ever widening circles so that you do not again touch the lesion with the swab that may now have picked up microorganisms from the skin. Repeat this with a fresh swab. Place skin towels so that you can extend the incision if necessary.

KEY POINTS Final examination

- You cannot be too sure about the lump; recheck its relation to the skin and surrounding structures.
- Re-examine it now – preferably with the patient in the position ready for operation.

Access

1 If there are no other considerations prefer a straight line parallel to the skin creases.

2 If the lump is a cyst such as a sebaceous cyst, make your incision curve just off centre of the punctum or blocked duct leading to the surface – which is not always evident. In this way you hope to avoid puncturing the cyst and allowing the contents to escape. If the lump is a tumour within or attached to the undersurface of the skin, or is possibly attached to or invaded by a tumour, employ an elliptical incision encompassing the tumour, with the margins clear of it (Fig. 5.1).

3 Before you proceed, achieve perfect haemostasis using patiently applied pressure, diathermy coagulation, or ligatures.

KEY POINT Haemostasis

- In your anxiety to 'get on with it,' do not proceed until you have secured a dry field. You cannot practise safe surgery in a pool of blood.

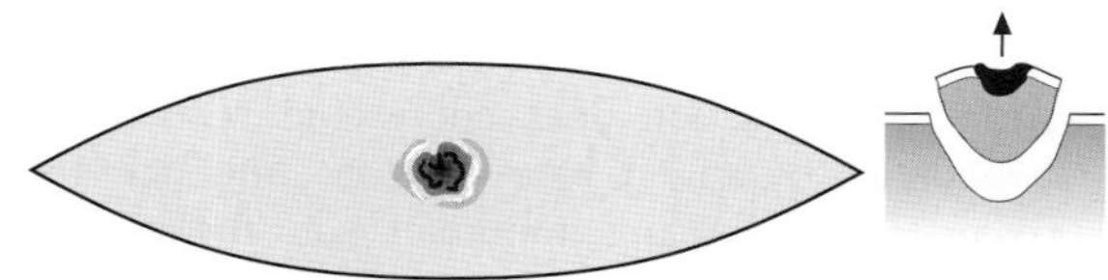

Fig. 5.1 If the lump is suspicious, keep clear not only in the horizontal plane but also in the depths, as indicated on the right in transverse section.

Assess

1 Identify and reassess the lump. It may feel different on direct palpation from expectation after feeling it through the skin. If it has a well-defined surface it is more likely to be benign than if the limits of the tumour are difficult to define, although this is by no means always reliable.

2 There are several possible courses of action, so consider them before proceeding. Decide whether it is safe to remove the lump while dissecting close to its surface if this is well defined; otherwise you may excise it radically (Latin *radix* = root; hence, by the roots), including a covering of normal tissue – an extracapsular excision. Alternatively, should you remove a biopsy specimen incorporating the edge of the lump meeting normal tissue, and have this examined immediately while you await the result, or close the wound because the report cannot be given immediately?

3 Remember that if you need to excise the lump totally, you must leave a generous margin not only horizontally but also in depth (Fig. 5.1).

4 Having gained all the necessary information should you close the wound and carefully record your findings?

▶ KEY POINTS Advice or help?

- If you struggle to make a decision ask yourself how you will justify it if there is an unfavourable outcome.
- Do not be too proud to ask an experienced person for advice and assistance.

Action

1 An obviously benign, encapsulated tumour, such as a simple cyst, can be removed safely by working along its surface and thereafter remaining in contact with it as you encompass it. If you are removing it under local anaesthesia and have injected around it, the injection fluid has partially separated the cyst and you need only to work round it, using mainly blunt dissection. Insert the rounded tips of haemostatic or non-toothed dissecting forceps in the junction of the cyst surface and adherent tissue, open or allow to spring open the blades and be prepared to cut the bridge of tissue you have put on stretch after confirming that it is simply connective tissue.

2 Remember that the blood supply of many lumps you encounter enters from the deep surface.

3 Be flexible and versatile in your choice of dissecting method. In case of doubt employ gentle separation of the tissues to displace them and reveal what lies beneath. Use sharp dissection only when you have completely identified the whole structure; if it contains blood vessels seal, ligate them or be prepared to control them immediately if you divide them.

4 The most dangerous moment is just as you are about to separate the lump. Very often you have applied traction and this produces the risk of distorting the anatomy. The deep connection is likely to include the blood supply. Check by relaxing tension, moving the lump from side to side. Only when you are certain that it is safe, carefully cut the connection.

? DIFFICULTY

1. Unexpected calamitous bleed? Do not rush to grab structures with clamps. Apply a finger or a swab, and press just sufficiently to control the bleeding. Maintain the pressure for 5 minutes checked by the clock. During this time use your head and not your fingers. Which major vessel may you have cut? Are you capable of dealing with it or should you call for senior advice or help? This is no time for pride or over-confidence. Do you need to have more swabs, a powerful sucker, vascular clamps or sutures available? When you have prepared your equipment, back-up – and yourself, gently lift the edges in turn until you have fully exposed the area. As a rule the bleeding has stopped and will remain stopped. Remember, though, that the patient's blood pressure may be low now but may recover. Straining raises intravascular pressure. In both circumstances the clot may loosen, resulting in reactionary bleeding. If you can identify the vessel, clip it and ligate it. This is difficult if the muscle contraction

that closed the lumen also causes it to retract into the tissues.
2. Cannot find the lump? It is quite possible for the lump you felt to change its position if the patient's posture has changed, or previously firm background muscles are now relaxed. If you are exploring in the neck or other areas containing closely packed vital structures, do not proceed unless you are intimately certain of the anatomical structures around the site.
3. Lump stuck? Not infrequently what felt like a mobile lump is discovered to be attached to a neighbouring structure. Make sure you can confidently identify the structure and that you can separate it without damaging the standing tissue.
4. Lump larger than anticipated? If a relatively small lump is palpable deeply within the tissues, you may not appreciate that it is the tip of a larger mass, or an extension from it. If you are a trainee, carefully determine its situation, size, surface, consistency, attachments, fixation, preferably dictating these to someone unscrubbed, who can write them down. Either ask a responsible person to contact a senior colleague or cover the wound and telephone yourself, for advice and help.
5. It is dangerous to embark on an extensive resection in an unprepared patient. Not only may the patient be in danger of immediate complications but also you may prejudice a radical, potentially curable resection of a malignant tumour by inexpert attempts to remove it.
6. Is the lump not singular but one of a group? An example of this is the discovery that what felt like a single lymph node turns out to be one of many, as occurs from time to time in Hodgkin's disease. The size and number of the resultant glands resected bears no relationship to the diagnostic value. A single gland, gently and perfectly removed without damage, is far more valuable than a mass of roughly excised, damaged glands.

Closure

1 Check that you have not caused any unnoticed injury.

2 Obtain perfect haemostasis.

3 Close the wound in a routine manner.

4 It may not be necessary to apply a conventional dressing but merely spray the closure with a plastic spray or support it with a simple adhesive strip.

Postoperative

1 Carefully write a detailed report of the incision, findings, actions and result.

2 Make absolutely certain that the specimen has been dealt with correctly and has been sent to the appropriate department for reporting.

3 Write up postoperative monitoring requirements and any medication you wish to be administered.

4 Inform your senior supervisor to report that the successful procedure or to report any adverse happenings.

5 Inform your patient of the findings and their implications.

SPECIAL SITES

NECK

Appraise

1 The neck is commonly affected with lumps of wide variety. Block dissection of neck nodes is discussed in Chapter 37. The most common lump you will be asked to remove is a lymph node. Dissection in the neck is complicated because the neck is packed with varied and important structures (see Fig. 37.3). Diligently identify the anatomical structures at the site of the lump related both to the surface and in depth. In particular distinguish any structures to which the lump is attached.

2 Do not embark upon the removal of any lump unless you have made every effort to make a firm diagnosis. Neck lump diagnosis is challenging but do not fail to exploit the wealth of excellent clinical tests that are available. Make sure you know the anatomical implications.

> **KEY POINTS Traps for the ignorant, incompetent and indolent**
>
> - It is negligent to remove any lump that could be a lymph node without a complete examination of possible local sources and exclusion of generalized glandular enlargement.
> - Assume any lump in the triangle occupied by the parotid gland is within the gland, however superficial it seems.
> - Remember the presence of the external jugular vein – it should be empty and therefore not visible if the patient is placed with head raised to avoid venous congestion.
> - Remember that a subcutaneous lump in the posterior triangle may be a solitary lymph node sitting on the accessory nerve as it leaves the junction of the upper and middle third of the sternocleidomastoid muscle, crossing to pass under the anterior edge of the junction of the middle and lower thirds of the trapezius muscle.
> - There are certain lumps which are susceptible to specific tests. For example, lumps in the thyroid gland, and branchial cysts, may be diagnosed using fine-needle aspiration cytology, or by ultrasound imaging scan.

Access

1 Carefully consider the underlying anatomy when planning the incision. What lies over the lump, what lies beneath it? A carelessly planned incision may result in transection of the external jugular vein. A badly sited submandibular incision may sever the mandibular branch of the facial nerve, denervating the muscles of the lower lip and chin.

2 Whenever possible place your incision along the lines of tension. These tend to be circular in the neck but if you extend onto the face, plan it after asking the patient to grimace beforehand, while you watch. Apart from the midline area you should see the platysma (Greek *platys* = flat, broad) muscle. The external jugular vein is superficial to the deep fascia except where it pierces it to enter the subclavian vein but the main structures lie deep to it.

Closure

1 Make sure that you have achieved perfect haemostasis. Because the skin of the neck tends to be loose, any oozing may produce a large haematoma beneath it. It may be valuable to have the patient lower the head so that any cut but collapsed veins will fill and reveal themselves.

2 Repair each layer, including platysma muscle, with finest absorbable synthetic sutures. You may close the skin with sutures, staples or with adhesive strips after drying it, applying a plastic coat or tincture of benzoin and allowing this to dry.

GROIN

Appraise

1 Like the neck, the groin contains important structures that need to be preserved. Mark the lump and carefully identify its relationship to the femoral artery, vein, nerve, the saphenous opening, vein and its tributaries, and other structures such as the pubic tubercle, inguinal ligament and rings. Remember that if the posture of the patient during the examination is different from the posture on the operating table, the anatomical relations of the lump may change.

2 Never forget to examine the scrotum and its contents in the male. Are they all normal and in their rightful position?

3 If you are operating above the inguinal ligament be aware of the deep fascia of the abdominal wall, described in 1809 by Antonio Scarpa (1747–1842) who was Professor of Anatomy in Padua. It is well developed in infancy and is easily mistaken for the external oblique aponeurosis. Below the inguinal ligament, apart from the defect at the saphenous opening you can easily identify the fascia lata.

KEY POINTS Take nothing for granted

- In an obese person many of the structures are embedded in fat. Do not assume that what appears to be a fatty lump is composed of fat throughout.
- Many femoral hernias are covered with extraperitoneal fat and the sac is easy to miss – but may contain a knuckle of bowel.
- In dissecting out a single lymph node from within a mass of fat, stay in contact with the surface of the node. If you wander away from it; you may damage an important structure.

AXILLA

Appraise

1 Although the commonest lump in the axilla requiring removal is likely to be a lymph node, a blocked apocrine gland and other skin and subcutaneous lumps may be difficult to differentiate.

2 Particularly in this site, the position of the arm when you examine the patient may be different from the position of the patient at operation. Make sure you examine the axilla with the arm positioned as it will be when you remove the lump.

Access

1 If you need to shave the axilla leave it as late as possible. Shaving is necessary only for access, not for reasons of sterility.

2 The axilla is very sensitive, so when injecting local anaesthetic and manipulating the tissues, take especial care not to handle them roughly.

3 If the arm is raised, the axillary vessels and nerves become quite superficial as the head of the humerus lifts them from behind. Identify the pulsations of the axillary artery to remind you of their closeness to the surface.

4 An incision parallel to the skin tension lines is around the joint, not longitudinally.

Closure

1 Since the patient's arm is adducted after operation, there is no tension on the suture line.

2 The axillary skin is often moist and the suture line then becomes soggy. Apply cotton wool over the gauze wound dressings to absorb perspiration, and also to apply gentle pressure into the axilla to prevent any blood from oozing under the loose, relaxed skin.

6

Superficial surgical infections

R. M. Kirk, M. C. Winslet

Appraise

Because major, life-threatening infections often begin as apparently superficial and even trivial, this description includes mention of dangerous conditions you should detect early.

Some specific infections are described in appropriate chapters, such as perianal and ischiorectal (Ch. 21), breast (Ch. 28), hands Ch. 40), styes (Ch. 51). However, you encounter infections almost anywhere in the body.

> **KEY POINTS Susceptibility?**
>
> - Diabetes? Always bear this in mind – it is increasing in incidence.
> - Immune deficiency? Generated by disease, or treatment of some diseases.

Infected sebaceous cysts occur especially on the scalp, scrotum and back. Carbuncles, usually on the back of the neck, are infections of adjacent hair follicles spreading in the subcutaneous tissues, often with multiple openings. Axillary abscesses usually arise in the sweat glands – hidradenitis (Greek *hidros* = sweat + *aden* = gland + *-itis* = inflammation).

Identify superficial infections that do not require surgical management, such as impetigo (Latin *impetere* = to rush upon), usually associated with *Staphylococcus aureus*, less often with group A β-haemolytic streptococci. It often occurs around the nose and mouth and on the legs in children during the summer months. An itch proceeds to a red macule, papule, vesicle which bursts and weeps, producing a tan or yellowish-brown crust. If it ulcerates it is called ecthyma (Greek *ekthyma* = a pustule). It usually responds to mupirocin 2% cream (Bactroban) applied three times a day for 3–5 days. If not, resort to systemic antibiotics.

Cellulitis is particularly associated with group A β-haemolytic streptococci which spread by producing hyaluronidase (Greek *hyalos* = glass), although other organisms including *Staphylococcus aureus* may be involved. It is characterized by hyperaemia and oedema but without cellular necrosis. There may or may not be an identifiable site of entry. The overlying skin is red, painful, oedematous, often showing *peau d'orange* (orange skin appearance); proximally, fine red streaks of lymphangiitis may be discerned and the regional lymph nodes may be tender. Pyrexia, toxicity and leucocytosis are variable.

Erysipelas (Greek *erythros* = red + *pella* = skin) from β-haemolytic streptococcus affects the dermis, subcutaneous tissues and lymphatics, producing a painful, spreading, intense red, indurated, well-demarcated border. It affects the face, arms, legs, usually in adults, producing pyrexia. Treat it with phenoxymethylpenicillin or erythromycin.

Necrotizing fasciitis

Several names are associated with this rapidly spreading and dangerous cellulitis of the subcutaneous tissues and deep fascia. The Parisian dermatologist Jean Fournier (1832–1914) described fulminating streptococcal gangrene; his name is reserved for male genital involvement. The New York surgeon Frank Meleney (1889–1963), described chronic skin ulcers caused by synergistic (Greek *syn* = together + *ergon* = work; working together) organisms. Type I is polymicrobial with microaerophilic and anaerobic organisms. The more common type II is monomicrobial group A streptococcus.

> **KEY POINT Apparently superficial is not trivial**
>
> - Be alert to the possibility that cellulitis may be life-threatening.

It may develop following an apparently simple cut, bite, scratch or a surgical procedure. In nearly two-thirds of patients there is co-morbidity such as diabetes, immune suppression, drug or alcohol abuse. Although it commonly develops in a limb, the perineum is the second most common site.

It starts in the superficial fascia, spreading rapidly and causing liquefactive necrosis and angiothrombosis in the subcutaneous fat. The skin is initially normal until deprivation of its blood supply causes necrosis. Erythema and swelling may initially suggest common cellulitis. but pain is a prominent feature. The skin colour often becomes violaceous allied to systemic upset so that the patient is sweaty and pale. In cellulitis the pallor following compression rapidly changes back to red as the vessels refill. In necrotizing fasciitis there is no capillary refilling and fixed staining develops in the skin.

KEY POINTS Distinguish necrotizing fasciitis from common cellulitis

- Look for early discriminatory features: severe pain and tenderness beyond the apparent extent of cellulitis; bullae and blisters.
- Do not wait for skin anaesthesia, dusky discoloration, fluctuance, gangrene.
- If the features are equivocal meticulously record them, mark out their extent and reassess them in one hour.
- If there is any deterioration, start intravenous benzylpenicillin 1–2 g 2-hourly, take the patient to the operating theatre without delay and explore the area – see below.
- Mortality varies between 20% and 80%.

If you are in serious doubt, take the patient immediately to the operating theatre, make a 2-cm incision over the area under local anaesthetic, down to the deep fascia and insert a finger. The diagnosis is confirmed if there is no bleeding, you can run your finger underneath the skin because the subcutaneous fascia is no longer present, and there is foul 'dishwater' pus (see Fig. 6.1, Ch. 42). Gram staining of the pus helps clarify which antibiotic to give. Meticulously excise all affected skin until you reach healthy subcutaneous tissue and send it for histology, culture and determination of sensitivity to antibiotics. Simply cover over the wounds, nurse the patient in an intensive care unit and return the patient to the operating theatre for re-exploration and re-excision as necessary.

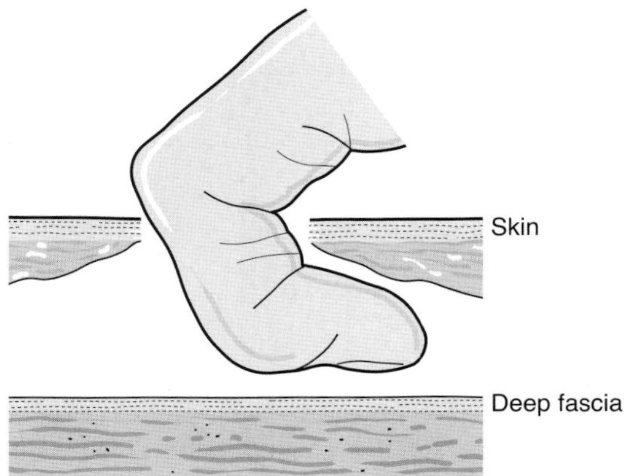

Fig. 6.1 Confirm suspected necrotizing fasciitis. Make an incision through the skin and insert your little finger. If you can rotate it in a free space between skin and deep fascia, the diagnosis is confirmed.

Clostridial gas gangrene

Clostridial gas gangrene is usually caused by the microaerophilic *Clostridium perfringens* (Greek *kloster* = spindle + Latin *perfringere* = to shatter), previously named *welchii*, named for the American pathologist William Henry Welch (1850–1934) who described it in 1892 (see Chs 9, 39). It is a spore-forming, gas- and toxin-producing organism found in cultivated soil but also in normal human skin, colon and vagina. Incubation usually takes about 12 hours but rarely develops within 1 hour – or is delayed for days or weeks. The toxins, which may spread at as much as 2 cm/h, cause myonecrosis, intense shock, often with renal failure, and death.

Infection results from inoculation into tissues with lowered oxygen tension, especially if they are traumatized, in the presence of diabetes, peripheral vascular insufficiency, drug abuse, and in immunocompromised patients.

KEY POINTS Diagnose gas gangrene early, not late

- Is the overlying skin discoloured, bronzed, brawny, black and with bullae?
- Is the area extremely tender?
- Is the patient more toxic than expected for the extent of the lesion?
- Do you detect crepitation?

If there is a discharge from a wound or ruptured bulla, it resembles dishwater and has a 'mousy' smell.

If you obtain any material send it immediately to the laboratory for confirmation of the diagnosis.

Give benzylpenicillin 0.6–1.2 g intravenously and metronidazole, and supplementary oxygen; restore circulating volume and take the patient to the operating theatre to excise all the affected tissue, after sending a specimen of the sweet-smelling pus for Gram staining. Affected muscle appears dull, pink, then red, purple and grey-green. In order to clear diseased necrotic tissue totally you may need to amputate a limb – but life is more important than limbs. Do not close the wound and be prepared to return the patient to the operating theatre for further excision if necessary.

Abscess

Abscess (Greek *apo* = from + *istemi* = to stand; Latin *ab* = from + *cedere* = retreat; a throwing off – of bad humours) is particularly associated with *Staphylococcus aureus*, which produces toxins causing cellular degeneration and death. The site is invaded by neutrophils many of which are killed and undergo autolysis to form pus by the leucocidins (Greek *leukos* = white [cells] + Latin *caedere* = to kill), of the pyogenic (Greek *pyon* = pus + *genesis* = producing) organisms. The resulting abscess cavity is lined with a fibrinous membrane heavily infiltrated with neutrophils beyond which are proliferating fibroblasts and new capillaries – granulation tissue, forming a barrier. The enclosed pus tends to track in the line of least resistance until it reaches a free surface where it may drain spontaneously or be released surgically. If it remains undrained the wall thickens, the contents become inspissated and eventually may calcify.

A superficial abscess presents the four cardinal (Latin *cardinis* = hinge; on which the diagnosis hinges) features of inflammation; tumor, rubor, calor, dolor (Latin = swelling, redness, heat, pain). The patient has a raised, swinging temperature. The tension from blood pressure with each arterial pulse makes the pain throbbing in nature. As the tension rises, blood vessels at the apex are compressed and the skin becomes white. As a result of the ischaemia, the skin becomes rapidly necrotic and turns black. If the necrotic skin falls out or if the abscess is surgically drained, the pus is released with a fall in tension and the swinging temperature settles.

A *boil* (Old English *byl*) or *furuncle* (Latin *furunculus* = little thief), is a localized abscess usually resulting from infection of a hair follicle or sweat gland. It may resolve without pointing – a 'blind boil', discharge spontaneously, or require surgical drainage.

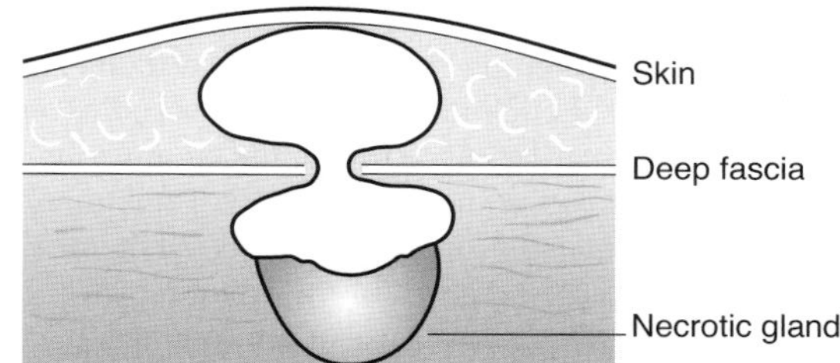

Fig. 6.2 Collar-stud abscess.

A *collar-stud* abscess may appear superficial but infection entering at a surface such as the mouth, teeth or lungs may drain to the lymph nodes beneath the deep fascia, such as the deep cervical fascia, and form an abscess which subsequently bursts through the deep fascia, presenting subcutaneously (Fig. 6.2).

Empyema necessitans may appear superficial when an abscess develops in the depths and tracks through to the surface as from the lungs or thorax to chest wall to appear as a superficial swelling. If there is no obvious local cause, it would be incompetent of you to fail to X-ray the chest before planning treatment.

Chronic abscess develops if there is a continuing cause, in spite of treatment. Tuberculosis, the presence of foreign material, dead tissue, ischaemia, immunosuppression are common causes of infection and abscesses that fail to resolve with routine measures.

Prepare

1. Exclude or stabilize any co-morbidity.
2. Discuss with the patient the diagnosis and proposed treatment so you can obtain informed consent.
3. If you suspect that management may be complex, do not hesitate to ask advice from a senior colleague.
4. Especially if the patient is at exceptional risk from the infection, be willing to give a versatile antibiotic whether or not you need to perform a surgical procedure.

Decision

1. Certain superficial abscesses resolve spontaneously and either settle or discharge. Provided they appear to be pointing spontaneously and locally, are not causing

constitutional symptoms, are not painful or spreading within the tissues, do not rush to drain them. A boil that looks as though it is pointing but becomes rather static can often be helped to drain by applying wet dressings, replacing them as they dry. These macerate (Latin *macerare* = to steep, soak) the overlying skin, facilitating the breakdown of the retaining cover over the pus. We deprecate the use of hot compresses.

2 Be cautious about carrying out any manipulative procedure on localized infections in the danger triangle of the face – between the nasolabial fold and upper lip; there is a danger of organisms entering the facial venous system, travelling retrogradely to the cavernous sinus, and causing septic thrombosis. If possible prefer to rely on systemic antibiotics.

3 Drain an abscess if it is painful, if it shows signs of pointing but does not burst, if it is tracking in the direction of sensitive tissues at risk, if the inflammation and swelling are increasing, and especially if the patient becomes pyrexial and toxic.

4 In some cases the skin overlying the abscess undergoes a series of colour changes. At first it is hot, red, shiny, then as tension rises it becomes first white, then black and necrotic. At this stage it usually bursts but sometimes the necrotic skin is hard and you may need to incise it.

5 Be suspicious of skin overlying a soft, fluid swelling that is discoloured, bluish, and thinned. Especially in the absence of signs of acute inflammation, in a patient with a possible susceptibility to tuberculosis, try to avoid opening what is probably a 'cold' abscess. Prefer to aspirate it using a long needle, inserted through healthy skin at a distance from the abscess. Send the aspirate for bacterial culture and examination, giving good clinical notes.

Access

1 Do you need to inject local anaesthesia? If your incision is through necrotic skin, sensation is lost and no anaesthetic is needed provided you stay within the necrotic area, use a pointed knife and perform it gently without raising the pressure too steeply within the abscess. A freezing spray with ethyl chloride may suffice. In many sites, it may suffice to apply a cream containing lidocaine and prilocaine (eutectic mixture of local anaesthetics, EMLA) provided you apply it 2 hours beforehand. It is especially effective on thin skin such as the scrotum.

2 If you intend injecting local anaesthetic (see Ch. 2), do not initially inject it into the site of the incision, which is very sensitive. Instead, raise a small intra-cutaneous bleb using the finest needle, into normal skin close by. Leave it for 5 minutes, then insert a longer needle through that spot and inject as you slowly advance the needle towards and into the intended incision site. Do not be impatient. Allow time for the anaesthetic to take effect. It may be valuable to add an ampoule of 1500 iu hyaluronidase (Hyalase), which improves the spread of the anaesthetic, reducing the likelihood of increasing the tension.

KEY POINTS Dangers of local anaesthesia

- Beware of over-casual use of local anaesthesia. The tissues are already under increased tension.
- If you inject local anaesthetic at high pressure you risk causing necrosis.
- A classic danger is a ring-block injected into a proximal finger in preparation for incising a distal pulp infection.
- Do not include adrenaline (epinephrine) which, because of its vasoconstrictive effect, is likely to cause tissue necrosis

3 Especially if you think the abscess may be deep-seated, loculated, containing foreign material that must be removed, of collar-stud type, requiring exploration, possibly neoplastic and therefore demanding biopsy, it may be wise to employ general anaesthesia.

Action

1 Under sterile conditions make an incision directly over the abscess. In the past there was a vogue in certain situations, especially the hand, to approach the abscess indirectly but there are few justifiable reasons for opening up previously healthy tissues.

2 As pus exudes from the abscess obtain a specimen for culture.

? DIFFICULTY

1. No pus? Is this a tumour, or cellulitis? Should you remove a specimen for histological examination and a culture swab in case this is a brawny cellulitis with organisms present?
2. Is the abscess deeper than it appeared? If this is a possibility, do not immediately extend the incision. Take a syringe and needle and carefully explore the area, aspirating the syringe to identify the pus before opening up the intervening tissues.

3 Except in the case of obvious local conditions such as a boil, gently explore the cavity with a gloved finger if it is sufficiently large or with a probe if it is smaller. Gently break down the partitions of a loculated abscess so that all parts can drain. Extract any foreign material. Search for a deep connection and gently pass a probe through into the deeper loculus, carefully widening the track to empty and drain the deep part; try and determine its cause. Can you obtain a further culture specimen and also a biopsy specimen? Have you seen, felt directly or felt through the probe, the lining of the cavity?

4 Create the best possible drainage. An opened boil requires no further action. It is possible to insert a wick of material but this usually just plugs the mouth of the abscess. A larger abscess demands a wide enough opening that will be prevented from closing until it is fully drained. Insert a plastic drain or tube if necessary, which also helps keep the mouth of the abscess open. If there is an ongoing cause of discharge, create appropriate drainage using a sump drain or suction drain.

5 A carbuncle often demands extensive removal of chronically undermined skin with wide exposure but once the surface has been cleaned, it may heal spontaneously with surprisingly little disability.

6 Axillary abscesses arising in the sweat glands frequently recur and although they are usually not acute, they cause deformity and scarring. Incise them; the pus is often offensive, suggesting the organisms are anaerobes, so always send it for aerobic and anaerobic culture.

▶ KEY POINTS 'Superficial' is not necessarily 'trivial'

- If you discover a serious infection at an early stage, do not vacillate.
- If you act promptly and effectively you may avoid a life-threatening deterioration.

7

Laparotomy: elective and emergency

R. C. N. Williamson, R. M. Kirk

CONTENTS

INTRODUCTION

The Greek word *laparos* (= soft or loose) was used for the soft part between the ribs and hips, thus the flanks or loins. There were objections in 1878 to the use of 'laparotomy' for incisions through the anterior abdominal wall. Although the term defines only the incision, used on its own it often implies 'exploration of the abdomen'.

Formerly, surgeons carried out a thorough exploration whenever possible to confirm the diagnosis and extent of the disease but also to exclude coexistent disease. This has changed because of improvements in diagnostic imaging, laboratory tests and technical facilities. Many operations are now carried out through restricted incisions and certain procedures are routinely performed by the technique of 'minimal access' (see Ch. 8). Laparoscopy is not only a therapeutic but also a diagnostic tool, particularly for the acute abdomen. Never forget that most diseases of the gastrointestinal tract primarily affect the mucosa; examining the hollow viscera from within the abdomen laparoscopically or at laparotomy does not replace endoscopic examination where this is possible.

An increasing number of conditions previously treated by operation can now be managed by alternative methods. Uncomplicated chronic peptic ulcer is usually amenable to medical treatment. Selected patients with perforated peptic ulcer can be managed conservatively. Gastrointestinal bleeding can often be successfully treated by endoscopic or radiological methods. Strictures can be dilated effectively with single or repeated balloon dilatation with additional stenting if necessary.

Not only may intra-abdominal examination of hollow viscera fail to reveal intraluminal disease, but you may also miss disease processes that are deeply placed in solid organs. However, intraoperative, high-resolution ultrasound scanning promises to be a valuable diagnostic tool. Vascular blockage or constriction from atheroma is often difficult or impossible to detect in mesenteric vessels at laparotomy because of pulsatile backflow from patent vessels. Undoubtedly, the best time to make the diagnosis is before operation; this knowledge allows you to plan the best treatment. In some cases adequate preoperative investigation may spare the patient the need for operation, for example by showing advanced neoplasia for which surgical management would be ineffective.

Do not place too much reliance on tests. Results expressed numerically have a sometimes spurious appearance of objectivity. Imaging techniques are operator-dependent and generally have an accuracy of only 80–90%. The most certain method of making a diagnosis remains the taking of a good history, carrying out a careful and thorough examination, followed by carefully selected and interpreted investigations. If these methods fail, the next step is not necessarily exploratory laparotomy. Whenever possible, it is better to repeat the diagnostic process from the start, after an interval. Alternatively, ask a trusted colleague to take a completely fresh view of the problem. Computer-aided diagnosis has improved accuracy in dealing with the acute abdomen. Perhaps the general application of this technique will be valuable in elective surgery to prevent inappropriate laparotomy.

AVOIDING ADHESIONS

There have been a number of studies of postoperative adhesions and, particularly, of their consequences. Well-known technical factors are extensive trauma, bleeding, infection, foreign material, intraperitoneal chemotherapeutic agents and, especially, ischaemic tissue. In Britain there are 12000–14400 admissions each year resulting from abdominal adhesions, and in the USA they account for approximately 950000 patient-days in hospital.

One of the most frequently identified causes is the use of starch glove powder. Swedish hospitals admit at least 4700 patients each year with adhesive small-bowel obstruction, and of these 2200 were operated on to relieve the obstruction. Only a quarter of the responders to a questionnaire used powder-free gloves and less than half of them ever washed their gloves. Those who did wash their gloves used ineffective methods. The Swedish authors also indicated suturing of the peritoneum as a probable cause of adhesion formation. Prefer powderless gloves. If you use starch-powdered gloves, put on the gloves, and carry out a 10-minute surgical scrub using 10 ml of povidone-iodine 7.5% in a non-toxic detergent base (Betadine), which combines with the starch. Now rinse in 500 ml of sterile water for 30 seconds. It is likely that the increasing use of minimal-access techniques will reduce the incidence of adhesions, although the technique has not abolished the problem. Liberal irrigation of the peritoneal cavity with Ringer's lactate solution, before abdominal closure, is said to reduce adhesion formation. In the last few years, adhesion-prevention barriers have been developed that prevent the formation of fibrin bridges. They can be laid between surfaces that are potentially adhesiogenic and are subsequently absorbed. Two cellulose-derived membranes have been approved for clinical use: Interceed (Johnson & Johnson) and Seprafilm (Genzyme).

OPENING THE ABDOMEN

Prepare

1 Preferably see the patient in the ward before the premedication is given, or in the anaesthetic room while he or she is still awake. Check that this is the correct patient by visual identification and inspection of the identity bracelet. Inspect the case notes and make sure that any relevant X-rays are available in theatre. If the lesion is unilateral, be quite certain that the operation will be carried out on the correct side (this should have been marked beforehand). It is inexcusable to neglect these elementary precautions.

2 If the bowel will be opened, or if necrotic or infected tissues are likely to be encountered, ensure that a prophylactic injection of an appropriate antibiotic is given at this stage. The choice depends on the nature of expected organisms, whether aerobic or anaerobic. Remember that facultative organisms must be considered in seriously ill patients.

3 Carefully palpate the relaxed abdomen of the anaesthetized patient before making the incision.

4 Make sure that the anaesthetist is prepared for the operation to start. Laparotomy is nearly always performed under general anaesthesia, with endotracheal intubation and an intravenous cannula in situ.

5 Cleanse the skin of the operation area with an antiseptic solution applied on gauze held in long sponge-holding forceps. Appropriate solutions include chlorhexidine (Hibitane) 1:5000), povidone-iodine 10% in alcoholic solution (Betadine), cetrimide 1% and 95% white spirit. Apply the solution along the line of the incision and continue to apply it in a centrifugal manner of increasingly wide circles over a wide area. Do not use an inflammable agent, such as white spirit, if you intend to employ diathermy to the skin or immediate subcutaneous tissues.

6 Apply sterile sheets or drapes and secure them to the skin with towel clips, unless local anaesthetic is being used. Leave exposed a limited extent of the abdomen on either side of the proposed line of incision. Alternatively, clip the drapes to each other, or apply an adhesive plastic sheet over the area, which seals off the skin over the proposed incision, extending over and securing the drapes. The incision will be made through the sheet.

Access (Figs 7.1, 7.2)

Plan the incision with care to give good exposure of the target area and versatility; it may be necessary to extend it. Aim to minimize damage to intervening structures and permit sound, cosmetically acceptable repair.

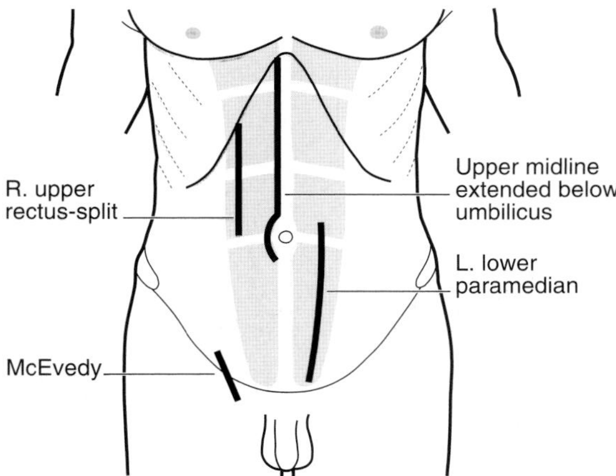

Fig. 7.1 Some vertical laparotomy incisions.

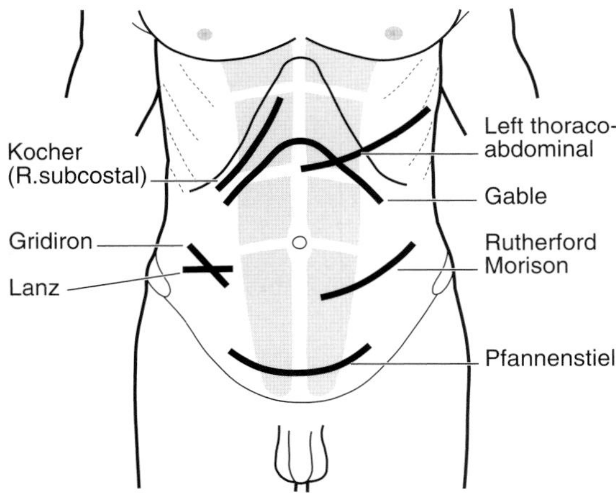

Fig. 7.2 Some transverse and oblique laparotomy incisions.

Midline incisions transgress the linea alba, the tough and relatively avascular cord that unites the anterior and posterior rectus sheaths. They therefore have the advantages of being relatively quick to make and to close and of provoking less bleeding than incisions that divide muscle fibres. Midline incisions can provide access to most abdominal viscera (Table 7.1). In the upper abdomen you can avoid the falciform ligament by keeping just to one or other side of the midline when entering the peritoneal cavity. In the lower abdomen remember that the linea alba is less well developed, so take corresponding care to close the wound securely. When necessary, bypass the umbilicus by curving the skin incision and bevelling the underlying cut to regain the midline of the aponeurosis below it.

Paramedian incisions provide very similar access to the upper, central or lower abdomen. All layers are divided in the line of the vertical skin incision, placed 2 cm to the right or left of the midline, except that the rectus muscle is dissected free and is drawn laterally, thus remaining intact. At the end of the operation allow the rectus muscle to fall medially, covering the line of closure of the peritoneum and, in the upper abdomen, the posterior rectus sheath.

Rectus-splitting incisions are made 3–4 cm lateral to the midline and divide all the tissues in this line, splitting the rectus muscle and its intersections. They avoid the time-consuming dissection required to free the muscle belly. In theory the medial part of the rectus muscle is denervated and thus rendered atrophic, but in practice the wounds heal strongly. A right upper rectus split provides good access to the gallbladder. Nowadays midline incisions are generally preferred to paramedian or rectus-splitting incisions because they are quicker to create and to close.

Oblique incisions can sometimes provide good access. The incision described by the Nobel prize-winning Swiss surgeon Theodore Kocher (1841–1917) extends 2 cm below the right costal margin from the midline to the lateral edge of the rectus muscle and exposes the gallbladder. The equivalent left subcostal incision can be used to approach the spleen. In the lower abdomen the incision of Rutherford Morison (1853–1939), who trained with both Lister and Billroth, starts just above the anterior superior iliac spine and divides all tissues in the line of the external oblique muscle and aponeurosis. The gridiron incision splits each of the three muscle layers of the abdominal wall in the line of its fibres; it therefore seldom gives rise to an incisional hernia. It provides an excellent approach to the appendix and can be enlarged by extending the skin incision in either direction and by dividing the internal oblique and transversus muscles, converting to Rutherford Morison's incision.

Transverse incisions usually leave the best cosmetic scars and provide adequate exposure, provided they are made long enough. They are therefore best suited for limited exposure in a planned procedure. Ramstedt's pyloromyotomy or transverse colostomy may be performed through a short transverse incision. Transverse laparotomy is useful in children, in certain obese patients and in the upper abdomen when the costal angle is broad. The incision described by Otto Lanz (1865–1935) of Amsterdam is a

TABLE 7.1 Incisions to expose the abdominal viscera

Midline	Upper	Hiatus, oesophagus, stomach, duodenum, spleen, liver, pancreas, biliary tract
	Central	Small bowel, colon
	Lower	Sigmoid, rectum, ovary/tube/uterus, bladder and prostate (extraperitoneal)
	Throughout	Aorta
Paramedian (incl. rectus split)	Upper	Biliary tract (right), spleen (left), etc.
	Central	Small bowel, colon
	Lower	Pelvic viscera, lower ureter (extraperitoneal)
Oblique	Subcostal	Liver and biliary tract (right), spleen (left)
	Gable (bilateral)	Pancreas, liver, adrenals
	Gridiron	Caecum–appendix (right)
	Rutherford Morison	Caecum–appendix (right), sigmoid (left), ureter and external iliac vessels (extraperitoneal)
Morison	Posterolateral	Kidney and adrenal (extraperitoneal)
Transverse	Right upper quadrant	Gallbladder, infant pylorus, colostomy
	Mid-abdominal	Small bowel, colon, kidney, lumbar sympathetic chain, vena cava (right)
	Lanz	Caecum–appendix (right)
	Pfannenstiel	Ovary/tube/uterus, prostate (extraperitoneal)
Thoracoabdominal	Right	Liver and portal vein
	Left	Gastro-oesophageal junction, enormous spleen

horizontal modification of the gridiron incision for appendicectomy and provides the least obtrusive scar at the expense of slightly inferior access. The incision of the Breslau gynaecologist Pfannenstiel (1862–1909) runs transversely above the pubis but just below the hairline. The aponeurosis is divided transversely and reflected above and below, allowing the rectus muscles to be separated vertically in the midline. Gynaecologists then open the peritoneum to gain access to the female reproductive organs, whereas urologists stay in the extraperitoneal plane for retropubic approach to the bladder and prostate.

Angled incisions provide not a mere slit that can be pulled into an ellipse but a space in the abdominal wall. Combined right and left subcostal incisions joining at the xiphisternum (the 'high gable' incision) enable a large flap to be turned down and provide excellent access for hepatectomy, pancreatectomy and bilateral adrenalectomy. A vertical incision with a T-shaped transverse extension (or vice versa) allows two flaps to be turned back. These incisions take longer to make and repair but can be invaluable for difficult or very extensive operations.

Thoracoabdominal incisions usually follow the line of a rib and extend obliquely into the upper abdomen. They make light of the cartilaginous cage protecting the upper abdomen. Alternatively, a vertical upper abdominal incision is sometimes converted into a thoracoabdominal approach by extending a thoracic incision in the line of a rib across the costal margin, to join it. Radial incision of the diaphragm towards the oesophageal hiatus (left) or vena cava (right) throws the abdomen and thorax into one cavity and provides unparalleled access for oesophagogastrectomy and right hepatic lobectomy. Thoracolaparotomy may be indicated for removal of an enormous tumour of the kidney, adrenal or spleen.

Posterolateral incisions for approach to the kidney, adrenal and upper ureter are described in the relevant chapters.

Making the incision

1 Incise the skin with the belly of the knife. Cut cleanly down to the aponeurosis or muscle. Discard the knife.

2 Stop the bleeding. Firmly press each bleeding site with a swab, then remove the swab quickly and pick up the vessel with the minimum surrounding tissue. Use fine-toothed or non-toothed dissecting forceps, which are touched with the diathermy electrode to coagulate the vessel. Alternatively, use diathermy forceps. Bipolar diathermy ensures that current passes only between the two tips of the grasping forceps. In either case, be careful not to burn the skin when coagulating superficial vessels. Capture larger vessels with artery forceps and ligate them with fine absorbable suture material. As you tighten the first half-hitch, have your assistant smoothly release the forceps, removing them when he is confident that you have safely secured the vessel. Complete a reef knot. Have the ligature cut 2–3 mm beyond the knot for small vessels, and 4–5 mm beyond when tying larger vessels.

3 Apply wound towels to the skin edges, if these are to be used. Fix the towels with clips or stitches. Wound towels help to prevent contamination of the wound by the fluid contents of abdominal viscera. If you use them, make sure that, if they become contaminated, they are immediately removed and replaced with fresh sterile towels.

4 Incise the aponeurosis with a clean knife in the line of the skin incision. Cut, split or displace the muscles of the abdominal wall. Cut the muscles with a knife or diathermy blade. When cutting the rectus muscle transversely, it helps to insinuate a pair of curved artery forceps beneath the muscle and then divide the fibres on to the forceps. Your assistant picks up vessels running vertically so that they can be ligated or coagulated. Split the muscles if the fibres run in the line of the incision or in the gridiron and Lanz incisions. In a paramedian approach displace the rectus muscle laterally within its sheath. Cut the tendinous intersection free from the medial part of the sheath and draw the muscle belly laterally. Stop the bleeding with diathermy coagulation or fine ligatures. Control persistent muscle bleeding by inserting a 2/0 absorbable stitch on a round-bodied needle, tying it just tightly enough to stop the bleeding and not so tight that it cuts through the muscle.

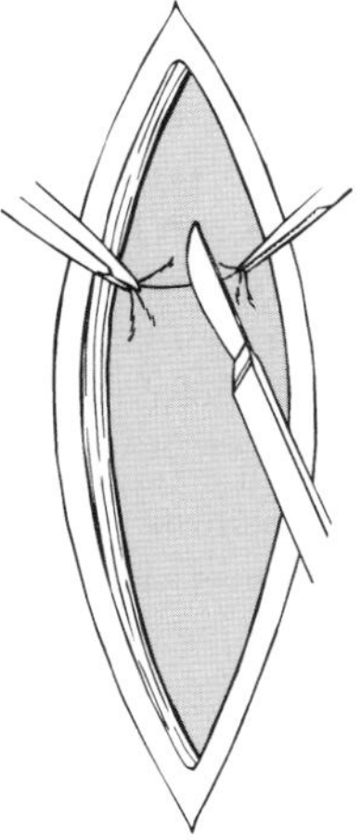

Fig. 7.3 Incising the peritoneum.

5 Open the peritoneum (Fig. 7.3). Pick it up with toothed dissecting forceps and grip the tented portion with artery forceps. Release the artery forceps and reapply to the peritoneum. The change of grip allows the viscera to escape if they are caught by the first application of the forceps. Incise the peritoneum with the belly of the knife. Air enters the abdomen and the viscera fall clear. Insert the blades of non-toothed dissecting forceps and use them to lift the peritoneum clear of viscera. Complete the peritoneal opening with scissors with the deep blade protected between the blades of the dissecting forceps, taking care not to injure the abdominal contents.

REOPENING THE ABDOMEN

Does the previous incision coincide with the site you would have chosen for present access? If so, reopen it. If not, ignore it and make a new incision in the correct site. Remember that you may require a longer incision than would be necessary for an initial operation. If the previous incision is convenient there is little advantage in creating a fresh incision. As a rule you will need to dissect off adhesions from within. From a fresh incision you will see them only from one side. Moreover, if the new incision is parallel to the first, there is an intervening denervated panel.

Access through the old incision

1 Make an incision down the centre of the old scar. If the scar is ugly or stretched, excise it as an elongated ellipse. Do not attempt to dissect out a previous paramedian incision, but cut through all the tissues in the line of the skin wound. Do not cut too boldly, because the deeper layers may be defective and you might quickly enter the cavity or even the contents of the abdomen.

2 When opening the peritoneum in the line of the previous incision, remember that viscera may be adherent to its undersurface. Entering the abdomen is greatly facilitated if you extend the wound at one end, so that unscarred peritoneum can be incised first. Alternatively incise the peritoneum slightly to one side of the old incision line. Once the abdomen is opened, carefully extend the incision little by little. Ensure that you identify every structure you cut. Ensure that you leave the abdominal wall and, if possible, the peritoneal lining, intact so that you can achieve a satisfactory closure.

? DIFFICULTY

1. Do not inexorably separate firmly fixed structures through an incomplete incision. Either skirt around them so that they now remain attached to one side of the wound, or open the other end of the wound and approach them from a different direction.
2. Have the wound edge lifted with tissue-holding forceps and encircle the adherent structures to estimate the degree of fixity and the plane of cleavage between them and the original parietal peritoneum. At intervals in the dissection allow the structures to relax, assess progress and start again, possibly from a new approach. Use a scalpel or scissors, remembering never to cut what cannot be seen. If you damage a structure, assess and repair the damage now. Check the repair at the end of the operation.

Access through a new incision

Although this approach may be initially easier, remember that, after a previous operation, viscera may be adherent to the parietal peritoneum anywhere. Once the abdomen is opened at a distance from the previous incision, have the intervening abdominal wall lifted with retractors. Arrange for the light to be directed towards any structures attached to the previous scar. If necessary, roll the patient slightly to one or other side, to improve access. Dissect adherent viscera from the undersurface of the old scar, frequently feeling around the other side.

Division of adhesions

Separation of adherent viscera from the wound edge has already been described. It can be an arduous and hazardous task, and the small bowel is particularly vulnerable to injury. If you enter the lumen of the small bowel inadvertently, close the defect with two layers of fine absorbable sutures immediately, pausing only to free the damaged loop of bowel to facilitate closure. Try and limit contamination of the wound with intestinal contents by prompt use of the sucker and gauze swabs. If contamination occurs nevertheless, consider lavage of the wound and peritoneal cavity with warm saline.

It is not necessary to divide every single adhesion between viscera during every laparotomy; indeed such a policy would often be counterproductive. On the other hand, when the viscera are tangled together it can be difficult to progress with the operation until the normal anatomical relationships have been restored. Learn to recognize thick, fleshy band adhesions that could distort the small bowel and give rise to future symptoms. When operating for adhesion obstruction, it is usually best to take down the adhesions completely and replace the small bowel in an orderly fashion.

When dividing intra-abdominal adhesions, vary the point of attack but do not become aimless. Keep in mind the objects of the dissection: allow adequate exploration, permit safe closure without fear of damaging the viscera, and prevent subsequent kinking or herniation of the bowel.

EXPLORATORY LAPAROTOMY

Full exploration of the abdomen was in the past considered a normal part of most operations, provided that it did not result in the spread of infection or malignant disease. If a standard procedure was to be performed, then careful surgeons routinely explored the whole abdomen to ensure that the diagnosed condition was really the cause of symptoms and to exclude incidental conditions that might be noted or demand treatment. The improvement of diagnostic capability (in particular endoscopy) and imaging methods (in particular computed tomography, CT) have eroded this principle. In procedures deliberately planned to be carried out through restricted access, wide exploration is impossible. For example, confidently diagnosed acute appendicitis, perforated peptic ulcer, the creation of a colostomy, the drainage of a localized abscess and the relief of biliary obstruction in patients with advanced pancreatic carcinoma are normally performed through limited incisions.

In dealing with emergencies you may not be able to make a clear-cut preoperative diagnosis; the decision is limited to the need for operation. In this case, exploration may be required to determine the cause of the presenting clinical features.

KEY POINTS Full abdominal examination

- In general, carefully explore the abdomen whenever possible. However, intraoperative use of high-frequency, high-resolution ultrasound promises to be a valuable diagnostic tool, even if the exploration has to be limited. In this way you will acquire a familiarity with the feel of normal structures. One of the most testing clinical decisions is to state that something is normal, so you must know what is the range of normality.
- Once an operation has been carried out, if symptoms continue or fresh features emerge, it is reassuring to know that other serious disease has been excluded.

In patients who have extensive carcinoma, adhesions that are unlikely to cause obstruction or a localized abscess that has been adequately drained, obsessive exploration is detrimental.

Intraoperative ultrasound scanning promises to be a valuable diagnostic tool. Solid organs such as the liver may contain lesions that are impalpable. Lesions that have been detected by preoperative tests may not be located at operation. Intraoperative ultrasound scanning aids the display or biopsy of such lesions. Within diseased tissues it may be difficult to identify vital structures by conventional means.

Exploration of the abdomen is still occasionally carried out as an elective 'final' diagnostic procedure when patients have had inexplicable distressing or sinister symptoms. One such example is a small bowel tumour. Improvement in diagnostic techniques has drastically reduced the indications, but occasionally they are equivocal. The introduction of laparoscopy has reduced the need for diagnostic laparotomy.

Remember, access to the abdominal cavity does not provide direct access to the site of many disease processes, such as the lumen of the bowel, visceral ducts or blood vessels. For this reason do not try to replace careful endoscopy, radiology and other imaging techniques with laparotomy. Some diseases affect the peritoneal surfaces, and some of these can be studied by peritoneal tap or diagnostic laparoscopy.

Sadly, patients are still occasionally explored for pain that is referred or which arises in the abdominal wall. Make sure that you have excluded sources of referred pain. If you suspect that the pain arises in the abdominal wall, try the effect of testing for tenderness with the abdominal wall relaxed and then tensed. The tensed muscles protect an internal source of pain from pressure. Tenderness remaining, or even increased, when the muscles are tensed strongly suggests an abdominal wall cause. The diagnosis is strengthened if the injection of local anaesthetic into the tender site gives relief, but warn the patient that the relief will be short-lived.

In the presence of unrevealed but clinically suspected intra-abdominal sepsis, time spent waiting for a series of increasingly complex investigations can be wasteful. However, CT is invaluable for delineating abdominal abscesses (see Ch. 11).

KEY POINT The need for laparotomy

- In emergency circumstances, if you are in doubt, use the time during which you are resuscitating the patient to repeat the taking of the history and examination. The features may change! When in doubt, trust your clinical acumen rather than 'suggestive' results of investigations, or the results of investigations that are at odds with your clinical findings.

Access

Choice of incision

1 Never forget that the prime function of an incision is to provide safe access. Although important, unsightliness, liability to herniation and discomfort are side issues. Remember that incisions heal from the sides and not the ends. Open the abdomen over the site of the suspected lesion, so far as the costal margin and iliac crest allow. Use one of the established types of laparotomy incision. Remember that the incision may need to be extended, particularly if you do not have a confident preoperative diagnosis.

2 The choice of incision for a particular operation is listed in Table 7.1 and discussed in the chapter devoted to the relevant organ. The choice may vary according to circumstances. For example, a long incision is appropriate when there is a confident preoperative diagnosis of acute appendicitis, whereas a vertical midline incision provides greater flexibility if the diagnosis is in doubt. In emergency colonic surgery, bear in mind the possible need for an intestinal stoma when selecting the laparotomy incision.

3 At emergency laparotomy for unexplained peritonitis or abdominal trauma, use either a right paramedian incision or a midline incision that skirts the umbilicus. Place the incision more above or more below the umbilicus, depending on the probable site of disease or damage. Incisions that extend on either side of the umbilicus can readily be extended in either direction once the pathology is revealed.

4 Midline incisions are quicker to create (and close) than paramedian incisions, so prefer them in cases of rapid bleeding, such as ruptured spleen or leaking aortic aneurysm.

5 Be prepared to use a previous laparotomy incision if it is conveniently placed or can readily be extended to allow appropriate access. The technique of abdominal re-entry is described in the section above.

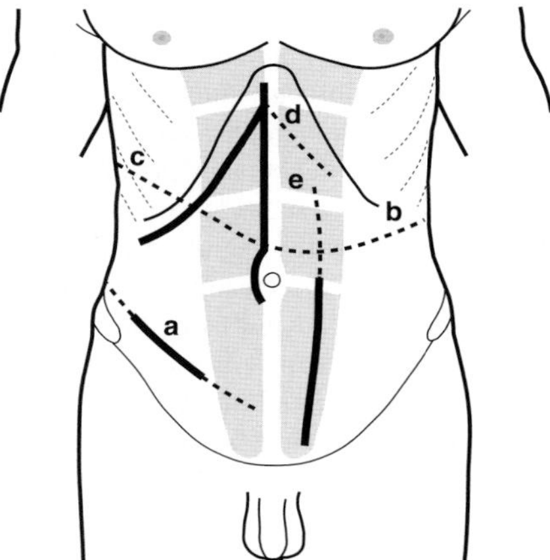

Fig. 7.4 Methods of extending certain abdominal incisions: a, gridiron incision extended laterally and (to a greater extent) medially; b, midline incision with T extension into left upper quadrant to deal with profuse splenic haemorrhage; c, midline incision with T extension into the right chest for ruptured liver; d, Kocher incision with left subcostal extension for major hepatic procedures; e, left lower paramedian incision extended upwards for mobilization of left colic flexure.

Access within the abdomen

1 If, on entering the peritoneal cavity, you find that the incision is likely to provide inadequate exposure, do not hesitate to extend it. If the incision proves to be inappropriate, such as a right Lanz incision for perforated peptic ulcer, close it and start again. Never be too proud to perform one or other of these manoeuvres. Disasters tend to occur when inexperienced surgeons struggle to complete an operation through the wrong incision. Figure 7.4 illustrates ways in which certain common incisions can be extended to deal with unexpected lesions or intraoperative difficulties.

2 Remember that the position of the patient on the operating table can greatly affect exposure, particularly of organs at either end of the abdominal cavity. To approach the pelvic viscera, ask the anaesthetist to tilt the table head-down, a procedure popularized by the Leipzig surgeon Friedrich Trendelenburg (1844–1924). Have the patient tilted head-up (reversed Trendelenburg) for access to the lower oesophagus and diaphragmatic hiatus. Rotating the table away from yourself facilitates an extraperitoneal approach to the ureter or lumbar sympathetic chain on your side. Rotation towards yourself when operating from the patient's right may improve access to the spleen. If you anticipate steep tilts in any direction, secure the patient adequately beforehand, using a pelvic strap and/or a support beneath the heels.

3 Nearly every laparotomy requires some retraction of the abdominal wall and adjacent viscera to expose the

organ(s) in question. Retraction of the wound edge will assist the initial exploratory laparotomy. When you have assessed the abdominal viscera and determined your operative strategy, insert retractor(s) and instruct your assistant(s) how to hold them. Pack away 'unwanted' organs, principally small-bowel loops, using large gauze swabs to which metal rings have been sewn or large artery forceps attached, to minimize the risk of their being left in the abdomen during closure. The rings or forceps are attached to the packs by tapes, so that they can always hang outside the wound. These packs should be wrung out in warm physiological saline, and they are more effective at restraining the bowel if they are not completely unfolded.

4 Marshal the forces at your disposal carefully. Use of a self-retaining retractor may release an assistant to provide more direct help. Instruments of the DeBakey pattern have an optional third blade, which may help to keep the small bowel out of the pelvis. A sternal retractor is invaluable in operations on the abdominal oesophagus and upper stomach. The instrument hooks under the xiphisternum and is connected to a gantry over the patient's head.

5 Specific manoeuvres are either essential or extremely helpful in the exposure of certain organs. For access to the oesophagus and hiatus, mobilize the left lobe of liver by dividing its peritoneal attachment to the diaphragm. To examine fully the back wall of the stomach and the body of pancreas, you must enter the lesser sac, usually by dividing part of the gastrocolic (greater) omentum. For thorough examination of the duodenum, divide the peritoneum along the convexity of its loop (Kocher's manoeuvre). Displace the small bowel into the upper abdomen to approach the pelvic viscera and out of the abdominal cavity into a plastic bag for operations on the aorta.

Assess

1 If you are not wearing powder-free gloves, wash off the starch powder. Wash blood from the gloves. Deal with established adhesions. Make sure that there are no instruments near the wound except for a retractor for your assistant and a sucker tube available for yourself. It is helpful to have someone in attendance to adjust the theatre light as necessary.

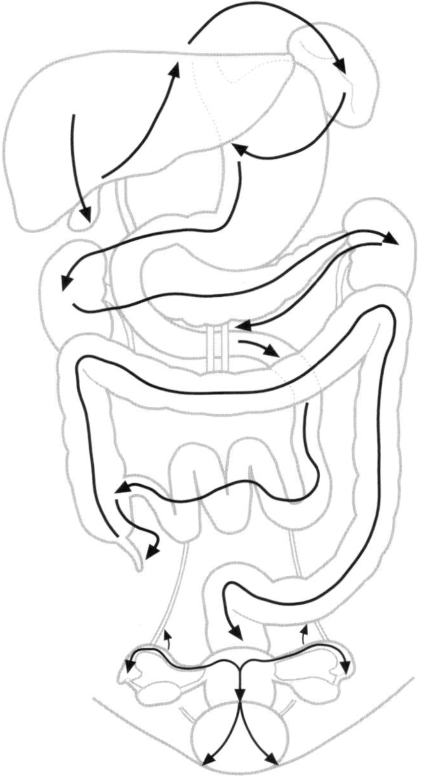

Fig. 7.5 The order of examining the abdominal contents at exploratory laparotomy.

2 Carry out a methodical examination of the abdomen and its contents by feel and, whenever possible, by sight. Always follow the same sequence (Fig. 7.5):

a. Right lobe of liver, gallbladder, left lobe of liver, spleen, diaphragmatic hiatus, abdominal oesophagus and stomach: cardia, body, lesser curve, antrum, pylorus and then duodenal bulb, bile ducts, right kidney, duodenal loop, head of pancreas.

b. Now draw the transverse colon out of the wound towards the patient's head. Examine the body and tail of pancreas, left kidney, root of mesentery, superior mesenteric and middle colic vessels, aorta, inferior mesenteric artery and vein, small bowel and mesentery from ligament of Treitz to ileocaecal valve, appendix, caecum, the rest of the colon, rectum.

c. In the pelvis examine the peritoneum, uterus, tubes and ovaries in the female, bladder, then the hernial orifices and main iliac vessels on each side. The ureters can sometimes be seen in thin patients, or if they are dilated.

3 In most *elective* cases, aim to carry out a thorough examination (as above), and record your findings carefully and in detail. These principles are particularly important when laparotomy is the last of a series of investigations to identify the cause of symptoms. Sometimes the incision chosen precludes a complete exploration, for example in interval appendicectomy or pyloromyotomy in infancy. Sometimes the condition found makes further exploration pointless, for example in carcinomatosis peritonei. In this circumstance make a gentle search for the primary tumour, obtain a biopsy from one of the deposits, make sure no palliative procedure (e.g. intestinal bypass) is required and close the abdomen. As a general rule do not touch a malignant tumour more than is essential, for fear of dissemination.

4 In *emergency* laparotomy, immediate action may be required, for example to stop bleeding or close a perforation. Thereafter, proceed to a methodical examination of the other viscera as before, unless the patient's general condition is poor or there is localized infection. Drainage of an abscess should usually be treated as a local condition. Do not forget to note the nature and amount of any free fluid, collecting some for chemical, cytological and microbiological examination. Obtain swabs for bacteriological culture of any potentially infected collection.

Action

1 In deciding the definitive procedure now to be undertaken, you will be guided by your preoperative knowledge of the patient, the extent of disease as revealed at laparotomy and the patient's age and general condition. Options include partial or total resection of an organ, bypass, drainage, exteriorization, closure of perforation, removal of foreign body, biopsy or perhaps no active procedure. In elderly or sick patients, control of the emergency or major elective condition should take precedence over the complete eradication of disease. Once you have formulated a plan of campaign, discuss your intentions with the anaesthetist and intimate how long you are likely to take to carry them out.

2 Be wary of tackling incidental procedures, such as prophylactic appendicectomy, without a clear indication. The chance finding of conditions such as gallstones, diverticula, fibroids or ovarian cysts does not automatically call for action unless they pose an immediate threat to health or offer a better explanation for symptoms than the condition originally diagnosed. The patient's prior consent is unlikely to have been obtained, so any adverse outcome may be more difficult to defend. By contrast, an unsuspected neoplasm should ordinarily be removed, if necessary through a separate incision, provided the patient's condition allows. Whatever course you adopt, be sure to record all your findings in the operation notes.

3 Remember that the interior of the distal small bowel and the entire large bowel are unsterile. Contents of hollow viscera that are normally sterile such as bile, urine, gastric juice, may also become infected as a result of inflammation and obstruction. Before opening the bowel or other potentially contaminated viscera, isolate them from contact with the wound and other organs. Consider using non-crushing clamps to occlude the lumen, and make sure that you have an efficient suction apparatus to remove any contents that spill. Pack away other structures before opening the viscus and discard the packs once it is closed. Remember that all the instruments used on opened bowel become unsterile; they must therefore be isolated and subsequently discarded. Likewise, change your gloves before closing the abdomen.

4 The danger of infection is one of degree. Healthy tissues can normally cope with a small number of organisms but are overwhelmed by heavy contamination or re-infection. 'It should be axiomatic that reducing bacterial contamination reduces infection.' In patients with impaired local host defences, be sure to obtain culture specimens because they may be growing facultative organisms, particularly if they have had previous antibiotics. *Enterococcus* and *Candida* may be pathogens. Generally, wounds are more susceptible to infection than the peritoneal cavity itself. If there has been gross spillage of infected visceral contents, wash out the abdominal cavity with warm saline and start broad-spectrum antibiotic therapy, but be guided by the microbiologist in case of doubt.

5 Intestinal clamps are of two types: crushing and non-crushing.

Crushing clamps are applied to seal the bowel when it is cut. Payr's powerful double-action clamps are most frequently used, but Lang Stevenson devised a similar clamp with narrow blades. Cope's triple clamps allow the middle clamp to be removed, so that the bowel can be divided through the crushed area, leaving its ends sealed.

Non-crushing clamps have longitudinal ridges and control the leakage of bowel contents without causing irreversible damage to the gut. Lane's twin clamps, which can be locked together, allow two pieces of gut to be occluded and held in apposition for anastomosis. Pringle's clamps hold cut ends of bowel securely, and the lightly crushed segment is so narrow that it can safely be incorporated in the anastomosis.

6 The danger of leaving articles in the abdominal cavity is ever-present, but to do so is inexcusable. Unfortunately, there is no single routine that will entirely guard against this mishap. Always use the minimum number of instruments and the largest swabs, which should remain attached to large instruments lying outside the abdominal wound. Make sure that they are never out of sight. As far as possible, use long-handled instruments for long-term holding, so that the handles protrude from the wound. Involve all your team in guarding against leaving an instrument or swab, even though you must accept the responsibility personally. If the scrub nurse reports a missing swab or instrument while you are closing the abdomen, check the peritoneal cavity once again. If all else fails, obtain an abdominal X-ray before letting the patient wake from the anaesthetic.

KEY POINT Avoid needless procedures

- If this is an exploration for undiagnosed acute or chronic symptoms, or if the expected diagnosis is not confirmed and no cause is found, do not carry out any procedure. Resist the desire to 'do something'. You may give yourself a false sense of security, cause further complications or confuse the diagnosis. Having made sure you have overlooked nothing, close the abdomen and determine to record all your findings.

CLOSING THE ABDOMEN

Before starting to close, make sure that the swab and instrument counts are both correct. Check for haemostasis. Decide whether you need to drain the abdomen (see below). Remove any odds and ends of suture material and replace the viscera in their correct anatomical position.

KEY POINT Avoid needle-stick injury

- Many needle-stick injuries are sustained during abdominal wall closure. Avoid using hand needles. However, even when using curved needles held in a needle holder, there is a danger of injury. A valuable development is the introduction of blunt-tipped (often called 'taper-point') needles, which pass through the tissues but penetrate gloves and skin only if pressed fairly hard against them. Protect yourself. Do not risk acquiring a transmitted viral disease.

There are several different techniques for abdominal closure; three are described in the section below. The choice depends upon the type of incision, the extent of the operation, the patient's general condition and your preference. If you are a trainee, as you assist different surgeons, you will learn various technical modifications and develop your own methods of closing the abdomen under differing circumstances. It is a common error among surgical trainees to sew up the abdomen too tightly, for fear it will fall apart. Remember that wounds swell during the first 3–4 postoperative days, oedema will make the sutures even tighter and there is a risk of tissue necrosis and subsequent dehiscence.

The most popular method of closure is now a continuous, spiralled, unlocked mass closure of the abdominal wall except for the skin and superficial fascia. The length of suture material used for the aponeurotic layer(s) should be at least four times the length of the incision, although this does not seem critical for lateral paramedian incisions. Place each suture 1 cm from the edge of the wound and 1 cm away from the previous 'bite'.

Select a strong non-absorbable suture material for closing the deeper (aponeurotic) layers of the abdominal wall; 1

monofilament nylon on a taper-point, round-bodied needle is very satisfactory in adults. Some surgeons use a doubled length of finer material such as 0 nylon, and run the first stitch through the loop to avoid having a knot at the end of the wound. Synthetic polyglactin 910, polydioxanone or glycomer 631, which are absorbable, have many advocates because they are less likely to produce chronic sinuses than non-absorbable nylon. With a long wound or an obese patient, it may be more convenient to use two lengths of suture, starting at each end and meeting in the middle.

There is strong disagreement about the use of tension sutures. Proponents use them if the abdomen is distended or obese, if the wound is infected or likely to become so, if the patient is malnourished, jaundiced, suffering from advanced cancer or has a chronic cough – in short, in any situation where wound healing is prejudiced. It is likely that these sutures have gained a poor reputation because the term 'tension' is often transferred to the tightness of the stitches, albeit that the suture is designed to withstand tension not to create it.

Remember that the abdominal wound is the only part of the operation that the patient can see, so take care to produce a neat result. Bury the knots used to tie off the deep sutures, especially in a thin patient. In an uncontaminated wound, aim for close apposition of the skin and a fine linear scar; therefore consider using subcuticular sutures.

Action

Layered closure

1 Some surgeons do not bother to close the peritoneum, especially in a midline incision. There is a view that suturing the peritoneum encourages adhesions in response to the foreign material. Certainly there is little strength to this layer, and a new mesothelial lining develops to cover the defect from within. Where the posterior rectus sheath exists as a separate layer, as in paramedian, transverse and oblique incisions in the upper abdomen, the peritoneum can also be incorporated in the deepest layer of sutures. Use a continuous, unlocked spiral stitch so that the tension can be evenly distributed along the whole suture line.

2 Pick up the edges of the peritoneum and posterior rectus sheath, and apply one pair of artery forceps to these combined layers on each side of the wound and at each end. Make sure that the bowel is not caught. Have the assistant hold up the artery forceps, so that the peritoneum is lifted clear of the viscera as you insert each suture.

3 Starting at one or other end of the incision, take a bite on each side close to the apex and tie the knot securely. Make sure that the needle does not pick up bowel or omentum. Take generous bites with each stitch, and pull up snugly but not tightly, passing it to your assistant to maintain the tension while the next stitch is inserted. Repeated tightening and loosening of the suture has a sawing effect on the tissues and also tends to fray the stitch. After placing four or five stitches and gently and evenly tightening them, insert a finger to confirm that the bowel is free. Tie the knots securely, and do not have the ends shorter than 5 mm.

4 When muscles have been cut or split, unite them with interrupted 2/0 polyglactin 910, polydioxanone or lactomer 9-1 sutures. Tie the sutures just tightly enough to appose the edges. When the rectus muscle is cut transversely, it is not necessary to repair it with sutures because the tendinous intersections limit retraction. Similarly, in a paramedian incision, the rectus muscle falls back into place after closing the peritoneum and no sutures are required. If the muscle does not cover the posterior suture line, draw it medially by inserting stitches through the fibrous intersections and through the medial edge of the rectus sheath.

5 Repair the aponeurosis of external oblique or the anterior rectus sheath using slowly absorbed synthetic or non-absorbable suture such as polyamide. After tying the knot at the end of the incision, cut the end of suture material short and take the next bite from within to without; this manoeuvre will help to bury the knot. Once again, have the assistant maintain an even tension on the thread and avoid pulling up each suture so tightly that you strangle tissue. Ensure that there is no oozing of blood in the superficial layers. Ligate or coagulate any residual bleeding vessels. If the subcutaneous tissues are deep, consider using a few interrupted fine 4/0 absorbable sutures to appose them.

6 Appose the skin edges, using one of several standard techniques. Interrupted sutures are preferable in a contaminated or irregular wound. Mattress sutures help to evert the skin edges slightly and bring together the deeper layers. Suitable suture materials include 2/0 black silk, 2/0 or 3/0 monofilament polyamide or polypropylene; skin clips and adhesive skin strips are

alternatives. Some surgeons use a continuous over-and-over or continuous mattress suture routinely.

7 In a clean and straightforward wound, a very acceptable scar results following subcuticular suture, using 2/0 polypropylene. Insert the needle in the line of the incision about 1 cm away from its apex and bring it out through the apex in the subcuticular plane. Now continue along the incision taking small and frequent bites of the subcutis; avoid piercing the skin. When you reach the other end, bring the needle out through the skin about 1 cm beyond the apex of the incision. Tighten the suture material to close the wound and make sure that it runs freely. Fix the suture at each end with tiny lead weights, or tie the ends in a slack loop.

Mass closure

1 This simple, rapid technique can be used routinely or reserved for difficult cases. It is particularly useful when closing an incision through a previous scar, when the layers are often partly fused. The peritoneum and rectus sheaths are closed together, or the linea alba may be closed in one layer without suturing the peritoneum.

2 Insert a continuous running stitch of 1 monofilament nylon mounted on a taper-pointed needle. Place the stitches 1–2 cm from the edges, 1–2 cm apart, catching all the included layers. Monofilament synthetic, slowly absorbable sutures may be successfully used.

3 Gently tighten the stitches as you proceed, checking that the bowel is free beneath. Do not let the stitch slip afterwards by getting your assistant to follow-up, but avoid undue tension. Make doubly sure that the bowel is free before tightening and tying the last stitch. Cut the bristly ends of nylon short.

4 Close the skin as for layered closure.

Closure with tension sutures

1 Tension sutures usually pass through all layers of the abdominal wall, including the skin, so they can be removed subsequently. Alternatively, they may be placed subcutaneously, where they remain permanently. Insert all the interrupted through-and-through sutures and tie them at the end. Use them to supplement a standard closure in poor-risk patients. Use a strong non-absorbable suture material, such as 1 monofilament nylon, swaged to a curved taper-point needle. Take deep bites about 3 cm away from the edge of the wound, incorporating all layers. Be very careful neither to prick the bowel when inserting the stitches nor to trap it when tightening them. If possible, always interpose the greater omentum between the wound and the small intestine to lessen this risk.

2 After inserting each deep tension suture, leave artery forceps attached to both ends of the suture while closing the deeper layers of the abdominal wall. Then tie the tension sutures to appose the skin and subcutaneous tissues. If skin is included, thread each suture over a length of polyethylene or rubber tubing to prevent it cutting in, and be particularly careful not to tie it too tightly. Complete the closure with a limited number of interrupted skin sutures.

3 If healing proceeds satisfactorily, remove the skin sutures 7–10 days postoperatively but leave the tension sutures for a further 2–4 days.

? DIFFICULTY

Closure of the deepest layer may be difficult because the abdominal contents keep bulging through the wound. Inadequate anaesthesia, obesity or intestinal distension are usually to blame. Even after successfully inserting your stitches, they may cut out. Be patient and do not despair.

1. Ask the anaesthetist if the abdominal muscles can be further relaxed.
2. Insert the stitches 2–3 cm from the edges, using a continuous over-and-over or mattress technique. Do not tighten the thread until you have inserted three or four stitches loosely. Now pull up slowly in the line of the incision, while the assistant compresses the abdomen from each side. The assistant should maintain the tension while you insert the next batch of sutures. As the closure proceeds it becomes easier.
3. The bowel is doubly at risk during difficult closures. Consider using a swab on a holder, a length of rubber drain or a 'shoe-horn' depressor laid in the wound to protect the bowel; remove it before completing the closure. Remember to avoid the bowel when placing the final sutures.

4. Brute force brings disaster: dragging the stitches through the tissues under tension acts like a saw, cutting out the stitch. Gentle persistence is most likely to succeed.
5. If a stitch tears out, remain phlegmatic. Insert a mattress suture from within the abdomen, 3–4 cm from the edge, taking a deep bite of tissue.
6. To cover abdominal wall defects or if the edges cannot be apposed without tension, absorbable polyglycolic acid (Dexon) and unabsorbable polypropylene mesh have been inserted to bridge the defect, even in the presence of infection.
7. If the intra-abdominal contents will later reduce in volume, do not fight to close the wound. Prefer to wait and perform delayed closure.

Delayed closure

1 If the abdominal cavity is grossly contaminated, as in faecal peritonitis, some degree of wound sepsis is almost inevitable. One option is to close the superficial tissues lightly around a drain. Another is delayed primary suture, leaving the skin and subcutaneous tissue widely open. In either case give parenteral antibiotics and drain the peritoneal cavity. Consider also the possibility of postoperative lavage. Close the musculo-aponeurotic layers of the abdominal wall with a continuous monofilament nylon suture. Be particularly careful not to draw the edges together too tightly, because considerable swelling can be anticipated. Superficial to this layer, loosely pack the wound with gauze swabs wrung out in saline.

2 Change the packs and inspect the wound daily. Delayed primary suture can be performed when the patient's condition improves and any wound sepsis has abated.

3 If peritonitis is particularly severe, for example after a major colonic perforation or resulting from infected pancreatic necrosis, it may be appropriate to leave the abdomen completely open as a 'laparostomy'. Make no attempt to close the abdominal wall. Cover the exposed viscera with moist gauze swabs on a polythene (Bogota) bag, and change them every 24–48 hours. In patients who survive, the wound will shrink with time. Late closure of the large incisional hernia may be needed.

4 An alternative to attempted coverage with skin is to apply a clear, sterile plastic sheet after drawing down the omentum, if possible. Over this are laid sump drains. The whole is covered by a double layer of iodophor-impregnated adhesive sheet. This has been successfully used following trauma. Yet another method is to use a zipper, with daily irrigations.

ABDOMINAL COMPARTMENT SYNDROME

Compartment syndrome is a rise in intra-abdominal pressure from a wide variety of causes. It is a potentially fatal condition unless it is correctly diagnosed and managed. Peritonitis, intra-abdominal abscess, intestinal obstruction or paralytic abscess, tension pneumoperitoneum, mesenteric venous thrombosis, acute gastric dilatation, intra-abdominal haemorrhage, ascites, large neoplasm, peritoneal dialysis, laparoscopic procedure or abdominal wound closure under tension may all provoke changes labelled 'abdominal compartment syndrome'. Other causes are massive visceral oedema, retroperitoneal haematoma and the need to pack the abdomen as a haemostatic measure. The physiological consequences are a rise in pulse rate and inferior vena cava pressure, with a fall in cardiac output, venous return and glomerular filtration rate. Blood pressure is not usually affected. Intra-abdominal pressure can be estimated via a catheter within the bladder.

Action

1 Do not attempt to close the abdomen formally, or be prepared to reopen it, if features develop of rising intra-abdominal pressure. If possible, close the skin after drawing the greater omentum down over the viscera. An alternative is to leave the fascia and skin open and cover the viscera with an absorbable or non-absorbable sheet. One such method is to use a Velcro-like closure (HIDIH Surgical, Doerrebach, Germany). If the underlying condition can be corrected, the abdomen may be formally closed in 2–14 days.

2 A longer delay may result in a defect requiring reconstruction, for example by bilateral advancement of the rectus muscles and fascia and by skin-relaxing incisions to complete the closure.

Drains and dressings

1 Tubular or corrugated drains of plastic or rubber may be inserted either through the end of the wound or through a separate stab hole in the abdominal wall. Place the inner end of the drain in the region of the operation site to evacuate blood and any other fluid contents from the peritoneal cavity. Fine-bore polyethylene tube drains can be screwed to a special trocar for insertion through the abdominal wall. They have many tiny drainage holes; ensure they all lie within the peritoneum; they can be connected to a vacuum bottle or bag to maintain suction. Alternatively insert a silicone tube drain without suction. Tubes can drain viscera to the exterior postoperatively; insert them through a separate stab incision. Examples are a T-tube into the bile duct, a gastrostomy or suprapubic cystostomy catheter and a feeding jejunostomy tube. Stitch the drain to the skin. When possible, insert a large safety pin through the drain to prevent loss within the abdomen, especially when it is shortened prior to removal. If a drainage tube is attached to a closed bag or suction apparatus, tie the stitch securely around the tube. Apply separate dressings over the drain wound, which can be re-dressed, shortened and removed without disturbing the main wound.

2 The use of drains following laparotomy is controversial and is no substitute for good technique, but they rarely do harm when properly inserted, and removed after about 48 hours if there is no discharge. A closed drainage system should not introduce infection. Some generally accepted indications for draining the peritoneal cavity are as follows:

a. After operations on the gallbladder, bile duct or pancreas, in case there is leakage of bile or pancreatic juice.

b. When there is a localized abscess.

c. After suture of a perforated viscus, such as stomach, duodenum or colonic diverticulum, when the tissues are friable. Consider if another operative manoeuvre would give greater safety.

d. When there is a large raw area from which oozing can occur. However, do not make insertion of a drain an excuse for failure to control bleeding.

e. After operations for severe general peritonitis, even if you have removed the cause.

3 Wound drains are occasionally indicated in very obese patients or grossly contaminated wounds. Insert a thin corrugated drain or tube suction drain deep to the skin and subcutaneous tissue, to be removed after 2–3 days or when it ceases to discharge.

4 Dressings are also controversial. From a bacteriological standpoint it probably makes little difference whether the wound is occluded by a dressing or left open to the atmosphere. Transparent adhesive dressings have the advantage of allowing the surgeon to inspect the wound repeatedly without disturbing the dressing. If much discharge is anticipated, use dressing gauze and wool. Remember that some patients are sensitive to adhesive strapping.

5 If primary closure of the superficial layers is not possible or is inadvisable because of tension, skin loss or contamination, avoid applying hydrocolloid dressings if the wound could be contaminated with anaerobic organisms.

Lavage

1 The peritoneal cavity has a remarkable ability to combat sepsis. None the less, spillage of contaminated contents, such as faeces or infected bile, may lead to early septicaemia and late abdominal abscess. When local peritonitis is marked, scrupulously remove all pus and debris from that part of the abdomen. Consider washing out the area with aliquots of warm saline (about 500 ml in toto), sucking out the fluid and inserting a drain. The theoretical risk of disseminating the infection through the peritoneal cavity does not appear to hold true in practice.

2 In generalized peritonitis, thoroughly clean the abdomen with warm saline (1–2 litres or more) at the end of the operation. In very severe cases (e.g. pancreatic necrosis, faecal peritonitis), consider inserting one or two delivery tubes and one or two drainage tubes for postoperative lavage. One drainage tube is placed in the abscess cavity and one in the pelvis; soft, wide-bore, silicone tubes or sump drains are appropriate. Use warmed (37°C) peritoneal dialysis fluid (Dialaflex 61) with added potassium for lavage, irrigating between 50 and 200 ml/hour depending on the extent of sepsis. Try and obtain a watertight closure of the abdominal wound and start with small amounts of dialysate (50 ml/hour) overnight, until the peritoneum seals the defects. Postoperative lavage is well tolerated and does

not seem to interfere with intestinal motility. Continue the treatment for up to 2 weeks and remove the drains when the return fluid becomes clear.

3 As an alternative to abdominal closure with lavage, the laparotomy incision can be left open in patients with necrotizing pancreatitis or severe faecal peritonitis. The technique of 'laparostomy' is described under laparotomy for acute pancreatitis (Ch. 24).

BURST ABDOMEN

Wound dehiscence results from poor healing, excessive strain on the wound or poor closure technique. In addition, septicaemia, abdominal wound contamination, haematoma or seroma, advanced neoplasia, diabetes, uraemia, jaundice, hypoproteinaemia, steroid or cytotoxic therapy can all impair healing. Abdominal distension from intestinal obstruction, intraperitoneal ascites, unresectable tumour or following loss of abdominal wall may place an excessive strain on the wound closure. However, the remarkably low rate of wound dehiscence reported by some surgeons tends to discount the importance of impaired healing or excess strain. Indict technical failure. The suture material may be incorrectly selected, damaged by crushing or abrasion, imperfectly inserted, overtightened, improperly knotted or trimmed too short at the knots. Layered closure appears to be associated with a higher incidence of burst abdomen than mass closure.

Suspect impending wound dehiscence if the patient's abdomen remains silent in the absence of an obvious cause, often accompanied by a low-grade unexplained pyrexia. A premonitory sign is the discharge of slightly bloodstained serous fluid from the wound. Dehiscence usually declares itself 7–14 days postoperatively following straining or the removal of the sutures. The patient feels something 'give' and may partially eviscerate. Burst abdomen is rarely painful; the patient is apprehensive but seldom shocked. The skin may remain healed, but as the patient strains the wound bulges. If the patient is managed conservatively, the skin may remain healed, leaving an incisional hernia.

Prepare

1 Reassure the patient; explain that the wound has given way but can be repaired. Cover the wound with large sterile packs held in place with an encircling bandage or corset or using adhesive, elastic strips. For most patients immediate reoperation is indicated, in which case give the premedication now and pass a nasogastric tube to aspirate the stomach.

2 If there is gross abdominal sepsis with contamination of the wound edges, plan to explore the abdomen, carry out corrective procedures, then pack the wound. Delayed re-suture can be carried out when sepsis is controlled by drainage, further operation, appropriate versatile antibiotics and supportive management of the patient. Alternatively, close the deep part of the wound, leaving the skin closure for later.

Access

1 Have the dressings removed, and make sure they are kept separate from the operative swabs. Have any skin sutures that remain in place removed. Open up the whole incision after preparing the skin and towelling off the area. Remove all suture material while carefully observing whether it has broken or cut out. How large are the suture holes?

2 Change your gloves.

Assess

1 Why has this wound broken down? Collect a bacteriological specimen for aerobic and anaerobic culture. Is the peritoneum partly intact? Where are its edges? Is there any cause for abdominal distension such as free fluid, abscess, blood or other fluid? Determine the cause. Remember that the tissues may be abnormally fragile. Are the abdominal contents normal? Is the underlying small bowel breached or dilated? If free fluid or pus are present or if the bowel is grossly dilated, check the cause.

2 It is inappropriate to re-suture the abdomen unless distended bowel is decompressed, obstruction relieved, ischaemic and necrotic viscera or other tissues excised, septic and foreign material removed and pus drained. If immediate correction is impossible in a very ill patient, consider carrying out what can be achieved now before packing the wound and re-examining the contents after 24–48 hours.

Action

1 Dissect the skin and subcutaneous tissues from the aponeurotic layer on each side to clear 2 cm of aponeurosis or muscle. Similarly, free the omentum and bowel

for a short distance on the deep aspect of the wound on each side.

2 Insert deep tension sutures, as described in the previous section. Pass each suture through all layers of the abdominal wall, including the skin. Allow 3–4 cm between tension sutures.

3 Now proceed with mass closure of the peritoneum and rectus sheath or the linea alba. Some surgeons prefer to use interrupted stitches of a strong non-absorbable material. Be certain to take deep bites of tissue, using plenty of suture material, and again avoid tension on the wound. Although recurrent burst abdomen is rare, pulling too tightly on strong thread passed through damaged tissue provokes stitches to cut out.

4 Whether you use continuous or interrupted sutures, take great care not to incorporate the viscera in any of the stitches. If possible, draw the omentum down over the abdominal contents.

5 Now loosely tie the deep tension sutures, once more remembering that they are there to resist tension, not to cause it.

6 Close the skin fairly loosely and consider using a superficial wound drain. In the presence of gross wound sepsis, leave the skin unsutured and place sterile packs on the deep wound closure. Carry out delayed suture when the wound is clean, graft the area, or allow the wound to heal by granulation.

7 A many-tailed bandage or an elastic corset provides extra support.

LAPAROTOMY FOR ABDOMINAL TRAUMA

See Chapter 3.

LAPAROTOMY FOR GENERAL PERITONITIS

The parietal peritoneum is locally irritated by contact with inflamed organs such as the appendix, gallbladder, colon with a segment of diverticulitis, or uterine salpinx. It is irritated by chemical contact from gastric acid, urine, bile, activated pancreatic enzymes, bowel content, blood or foreign materials such as talc and starch. It becomes intensely inflamed by contact with pus or material infected with microorganisms such as infected bile, faecal leakage and bowel content exuding from gangrenous bowel. The features develop over the inflamed area and so may be local or generalized. Adhesion of intestinal loops and omentum may confine the peritonitis so that a localized abscess develops; otherwise the irritant and infected material spreads widely. The magnitude of the contamination is crucial. In a previously healthy person resolution may be rapid and complete, provided the cause does not continue.

Peritonitis is easily diagnosed and assessed if it presents conventionally with sharp abdominal pain, worse on moving and breathing, accompanied by tenderness, guarding and rigidity, absent bowel sounds, tachycardia, tachypnoea and pyrexia. The blood granulocyte count rises and there is a shift to the left. There is frequent disturbance of the serum electrolytes. Plain X-ray of the abdomen often shows some dilated bowel loops and, if there has been a leak, free air is usually visible. When intraperitoneal fluid is much increased it produces a ground-glass appearance. Imaging techniques such as ultrasound scan may be helpful in localizing a cause or a mass.

The findings are affected by the delay between the onset and your examination. The pain and rigidity often pass off, though the tachycardia and pyrexia continue to rise while blood pressure falls. Always pursue the history of onset of the symptoms. For example, when you see a patient the pain may be generalized, but it may have started suddenly in the epigastrium if a peptic ulcer perforated, then radiating as the released gastric contents spread through the abdomen. When you first see the patient, the pain and tenderness may be maximal in the right iliac fossa if the contents have tracked down the right paracolic gutter to this site; appendicitis may wrongly be diagnosed unless you ask, 'Where did the pain start?' If the patient becomes septicaemic, the temperature may fall and multisystem failure can develop. Features often change rapidly, so be prepared to repeat the assessment at intervals in case of doubt. Immunocompromised patients such as those suffering from AIDS present particular diagnostic problems including toxic megacolon, which may perforate, or appendicitis caused by cytomegalovirus (CMV). Atypical mycobacterial infection is also reported. Exclude medical conditions that confuse the diagnosis, such as diabetic ketoacidosis, uraemia, sickle cell crisis, Henoch–Schönlein purpura or porphyria. Difficulty is increased when patients who are seriously ill from a medical condition, following trauma or major surgery, develop acute abdominal features. A condition that seems to be increasing in incidence, especially in the intensive care unit, is acalculous cholecystitis. If this is missed, the gallbladder may perforate and produce biliary peritonitis. Ultrasound scan should be diagnostic.

Very occasionally generalized peritonitis develops in the absence of any overt visceral disease. Primary peritonitis can occur spontaneously in children and is more common in patients with ascites or nephrotic syndrome or in patients with continuous ambulatory peritoneal dialysis (CAPD). The pneumococcus is one of the more common infecting organisms. Computer-aided diagnosis of the acute abdomen is a valuable and proven method of improving accuracy. It encourages us to try and be specific and not make treatment decisions without defining what we are treating. It acts as an educational tool when we look back on our diagnosis, management and the outcome. Fine-catheter aspiration cytology has been recommended for distinguishing between acute inflammatory causes of peritonism and non-specific abdominal pain. A high leucocyte count in the aspirate signals a definite inflammatory lesion. Laparoscopy can also help in equivocal cases of suspected peritonitis but is unnecessary if there is clear evidence of generalized peritonitis. A laparoscopic approach can be used for appendicectomy and closure of perforated peptic ulcer.

Decide

In the past, many surgeons made only one decision: whether or not to operate on the acute abdomen. We frequently still have to fall back on the aphorism, 'It's better to look and see than wait and see'. There are times when delay is vacillation and others when precipitate action offers an excuse for not thinking the problem through. When your clinical findings and laboratory investigations are at odds with each other, you must ultimately trust your clinical judgement.

Prepare

1 Restore the patient's fluid, electrolyte and acid–base balance intravenously. Pass a nasogastric tube and aspirate the stomach.

2 As far as possible, assess and correct incidental medical conditions, in particular cardiorespiratory disease.

3 Start parenteral antibiotic therapy with a third-generation cephalosporin together with an aminoglycoside and metronidazole. The organisms found within the abdomen are often not those expected, particularly in critically ill patients. *Candida albicans, Enterococcus* sp. and *Staphylococcus epidermidis* are more common than most surgeons suspect, so the antibiotic range may need to be broadened.

4 Make sure that the assistance and the instruments available are adequate for the proposed procedure.

5 Examine the abdomen under anaesthetic – an unsuspected mass may help you place the incision. Plan to use a midline or right paramedian incision placed half above and half below the umbilicus if there are no localizing signs,. Be prepared to extend it in either direction once the lesion is revealed. Since acute appendicitis is the commonest cause of peritonitis, use a Lanz or gridiron incision if the diagnosis seems at all likely; it can be extended medially or laterally to deal with nearby conditions if the diagnosis proves wrong, or it may be closed and a fresh incision made. Remember that irritant fluids, such as gastric juice, blood and bile, may track around the abdomen. Make sure you had established where the pain first started. If peritonitis follows a recent operation, reopen the previous incision.

Action

1 Note any free fluid or pus and save a specimen for laboratory examination. After a rapid preliminary examination of the abdomen, carry out a methodical exploration.

> **KEY POINT Keep the main goal in mind**
>
> - In all emergency operations and operations carried out on ill patients, never lose sight of the object of the procedure. You are operating for a specific reason. Do not indulge in unnecessary 'heroic' procedures – it is not you who is being heroic. It is the patient who will need to be courageous afterwards. Nevertheless, remember that you must assiduously and fully correct the cause of the condition, though by the simplest and most effective means.

2 Resect an inflamed appendix, gallbladder, segment of gangrenous or damaged bowel, perforated neoplasm or diseased Meckel's diverticulum. Repair ruptured small

bowel or a leaking suture line from a previous operation. Close a perforated peptic ulcer. Consider definitive procedures such as proximal gastric vagotomy or vagotomy and pyloroplasty only in appropriate patients with a long history of indigestion who are fit and would merit elective surgical treatment before the perforation occurred. Such patients are now rare.

3 Resect a specimen of perforated colon, but be very cautious about restoring intestinal continuity without a proximal diverting colostomy. Resection with exteriorization of the bowel ends is an even safer option. Closure of a perforated sigmoid diverticulum with or without transverse colostomy may be appropriate in a few selected cases, but resect perforated carcinomas if possible.

4 Make sure no dead or ischaemic tissue remains.

5 Remove any foreign bodies from the peritoneal cavity. Consider saline lavage and postoperative drainage if there is gross infection or contamination with intestinal contents. Drain an abscess.

6 Normally take no definitive action if you encounter acute pancreatitis, acute salpingitis, uncomplicated ileitis or primary peritonitis. Consider whether a biopsy (e.g. of a lymph node in Crohn's disease) or bacteriological culture swab from the uterine tube might provide useful information. Recognize acute pancreatitis by a bloodstained effusion, retroperitoneal discoloration and whitish patches of fat necrosis. Both uterine tubes are reddened, swollen and oedematous in salpingitis. Regional ileitis produces an inflamed, thickened bowel and mesentery, often covered with exudate. In primary peritonitis no cause can be found; the pus tends to be odourless, and a Gram film may reveal cocci.

7 If there has been extensive contamination, carefully wash out the peritoneal cavity using sterile normal saline at body temperature, repeating this until the aspirate is clear. Drains usually drain for a few hours so you may decide to continue lavage after operation by inserting an inflow catheter and a pelvic sump drain – but carefully chart and monitor fluid balance.

8 Have you achieved the purpose of the intervention? If you have not, and require to reoperate to accomplish something that should have been completed now, the patient's chance of recovery is seriously prejudiced.

LAPAROTOMY FOR INTESTINAL OBSTRUCTION

The diagnosis of intestinal obstruction is not always easy to make, nor is it an automatic indication for operation. The features may be indefinite and sometimes fleeting, so that a once-and-for-all history-taking and examination are often misleading. Classically there are four cardinal features – colic, distension, vomiting and constipation – but the prominence of each of these is affected by the site and type of obstruction.

KEY POINT Repeated examination of a patient with obstruction

- Intestinal obstruction is not a once-and-for-all diagnosis. Examine the patient generally, locally and rectally at intervals to identify localizing features and indications that there may be strangulation, sepsis, perforation or other associated conditions in what appeared to be straightforward mechanical obstruction.

Vomiting is early, distension often absent and constipation late if the obstruction is high. The small bowel is most frequently obstructed from adhesions and external hernia. Aerobic and anaerobic microorganisms rapidly flourish as soon as the normally sterile upper intestinal content stagnates. Mesenteric vascular occlusion often presents insidiously with pain, paralytic ileus, diarrhoea or gastrointestinal bleeding. Colonic carcinoma is the commonest cause of large-bowel obstruction classically with distension and early constipation but occasionally resembles small-bowel obstruction – so never fail to perform a rectal examination and sigmoidoscopy. Plain abdominal X-rays are very helpful.

Classically, it is possible to distinguish strangulation from simple obstruction because there is residual pain between bouts of colic. Of course there may also be tenderness, but this is often detectable at the site of simple obstruction. There may also be guarding and rigidity in strangulating obstruction but this is frequently a late sign, as are increasing tachycardia, pyrexia, hypovolaemic shock, gastrointestinal bleeding and a rising white cell count. These features may also be produced by perforation and infection. Do not delay. Carry out a rapid assessment of the likely cause, correct the patient's fluid, electrolyte and acid–base balance, administer versatile antibiotics intravenously and proceed with exploratory laparotomy.

Perhaps the most difficult diagnostic problem is postoperative obstruction following abdominal surgery. The history and physical signs are atypical because they are added to the expected postoperative delay in function, discomfort, wound pain, tenderness and a tensely held abdominal wall. Call in a trusted colleague for a second opinion if you remain in doubt.

Prepare

1 It is rarely beneficial to embark on immediate operation. Some conditions respond to conservative treatment, some require further assessment. Restore the patient's condition both from the effects of the obstruction and from any underlying disease. Pass and aspirate a nasogastric tube.

KEY POINT Did you miss the onset?

- It is sometimes said that early intestinal obstruction is usually less important than later obstruction. Too often the more serious late obstruction is the continuing missed early obstruction.

2 Institute appropriate antibiotic therapy if the patient is pyrexial; or, as soon as operation is decided upon, at once administer a versatile cephalosporin or an aminoglycoside together with metronidazole.

Access

Make a midline incision half above and half below the umbilicus and at least 15 cm long, unless the site of obstruction is known (e.g. strangulated femoral hernia; see Ch. 9). Alternatively, use a right paramedian incision of similar length. If the patient has had a previous operation, incise through the old scar, if it is convenient. Extend one end of the incision so that the peritoneum can be opened where it is unlikely to be adherent.

Assess

1 Aspirate any free fluid after obtaining a bacteriological specimen. Insert your hand and gently explore the abdomen. Identify the caecum; if it is collapsed, the obstruction lies within the small bowel. Trace the dilated bowel distally to identify the cause of the obstruction, dividing any major adhesions that you encounter.

2 If the abdomen is grossly distended, lift out all the dilated loops of bowel and wrap them in warm, moist packs. Avoid any drag on the mesentery which could render the exteriorized bowel ischaemic. Have the assistant support the heavy distended coils of bowel.

Action

Small-bowel obstruction

1 Release the obstruction if possible. Divide adhesions and bands. Reduce an internal hernia or overlooked external hernia or volvulus of the small bowel. If the bowel is grossly distended, empty it before closing the abdomen. In high obstruction a pernasal or peroral tube can often be manipulated into the bowel from within the abdomen and can be attached to a sucker. Sometimes distal contents can be gently milked proximally and aspirated, after which the tube is withdrawn. Alternatively, insert a seromuscular purse-string suture on the antimesenteric border of the bowel. Insert a sucker through a small stab wound within the purse-string. After emptying the bowel, remove the sucker and tighten and tie the purse-string suture. Reinforce this suture with a second suture.

2 Pause after releasing strangulated bowel. When the blood vessels are constricted the low-pressure veins are occluded first; as arterial blood pumps in, the small vessels distend with blood that stagnates, losing its oxygen. If the constriction is released now, the dark, congested bowel rapidly improves in colour. If constriction continues, however, the distended small vessels rupture and blood leaks into the interstitial tissues, including the subserosa. Do not then expect the colour to improve greatly when the vascular occlusion is released; it will take days for the extravasated blood to be removed. The bowel may still appear purple or black. Provided it retains its sheen and the supplying blood vessels pulsate, it usually survives, although the most

metabolically active layer, the mucosa, may ulcerate and possibly form a stricture when it heals. The critical site to examine is the bowel wall where it has been included in the constricting band or ring. It is usually white from ischaemia, but if it soon regains its colour it may safely be left. Any small doubtful area can be invaginated with a few seromuscular stitches. If the colour of the constriction rings fails to improve at all, or if they are green or purple in colour, excise the segment, ensure the remaining bowel ends are well supplied with blood and carry out an anastomosis.

3 Sometimes a knuckle of small bowel that has been trapped in an internal or external hernia will spontaneously reduce itself. If you observe constriction rings, look for the possible site of hernia and try to close the defect. Constriction rings that remain slightly ischaemic may be invaginated by Lembert sutures.

4 Resect the obstructed bowel if there is a neoplasm or if the bowel or its blood supply are damaged. Massive resection may be necessary if the main vessels are blocked; consider embolectomy in selected patients (Ch. 32).

5 Bypass the obstruction if it cannot be removed. Gastroenterostomy relieves pyloric or duodenal obstruction. Duodenojejunostomy bypasses annular pancreas or duodenal atresia. An enteroanastomosis short-circuits an irresectable primary or secondary tumour of the jejunum or ileum (Ch. 17). Obtain a biopsy specimen in all irresectable cases. Break up, push on or remove intraluminal obstruction such as a food bolus, gallstone or collection of worms.

6 Reduce an intussusception (Chs 17, 43). Resect a polyp or other pathological lesion at the apex of the intussusception (usually in adults).

7 Stricture resulting from Crohn's disease is conventionally treated by resection and anastomosis. Unfortunately, you can never be certain that further resections are avoidable. Indeed, some of the patients presenting with obstructive disease have already had previous extensive resections. In recent years a much more conservative policy has become popular, supported by the fact that what appear to be unaffected healthy segments of bowel are already histologically diseased. For this reason, resection of strictures is kept as short as possible, transgressing macroscopically diseased but unstrictured bowel. For short segments, strictureplasty seems to be satisfactory. The procedure is particularly indicated if the stricture is short, if the disease process is not florid – indicating possible 'burned-out' disease – and if the bowel is already short or will be made short by resecting a large length of strictured bowel (Ch. 17). The operation is performed after the fashion of a Heineke–Mikulicz pyloroplasty; the bowel is incised longitudinally throughout the length of the stricture and opened out so that the incision can be closed to produce a horizontal suture line.

8 If you can offer no other relief be prepared on occasion to create a proximal stoma as a terminal palliative measure, rather than leave a patient obstructed and vomiting without relief.

9 The management of neonatal obstruction is described in Chapter 43.

10 Recurrent adhesive obstruction can sometimes be prevented using a modification of Noble's operation; lengths of bowel are folded back and forth in a boustrophedon (Greek *bous* = ox + *strophe* = a turning), like the course of the plough in successive furrows or the folds of a 'jumping jack' cracker, and secured.

Large-bowel obstruction

1 Release an external cause of obstruction. Sometimes a loop of small bowel is adherent to an inflammatory diverticular mass and requires release.

2 A diverticular mass may totally obstruct the sigmoid colon. Conventionally a loop transverse colostomy, subsequent resection of the diseased segment and colostomy closure were performed in three stages. You may decide to resect diseased bowel initially. Following sigmoid colectomy you may create a temporary terminal iliac colostomy, closing and dropping back the lower cut end for later reconstruction (Hartmann's procedure).

3 Resect an obstructing carcinoma of the caecum, ascending colon or transverse colon, and restore continuity by end-to-end ileocolostomy. Although three-stage removal of sigmoid carcinoma is conventional, Hartmann's procedure may be appropriate. If obstruction is not gross, consider primary resection and anastomosis, protecting the anastomosis with a loop transverse colostomy or caecostomy. Resection and anastomosis can be safely achieved if faeces can be cleared by washing them out by running in physiological saline through a Foley catheter. In gross obstruction, always

inspect the caecum for overdistension, perforation or gangrene. In case of doubt perform a caecostomy.

4 Bypass an irresectable carcinoma of the right colon by ileotransverse colostomy and irresectable carcinoma of the left colon by colocolostomy if possible. Relieve unresectable obstructing carcinoma of the distal colon or rectum by means of a left iliac end colostomy. If you carry out a colostomy above the tumour, bring the lower cut end to the surface as a mucous fistula. If you close it, you have left a closed loop above the obstructing carcinoma.

5 Always obtain a biopsy specimen if you do not resect the carcinoma.

6 Untwist a volvulus. Have a rectal tube in place so that the distended bowel can be deflated. Move on, break up or remove intraluminal obstruction such as a faecalith. Ischaemic colitis that causes obstruction is best resected and the ends brought to the surface, because it is difficult to be sure how much of the colon will survive.

7 Never forget the purpose of this emergency operation. Do not perform any procedure that does not fulfil this purpose.

Closure

This can be difficult if the abdomen is distended. Take care to avoid injuring dilated loops of small bowel. Consider inserting tension sutures if abdominal distension is gross.

? DIFFICULTY

1. In the presence of grossly distended bowel, do not flounder within the abdomen through an inadequate incision. Extend the incision and gently deliver the entire small bowel. Consider decompressing the small bowel by means of a special sucker (p. 78). Decompress the upper small bowel by milking contents back up to within reach of the nasogastric tube, and try to manoeuvre this tube through the pylorus into the duodenum or jejunum.
2. Sometimes adhesions prevent easy delivery of the small bowel or produce an apparently inextricable tangle. Such cases can be very testing. Settle down to a prolonged dissection. Make sure that the incision is adequate for you to visualize the restraining bands, which should then be divided. Patiently disentangle all adherent loops and run the whole small bowel through your hands to make sure it is unravelled, and intact.

Aftercare

1 Monitor fluid, electrolyte and acid–base balance in order to determine the intravenous requirements. Wait until the nasogastric aspirate falls to less than the intake after oral fluids have started and/or until the patient passes flatus per rectum.

2 Examine the abdomen frequently to ensure that it is soft, not distending and not tender. Listen for returning bowel sounds. Monitor the passage of flatus and faeces.

3 If there was contamination, continue antibiotics until the swab cultures are reported, then make a decision about stopping or changing them.

LAPAROTOMY FOR GASTROINTESTINAL BLEEDING

Appraise

Ideally, manage patients with gastrointestinal bleeding jointly with a gastroenterological physician with whom you have an agreed policy. A high proportion of affected patients are over 60 years of age and many suffer from concomitant disease. Approximately one-third will have taken aspirin or other non-steroidal anti-inflammatory drugs within a few days of the onset of bleeding.

Never fail to carry out a thorough examination, including rectal examination, proctoscopy, sigmoidoscopy and upper or lower bowel flexible endoscopy. The availability of more complex methods of investigation sometimes beguiles clinicians into forgetting basic manoeuvres. Consider bleeding or clotting disorders, parasitic infestation, Peutz–Jeghers syndrome, drug therapy and AIDS.

There is a wide range of endoscopic and radiological methods of controlling bleeding. For bleeding from oesophageal varices see Chapter 25. Do not, however, vacillate in patients with bleeding peptic ulcer if they are over the age of 60 years, have concomitant disease, are shocked, have a visible vessel or are bleeding at endoscopy, continue bleeding, or have recurrent bleeding. Such patients need an operation.

Operations for the control of severe gastrointestinal bleeding require to be performed by experienced surgeons backed by expert anaesthetists and a trained team of assistants. If you are not experienced in this very demanding field, seek help urgently.

Prepare

1 As you assess the patient, initiate appropriate resuscitation. Do not place too much reliance on the initial haemoglobin and haematocrit results because they are affected by physiological blood dilution.

2 Give appropriate drugs in peptic ulcer bleeding.

3 Do not take a patient to the operating theatre without also taking the endoscope. Be willing to pass it when the patient is anaesthetized, to confirm the lesion – and confirm that it is still bleeding. On occasion an unnecessary operation can be cancelled or deferred if the bleeding has stopped. Intraoperative endoscopy can be invaluable, including operative guidance of an endoscope passed perorally or peranally to localize small-bowel bleeding.

Access and assess

1 Make a midline or right paramedian incision, sited in the upper or lower abdomen according to the preoperative diagnosis or midway if this is uncertain.

2 Recognize blood in the lumen from the bluish-black coloration of the gut. The distribution of blood in the stomach, small bowel and colon may roughly localize the site of bleeding, but remember that blood can travel for a considerable distance proximal as well as distal to the lesion.

3 Inspect and palpate the alimentary canal from oesophagus to rectum. Note any abnormality, particularly an ulcer crater, tumour, inflammation, petechiae, scarring or a local increase in vascularity. Examine the liver and spleen. Cirrhosis raises the possibility of variceal haemorrhage; splenomegaly might be associated with a clotting defect. If the gut appears normal, remember that haemobilia and pancreatic cysts are rare causes of gastrointestinal haemorrhage.

Action

1 If there is evidence of *upper* gastrointestinal bleeding, concentrate on the stomach, duodenum and jejunum.

2 If there is evidence of *lower* gastrointestinal bleeding, concentrate on the colon and ileum. The site of bleeding can be difficult to identify in the intestine.

3 There is no indication for 'blind' procedures, such as partial gastrectomy. If you have done all you can to find the site of bleeding, close the abdomen, carefully record your findings and determine to carry out appropriate further investigations.

KEY POINT Never forget the purpose of the operation

- The purpose of the operation is to control life-threatening bleeding and prevent it from recurring. Do not perform any procedure outside this purpose.

LAPAROTOMY FOR EARLY POSTOPERATIVE COMPLICATIONS

This can be one of the most daunting surgical challenges that we face. Reopening the abdomen is associated with a sense of guilt and failure. We feel that, if the first operation had been better performed, or if we had chosen a more appropriate procedure – or even, occasionally, an alternative to operation – or prepared the patient better, a second operation would be unnecessary. Having failed once, how can we hope to succeed from a less advantageous position? Very often complications result from infections and leakage, and effective drainage of pus or hollow visceral content is vital (Figs 7.6, 7.7).

As a trainee do not embark on such an operation without taking advice or senior assistance, because the interpretation of the findings, the decisions required and the technical skills demand an experienced surgeon.

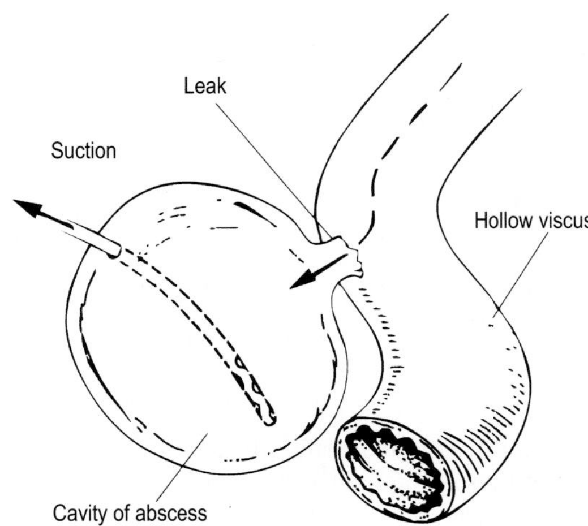

Fig. 7.6 How not to drain an abscess following a leak. The abscess will continue indefinitely unless you drain the leak directly, excise or exteriorize it. (Adapted by permission from Hospital Update.)

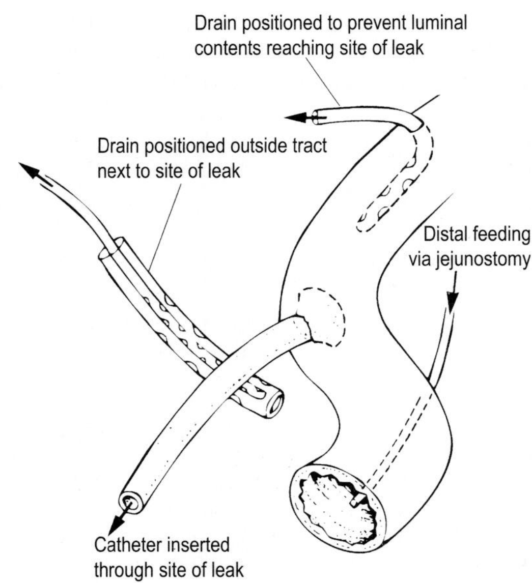

Fig. 7.7 Draining a leak from bowel that cannot be closed, exteriorized or excised. (Adapted by permission from Hospital Update.)

In dealing with minor complications that are delegated to you, do not feel defeated before you begin; this is a testing time, but success will bring all the more sense of accomplishment.

FURTHER READING

Jones PF, Krukowski ZH, Young GG 1998 Emergency abdominal surgery, 3rd edn. Chapman & Hall, London

Kaufman GL 2000 Acute abdomen. In: Corson JD, Williamson RCN (eds) Surgery. Mosby, London, pp 3.1–3.13

O'Dain GN 2000 Leaper DJ 2003 Sequential physiology scoring facilitates objective assessment of revisitation in patients with an intra-abdominal emergency. British Journal of Surgery 90:1445–1450

Silen W 1996 Cope's early diagnosis of the acute abdomen, 19th edn. Oxford University Press, London

Wheatley KA, Keighley MRB 1990 Peptic ulcer haemorrhage. In: Williamson RCN, Cooper MJ (eds) Emergency abdominal surgery. Churchill Livingstone, Edinburgh, pp 95–109

Williamson RCN, Cooper MJ (eds) 1990 Emergency abdominal surgery. Churchill Livingstone, Edinburgh

8

Principles of minimal access surgery

P. A. Paraskeva, A. Darzi

GENERAL PRINCIPLES OF LAPAROSCOPY

Minimal access surgery is intended to cause the least anatomical, physiological and psychological trauma to the patient. The rapid advancements in this type of surgery since the late 1980s have seen the dawning of an age of surgical technological innovation. It would not have been possible without the simultaneous development of improved methods of imaging to replace the traditional 'hands-in' method of open surgery assessment.

Success has been achieved from the recognition that adequate education and training in minimal access techniques combined with well-considered pre- and postoperative care are essential for the application of these new approaches. Many surgical and gynaecological procedures are regularly performed using a minimal access approach (Table 8.1). Discussion in this chapter is related to the basic principles of laparoscopy.

Minimal access surgery has implications for the economics of hospitals offering surgical services. Capital equipment is expensive and requires regular servicing to ensure good working standards. Consumables are particularly expensive, and reused equipment may prejudice performance. Theatre times increase initially, although they decrease as surgeons gain experience. Short-stay and 5-day wards with rapid turnover reduce 'hotel' costs, freeing main ward beds to reduce waiting lists.

All members of the surgical team need adequate training in the techniques and care of the equipment, leading to the establishment of minimal access therapy training units (MATTUs) offering basic and higher training courses accessible to senior surgeons trained in open surgery. The theatre team also needs to be trained and efficient, with knowledge of how the equipment functions.

Advantages

a. Smaller incisions
b. Procedures are less painful and disabling
c. Decreased wound-related pathology, such as wound infection
d. Decreased tissue trauma
e. Decreased physiological insult to the patient when compared to open surgery
f. Earlier return to full activity
g. Significantly reduced stay in hospital postoperation, leading to cost-effectiveness
h. Cosmetic acceptability
i. Decreased contact with pathogens such as human immunodeficiency virus (HIV) and hepatitis B virus (HBV)
j. The use of video records aid in the art of communication between doctors and with patients and their families. It may also help improve clinical decision-making.

Disadvantages

a. Lack of tactile feedback from tissues
b. Bleeding is difficult to control
c. Procedures may take longer, especially on the initial slope of the surgical learning curve
d. Technical expertise, advice and specialist equipment are required
e. Iatrogenic damage has been a greater problem following minimal access surgery than following traditional

TABLE 8.1 Examples of minimal access operations

General surgery	Gynaecology	Others
Diagnostic laparoscopy	Oophorectomy	Arthroscopy
Cholecystectomy	Treatment of ectopic pregnancy	Minimal access urology
Choledochoscopy	Hysterectomy	
Hernia repair	Diagnosis and ablation of endometriosis	
Adhesiolysis	Ovarian cystectomy	
Nissen fundoplication	Myomectomy	
Repair of perforated duodenal ulcer	Tubal surgery	
Appendicectomy	Infertility treatment	
Excision of Meckel's diverticulum		
Rectopexy		
Splenectomy		
Vagotomy		
Colectomy		

open techniques (e.g. bile duct injuries during laparoscopic cholecystectomy).

As surgeons become increasingly familiar with laparoscopy it can be successfully used in many situations previously contraindicated. However, laparoscopy is contraindicated in the presence of generalized peritonitis, intestinal obstruction, clotting abnormalities, liver cirrhosis, failure to tolerate general anaesthesia, and refusal by the patient. Some conditions are relative contraindications to laparoscopy, such as pregnancy, abdominal aortic aneurysm and organomegaly of, for example, liver or spleen. Overweight patients are likely to suffer fewer postoperative respiratory complications than they would following open operation but gross obesity may rule out laparoscopy. Multiple abdominal adhesions may prevent safe entry, but provided the first instrument can be introduced by an open technique, the procedure may be performed in the presence of moderate adhesions.

Prepare

1 Patients can be admitted on the day of planned surgery. Evaluate and investigate them beforehand to decide whether they can be managed on a day-case basis. Obtain informed consent, including permission to convert to open operation if necessary and quote the likely percentage of conversions to open operation. Warn patients of the possibility of experiencing postoperative shoulder tip pain and of developing surgical emphysema. Explain not only the likely benefits of minimal access techniques but also the commonly occurring risks, how they present and how they are managed.

2 In the absence of contraindications, arrange antithrombotic prophylaxis such as low-dose heparin and compression stockings. Give prophylactic antibiotics if organs such as the gallbladder are to be removed. Bowel preparation is unnecessary.

3 Some anaesthetists prefer non-steroidal anti-inflammatory drugs rather than opiates as premedication, if necessary with the addition of short-acting benzodiazepines. General anaesthesia is usually augmented with muscle relaxation, intubation and ventilation so that pneumoperitoneum can be induced without causing cardiorespiratory embarrassment. The anaesthetist monitors abdominal distension and its effect on blood pressure and airways pressure throughout.

4 Check your equipment. Prefer large monitors, with good-quality, high-resolution screens, mounted on mobile trolleys, also containing the light source, insufflator and camera. The video camera head, either a single microchip or a superior three-chip instrument, is attached to the laparoscope to form an electrical–optic interface. The camera is connected by cable to a video processor which interprets and modifies the signal and transmits it to the monitors. Most systems

incorporate a 'white balance' function, which can be calibrated to represent the colours accurately.

5 Place the monitors on either side of the patient, allowing you and your assistants to view them (Fig. 8.1). You should be able to see the light source, usually xenon or halogen, and monitor the light intensity. Ensure that the patient is not at risk of burning.

6 Suction and irrigation are carried out through a probe connected to a pressurized reservoir and a suction source, controlled by buttons. The rapid-flow insufflator supplies carbon dioxide to create and maintain the pneumoperitoneum. Have it placed so you can see the display of the intra-abdominal pressure and gas flow in response to preset pressure values. It may also incorporate a gas warmer.

7 Make sure the camera operator will follow your movements and keep the area of interest centred in the field of view.

8 Warm the laparoscope to prevent fogging of the lens. For the same reason do not insufflate cold carbon dioxide through the same port as the camera.

9 The ports for insertion of instruments can be disposable or reusable. More expensive disposable ports have the advantage of being sharp, radiolucent and sterile. They may have blunt ends for open induction of pneumoperitoneum, or be fitted with a sharp, spring-loaded trocar with a plastic guard that projects beyond the point as soon as the trocar enters the peritoneal cavity. They are of a range of sizes to accommodate various instruments, but large ports can be fitted with sizers to reduce the lumen. All have attachments to allow insufflation, and valves to prevent gas leaks. Some have collars, allowing them to be secured in position (Fig. 8.2).

10 In the closed method of insufflation a Veress needle is inserted. This incorporates a spring-loaded obturator that covers the sharp needle-tip as soon as it enters the peritoneal cavity. It incorporates an attachment to the gas supply (Fig. 8.3).

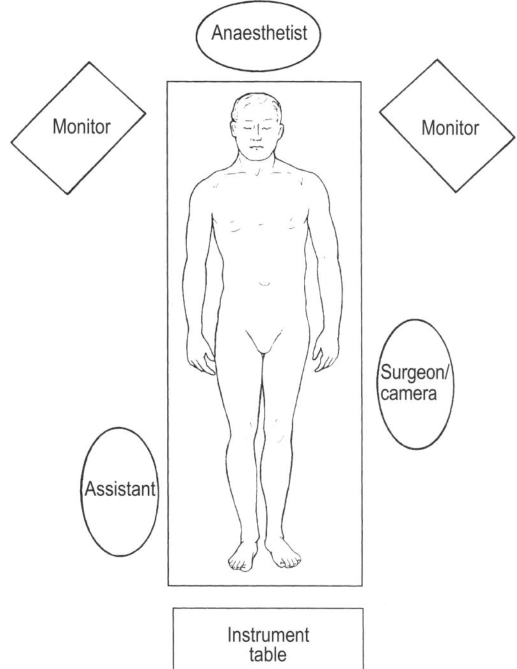

Fig. 8.1 Diagram showing the positioning of the patient, surgeon, assistant and video monitors for a laparoscopic cholecystectomy.

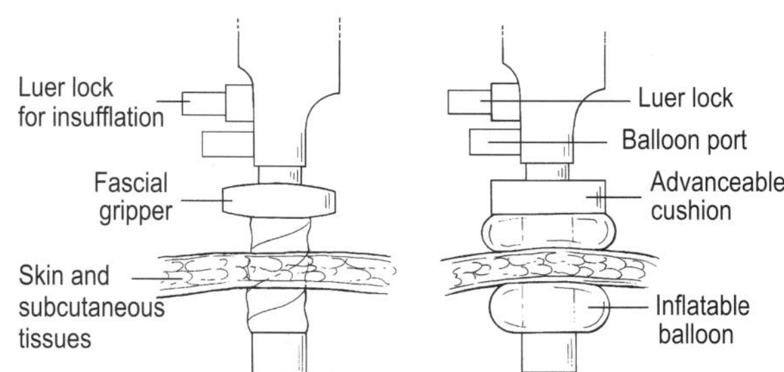

Fig. 8.2 Diagram of two types of laparoscopic port, one with a screw collar and the second with inflatable balloons. Both help to prevent gas leaks around the ports.

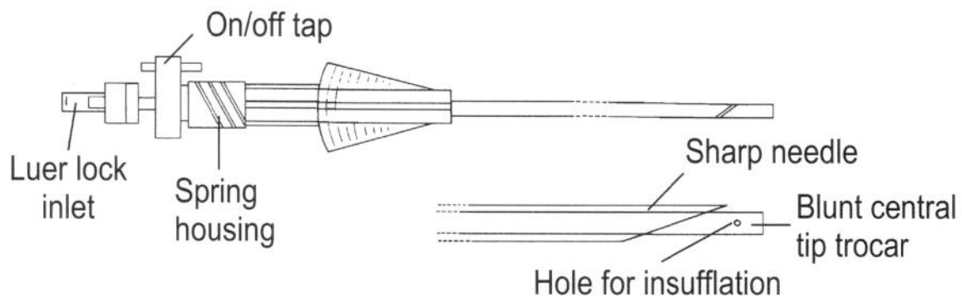

Fig. 8.3 Diagram of a Veress needle showing the device in its entirety, and the spring-loaded tip.

11 A large range of graspers, staplers, dissectors, scissors and diathermy applicators have been developed – either reusable or disposable.

Access

1 Induce a pneumoperitoneum. The initial penetration of the abdominal cavity to produce a pneumoperitoneum can be a hazardous task in laparoscopic surgery; you may injure underlying viscera such as bowel or bladder, or even deeper structures such as the aorta and the vena cava. Once you have established the first port you can insert additional ports in relative safety.

2 There are open and closed methods of producing a pneumoperitoneum.

Prefer the safe, open (Hasson) method of port insertion, especially if there has been previous surgery. Make a 1–2-cm infra-umbilical incision, deepening it to the linea alba. Incise the linea alba between two stay sutures and open the peritoneum under direct vision. The stay sutures can be tied together to close the port site at the end of the procedure, by using a box stitch (Fig. 8.4). If you have difficulty locating the linea alba in an obese patient, evert the base of the umbilical stalk upwards, using a clip. This brings the linea alba to the surface (Fig. 8.4a). Insert a finger to sweep away any adhesions around the insertion site before introducing a blunt-tipped trocar. Connect the gas supply and establish a pneumoperitoneum. The main disadvantage of this method is the increased incidence of gas leaks around the port. Special ports with sealing balloons have been developed to prevent this.

The closed (Veress needle) technique is most commonly used. As before, make an infra-umbilical skin incision. Apply a 20–30° Trendelenburg tilt to the patient. Together with your assistant grasp the anterior abdominal wall and lift it up. Insert a Veress needle (Fig. 8.5) perpendicular to the abdominal wall until it penetrates the linea alba and the peritoneum. As soon as a 'give' is felt as the needle enters the peritoneal cavity, direct the needle downwards towards the pelvis to avoid damaging the great vessels.

3 Is the needle freely mobile? Place a drop of saline on the Luer connector of the Veress needle. It should fall freely into the abdomen, where the pressure is subatmospheric. Aspirate to check that you do not obtain bowel content or blood. Inject 5 ml of saline; it should flow freely through the needle. Insufflate gas slowly; if the tip of the needle is within the peritoneal cavity, this should not produce a significant rise in the pressure reading.

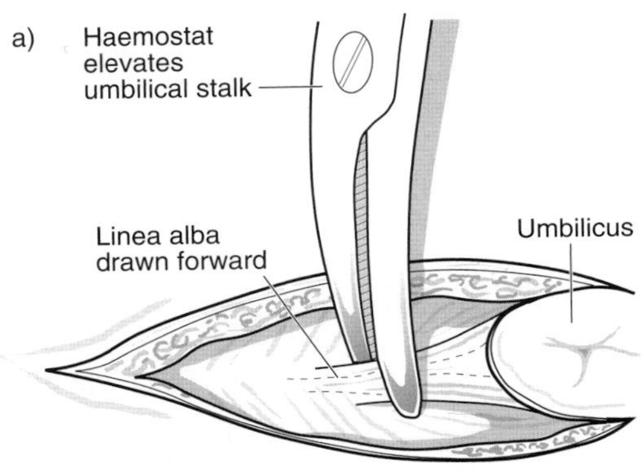

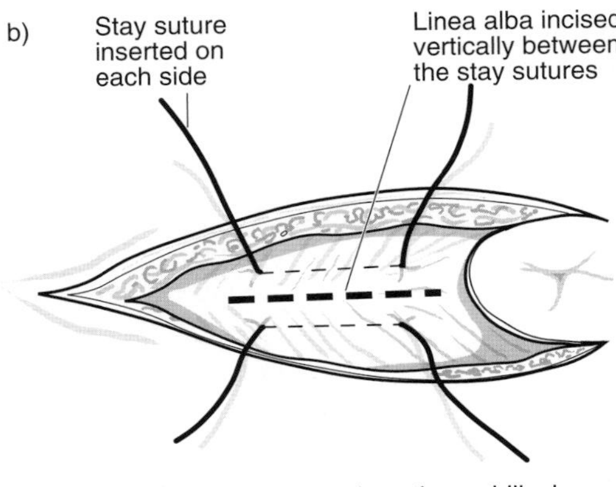

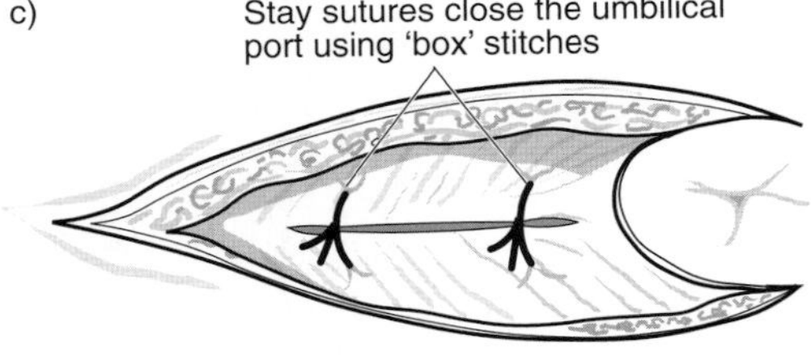

Fig. 8.4 Insertion of a Hasson port just below the umbilicus. (a) Shows the vertical incision made just below the umbilicus, dissected down to the linea alba. (b) Longitudinal absorbable stitches (Vicryl) have been inserted on each side of the midline; the vertical midline incision will be made between them through which the Hasson port will be inserted. (c) On completion and removal of the port, close the defect by tying the sutures across to produce a 'box' or 'mattress' stitch.

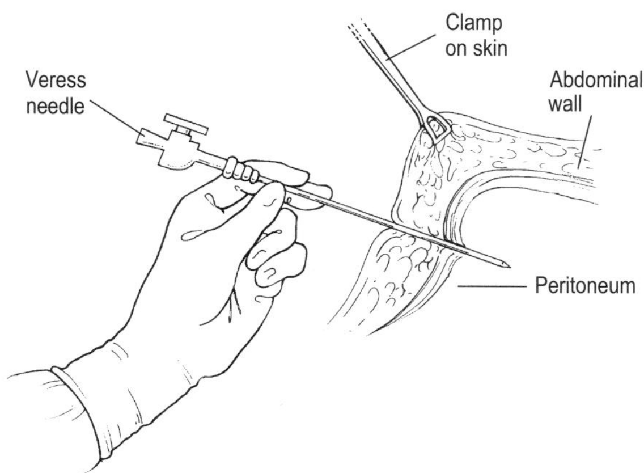

Fig. 8.5 Diagram showing a technique for inserting the Veress needle into the abdominal wall and the layers the needle passes through.

> **? DIFFICULTY**
>
> If the intra-abdominal pressure rises above the preset level, an alarm usually sounds. At this point:
>
> 1. Stop insufflation, check port/needle positioning and check that the gas tubing is not obstructed and that the control taps are on.
> 2. If there has been too much gas introduced into the abdomen, let some gas out via one of the ports.
> 3. Liaise with the anaesthetist in case there has been a loss of muscle relaxation.

4 When the abdomen is fully distended and tympanitic to percussion, withdraw the Veress needle and enlarge the superficial part of the incision to accommodate the cannula. Insert a 10-mm trocar and cannula, aiming the tip anterior to the sacral promontory, parallel to the aorta. Use a drilling action from the wrist while lifting up the abdominal wall below the insertion site. Withdraw the trocar, insert the laparoscope and connect it to the insufflator. Observe the view as you insert it to ensure the viscera are not at risk. Inspect the abdomen to identify structures that could be potentially damaged when the other ports are inserted. Secure the port either using a threaded collar or with stay sutures.

5 Insert additional ports under direct vision. You may first infiltrate the tissues with local anaesthetic prior to incision. The sites, size and number are determined by the intended procedure. Each trocar and cannula is inserted while your assistant moves the camera to provide a view so you do not spear the viscera or vessels. Secure the ports with threaded collars or stay sutures.

Assess

1 Now survey the abdomen prior to performing the procedure. Be systematic in identifying landmarks and inspecting the relevant area. Locate the ligamentum teres and falciform ligament. In the right upper quadrant visualize the liver, gallbladder and the underside of the right hemidiaphragm. Manipulate the laparoscope under the ligamentum teres to look at the left lobe of the liver and the spleen. Change the patient's position to aid visualization by moving the bowel. Inspect both the left and right paracolic gutters, facilitating the exposure by inserting a probe or grasper to manipulate the bowel if necessary.

2 Place the patient in the Trendelenburg position to locate the caecum and appendix. Insert an endoscopic grasper to manoeuvre the bowel while you examine it from distal to proximal. While the patient is in the head-down position examine the pelvis; this is especially important in female patients when they have lower abdominal pain of unknown cause. You can directly visualize the ovaries, uterus and vermiform appendix.

3 In order to inspect organs such as the pancreas, additional manipulation and dissection may be necessary. Diseases such as Hodgkin's can be staged, and masses biopsied.

Diathermy

Diathermy used during laparoscopic surgery to achieve haemostasis, along with sutures and clips, can cause unrecognized, inadvertent, even fatal injury. Carefully identify the correct structure. The most common injury results from misidentification and hence burning the wrong structure. Inadvertent activation of the diathermy pedal risks damaging other structures in the abdominal cavity, especially when the electrode is outside the field of view.

Faulty insulation, especially when using old instruments subjected to abrasive cleaning, creates a conducting surface other than the electrode to come into contact with a viscus.

TABLE 8.2 Some complications common to laparoscopy and pneumoperitoneum

During pneumoperitoneum induction	Related to port placement	During procedure	Patient-related complications
Damage to viscus or vessels	Damage to underlying structures	Diathermy-related injuries	Obesity: makes operation more difficult, increasing operating time, and may require special instruments
Misplacement of the gas	Be poorly placed	Inadvertent organ ligation or division	Ascites causes oozing from port sites, increasing the risk of port-site damage
Insufflation of the bowel lumen	Haemorrhage	Unrecognized haemorrhage	Organomegaly increases the risk of organ damage
Carbon dioxide embolus and metabolic acidosis may complicate pneumoperitoneum	Herniation		Clotting problems may result in haemorrhage, or conversely in deep vein thrombosis
Over-insufflation of the peritoneal cavity may cause cardiorespiratory problems			Following operation for malignant disease, cancer cells may be transferred to the port site, resulting in metastases

If burning does not directly cause a perforation, it may lead to autodigestion and perforation at a later date.

Current may flow from the active electrode to a contiguous conducting instrument; this is an example of direct coupling. The result is poor function at the active electrode and an unnoticed burn from the second instrument. After use, diathermy electrodes can remain sufficiently hot to cause burns so withdraw the electrode or keep it in view. As in open surgery, diathermy of a pedicle concentrates the current density and so can lead to inadvertent perforation of structures, such as the common bile duct, during laparoscopic cholecystectomy.

Alternating currents can pass through insulating materials, as occurs in devices called capacitors. During laparoscopy a capacitor may be inadvertently formed so current induced in a metal port then flows into neighbouring bowel and causes a burn. Avoid capacitative coupling by using a non-conducting electrode. If you are using a metal port ensure that it makes good contact with the abdominal wall. Avoid open-circuit activation, and high-voltage diathermy, such as fulguration.

Closure

1 Before removing the ports, ensure that haemostasis is complete and that there are no free bodies in the abdomen such as spilt gallstones. Remove all laparoscopic instruments and ports under direct vision while checking for port-site bleeding. Make sure no intra-abdominal structures have become trapped in the ports or port sites. Remove the final port slowly, with the laparoscope still inside to finally check.

2 Palpate the abdomen, helping to expel any remaining carbon dioxide, then close the port holes. Identify and grasp the fascia with toothed forceps. Use interrupted

absorbable synthetic sutures such as polyglactin 910 (Vicryl) or polydioxanone (PDS). Take care not to pick up bowel with the stitch. Close the skin with either absorbable or non-absorbable sutures.

Postoperative

Monitor all patients as following an open laparotomy, with regular observations. Remind them of referred shoulder tip pain from stretching of the peritoneum lining the hemidiaphragms following pneumoperitoneum. Mobilize patients early and encourage them to eat and drink.

Most patients can be discharged within 24 hours of laparoscopy; the length of stay increases with more extensive procedures. Some surgeons now perform day-case laparoscopic cholecystectomy.

Complications

Since laparoscopic surgery usually requires a general anaesthetic, patients are susceptible to the usual complications related to this. Table 8.2 lists complications common to laparoscopy and pneumoperitoneum.

FURTHER READING

Darzi A 2004 Minimal access surgery. In: Kirk RM, Ribbans WJ (eds) Clinical surgery in general, 4th edn. Churchill Livingstone, Edinburgh, pp 237–240

Darzi A, Monson JRT 1994 Laparoscopic inguinal hernia repair. ISIS Medical Media, Oxford

Darzi A, Talamini M, Dunn DC 1997 Atlas of laparoscopic surgical technique. Saunders, London

Hasson HM 1971 Modified instrument method for laparoscopy. American Journal of Obstetrics and Gynecology 110:886–887

9

Hernias and abdominal wall

D. F. L. Watkin, G. S. M. Robertson

CONTENTS

GENERAL ISSUES IN HERNIA SURGERY

Groin pain may arise from hip osteoarthrosis or groin strain, rather than the obvious inguinal hernia. Epigastric pain may be biliary colic or from peptic ulcer, not from an epigastric hernia.

Thoroughly check those admitted for operation the same day, confirming they have fully consented to operation, understand the circumstances under which it will be performed and the discharge arrangements.

The hernia may not be evident in the anaesthetized patient so it is essential that the site (and side) are marked preoperatively.

If prosthetic mesh will be inserted, you may give a prophylactic dose of antibiotic at induction and apply topical antibiotics. Always do so when operating for strangulated hernia, because the wound may be contaminated.

Local anaesthesia is suitable for the repair of many groin hernias and some other hernias but is less well tolerated in young adults, who may require the addition of sedation. It is economically beneficial, particularly for day-case operations and in the elderly, but it is not devoid of risk so monitor blood pressure, pulse rate, oxygen saturation, and make sure you know the appropriate procedures for resuscitation in case the patient develops an adverse reaction. For effective anaesthesia use a sufficient volume; our preference is for 0.5% lidocaine with adrenaline (epinephrine) 1 in 100000. Alternatively use bupivacaine (0.25%) but it acts more slowly. You may use a mixture of lidocaine and bupivacaine. Stick to a chosen local anaesthetic to avoid confusion and do not exceed the safe dose of local anaesthetic; for lidocaine with adrenaline (epinephrine) this is 7 mg lidocaine per kg, approximating for an average adult to 500 mg, equivalent to 100 ml of a 0.5% solution. Clearly record the dose of local anaesthetic and other drugs in the notes.

Non-absorbable sutures on curved, round-bodied, eyeless needles should always be used for the repair. Monofilament materials minimize the risk of persistence of a wound infection, polyamide (nylon) and polypropylene being the most popular. Remember that monofilament sutures require extra knots for security and handle them carefully since they are weakened by jerking them when tying knots or grasping them with instruments. Dragging fine sutures through the tissues cuts them, enlarging the holes. Too tight sutures cut out or strangle the tissues, and increase the risk of troublesome neuralgia. Even bites of the tissues look neat but tend to detach a strip of aponeurosis, so take successive bites at differing distances from the edge. Close skin with sutures, clips, staples or adhesive strips but a continuous subcuticular absorbable stitch (e.g. polyglactin 910) is neat and avoids the discomfort and cost of suture removal.

Postoperative analgesia is important in day-case work and for patients discharged the following morning. Rectal diclofenac inserted in theatre, with patients' prior consent, is effective in those not suffering from asthma or peptic ulcer. Postoperatively give regular oral diclofenac 50 mg t.d.s. for 2 days.

Wound complications include bruising and haematomas – avoid by meticulous haemostasis and judicious use of suction drains. Wound infection rarely requires more than drainage of any collection. Sinus formation is rare with the use of monofilament sutures but occasionally requires removal of suture knots or mesh. Technical failure risks recurrence, including missed hernia sac and inadequate placement or size of mesh. Outpatient follow-up reveals late wound infections and local numbness or pain.

Prosthetic biomaterial meshes are now commonplace; they are quickly inserted and have proved to be effective worldwide. There is little doubt that they often make hernia surgery quicker and easier, reducing recurrence rates as fibrosis invades the pores, provided the mesh extends 2–3 cm to allow for shrinkage. Some meshes incorporate antimicrobial agents.

INGUINAL HERNIA

Formerly, indirect hernias were usually repaired, diffuse direct hernias were treated with a truss but most are now operated upon except for trivial direct hernias; those with cardiovascular and respiratory disease can be given epidural anaesthesia or local anaesthesia which is safe, effective and low cost, allowing shorter stay. Defer operation for gross obesity or consider laparoscopic repair (Ch. 10), and as a trainee do not embark on such operations. Bilateral hernias can be repaired at the same time although the results are slightly better following separate repairs; local anaesthesia requires an excessive dose but an option is laparoscopic repair. As a trainee avoid attempting repair of recurrent diffuse hernias in obese patients with stretched, fat-infiltrated tissues or with chronic coughs since they are not at risk of strangulation and recurrence is likely.

The open anterior approach can be performed under local anaesthesia; laparoscopic repair has advantages for repairing bilateral and recurrent hernias. Our, conservative, view is that the majority of primary groin hernias should continue to be repaired by the anterior approach but some patients may choose laparoscopic repair in the interest of a more rapid return to work.

Surgeons often attribute their excellent results to particular details of their technique, but the common factor that produces success is the perfection with which the procedure is accomplished. For this reason, do not attempt to acquire mastery of all the techniques but become familiar with a small range that will deal with most demands. We shall describe two methods.

Inspect

The diagnosis of groin swellings is notoriously difficult. Experienced as well as inexperienced surgeons make frequent mistakes. Do not accept the diagnosis of the referring doctor, but take a fresh history and carry out a complete examination. Is there another possible cause for the patient's symptoms apart from the hernia? If a clear history of a reducible intermittent lump in the groin is accompanied by a negative examination, a hernia will be found on exploration; if in doubt consider herniography using ultrasound or radiology following intraperitoneal injection of non-ionic contrast.

Palpation is not the only, or even the most important, method of examination. Look with the patient standing and again with the patient supine. If you see a lump, ask yourself 'Where is it?' If it is reducible, where does it first reappear on coughing or straining? Apart from obstructed and strangulated hernia, a cough impulse may be absent, especially over a femoral hernia in which a small sac is covered by much fatty extraperitoneal tissue. Conversely, a cough impulse is present over Malgaigne's bulgings or a saphena varix.

Never fail to examine the scrotum and its contents in male patients. If there is a swelling, ask yourself the fundamental question, 'Can I get above it?' Occasionally undescended testes will be diagnosed and should be addressed at the same procedure.

Finally, examine the other hernial orifices.

Prepare

Many operations can be performed on a day-case basis in fit people who have good home circumstances. Bilateral procedures (unless done laparoscopically) and operations in unfit or elderly patients or those who live alone require overnight or 48-hour stay. Warn the patient of the possible complications of haematoma (especially for large inguino-scrotal hernias), ischaemic orchitis and persistent groin pain.

Local anaesthesia for inguinal hernia repair

Do not exceed the maximum dose, e.g. 100 ml of lidocaine 0.5% with adrenaline (epinephrine). Inject 20 ml along the line of the proposed incision using a fine needle to raise a continuous bleb within the epidermis. Replace the needle with a larger one to inject deeply and along the same line superficial to the anterior wall of the canal. Blunt the needle to improve the 'feel' of passage through the aponeurosis and inject 5 ml of fluid 2 cm above and medial to the anterior superior iliac spine deep to the external oblique to block the iliohypogastric and ilioinguinal nerves. Reserve about half the anaesthetic to inject under the external oblique, around the neck of the sac and into other sensitive areas during the operation.

Access

1 Start the incision a finger's breadth above the palpable pubic tubercle within the skin crease which is often present (as opposed to parallel to the inguinal ligament) and extend this to two-thirds of the way to the anterior superior iliac spine. Incise the fascia to expose the external oblique aponeurosis, ligating and dividing two or three large veins that cross the line of the incision. Avoid cutting into the hernial sac and spermatic cord at the medial end of the incision. Expose the glistening fibres of the external oblique aponeurosis and identify the external inguinal ring, which confirms the line of the inguinal canal.

2 Make a short split with a knife in the line of the fibres of the external oblique aponeurosis over the inguinal canal. Enlarge the split medially and laterally by pushing the half-closed blades of the scissors in the line of the fibres. At the medial end of the split, the external inguinal ring will be opened; be sure to enter the external ring and do not allow the curved blades of the scissors to skirt around outside its crura. Preserve the ilioinguinal nerve lying under the external oblique, to minimize the risk of postoperative numbness and pain.

3 Apply artery forceps to the edges of the aponeurosis and gently elevate each side. As the upper leaf is turned back, look for the arching lower border of internal oblique muscle, with the cord below it. As the lower leaf is everted, sweep loose tissue from the deep surface of the inguinal ligament.

Assess (Fig. 9.1)

▶ KEY POINT Confirm the diagnosis

- Do not rely on preoperative findings of the type of inguinal hernia; determine this during mobilization.

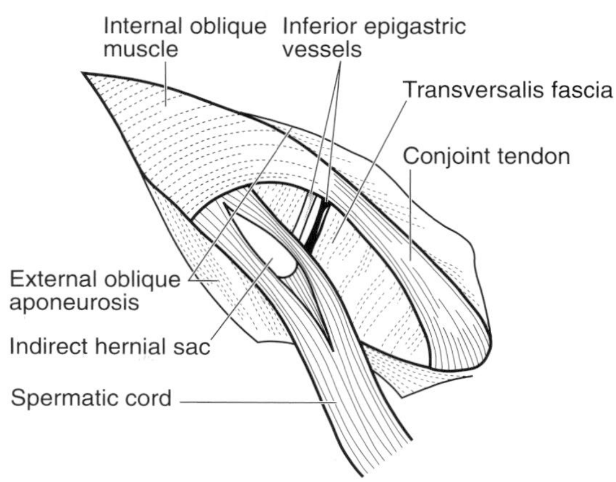

Fig. 9.1 Exposure of the right inguinal canal. The cremasteric fascia is split to show an indirect hernial sac.

1 Start to mobilize the cord by incising, just above and lateral to the public tubercle, the 'mesentery' of fascia and fibres of cremasteric muscle that extends downwards from the medial part of the conjoint tendon to envelop the cord. Deepen this small incision behind the cord, drawing the latter downwards while passing the index finger from below against the pubic tubercle, to develop a plane to encircle the cord and apply a hernia ring.

2 Now dislocate the cord laterally and downwards by incising the coverings along lines just above and below it. This exposes a direct hernia, which can be freed from the cord. Carefully divide the fibres of cremaster just distal to the internal ring, ensuring haemostasis.

3 Even though a direct hernia is evident, examine the cord. Normally it is about the thickness of a pencil. It is markedly distended by an unreduced, sometimes adherent, or sliding, hernia. A thickened sac results from a longstanding indirect hernia. Cord lipomata produce thickening, as does an encysted hydrocele of the cord (in females a hydrocele of the canal of Nuck). To exclude an indirect sac, open the spermatic fascia covering the cord and identify the edge of the peritoneum deep to the internal ring.

4 Identify the lower arching fibres of the internal oblique muscle, becoming tendinous at the conjoint tendon, and examine the posterior wall below this. A direct hernia may be a large bulge, a diffuse weakness of the

whole posterior wall or, less often, a funicular hernia through a small localized defect (Ogilvie's hernia). If you are in real doubt, ask the anaesthetist to temporarily increase intra-abdominal pressure while you watch for distension and bulging.

5 If you are concerned that a femoral hernia may be present, incise the transversalis fascia (as in a Shouldice repair) to expose the upper aspect of the femoral canal. If a femoral sac is present, deal with it as a Lothiesen procedure (see later).

6 The cremasteric vessels pass medially from the inferior epigastric vessels adjacent to the cord. If the internal ring is enlarged it may be necessary to carefully identify, isolate, ligate and then divide the cremasteric vessels to facilitate a snug repair at the internal ring. If they are injured more medially, ligate them proximally and distally to the damage.

Hernial sac

Indirect sac

1 With the left thumb in front, gently stretch the previously mobilized cord over the left index finger, which is placed behind the cord. Make a short split with a knife, in the line of the cord, through the cremasteric and internal spermatic fascial layers. Continue the split proximally to the internal ring using scissors, first with their blades on the flat, separating fascia from deeper layers, then splitting the fascia.

2 Look for the sac. A white curved edge may be seen if the hernial sac is small (Fig. 9.1); if it is large it will be obvious as the fascial layers are separated. Using the point of the scalpel, gently incise the fibres crossing the fundus or the side edges of the sac. Unless it is very adherent it will then be possible to peel the sac out of the cord, with the aid of a few further strokes of the blade. The sac is then dissected back to the level of the abdominal peritoneum, using a combination of wiping with a gauze swab and snipping firm attachments with scissors. Keep the dissection close to the sac and avoid damaging other structures in the cord.

3 Pick up the sac with two artery forceps and open it between the forceps with a knife. Note any contents of the sac and return them to the peritoneal cavity. Free, ligate and excise adherent omentum. While holding the empty sac vertically with artery forceps, transfix its neck with a polyglactin (Vicryl) suture. Tie the ends of the suture-ligature into a half hitch, completely encircle the neck of the sac and tie a triple-throw knot to ligate the neck of the sac. If contents tend to bulge into the sac, gently hold them back using non-toothed dissecting forceps, sliding them out as the ligature is tightened.

4 Do not let your assistant cut the ends of the ligature. First excise the sac 1 cm distal to the ligature. Examine the cut end to ensure that only sac is seen, it does not bleed and the suture is secure, then cut the ligature yourself. The stump of the sac should retract through the internal ring. Alternatively, after fully mobilizing the sac, simply invert it – the sac need not be ligated for this.

5 If there are large extraperitoneal lipomata, carefully isolate, ligate and excise them but do not try to dissect out all the fatty tissue

Large sac

1 Complete hernias, or scrotal funicular hernias, have no distal edge to the sac as seen at the level of the pubic tubercle. Attempts to dissect out the whole sac cause the scrotal part of the sac and the testis to be drawn into the wound, increasing the risk of haematoma or ischaemic orchitis. Purposefully divide the sac straight across within the inguinal canal. Isolate the proximal portion up to the internal ring, and leave the distal portion open. In this way the dissection is kept to a minimum.

2 If the sac is adherent, open the sac in front and place artery forceps at intervals round the inside as markers. Lift up two forceps, stretch the portion of sac between them, separate the sac from the cord and cut it distal to the forceps. Take the next two forceps and repeat the manoeuvre. Continue in this manner until the proximal circumference of the sac is completely sectioned, with the edges still held in the forceps. After stripping the proximal part of the sac to the inguinal ring, transfix and ligate the neck and leave the distal part of the sac open.

SLIDING HERNIA

In some hernias, retroperitoneal structures slide down to form part of the sac wall, chiefly the sigmoid colon, bladder or caecum. Always be on the look-out for sliding hernia; you discover it when you attempt to empty and free the sac. If the sac is intact, do not open it. If you have already opened it, mark the fringe of peritoneum on the viscus with artery forceps and carefully and completely close the sac.

Make sure that neither the organ nor its blood supply was damaged before the true situation was recognized. If the bladder was damaged, repair the wall and remember to insert an indwelling urethral catheter at the end of the operation. The entire hernia sac and sliding viscus should be fully mobilized from the cord and replaced in the abdomen. However, if the sac is inguinoscrotal, divide and close it below the sliding viscus and replace both in the abdomen, then carry out the best possible repair of the posterior wall of the inguinal canal.

HERNIA IN INFANTS

Infants' tissues are fragile, unsuitable for handling by impatient or rough surgeons.

Make an incision in the skin crease just above the superficial inguinal ring. The well-developed deep fascia is easily mistaken for the external oblique aponeurosis. The internal and external rings are almost superimposed in infants and it is therefore unnecessary to split the external oblique aponeurosis.

Isolate the cord just distal to the external ring, open the external fascial layers of the cord longitudinally and look for the sac. Pick up each layer with two pairs of fine artery forceps and open it between the forceps in the line of the cord. A short sac can be recognized by the white curved distal edge. The easy movement of the slippery internal surfaces of a large sac helps in identifying it. Make sure you are in the correct layer. When the sac is opened, the inner wall is shiny and the tips of the forceps can be passed into the peritoneal cavity.

Take great care in dissecting the fragile sac proximally; avoid tearing or splitting it or damaging the inconspicuous and adherent vas deferens. The sight of extraperitoneal fat confirms that the neck has been reached. If the hernia is complete (i.e. it extends down to the testis), do not dissect it distally. Carefully free it circumferentially just distal to the external ring, either from the outside if it is unopened or from within if it is open. Transect the sac, leave the distal end open and dissect the proximal sac. At the external ring, transfix, ligate and divide the neck of the sac. Do not twist the sac, because the vas may be inadvertently twisted with it and damaged.

If the external ring has been stretched by a large hernia, narrow it with one or two absorbable synthetic stitches. No other repair is necessary in an infant. Close the subcutaneous layers with fine absorbable sutures. Close the skin with a fine absorbable subcuticular suture.

INGUINAL HERNIA IN WOMEN

The approach is similar to that employed in men. The round ligament of the uterus lies in the position of the male spermatic cord. Ligate and excise it at the level of the internal ring to allow closure of the latter. Recognize and isolate the sac, then transfix, ligate and divide it at its neck.

If the hernial sac is small, herniotomy is sufficient, combined with closure of the internal ring. For a larger hernia, repair the posterior wall as in a male.

DIRECT HERNIA

Always look for an indirect sac.

If the direct sac is funicular (cord-like), resulting from a localized defect in the posterior wall, isolate it, empty it, then transfix, ligate and divide it at the neck. Define the margins of the posterior wall defect. If the hole is small and it can be closed without tension, suture it now, with non-absorbable material on a fine, curved, round-bodied needle.

More often the sac is diffuse and associated with a general weakness of the posterior wall; do not open it. If a Lichtenstein repair is to be employed, push it inwards and maintain the invagination by a running suture, of 2/0 polypropylene or polyglactin 910, carried across the stretched transversalis fascia so as to flatten the bulge without tension. The sutures must not bite deeply or the bowel or bladder may be damaged. If a Shouldice repair is to be used, excise any excess of transversalis fascia when preparing the flaps for overlapping. Carry out a suitable repair of the posterior wall of the canal.

COMBINED DIRECT AND INDIRECT HERNIA

Such hernias protrude on either side of the inferior epigastric vessels. They are sometimes likened to the legs of pantaloons. In a few cases, a direct funicular sac can be manoeuvred laterally so both sacs emerge lateral to the vessels and can be dealt with together. Do not struggle to achieve this, but deal with each sac separately.

? DIFFICULTY

1. If you cannot find the sac or recognize the tissues, first find the vas deferens, felt as a string-like structure towards the back of the cord. The testicular vessels lie near the vas and, once these are separated, the rest of the cord may be cautiously divided, starting at the front, while keeping in mind that abdominal organs may be encountered. If a structure seems to be the sac, cautiously open it after tenting a portion between two artery forceps. Look for a glistening inner surface and insert a finger to determine if the sac communicates with the peritoneal cavity.
2. *Torn neck of sac?* Carefully free peritoneum from the abdomen to form a new neck.

REPAIR

In an infant, child or adolescent with a small indirect hernia, herniotomy is all that is required.

If the margins of the internal ring have been stretched by an indirect hernia, narrow the gap in the posterior wall using a non-absorbable suture to approximate the attenuated margins of the transversalis fascia medial to the cord. This is one of the effects of a Shouldice repair.

Posterior wall repairs are of two types:

- Tissues are brought in from the margins to strengthen the posterior wall. In the classic Bassini repair, the lower fibres of the internal oblique and transversus abdominis muscles, with their medial aponeuroses, are sutured to the inguinal ligament behind the cord. The Shouldice repair is a development of this.
- Natural or artificial material may be inserted as a sheet to bridge the defect. The insert must be large enough to overlap normal tissue and form a strong fibrous union with it, otherwise the repair will fail. This is exemplified by the Lichtenstein repair. Additionally or alternatively, a mesh 'plug' may be inserted into the defect. Darns of nylon or polypropylene to reinforce the posterior wall have largely been abandoned because of a high recurrence rate.

LICHTENSTEIN REPAIR

The Lichtenstein repair[1] employs a sheet of polypropylene mesh covering the posterior wall of the inguinal canal and extending, for security, over adjacent structures, with a hole to transmit the cord. It is a 'tension-free repair'.

Action

1. Expose the inguinal canal and fully mobilize the cord. If there is an indirect sac deal with it as described previously. If there is a substantial direct bulge this may first be plicated so as to invert the excess, but place the suture line so as not to create tension.
2. The mesh should have overall dimensions of 11 cm × 6 cm. To accommodate this, the external oblique aponeurosis must be separated from the deeper layers superiorly and medially and from the muscular part of internal oblique laterally to create an adequate pocket to receive the mesh. Prepare the polypropylene mesh as indicated in Fig. 9.2a. The lower medial corner is slightly rounded, the upper medial corner rather more so. Then incise the mesh from its lateral margin, placing the cut one-third of the distance from the lower edge. The cut extends for approximately half the length of the mesh, depending upon the size of the patient; it may need to be extended when the mesh is in place. In small patients the upper edge may need to be trimmed slightly.
3. Place the mesh in its final position (Fig. 9.2b). Lift the cord and bring the narrow lower tail through under it, below the internal ring. Then tuck the lateral end under the external oblique; the lower edge of the mesh now lies along the inguinal ligament. Now insert the upper two-thirds of the mesh so that it lies under the external oblique aponeurosis superiorly and medially, ensuring that there is a good overlap on the rectus sheath medially. Tuck the wide upper tail under the external oblique laterally, with its lower edge over the lower tail. Insert your fingers under external oblique superiorly and laterally to ensure that the mesh lies quite flat in the peripheral part of the pocket, though there may be a slight bulge centrally.
4. Start the fixation by passing a 2/0 polypropylene stitch through the mesh and the tissues overlying the pubic tubercle and tying this. Use this to form a continuous suture between the lower edge of the mesh and the inguinal ligament, working from medial to lateral,

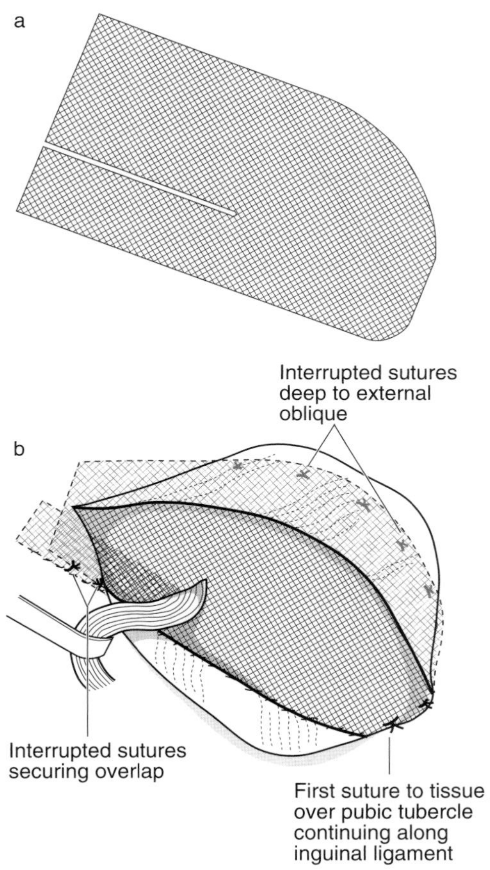

Fig. 9.2 Lichtenstein repair: (a) mesh cut to shape; (b) mesh sutured in place.

extending to at least 2 cm lateral to the internal ring. Take irregular bites of the inguinal ligament to avoid splitting it and do not allow the lower leaf of external oblique to roll in and be included in the sutures; if this happens, there will be no external oblique left to close. For the medial part of this suture line it is best to retract the cord downwards. Then as the suture approaches the internal ring, move the cord cephalad and pass the needle under it to continue laterally. When suturing immediately in front of the femoral vessels be careful to take only the ligament and not a bite of a major vessel!

5 If the slit in the mesh is too short, extend it so that the cord passes directly from the internal ring to the opening in the mesh. A bulky cord may be accommodated by making a small cut in the mesh at right angles to the slit. If your cut is too long, all is not lost; simply shorten the slit with one or two sutures. Overlap the tails of the mesh by bringing the lower edge of the upper portion in front of the lower tail and securing it to the inguinal ligament with two interrupted sutures (or by including it in the lateral part of the continuous suture). The resulting opening in the mesh should be a snug, but not a tight, fit around the cord (Fig. 9.2b).

6 Now secure the medial and upper margins of the mesh with about six interrupted sutures, avoiding the nerves (Fig. 9.2b). These are most conveniently placed 0.5 cm away from the edge, so that the mesh lies flat on the underlying aponeurosis or muscle. The medial sutures are particularly important as there is less overlapping of the mesh there, making it a potential site for recurrence. The mesh repair is now completed. It appears slightly redundant centrally but that does not matter.

▶ KEY POINT Sound repair?

- Provided there is sufficient overlap medially, superiorly and laterally, with a good suture line inferiorly, the fibrosis induced by the polypropylene (Prolene) mesh will produce a sound result.

7 Replace the cord in the inguinal canal. Close the external oblique aponeurosis with a synthetic absorbable suture, starting laterally and ending medially to re-form the external ring snugly but not tightly around the emerging cord. Once again, take care to take bites at unequal distances from the edges, otherwise you will pull from the cut edges a strip of aponeurosis. Appose the subcutaneous fascia with fine absorbable stitches and close the skin wound.

SHOULDICE REPAIR (Fig. 9.3)[2]

The results obtained at the Shouldice Clinic in Toronto are outstanding, with recurrence rates below 1%. It has generally been superseded by the Lichtenstein repair, but some surgeons still use it for young adults, or when mesh is unavailable or bowel resection is required.

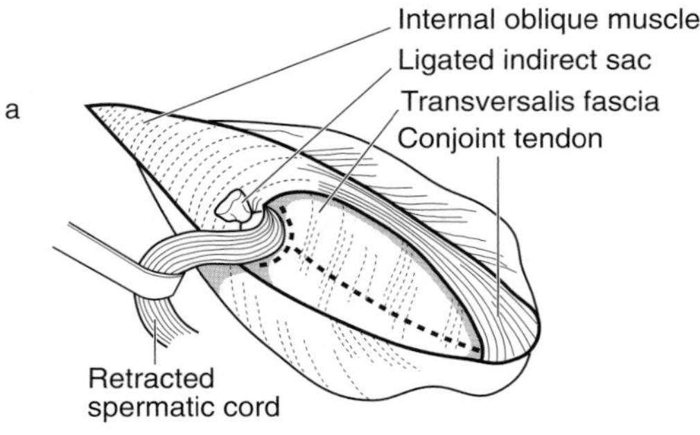

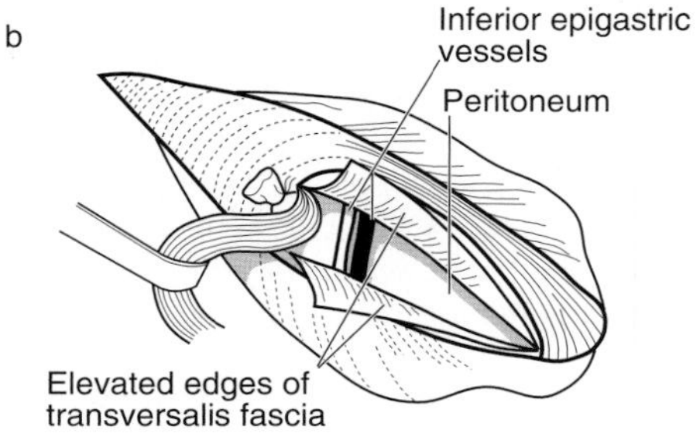

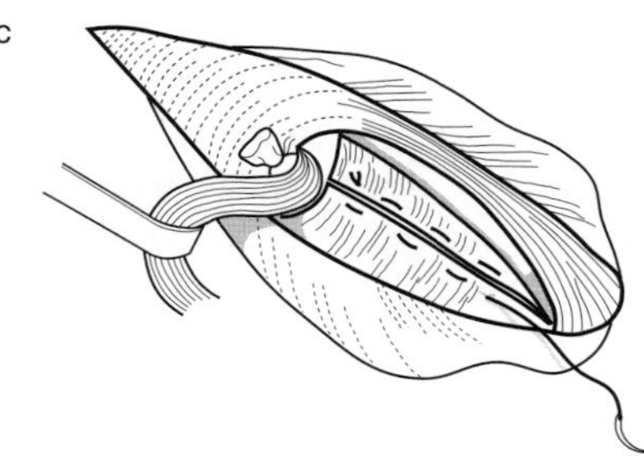

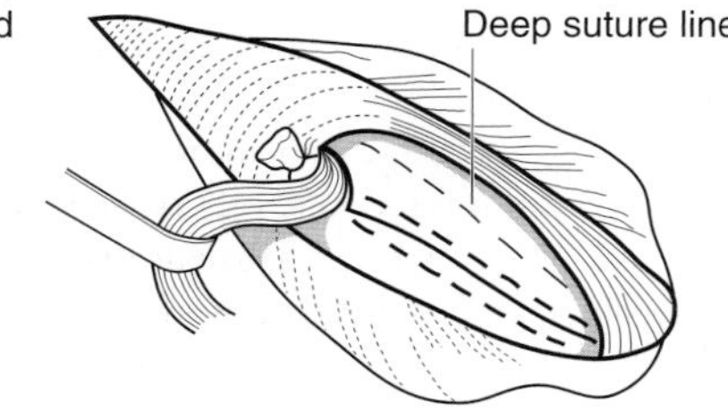

Fig. 9.3 Shouldice repair: (a) the broken line is the incision in transversalis fascia and around the internal ring; (b) the upper and lower flaps have been elevated; (c) the lower flap is sutured to the undersurface of the upper flap; (d) the upper flap is sutured over the lower flap. Finally, the conjoint tendon is sutured to the inguinal ligament.

Action

1 Expose the inguinal canal, mobilize the cord and divide its coverings; if there is an indirect sac deal with it, as described earlier.

2 If there is not a large direct hernia, gently insinuate the closed tips of non-toothed dissecting forceps under the medial edge of the internal ring and pass them medially towards the pubic tubercle, separating the transversalis fascia from the inferior (deep) epigastric vessels. Allow the blades of the forceps to separate by a small amount and insert the deep blade of slightly opened scissors beneath the medial edge of the internal ring, between the forceps blades. Divide the medial edge of the internal ring and continue medially, to split the transversalis fascia as far as the pubic tubercle, halfway between the conjoint tendon and the inguinal ligament (Fig. 9.3a). Bleeding from small vessels in the fascia often requires diathermy. If there is a large direct hernia, make a spindle-shaped incision in the transversalis fascia, judged so as to preserve suitably sized upper and lower flaps. The intervening, excess, portion of the fascia is then inverted with the hernia.

3 Elevate the upper flap of transversalis fascia from the underlying extraperitoneal tissue, brushing the fat away to expose its shiny white deep surface at the level of the conjoint tendon. If you have not already isolated, ligated and divided the cremasteric vessels close to their origin from the inferior (deep) epigastric vessels when you mobilized the cord, do so now. Separate the lower flap of transversalis fascia down to the inguinal ligament where it continues inferiorly as the femoral sheath (Fig. 9.3b). Take the opportunity to check that there is no femoral hernia.

4 Repair the transversalis fascia by overlapping the upper and lower flaps. Bulging of the extraperitoneal tissues into the wound can be prevented by inserting a small dry gauze swab into the extraperitoneal space, removing it just before the first suture line is completed (removal is your responsibility!). Alternatively, a flat retractor or closed sponge-holding forceps can be used to push back the extraperitoneal tissues, being gradually withdrawn as the repair is completed.

5 Lift the upper flap of transversalis fascia and bring to its undersurface the edge of the lower leaf (Fig. 9.3c). Start at the medial end, using a continuous 2/0 monofilament nylon or polypropylene suture. Insert the

sutures approximately 3 mm apart, at irregular distances from the lower flap edge. On the upper flap, pick up the more robust white transversalis fascia thickened at the level of the conjoint tendon. As you reach the lateral end, refashion the internal ring snugly around the thinned, emerging cord, taking exceptional care that a ligated indirect sac stump does not slip out.

6 Now fold down the upper flap of fascia transversalis and suture it into the lower flap where it thickens (the iliopubic tract) as it passes under the inguinal ligament (Fig. 9.3d). Suture it securely medially and, at the lateral end, carefully suture it around the medial aspect of the internal ring to reinforce the snug fit around the emerging cord. Further strengthen the posterior wall by suturing the conjoint tendon down to the inguinal ligament. Start medially at the pubic tubercle and work laterally, everting the internal oblique muscle in order to catch the tendinous portion. Take great care, when you reach the internal ring, to snugly enclose it. If the patient is a woman the internal ring and external oblique aponeurosis may be completely closed.

7 Lay the cord back into place and close the external oblique aponeurosis and the wound as described for the Lichtenstein operation.

Postoperative

Following repair of inguinal hernia under local anaesthesia, allow the patient to leave the operating theatre on foot, which is good for confidence. Patients should mobilize immediately after recovery from general anaesthesia. Inpatients generally go home the next day. Activities should be limited only by the patient's comfort.

Complications of inguinal hernia repair

In addition to the complications mentioned under general issues, some are specific to the groin.

Scrotal complications. Ischaemic orchitis uncommonly presents as pain and swelling within a few days and may result in testicular atrophy. Recognize and repair damage to the vas. Hydrocele, more common after transection of the sac, usually resorbs spontaneously as does genital oedema.

Nerve injury. Transient numbness is common below and medial to the incision; in at least 3% there is chronic residual pain.

Urinary problems. Recognize and repair bladder injury, inserting an indwelling catheter. Urinary retention usually resolves following a 24-hour period of catheterization.

Impotence does not appear to result from an organic cause.

RECURRENT INGUINAL HERNIA

Consider laparoscopic repair to avoid the adherent tissues. For open operations, with a mesh repair, orchidectomy is unnecessary but warn of the risk of ischaemic orchitis. A small direct defect may be protected by inserting a small piece of polypropylene mesh extraperitoneally, either as an underlay or as a 'plug'. For all other inguinal recurrences the Lichtenstein method is the best open repair.

REFERENCES

1. Amid PK, Shulman AG, Lichtenstein IL 1993 Critical suturing of the tension free hernioplasty. American Journal of Surgery 165:369–371
2. Glassow F 1984 Inguinal hernia repair using local anaesthesia. Annals of the Royal College of Surgeons of England 66:382–387

FEMORAL HERNIA

It is usually accepted that all femoral hernias should be repaired because of the high risk of strangulation, but there are no absolute rules in surgery. A very old, frail person with an incidentally discovered, longstanding femoral hernia can reasonably be left alone.

One reason for offering surgical repair freely is that the operation can be accomplished easily using local anaesthesia. Be aware of the prevascular femoral hernia; its neck extends laterally in front of the vessels. Try each of the three current open approaches for femoral hernia and identify a favourite (Fig. 9.4). They all have merits and are safe, provided you perform them skilfully. We use the low approach for elective operations and McEvedy's for strangulated hernias. They can be repaired laparoscopically, but if diagnosed preoperatively the benefits appear negligible as the low approach does not require muscle incision while laparoscopic dissection close to the femoral vein presents a risk.

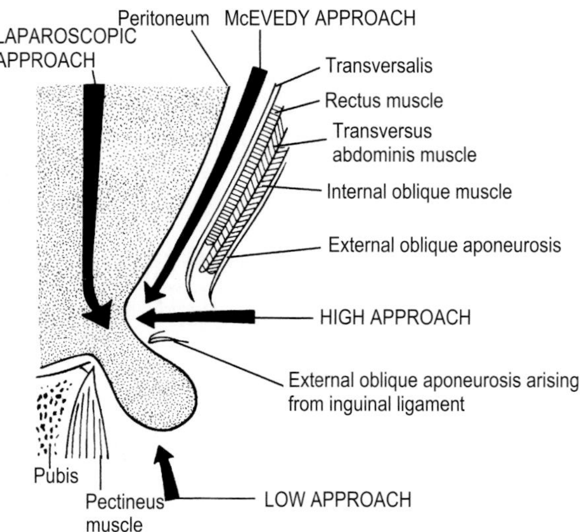

Fig. 9.4 Femoral hernia. A sagittal section through the hernial sac shows the various approaches.

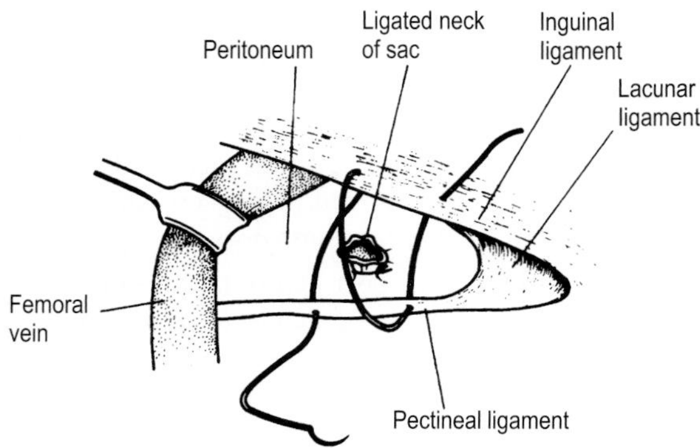

Fig. 9.5 Low approach to right femoral hernia.

LOW APPROACH (LOCKWOOD)

Access

Make an incision 4–5 cm long in the crease of the groin, below the medial half of the inguinal ligament. Cut the superficial tissues over the hernia in the line of the skin incision. Identify, ligate and divide the small veins running into the long saphenous vein as necessary.

Action

1 Expose the fat-covered hernial sac. Often, what appears to be a large swelling is mostly extraperitoneal fat, in which lies a small sac. Clean the sac so that it may be traced proximally beneath the inguinal ligament.

2 Cautiously open the sac by incising it while it is held up between two artery forceps. Remember that the bladder may form the medial wall of the sac. Recognize the inside of the sac by seeing free fluid, a glistening surface and contents that may be reduced into the main peritoneal cavity. Pick up the open edges of the sac with three equally spaced artery forceps, then sweep away the external fat to expose the neck, lying between the inguinal ligament anteriorly and the pectineal ligament posteriorly in the same horizontal plane. Note how deeply lies the neck of the sac. Identify the femoral vein lying just laterally and preserve it from damage. Empty the sac, transfix and ligate the neck with 2/0 absorbable suture; it should retract. Now excise the sac 1 cm distal to the ligature.

3 The inguinal and pectineal ligaments meet medially through the arched lacunar ligament. The object of the repair is to unite the ligaments for about 1 cm laterally, without producing constriction of the femoral vein (Fig. 9.5). Use 2/0 monofilament nylon or polypropylene, on a small needle. A standard 30-mm round-bodied needle can be shaped to fit into the available space, but avoid damaging the tip. Many use a J-shaped needle.

4 Place a small curved retractor over the femoral vein to protect it and draw it laterally. Insert a stitch deeply into the inguinal ligament and use this to draw the ligament upwards, while the needle is insinuated behind it, to take a good bite of the pectineal ligament. Avoid taking too deep a bite or the needle point will break as it strikes the pubic crest. One, two or three stitches may be used but, for ease of access, insert all the stitches before tying any. As the stitches are tightened, ensure that the femoral vein is not constricted.

5 Alternatively, occlude the femoral canal with a 'plug' of rolled mesh, secured with three sutures.

6 Unite the subcutaneous tissues with fine absorbable stitches and close the skin, preferably with an absorbable subcuticular suture.

? **DIFFICULTY**

1. *Can you not identify the sac in the fatty lump?* Remember that most of the lump may be preperitoneal fat. Gently and carefully incise it and separate it. When the peritoneum is incised you can usually see glistening visceral peritoneum or lobulated omental fat. If the sac contains free fluid it appears bluish and may be confused with the appearance of congested bowel. When the sac is carefully incised the fluid escapes, revealing the contents. If you inadvertently tear the neck of the sac, gently free peritoneum from the peritoneal cavity so that it can be drawn down to form a new neck.
2. If you tear the femoral vein, compress it with gauze packs for 5 minutes, while ordering blood, arterial sutures, tapes, bulldog clamps and heparin solution, and summon assistance. Expose the vein; do not hesitate to approach it from above and below the inguinal ligament. Apply bulldog clamps and tapes above and below the damaged segment. Insert fine 4/0 or 5/0 sutures set 1 mm apart, 1 mm from the torn edges to evert them and close the hole. Flush with heparin at intervals. Release, then remove the clamps and tapes.
3. It is not possible to suture the whole of a prevascular defect. Insert a piece of mesh and suture the opening medial to the vein.

HIGH APPROACH (LOTHIESEN)

The advantage of this approach is that it can be used for repairing coexisting inguinal and femoral hernias but for femoral hernia alone it has the disadvantage that it damages the inguinal canal and could lead to a subsequent inguinal hernia.

Expose the inguinal canal and dislocate the cord, as for operation for inguinal hernia. Incise the transversalis fascia, as in the Shouldice operation.

Action

1 Identify and isolate the neck of the sac and the external iliac vein and gently withdraw the fundus. If this is difficult, have the lower skin flap retracted downwards, incise the cribriform fascia and isolate, open and empty the sac from below. Ensure that the sac is empty and that the bladder is not adherent, then transfix, ligate and divide the neck of the sac. With your index finger, feel the margins of the femoral canal. In front is the inguinal ligament, medially the lacunar ligament, posteriorly the pectineal ligament and laterally the femoral vein.

2 Narrow the triangular gap by inserting non-absorbable sutures of 2/0 monofilament nylon or polypropylene between the pectineal ligament and the inguinal ligament.

3 If you selected the upper approach because there is also an inguinal hernia, deal with an indirect sac now. Either close the posterior wall as a Shouldice repair or close the incision in transversalis fascia with a non-absorbable suture and carry out a Lichtenstein repair.

4 Close the inguinal canal, subcutaneous tissue and skin as for an inguinal hernia.

MCEVEDY'S APPROACH

We prefer this approach for strangulated hernias as it provides excellent access for assessment of bowel and if necessary for resection. The original skin incision left an ugly scar; avoid this by placing it more horizontally.

Insert a catheter preoperatively, reducing the risk of damage to the bladder.

Action

1 Make an incision from 3 cm above the pubic tubercle running obliquely upwards and laterally for 7–8 cm, crossing the lateral border of the rectus muscle, which lies more vertically. Reflect the skin flaps so as to display the lateral part of the rectus sheath.

2 Incise the lower rectus sheath about 1–2 cm from, and parallel to, its lateral border. The lateral edge may tend to separate into its two anatomical layers. Lift the lateral edge of the sheath and incise the thin transversalis fascia from about 2.5 cm above the pubic tubercle to mobilize the lower lateral edge of the rectus medially. Ligate and divide the inferior epigastric vessels which cross this line low down. The neck of the hernia is now

in view as it enters the femoral canal. Retract the lower skin flap and isolate the sac.

3 Reduce the sac, manipulating it from above and below. Open and empty it, then transfix, ligate and divide the neck of the sac. For a strangulated hernia, which is the reason for using this approach, you may open the peritoneum above the neck so you can assess the bowel and carry out a resection if necessary.

4 Repair the canal from above, close the incision in the rectus sheath with 0 nylon or polypropylene, appose the subcutaneous layers, and close the skin.

STRANGULATED HERNIA

Most operations listed as strangulated hernia are carried out for painful, irreducible or obstructed hernias. Some hernias reduce spontaneously when the patient is sedated prior to operation, or when anaesthesia is induced. Strangulation results from venous obstruction, a rise in capillary hydrostatic pressure, transudation of fluid, exudation of protein and cells, and eventual arterial obstruction. Alternatively, the pressure of a sharp constriction ring at the neck of the sac may cause local necrosis of the bowel wall.

Try reassurance to relax the supine patient; head-down encourages spontaneous reduction. If you are experienced you may try reduction by gentle manipulation. Reduction en masse is a slight risk – the hernia remains within the peritoneal sac, the constricting neck remains, so the strangulation is unrelieved. If you can easily reduce the hernia, emergency surgery is unnecessary. Plan for early elective operation.

Do not rush patients with strangulated hernias to the operating theatre. Is there a reason, such as urinary outflow obstruction or a chest infection, why the patient has developed strangulation now? Identify coincidental disease that may make general anaesthesia and operation hazardous.

If strangulation has been present for some time, the patient requires fluid and electrolyte replacement. Some patients, especially with strangulated femoral hernias, do not reach hospital for a few days and by then have a severe biochemical disturbance. They may require up to 24 hours of resuscitation to correct the fluid deficit. This takes priority over the operation. It is likely, in such cases, that bowel in the hernia will already be irreversibly ischaemic, so little is lost by the delay.

The approach for inguinal and most other hernias is similar to that for an elective operation. For strangulated femoral hernias prefer McEvedy's incision as it provides better access to assess, and if necessary resect, bowel. If you use the low approach and bowel resection proves difficult, have no hesitation in opening the abdomen formally.

Assess

If the history was short, the sac is frequently empty by the time you expose it. The relaxation produced by the anaesthetic often succeeds when other conservative methods have failed; there is then no merit in exploring the abdomen. Repair the hernia as though this were an elective operation. If bowel is present in the sac, do not let it slip back into the abdomen but gently draw it down into view. The bowel is likely to have suffered the greatest damage where it was trapped at the neck of the sac. Feel the margins of the neck of the sac with a fingertip.

In Richter's hernia, most frequently associated with femoral hernia, a knuckle of the bowel wall is trapped. The bowel lumen is thus not obstructed but the knuckle may become gangrenous and perforate. Maydl's strangulation is very rare. Two loops lie in the sac but the blood supply to an intermediate loop within the abdomen may be prejudiced so that it is gangrenous.

KEY POINTS Is the bowel viable?

- If there is a sheen to the bowel wall, if it is pink or becomes pink after release, if the arteries pulsate, if peristalsis is seen, replace the bowel with confidence. If it is black, green or purple, with no sheen, if there is no pulsation in the mesenteric vessels or it is malodorous, resect it.
- If the bowel is congested, bluish or plum-coloured and still has a sheen, but vascular pulsations cannot be felt, then its viability is doubtful. Remember, however, that blood extravasated subperitoneally cannot be reabsorbed immediately so the colour may not change. Cover the bowel with warm moist packs for 5 minutes and re-examine it. If it has improved in appearance and mesenteric arterial pulsations are palpable it is probably viable.
- The critical areas are the constriction rings at the point of entrapment. These are white when the bowel is first drawn down but may

be greenish or black if they are obviously necrotic. Re-examine doubtful rings after an interval to see if the blood supply returns. If it does not, the bowel must be resected. Occasionally it is possible to invaginate and oversew a doubtful ring.

- Experienced surgeons probably resect bowel less frequently than those who are inexperienced. The mucosa is more vulnerable than the seromuscularis to the effects of ischaemia and, if the outer layers survive, the mucosa may slough to leave an annular ulcer. When this heals a constriction may develop. This is the intestinal stenosis of Garré. The patient presents after an interval of weeks or months with incipient small-bowel obstruction. Provided this is recognized, a simple elective resection can be carried out.

Action

1 If the neck of the hernial sac is constricted, first draw down healthy bowel, then place an index fingertip on each side of the contents, nails facing outwards. Gently dilate the neck of the sac (Fig. 9.6). Make sure the bowel does not slip back. Draw it out to ensure that there is no peritoneal constriction and to expose healthy bowel. If the bowel is viable, return it to the abdomen.

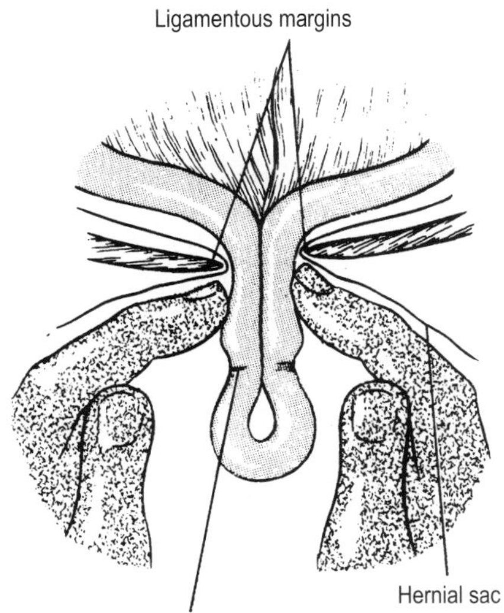

Fig. 9.6 Reducing a strangulated hernia. Healthy bowel is drawn down. The index fingers form a wedge to dilate the ligamentous margins.

2 If necessary, resect a gangrenous segment of bowel, performing an end-to-end anastomosis.

3 After opening the sac and dealing with the contents, repair the hernia as though this were an elective operation, but if possible avoid the use of mesh, for fear of infection.

? DIFFICULTY

1. Sometimes the bulk of tissues contained in the hernial sac makes reduction seem impossible. Provided the margins of the neck are defined, gentleness, patience and persuasion will succeed. If only a little at a time is reduced, do not despair because the reduction must get progressively easier.
2. The McEvedy approach avoids most of the difficulties in dealing with the bowel in a strangulated femoral hernia. When reducing a strangulated femoral hernia from below, it is not necessary to use a bistoury to incise the lacunar ligament; indeed, we find this illogical. Failure to reduce the hernia results from a tight sac neck, not from tight ligamentous margins, which are absent laterally. The femoral vein can be emptied and displaced, producing ample room to reduce the contents.
3. A large mass of fibrotic greater omentum may be adherent within the sac. Do not hesitate to excise the mass, provided the neck of the sac can be isolated, the bowel is not damaged and every blood vessel is safely ligated.
4. If gangrenous bowel slips back into the abdomen and cannot be recovered, repair the hernia, then open the abdomen through an appendix incision, following the terminal ileum proximally until the affected bowel can be delivered, wound protection applied and the gangrenous segment resected.

UMBILICAL HERNIA

ADULT UMBILICAL HERNIA

Most hernias in adults are para-umbilical, protruding adjacent to the cicatrix. The contents are most frequently omentum, which is often adherent to the interior of the sac. Some adults, especially of African origin, have true umbilical hernias that have been present throughout life.

Umbilical hernia is conventionally treated by early operation for fear of strangulation, but small para-umbilical hernias (less than 1 cm) can be left untreated if asymptomatic. Adjure patients who are grossly obese and elderly, with cardiovascular or respiratory disability and a longstanding hernia that has not been troublesome to lose weight – and hesitate about offering operation. Ascites may provoke umbilical hernia; find the cause and treat it. In some cases there is extensive malignant disease, when surgery is rarely indicated.

Operate on strangulated, painful, irreducible – but not necessarily painless irreducible – hernias and painful reducible hernias, especially those with small, hard margins.

The Mayo repair has been widely used, but a mesh repair placed at open operation or laparoscopically has been shown to be preferable. For large hernias which distort the entire umbilicus consider excising the umbilicus completely.

Access

1 Make a curved incision in the groove above or below the hernia. If necessary extend the cut transversely outwards on each side, for 2–4 cm.

2 Deepen the incision, identify the aponeurosis and expose it around the adjacent half of the circumference of the hernia.

3 If the hernia is small, preserve the umbilical skin by dissecting it off the hernia as a flap. If the hernia is large, make a spindle-shaped incision to include the umbilicus, excising the stretched skin.

4 Expose 2 cm of aponeurosis around the remainder of the margin of the hernia.

Action

1 Cut through the thinned-out edge of aponeurosis to expose the peritoneum and gradually work round to display the whole circumference of the neck of the sac. Clear the sac of fatty tissue and cut it right round, at least 2 cm distal to the neck if possible. The contents of the sac are less likely to be adherent here than in the fundus, but free them if necessary. Mark the peritoneal edges with artery forceps.

2 If the contents of the sac are free, reduce them. If they are adherent to the fundus of the sac, free them and return them to the peritoneal cavity. If there is a mass of fibrous omentum, excise it with the fundus of the sac but take care to ligate all the bleeding omental vessels and avoid damaging the transverse colon.

3 Separate the peritoneum from the undersurface of the rectus sheath all round, without tearing it.

4 Close the peritoneal neck of the sac with a continuous 2/0 synthetic absorbable suture, producing a transverse linear suture line.

5 Parachute a piece of polypropylene mesh, 2 cm larger than the defect in each direction, into the extraperitoneal plane and secure it, as described for the underlay repair of a small recurrent inguinal defect (p. 98).

6 If the skin over the fundus was preserved, pick up the undersurface of the navel with a synthetic absorbable stitch and sew it to the rectus sheath to produce a dimple. Suture the skin as a curved line above or below the newly fashioned umbilicus. If the umbilicus was excised, close the subcutaneous fat and the skin as a transverse suture line.

? DIFFICULTY

1. The hernia may be a true umbilical one, hidden within the cicatrix.
2. Divide the upper or lower edge of the cicatrix to find it.
3. If present, the congenital defect will be obvious and can be closed with interrupted non-absorbable sutures.

INFANTILE UMBILICAL HERNIA

Most infantile umbilical hernias protrude through the incompletely closed cicatrix. They appear to be more frequent in infants of African origin. Most of them close spontaneously without surgical repair, so wait for 1–2 years.

Repair them only if they increase in size. Infants infrequently develop a supra-umbilical hernia. It will not close spontaneously, so repair it locally through a transverse incision sited directly over the defect.

1 Approach the hernia through a transverse incision curved beneath the everted umbilicus. Preserve the umbilical skin by turning it upwards as a flap.

2 Expose the aponeurosis and the neck of the sac, which is within the cicatrix. The separation is much easier than in acquired hernias.

3 Open the sac, empty it, then close it by suture or transfixion ligature. Edge-to-edge repair of the aponeurosis is effective. Make sure the peritoneum is separated sufficiently to allow good bites of sheath to be taken, without piercing the peritoneum. Create a transverse suture line using polypropylene or nylon, inverting the knots. Suture the deep surface of the umbilical skin to the aponeurosis with fine absorbable synthetic material. Close the skin to leave a curved transverse wound, using an absorbable subcuticular stitch.

ABDOMINAL WALL SEPSIS

Wound infection arises from wound contamination with a variety of organisms often into a haematoma and perpetuated in the interstices of multifilament stitches. As prophylaxis, prefer monofilament materials for non-absorbable sutures, perioperative antibiotics, scrupulous haemostasis in the abdominal wall and covering the wound edges with Betadine (povidone-iodine)-soaked swabs or plastic wound protectors for potentially contaminated wounds. Infection may be a localized abscess, an abscess occupying the whole wound, with or without surrounding cellulitis, or there may be cellulitis without, as yet, an abscess. The wound is hot, red and swollen, the patient is pyrexial and may be toxic.

The mainstay of treatment is drainage, possibly on the ward by removing a suture from the softest part of the wound, followed by probing with forceps, or enlarging a wound discharging spontaneously. Always send a specimen for bacteriology. Do not routinely administer antibiotics unless there is cellulitis, the patient is already septic or at risk from immune deficiency, cardiac disease or prosthetic heart valves.

Sometimes when the wound is opened, severe tissue necrosis is discovered. Do not then make the error of leaving a small hole and inserting a drain (see necrotizing fasciitis, below).

Following drainage of a wound abscess, a chronic stitch sinus may persist. Explore the sinus with a pair of fine, sterile mosquito forceps, or a sterile crochet hook, to extract the stitch if possible. If the sinus persists, explore it under local or general anaesthesia to remove the suture material. Usually a knot of non-absorbable suture material is found; early removal of this may weaken the whole wound, so prefer to delay for up to a year.

Synergistic spreading gangrene is usually named after Meleney, the New York surgeon who described it in 1933. When it affects the scrotum it is called Fournier's gangrene. It may result from the synergistic effects of a number of microorganisms, or from a single organism. The nature of an operation or injury, and the patient's general condition, may predispose to the condition. Exclude diabetes, immunosuppression, uraemia and hepatic disease. It develops as a slowly extending area affecting the whole thickness of the skin. The advancing edge is typically serpiginous and leaves dead, sloughing skin that separates to expose unhealthy granulation tissue.

Immediately start broad-spectrum antibiotics, such as a cephalosporin and metronidazole, pending the result of bacteriology and excise all the necrotic tissue, exposing healthy, clean tissue. Leave the wound open and dress it frequently, repeating the excision of any developing necrotic tissue. When the infection has been completely controlled, plan to resurface the denuded area with partial thickness skin grafts.

Necrotizing fasciitis is a spreading gangrene primarily affecting the abdominal fascia. It may follow surgical operations or injury. It is predisposed to by general disease, particularly diabetes. Subsequently the overlying skin is also affected, but the skin involvement may not indicate the extent of the fascial infection. The mortality rate is 30%. Management is with broad-spectrum antibiotics and immediate radical excision of all the necrotic tissue to leave healthy living tissue (in the limbs this may involve amputation).

Gas gangrene is clostridial infection of abdominal wounds and is remarkably rare, considering that the organisms can be recovered from normal faeces. The patient rapidly develops pyrexia, toxicity and hypotension. The discoloured wound edges are crepitant and may discharge thin pus, described as smelling 'mousy'.

Administer 600 mg of benzylpenicillin and continue high doses thereafter, and as rapidly as possible correct the patient's general condition. Under general anaesthesia radically excise the whole area, back to clean, living tissue. Thoroughly wash the raw area with hydrogen peroxide (20 vols). Hyperbaric oxygen at 3 atmospheres has been recommended.

MISCELLANEOUS

Umbilical infections, tumours, fistulas and sinuses: Neglected or imperfectly treated umbilical sepsis, in infants, can progress to septicaemia, distant pyogenic infections, pylephlebitis, liver suppuration and fatal jaundice. An *enteroteratoma* is the remnant of the vitellointestinal duct forming a raspberry tumour. Cauterize it to destroy the mucosa. Persistent discharge from the umbilicus in infants, children and young adults is likely to be due to a congenital abnormality. *Congenital faecal fistula* results from persistence of the whole vitellointestinal duct. Patent urachus is persistence of the allantois, usually associated with membranous obstruction of the urethra. Aggregated keratin forms an 'omphalolith' within a deep umbilicus and may provoke infection and granulation tissue. Rarely pilonidal sinus may develop. Endometrioma at the umbilicus classically bleeds at the time of the menses. Squamous epithelioma can involve the inguinal lymph nodes. Secondary carcinoma from the liver or porta hepatis may reach the umbilicus along the ligamentum teres. This presents as Sister Joseph's nodule, first noticed by an observant nun. A port-site metastasis may occur after laparoscopic surgery.

Epigastric hernia results from a small knuckle of extraperitoneal fat insinuating itself through a vascular opening in the linea alba. It rarely has a peritoneal sac or contains bowel. *Port-site hernias* occur after laparoscopic surgery. Repair them by defining the margins, reducing the sac, usually without opening it, and closing the defect with non-absorbable stitches or with an overlapping polypropylene mesh.

Spigelian hernia occurs at the lateral margin of the lower rectus sheath and often expands beneath the external oblique aponeurosis. Repair may be by open operation or laparoscopically; the latter facilitates accurate diagnosis with sutures or polypropylene mesh placed extraperitoneally.

Haematoma of the rectus sheath results when a sudden strain ruptures one of the inferior epigastric vessels entering the lower rectus abdominis muscle, producing pain. It is more common in patients who are anticoagulated. On the right side, the localized pain and tenderness may be misdiagnosed as appendicitis but there are no systemic or gastrointestinal features and local tenderness in the right iliac fossa is greater when the patient puts the muscles under tension. Management is conservative. If you operate thinking the patient has appendicitis and discover a haematoma lying behind the lower rectus muscle, evacuate it. If there is a suspicion of continuing bleeding, isolate and ligate the inferior epigastric vessels in continuity.

Desmoid tumours are non-encapsulated tumours that develop in the muscle intersections. They are classified as fibromatoses; connective tissue hyperplasia infiltrates locally, but they do not metastasize. Most occur in women, especially those who have borne children. Remove abdominal wall desmoids completely or they recur. Patients with familial adenomatous polyposis may also develop desmoids within the abdomen; these generally surround the mesenteric vessels and so are irremovable. Excise the tumour with adequate clear margins and depth. Do not fail to cut through healthy muscle and connective tissue all the way round.

Carcinoma of intra-abdominal structures may directly invade the abdominal wall. If the tumour is otherwise resectable do not hesitate to excise a portion of the abdominal wall en bloc with the primary neoplasm.

Incisional hernia is a deep disruption of the abdominal wound while the superficial layers remain intact; if the superficial layers also separate then a burst abdomen results. Jaundice, malnutrition, obesity, postoperative distension, steroids and immunosuppression may be contributory. Repairs have a high recurrence rate, reduced by inserting mesh extraperitoneally or intraperitoneally.

Parastomal (Greek *para* = besides) hernias develop alongside stomas, and also with prolapse of the stoma. The stoma may be re-sited or after inserting a polypropylene mesh the stoma can be brought through a hole created in the mesh.

Non-hiatal diaphragmatic hernia presenting in a neonate may be diagnosed by ultrasonic scan before delivery and should be repaired immediately because the lungs cannot expand since the chest cavity is filled with abdominal viscera. The defect is the persistent pleuroperitoneal canal – the hernia of Bochdalek (see Ch. 43). Reduction from below is easy, unless the abdominal viscera are adherent within the chest. Hernia of the foramen of Morgagni passes between the costal and xiphoid diaphragm slips. Eventration is a bulge of the thinned central diaphragm with good muscle around the periphery; it can be folded and sutured. Traumatic rupture can usually be repaired satisfactorily.

Obturator hernia rarely occurs on the right side in females over the age of 50, usually presenting as intestinal obstruction, sometimes with pain radiating down the inner thigh and knee. It may be treated by open operation or laparoscopically. *Lumbar, gluteal* and *sciatic hernias* can occur respectively through the triangle of Petit bounded by the iliac crest, posterior edge of external oblique and anterior edge of latissimus dorsi; through the greater sciatic notch; through the lesser sciatic notch. *Pelvic floor and internal hernias usually* develop respectively following surgery of the pelvic floor; following abdominal operations causing adhesions or internal herniation – including the foramen of Winslow.

BLOCK DISSECTION OF GROIN LYMPH NODES

Radical groin dissection is carried out for resection of proven or suspected malignant lymph nodes and excision of metastatic melanoma deposits from primary sites in the leg, perineum and gluteal regions. The inguinal glands are excised through an incision parallel to the inguinal ligament.

The inguinal nodes may be involved by epidermoid carcinoma of the external male or female genitalia, or of the anal skin. In these cases the nodal dissection is usually accomplished in continuity with excision of the primary lesion. The iliac nodes can be removed separately by open repair or laparoscopically. A combined approach is usually through a vertical incision.

FURTHER READING

Fitzgibbon RJ, Greenburg AG (eds) 2001 Nyhus and Condon's hernia, 5th edn. Lippincott, Philadelphia
Kingsnorth AN 2003 Hernias: inguinal and incisional. Lancet 362:1561–1571
Kingsnorth AN, LeBlanc KA 2003 Management of abdominal hernias, 3rd edn. Arnold, New York
Macintyre IMC 2003 Best practice in groin hernia repair. British Journal of Surgery 90:131–132

10

Laparoscopic repair of groin and other abdominal wall hernias

J. M. Wellwood, M. G. Tutton

CONTENTS

GENERAL CONSIDERATIONS

Laparoscopic hernia repair is performed through three short abdominal wounds. The advantages include fewer wound complications, less postoperative pain and for incisional hernias shorter inpatient stays when compared to the open mesh repair. Long-term recurrence rates are similar for open and laparoscopic repair in experienced hands. The total extraperitoneal (TEP) approach should not involve entry into the peritoneal cavity, but the transabdominal preperitoneal (TAPP) approach and repair of other abdominal hernias carries a risk of damage to intraperitoneal organs. All inguinal hernias may be repaired laparoscopically. Bilateral hernias can be repaired through the same three ports used for unilateral repair. Recurrent hernias after open repair can be repaired laparoscopically without the need to dissect through scar tissue, reducing the risk of inadvertent injury to nerves and vessels.

Laparoscopic repair cannot be satisfactorily performed using local anaesthetic. Do not consider it for patients in whom local anaesthesia is medically desirable or requested by the patient. The repair may be more expensive for the hospital than mesh repair through a standard groin incision. Anticoagulant therapy is a relative contraindication to laparoscopic repair as bleeding can be more difficult to control than during the open operation. Significant obesity may also contraindicate laparoscopic repair.

TRANSABDOMINAL PREPERITONEAL (TAPP) HERNIA REPAIR

Create a pneumoperitoneum using either an open (Hasson) technique or a closed technique (see Ch. 8; Fig. 10.1). The Hasson technique is safer if there are intra-abdominal adhesions.

The synthetic mesh placed in the preperitoneal space should extend from the midline medially to a point close to the level of the anterior superior iliac spine laterally, thus covering the whole extent of the inguinal canal including the internal ring and the area medial to the inferior epigastric vessels where direct hernias originate. The mesh will also cover the internal opening of the femoral canal. Mesh, as opposed to sutures, ensures that the repair is tension-free (Fig. 10.2). The mesh is covered with peritoneum.

TOTALLY EXTRAPERITONEAL (TEP) HERNIA REPAIR

In order to fashion a preperitoneal space, pass a 10-mm trocar and cannula with a balloon at its tip into the rectus sheath and guide it downwards until it reaches the pubic symphysis and then angle the tip to a position just behind the symphysis (Fig. 10.3). Take great care not to angle the cannula in such a way that it might damage the peritoneum and enter the peritoneal cavity, as carbon dioxide gas entering the peritoneal cavity could lead to difficulty maintaining access for TEP repair. Insert a laparoscope into the cannula and maintain the tip of the cannula at a point immediately deep to the pubic bone. Gently inflate the balloon around the end of the cannula until the pubic bone is visible, thereby creating a space between the peritoneum

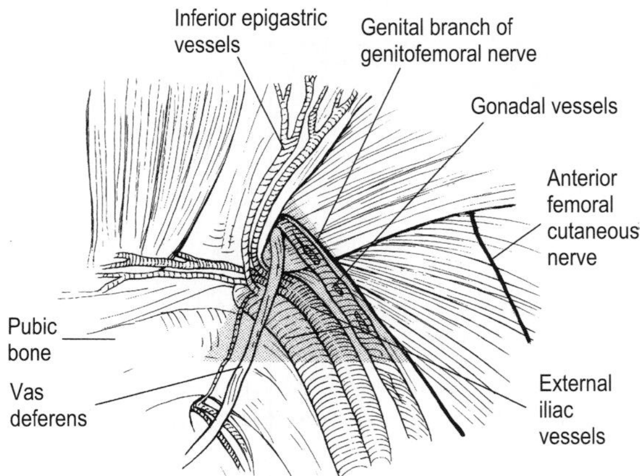

Fig. 10.1 The anatomy of the right groin in relation to TAPP repair. The shaded area has been called the 'triangle of doom' and is bounded by the vas deferens medially and the spermatic vessels laterally. In the floor of the triangle the external iliac vessels can be seen. The femoral nerve is not shown as it is on a deeper plane lateral to the vessels. The genitofemoral and anterior cutaneous nerve of the thigh are shown.

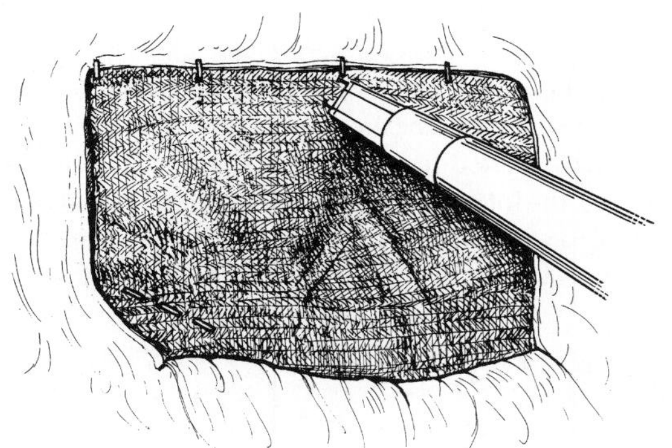

Fig. 10.2 The 15 cm × 10 cm mesh is being stapled into place. Note the three medial staples anchoring the mesh to Cooper's ligament and the pubic bone. Staples are also placed along the superior border of the mesh but nowhere else.

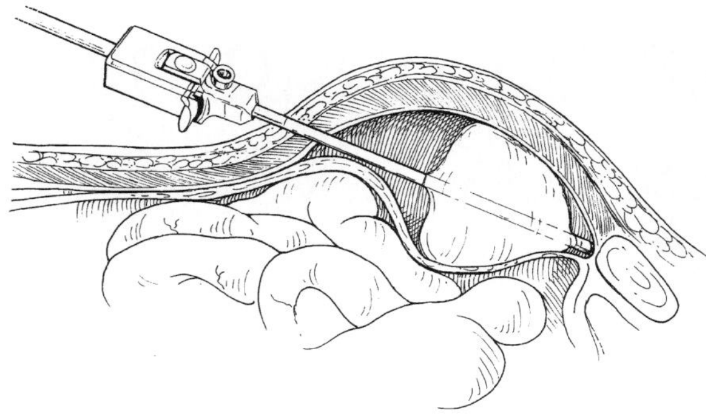

Fig. 10.3 A diagrammatic view of the initial dissection of the preperitoneal space.

posteriorly and the rectus muscle anteriorly. The lower edge of the posterior rectus sheath can be seen (arcuate line). Inflate the balloon under direct vision and resist the urge to pump the balloon up quickly as this will reduce the likelihood of bleeding. Ensure that the balloon inflates completely. Approximately 20 pumps will be required.

LAPAROSCOPIC INCISIONAL, UMBILICAL AND SPIGELIAN HERNIA REPAIR USING INTRAPERITONEAL ONLAY MESH

After obtaining access it is possible to repair incisional hernias although dense adhesions may make access difficult or impossible. Umbilical repair is possible as is herniation along the semilunar line, described by the Belgian anatomist Adrian van der Spieghel (1578–1625).

11

Appendix and abdominal abscess

R. C. N. Williamson, D. E. Whitelaw

CONTENTS

APPENDICECTOMY

The diagnosis of acute appendicitis is essentially clinical, based on a detailed history and careful examination rather than radiological investigations except to rule out alternative diagnoses. Appendicectomy is still the most common reason for laparotomy but remember that young children and the elderly may have atypical presentations of appendicitis and also have a higher mortality and morbidity from this condition. Females may have gynaecological rather than appendicular causes for pain and tenderness in the right iliac fossa, so order a pelvic ultrasound scan and consider carrying out a diagnostic laparoscopy in such cases, proceeding to laparoscopic appendicectomy if necessary (Ch. 12). Although elderly patients do develop appendicitis, also consider perforating carcinoma of the caecum and diverticulitis, so be prepared to use a midline incision to permit a full abdominal examination or in frail patients consider spiral computed tomography (CT).

Tend to treat conservatively a patient with symptoms for 5 or more days in whom you find a mass in the right iliac fossa. Give a 7-day course of intravenous antibiotics such as cefuroxime and metronidazole, withhold oral feeding and replace fluid intravenously. Perform an ultrasound scan to exclude the presence of a large abscess that can be drained percutaneously. Carefully monitor the patient and perform an operation only if the mass, judged by its initially marked margins, increases in size, or bowel obstruction, peritonitis, worsening toxaemia, or septic shock develop. When the mass has settled, consider barium enema X-ray or colonoscopy to exclude caecal carcinoma in those aged over 40 years. It was conventional practice to perform 'interval' appendicectomy 1–2 months later but the risk is small if operation is deferred indefinitely after fully informing the patients to seek advice if symptoms recur.

Avoid removing a normal appendix incidentally during other operations, such as cholecystectomy. It is a possible cause of complications such as wound infection and subsequent adhesive intestinal obstruction.

Prepare

1. Wound infection is the most common complication following operation for acute appendicitis, so routinely insert a 1-g metronidazole rectal suppository as soon as the decision is made to operate or give 500 mg of metronidazole intravenously at induction of anaesthesia.
2. In patients with clinically severe acute appendicitis who are elderly, have cardiac disease, an implant such as a hip joint replacement, or diabetes, also give cefuroxime prophylactically (1.5 g intravenously).
3. Patients who have a perforated appendix require a full 5-day course of cefuroxime and metronidazole.

KEY POINT Re-examine the abdomen when the patient is anaesthetized

- Intend to re-examine the abdomen when the patient is anaesthetized. You may feel a mass in the relaxed abdomen that was impalpable beforehand. Indeed, it is a valuable general rule before any abdominal operation, and may help you determine the best site for the incision.

Access

1 As a routine employ a Lanz incision in a skin crease. This modification of the gridiron incision transversely crosses McBurney's point – the junction of the middle and outer thirds of a line joining the anterior superior iliac spine and the umbilicus. The incision starts 2 cm below and medial to the right anterior, superior iliac spine and extends medially for 5–7 cm. It may be possible to site it lower in a young girl so that the scar lies below the waistline of a bikini swimming costume.

2 Use the traditional gridiron incision, 5–8 cm long, in line with the external oblique fibres if you anticipate the need to extend the exposure (Fig. 11.1). The incision crosses McBurney's point at right angles to the spino-umbilical line, one-third above, two-thirds below. If necessary, the external oblique muscle and aponeurosis can be split in either direction and the internal oblique and transversus muscles can be cut to convert the incision into a right-sided Rutherford Morison incision (see Ch. 7).

3 If appendicitis is but one of a number of likely diagnoses, prefer a lower midline incision.

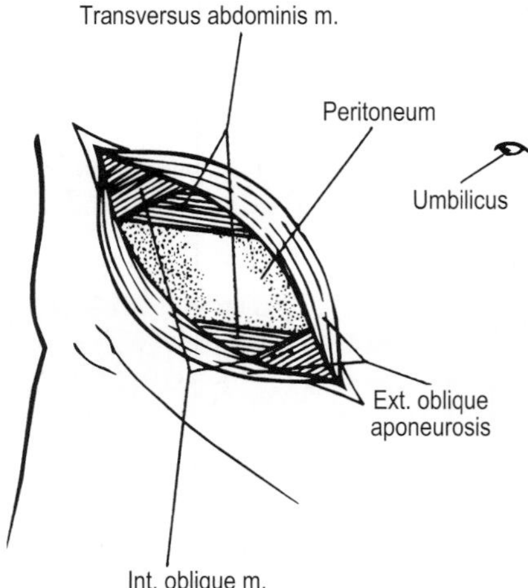

Fig. 11.1 Gridiron incision for appendicectomy. In the Lanz modification the skin incision is transverse but the abdominal muscles are similarly split in the line of their fibres.

Opening the abdomen

1 Incise the skin cleanly with the belly of the knife. Divide the subcutaneous fat, Scarpa's fascia and subjacent areolar tissue to expose the glistening fibres of the external oblique aponeurosis. In the gridiron approach these fibres run parallel to the skin incision.

2 Stop the bleeding. Incise the external oblique aponeurosis in the line of its fibres. Start with a scalpel, then use the partly closed blades of Mayo's scissors (Fig. 11.2) while your assistant retracts the skin edges.

3 Retract the external oblique aponeurosis to display the fibres of internal oblique muscle, which run at right angles. Split internal oblique and transversus abdominis muscles, using Mayo's straight scissors (Fig. 11.3).

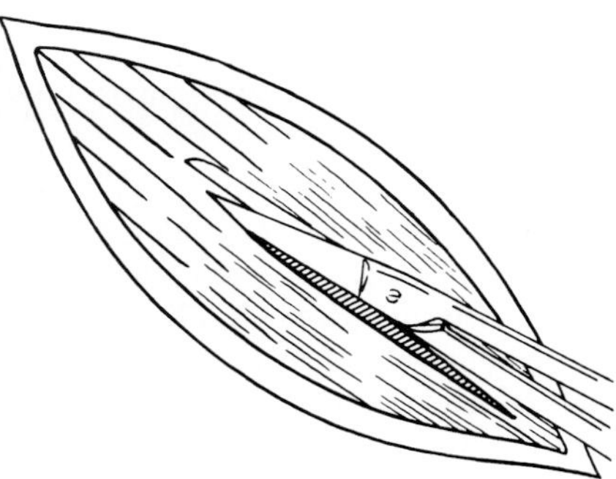

Fig. 11.2 Appendicectomy. Regardless of which skin incision is used, the external oblique aponeurosis is split by pushing partly closed scissors in the line of the fibres.

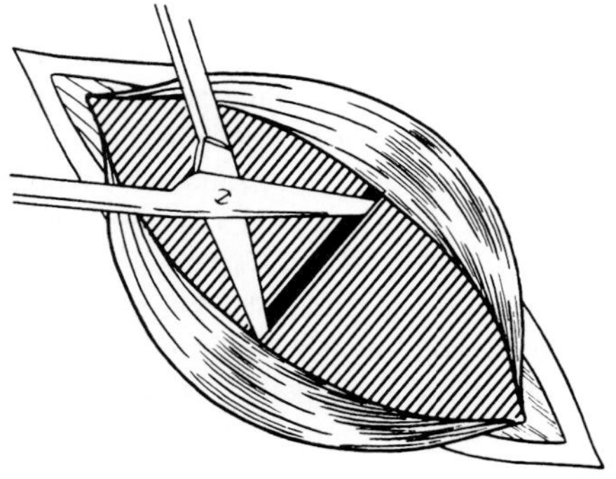

Fig. 11.3 Appendicectomy. The internal oblique muscle is split by opening Mayo's straight scissors in the line of the fibres.

Open the blades in the line of the fibres and use both index fingers to widen the split. Provided the scissors are not thrust in violently, the transversalis fascia and peritoneum are pushed away unopened.

4 Stop the bleeding. Have the muscles retracted firmly to display the fused transversalis fascia and peritoneum.

5 Pick up a fold of peritoneum with toothed dissecting forceps and grasp the tented portion with artery forceps. Release the dissecting forceps and take a fresh grasp to ensure that only the peritoneum is held. Make a small incision through the peritoneum with a knife. Allow air to enter the peritoneal cavity, so that viscera fall away. Use scissors to enlarge the hole in the line of the skin incision. Now protect the wound edges with swabs or skin towels.

Assess

1 Look. Is there any free fluid or pus? If so, take a specimen for microscopy and culture for organisms.

2 Find the caecum, identify a taenia and follow it distally to the base of the appendix. Insert a finger and lift out the appendix by pushing from within, not by pulling from without.

KEY POINT Manipulate the inflamed appendix with care

- **Never pull on the appendix if the distal end is stuck. If it is gangrenous it will tear and release infected material into the peritoneal cavity. Always improve your view, if necessary by extending the incision.**

3 If the appendix is not evident, push your index finger posteriorly until it comes to lie on the peritoneum over the psoas muscle. Then, maintaining contact with the posterior peritoneum, draw your finger to the right until it can go no further. The caecum should now lie between the 'hook' of your finger and the right limit of the iliac fossa, and may be gently pushed out onto the surface. In some cases you may need to mobilize the caecum by incising the parietal peritoneum in the paracolic gutter, in order to raise the caecum on its mesentery, especially if the appendix is adherently retrocaecal. If the caecum is not evident, remember that it sometimes lies quite high, under the right lobe of the liver.

? DIFFICULTY

There is no appendix? In a small number of patients there is no appendix, either because it did not develop or because it has been digested or has atrophied as a result of previous inflammatory disease. In this case, what is the cause of the patient's clinical features? Carry out a search for disease of nearby organs (see below).

4 Confirm the diagnosis: the appendix, or more usually its tip, is swollen, congested, inflamed, even gangrenous, often with fibrin deposition, turbid fluid or frank pus.

? DIFFICULTY

1. If the appendix is not inflamed? Examine its tip to exclude carcinoid tumour, which is usually a yellowish swelling at the tip, since appendicectomy may well be curative. Adenocarcinoma of the appendix demands right hemicolectomy.
2. Examine the caecum, since an ulcer, inflammation or cancer may present as appendicitis. Pass the distal 1.5 m of the ileum and its mesentery through your fingers to exclude mesenteric adenitis, Crohn's disease or Meckel's diverticulum. Palpate the posterior abdominal wall, ascending colon, liver edge and gallbladder fundus and the lower pole of the right kidney. Now feel below into the right rim of the pelvis, the bladder fundus, right iliac vessels and right inguinal region. In females examine the right ovary and fallopian tube, and attempt to feel the uterus and left ovary and tube.
3. Look for features of a distant cause such as bile-stained fluid tracking down from a perforated peptic ulcer, an inflamed gallbladder or a gynaecological cause. Be prepared to close a standard Lanz incision and make a fresh, well-placed incision, rather

than struggle to deal with the problem by extending or stretching the incision in the right iliac fossa. The presence of free purulent fluid is an indication to embark on wider examination of the abdominal contents.

Action

1 Mobilize the appendix from base to tip by gently moving or peeling away adherent structures. Remember that the artery enters from the medial aspect. If the tip is adherent, improve the view. Do not dissect blindly. If necessary, extend the incision. Apply Babcock's tissue forceps to enclose, but not grasp, an uninflamed portion of the appendix, to hold it so you can view the mesentery against the light and identify the artery.

2 Pass one blade of the artery forceps through the mesoappendix and clamp the vessels (Fig. 11.4). If it is thickened, take the mesoappendix in two bites. Divide the mesoappendix distal to the clamp and ligate the vessel gently but firmly with 2/0 polyglactin 910 or similar material, ignoring the slight backbleeding from the distal cut end.

3 Crush the base of the appendix with a haemostat then replace the clamp 0.5 cm distal to the crushed segment. Ligate the crushed segment with 0 polyglactin 910. Apply a haemostat to the ligature ends after trimming them.

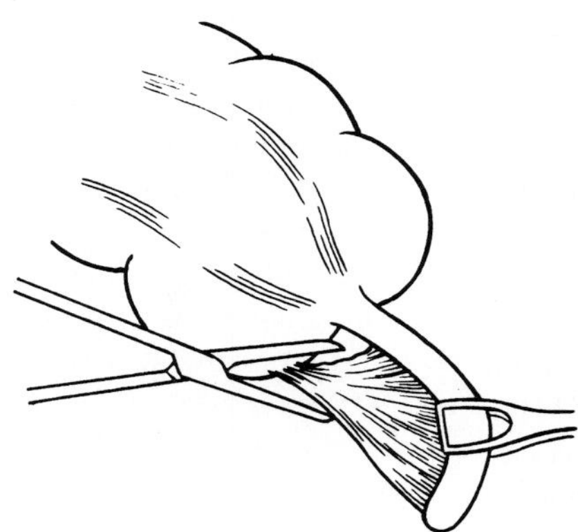

Fig. 11.4 Appendicectomy. Clamping the mesoappendix. The appendix is held up with tissue forceps.

4 Cut off the appendix just distal to the haemostat.

KEY POINT Sterility

- Stop! You have entered the bowel. Place the appendix, held by the Babcock's forceps, together with the knife, into a kidney dish for contaminated articles.

5 Insert a seromuscular purse-string suture of 2/0 polyglactin 910 or similar material, mounted on a round-bodied needle, in the caecum encircling the base of the appendix, at a distance of 10–15 mm from the base. Use the haemostat on the appendix stump ligature to push it in while tying the first half-hitch of the purse-string suture (Fig. 11.5). Gently remove the haemostat before tightening the first half-hitch and then completing the reef knot.

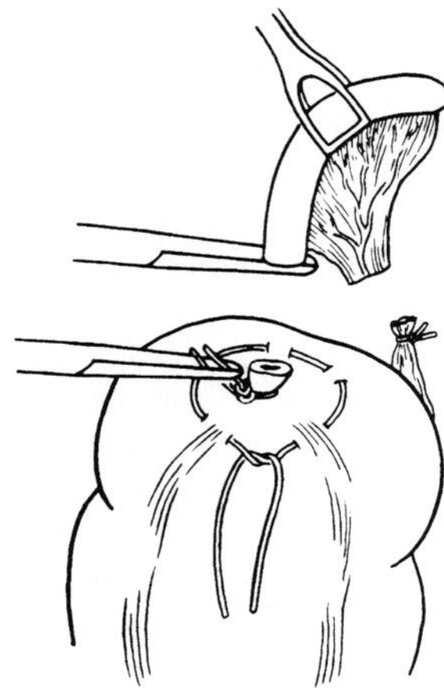

Fig. 11.5 Appendicectomy. The resected appendix, together with the haemostat at its base and the tissue forceps, is placed in a separate dish. The ligated stump of the appendix is invaginated while tying the purse-string suture.

? **DIFFICULTY**

1. If you cannot carry out the steps of the operation safely you must improve the exposure by extending the wound in the line of the skin incision laterally. Extension of the wound medially may encroach on the inferior epigastric vessels but once you enter the rectus sheath you can retract the rectus muscle medially.
2. If you cannot free the tip of the appendix, it is sometimes helpful to carry out retrograde appendicectomy. Crush, clamp and ligate the base of the appendix before dividing it. Now the base is free you will be better able to follow it to the tip.
3. If the appendix bursts in spite of gentle manipulations, remove it and look to see if a faecalith has escaped. Wash out any freed material using saline lavage and suction. If there has been any contamination, consider inserting a drain into the superficial tissues, since the peritoneal cavity usually copes well with contamination provided the cause is removed.
4. If the base of the appendix is oedematous and fragile, do not attempt to crush it. If possible, carefully ligate it and cut it off 5 mm distally. If it appears unsafe to insert a purse-string, look for a piece of omentum or other peritoneum to draw over the stump and stitch it to a healthy piece of caecal wall.
5. If gangrene extends on to the caecal wall, first apply a non-crushing clamp gently across the bowel to limit contamination. Resect the gangrenous part to reveal healthy wall that can be closed with a suture line. If the hole cannot be closed, insert a large tube drain into the caecum and suture the edges of the bowel to the skin as a caecostomy. The stoma will close spontaneously in most cases, when the tube is removed after a few days.
6. If there is Crohn's disease and the appendix is not inflamed, do not carry out any procedure.
7. If you find an abscess, drain it but do not explore further or pursue a search for a buried appendix within the cavity. It will most probably be destroyed by the inflammatory reaction.
8. In the presence of purulent peritonitis, carry out appendicectomy. Now gently remove pus and debris and drain the wound. Consider copious saline lavage to cleanse the abdomen (see Ch. 7).

Closure

1 Pick up the edges of the peritoneum around the entire incision with fine haemostats to allow easy and safe suturing of the opening with continuous 2/0 polyglactin 910 or similar material.

2 Insert loose interrupted stitches of the same material in the muscle with a continuous stitch to the external oblique aponeurosis to appose but not constrict the tissues.

3 Apply povidone-iodine solution to the wound once the peritoneum is closed.

4 Appose the subcuticular tissues with fine sutures in an obese patient and close the skin with a continuous subcuticular suture or clips.

Postoperative

1 In the absence of general peritonitis, start oral fluids and a light diet when the patient is fully awake, as tolerated.

2 If the appendix was perforated, and particularly in a high-risk patient, continue metronidazole suppositories for 5 days and add intravenous cefuroxime 750 mg, 8-hourly.

3 Remove any drain after 2–3 days unless there is still profuse discharge.

4 Monitor the wound if pyrexia develops, and exclude chest and urinary infection.

> **KEY POINT Explain to the patient what was done**
>
> - If you decided not to remove the appendix, ensure that you explain this to the patient. A future clinician, seeing a scar in the right iliac fossa, may wrongly assume that the appendix has been removed and attribute clinical features to other organs.

Complications

Wound infection develops occasionally in patients with mild appendicitis but has a higher incidence in those who have had a gangrenous or perforated appendix removed. Anaerobic *Bacteroides* and aerobic coliform organisms are usually responsible. Examine the wound regularly and remove some of the skin suture or clips if there is evidence of infection, to allow any pus to drain.

If pyrexia develops, always carry out a rectal examination. Pelvic infection produces localized heat, 'bogginess' and tenderness. Repeat the examination at intervals to detect if an abscess develops and 'points'. Ultrasound or radiological imaging may help if you are uncertain. Finger pressure may release pus but, if not, be willing to aspirate it using a needle inserted through the vagina or rectum. If needle aspiration confirms the presence of an abscess, gently thrust closed, long-handled forceps into the cavity to drain it into the rectum.

Reactive haemorrhage is infrequent, but occasionally the ligature falls off the appendicular artery. Return the patient to the operating theatre and reopen the wound to catch and re-ligate the artery.

Faecal fistula develops in two circumstances. Either the patient has unsuspected Crohn's disease or in florid appendicitis the appendicular stump or adjacent caecum has undergone necrosis. In the presence of necrosis do not over-optimistically rely on suturing the defect. Prefer to insert a large tube in the hole and suture the margins of the hole to the anterior abdominal wall where the tube emerges. The tube can be removed after a week and the fistula usually heals spontaneously.

APPENDIX MASS

This is usually a late presentation of acute appendicitis. It may result from the adherence of omentum and other viscera to the inflamed appendix. More usually the appendix has ruptured and an abscess has formed, its walls comprising the fibrin-lined omentum and adherent viscera.

Antibiotics are commonly given even when there are no clinical features of sepsis and the white cell count is not raised. Provided the patient is well, with no features of sepsis, toxicity or peritonitis, expectant treatment without operation is the preferred management. Mark out the margins of the mass and regularly monitor progress. Provided the marked margins of the mass do not extend and features of toxaemia or peritonitis do not develop, wait for the mass to resolve.

Ultrasound scanning or computed tomography (CT) are valuable to confirm the diagnosis and determine whether an abscess is present, which can then be drained percutaneously. If it extends into the pelvis it may be amenable to drainage transrectally under ultrasound guidance. Perform open drainage only if worsening toxaemia or peritonitis develops, or if percutaneous drainage is not feasible or fails.

The subsequent management of patients with a resolved abscess remains controversial. Conventionally, the patient is readmitted for interval appendicectomy after 1–2 months. However, at such operations one frequently finds no evidence of the appendix and, if no interval appendicectomy is undertaken, it is only rarely that recurrent appendicitis develops.

Access

1 Define the mass when the patient is relaxed under anaesthesia.

2 Employ a standard Lanz incision. You may encounter oedema as you reach the deeper layers of the abdominal wall.

3 Alternatively you may enter the abdomen and find the mass on the posterior wall.

Action

1 If you find on entering the abdomen that you are within the abscess cavity, do not rush to explore the wound. Take a specimen of the contents of the cavity for bacterial culture and to determine the antibiotic sensitivity of the contained organisms. Gently and thoroughly aspirate all pus and debris. Explore the cavity with your finger to decide whether it is safe to enlarge the opening

without damaging viscera or disrupting the cavity wall.

2 If you gain an improved view you may see the appendix and be able to remove it safely. Sometimes the terminal part has separated and you will need to remove it piecemeal.

KEY POINT The appendix looks normal

- Do not misinterpret the presence of a short, apparently normal appendix. This is the stump left after the distal part has dropped off after a perforation and is lying in the abscess cavity. Look carefully for it and for a causative faecalith and remove both.

3 Sweep your finger round the cavity to identify any loose contents and remove them. Thoroughly aspirate any pus.

4 If you cannot find the appendix or if it is unsafe to open up the abscess cavity, insert a drain, closing the wound layers loosely around it.

5 If, when you open the abdomen, you enter the peritoneal cavity and find a mass lying on the posterior wall, pack it off from the remainder of the abdomen and gently explore it to determine if there is a plane of cleavage into the interior. Remember, inflamed tissues are friable; respond to the findings and be willing to stop if you encounter difficulty.

6 The mass or abscess may lie retrocaecally, retroileally, or within the pelvis. Be prepared to pack off the rest of the abdomen and mobilize the caecum by incising the peritoneum in the paracaecal gutter, so you can gently lift it off the mass. Now explore the mass to decide whether to enter it or leave it.

7 Whether you open the mass or leave it, insert a drain into the peritoneal cavity to provide a track for any pus.

SUBPHRENIC AND SUBHEPATIC ABSCESS

An abscess may form following major surgical procedures, operations performed in the presence of infection, or sometimes spontaneously following perforation of a viscus. It could result from a retained foreign body, necrotic tissue, inadequate drainage of blood or contaminated fluid, or an anastomotic leak. The abscess may develop above the liver (subphrenic), below the liver (subhepatic), along either paracolic gutter, between loops of bowel in the mid-abdomen, or in the true pelvis.

Reserve the term 'subphrenic' for an abscess lying immediately below the diaphragm. On the right it lies above the right lobe of the liver, on the left it lies above the left lobe of liver, gastric fundus and spleen (Fig. 11.6). Right subhepatic collections may be anterior (paraduodenal) or posterior (suprarenal). Left subhepatic collections may lie anterior to the stomach and transverse colon, or posteriorly in the lesser sac.

Suspect the diagnosis if the patient develops rigors, swinging pyrexia, toxicity and leucocytosis. In the presence of a subphrenic abscess the hemidiaphragm may be elevated, as demonstrated on a chest X-ray, and a 'sympathetic' pleural effusion often collects above the diaphragm. You may see a fluid level with gas above if leakage from a viscus or anastomosis has developed, or in the presence of gas-forming organisms. Aspirate a specimen of pus for culture and determination of antibiotic sensitivity. CT or ultrasound scans are valuable means of confirming an abscess, and a radiolabelled white blood cell scan may reveal an occult abscess that is not detectable by other imaging methods.

Once an abscess is identified and localized by clinical signs or imaging methods, insert a percutaneous needle to confirm the presence of pus. Send aspirated material for culture and to be tested for antibiotic sensitivity. The

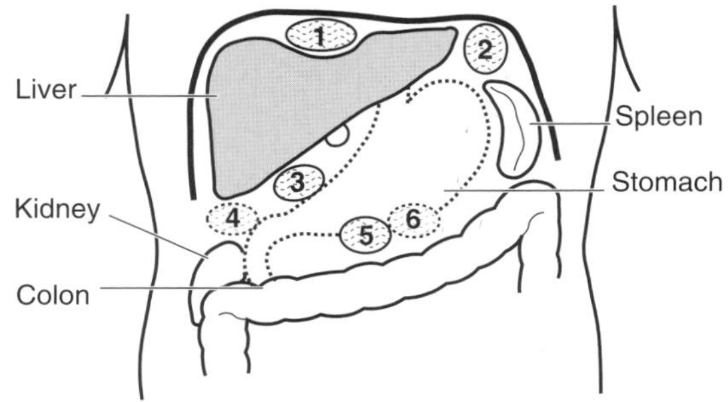

Fig. 11.6 Common sites of abscess above and below the liver: 1, right subphrenic; 2, left subphrenic; 3, right anterior subhepatic; 4, right posterior subhepatic (hepatorenal); 5, left anterior subhepatic; 6, left posterior subhepatic (lesser sac).

modern, first-line method of dealing with such an abscess should be percutaneous drainage. This is usually effective even for recurrent abscesses. A needle is inserted under ultrasound or CT guidance to avoid damaging adjacent structures. A flexible guidewire is then passed through the needle, which is withdrawn. A bevel-tipped catheter is passed over the guidewire into the cavity and the guidewire is withdrawn. This is the Seldinger technique. This technique may not be successful in obtaining drainage of multiloculated abscesses but these may be successfully drained laparoscopically.

Open operation is now rarely necessary for large, loculated or recurrent abscesses and those containing necrotic or inspissated material. The choice of approach depends on the site of the abscess. Ideally, an extrapleural, extraperitoneal approach avoids the possibility of contaminating the peritoneal or pleural cavities. As a rule this is possible only for posterior collections, although a right anterior subphrenic abscess can sometimes be approached extraperitoneally. Multiple or loculated abscess cavities usually demand a transperitoneal approach. Start antibiotic cover against the likely organisms before embarking on operation. Take advice from a clinical microbiologist, especially if you have managed to send a specimen of pus for study.

Posterior approach is through the periosteal bed of the excised 12th rib. Divide the origin of the diaphragm and displace the kidney forwards. Feel for the lower edge of the liver and explore below it, using a needle and aspirating syringe to seek out pus. To drain a subphrenic abscess, separate the peritoneum from the undersurface of the diaphragm. When you find it, open the cavity, suck out the pus and debris. Explore it with your finger to avoid leaving necrotic or inspissated material. Now insert a drain.

Anterolateral approach is through a lateral incision 1 cm below the costal margin and cut through all layers down to, but not including, the peritoneum. Strip the peritoneum from under the diaphragm until you reach the abscess. Open it, and drain it. If you cannot find pus, carefully explore with a needle and finger through the peritoneum and be prepared to enter the peritoneal cavity.

Transperitoneal approach: site the incision according to the site of the abscess derived from the preoperative ultrasound or CT scan. If you are unsure of the site or cause, be prepared to perform exploration of the abdomen (see Ch. 7) prior to opening the abscess, to avoid general contamination. Explore the right and left subphrenic and subhepatic spaces, and enter the lesser sac through an avascular part of the hepatogastric omentum. On encountering an abscess, pack off the area and open the abscess, suck out the contents and drain the cavity through a separate stab wound in the abdominal wall.

FURTHER READING

Cooper MJ 1990 Manifestations of appendicitis. In: Williamson RCN, Cooper MJ (eds) Emergency abdominal surgery. Churchill Livingstone, Edinburgh, pp 221–232

Jones PF 2001 Suspected acute appendicitis: trends in management over 30 years. British Journal of Surgery 88:1570–1577

Kirk RM 2002 Basic surgical techniques, 5th edn. Churchill Livingstone, Edinburgh, pp 161–173

Silen W 2000 Cope's early diagnosis of the acute abdomen. Oxford University Press, Oxford

12

Laparoscopic appendicectomy

S. J. Nixon, A. Rajasekar

DESCRIPTION OF OPERATION

Appendicectomy for appendicitis is the most common emergency abdominal operation. A detailed examination of the abdomen and pelvis is not possible. Postoperative morbidity includes wound infection, incisional hernia, deep infection, prolonged ileus, adhesive obstruction, infertility in females and subsequent right inguinal hernia. Laparoscopic appendicectomy requires general anaesthesia with endotracheal intubation and muscle relaxation.

Laparoscopic appendicectomy is increasingly used. Advantages claimed are decreased wound infection, reduced postoperative pain and accelerated recovery. Laparoscopy allows detailed pelvic and abdominal examination, particularly valuable in young women where preoperative diagnostic accuracy is low. Increased technical difficulty, longer operating times, increased risk of deep infection and increased cost offset these potential advantages. Routine use of laparoscopic appendicectomy is debatable on evidence from the surgical literature and depends on your experience. However, it may offer particular advantages in women of childbearing age and in obese individuals. The conversion rate and morbidity reported in the literature vary from 0% to 15% and 0% to 18%, respectively. There are no absolute contraindications, and relative contraindications are the same as for other laparoscopic procedures.

KEY POINTS Clinical diagnosis

- In patients with equivocal symptoms and signs, repeated clinical examination is the mainstay of diagnosis.
- Minimize negative laparotomy or laparoscopy rates.

Prepare

1. Obtain informed consent for both laparoscopic and open appendicectomy. Administer metronidazole as a 1-g rectal suppository 1 hour before the operation or give parenteral metronidazole and broad-spectrum antibiotics during anaesthetic induction.
2. Place the patient supine. In females, the lithotomy position allows peroperative vaginal examination. You and your assistant stand on the patient's left side with the nurse on the right and a monitor at the foot of the table. Catheterize the urinary bladder to reduce risk of injury if there is doubt regarding the recent micturition.

KEY POINTS Examine the abdomen again

- Re-examine the abdomen when the patient is anaesthetized.
- The presence of a mass suggests likely technical difficulty but does not contraindicate trial laparoscopy.

Access

Induce pneumoperitoneum (see Ch. 8), preferably using an open technique. Introduce a 10-mm port at the umbilicus. Insert a 10-mm telescope, inspect the peritoneal cavity and confirm the diagnosis. If you cannot visualize the structures in the right iliac fossa and pelvis, improve access by rotating the patient to the left side with some head-down tilt. Introduce two 5-mm ports, one in the right flank at a distance from the appendix itself and one in the lower midline above the pubic symphysis, avoiding the bladder.

Assess

Examine all other pelvic and abdominal organs to exclude ovarian cyst, ectopic pregnancy, pelvic inflammatory disease, cholecystitis, perforated peptic ulcer, Meckel's diverticulum, colonic diverticulitis, Crohn's disease and ischaemic bowel. Your ability to examine abdominal contents is much greater using laparoscopy than by open surgery through a small incision. Identify the appendix which, in early appendicitis, may appear normal if mucosal inflammation has not yet extended to the peritoneum. Plan to remove an apparently 'normal' appendix if you can find no cause for the patient's pain.

Action

1 Your intention is to separate the appendix from its mesentery using diathermy dissection, ideally bipolar if you have it available, starting at the tip and working towards the base where the appendix expands into the caecum, identified by the taenia coli. Do not remove the appendix mesentery. If this is a late presentation with advanced inflammation and oedema you may need to divide the appendix base and mesentery en masse, using a vascular stapler such as the EndoGIA II (Autosuture). Do not invaginate or diathermize the appendix stump.

2 Identify the appendix. Elevate its tip using the left-hand grasper and mobilize it, if necessary also mobilizing the caecum. Introduce a Vicryl Endoloop (Ethicon) through the lateral port and place it around the base of the appendix. Place two ties close to the caecum and the third tie approximately 1 cm distal to the first two. Transect the appendix, leaving two ties on the caecum. If the appendix base is friable and oedematous, divide it using a stapler, including some caecal wall if necessary.

3 Remove the appendix through the 10-mm umbilical port; to prevent contamination, use a retrieval bag if necessary.

Postoperative

In the absence of general peritonitis allow oral fluids on the first postoperative day. Mobilize the patient on the day of operation and usually discharge on the first postoperative day, continuing metronidazole and a parenteral antibiotic for 3–4 days if there was serious sepsis or contamination, especially in poor-risk patients. If pyrexia develops, check the wounds and exclude chest and urinary infection.

FURTHER READING

O'Reilly MJ, Reddick EJ, Miller WD et al 1993 Laparoscopic appendectomy. In: Zucker KA (ed.) Surgical laparoscopy. Update, St Louis, pp 301–326

Richardson WS, Hunter JG 1997 Complications in appendectomy. In: Ponsky JL (ed.) Complications of endoscopic and laparoscopic surgery. Prevention and management. Lippincott-Raven, Philadelphia, pp 171–176

Internet website

http://www.edu.rcsed.ac.uk/video_album_menu.htm

13

Oesophagus

R. Mason

CONTENTS

ENDOSCOPY

Endoscope every patient with dysphagia except when this is fully explained by the presence of neurological or neuromuscular disease. Endoscope patients with suspected disease in the oesophagus producing pain on swallowing (odynophagia), heartburn not responding to simple medication or arising de novo in patients over 50 years, bleeding, or if accidental and iatrogenic damage are suspected.

Prepare

Ensure that the endoscope, the ancillary equipment and necessary spares are available, function correctly and are appropriately sterile. The endoscope must be thoroughly prepared between procedures. Modern fibreoptic gastrointestinal endoscopes are slim, versatile, have remarkably flexible tips and can be passed with pharyngeal anaesthesia alone in most patients, allowing you to examine the oesophagus, stomach and duodenum. Use the end-viewing instrument routinely; through it can be passed biopsy forceps, cytology brushes, snares, guidewires for dilators and needles for injection. Argon plasma coagulation or Nd-YAG laser may be applied through it for the palliation of inoperable neoplasms or treatment of Barrett's oesophagus.

Obtain signed informed consent from the patient, remove dentures from the patient and, except in an emergency, have the patient starved of food and fluids for at least 5 hours.

Obtain a preliminary barium swallow X-ray if you suspect a pharyngeal pouch. If you sedate the patient attach a pulse oximeter probe to a finger. Spray the pharynx with lidocaine solution just before passing the endoscope which has been lubricated with water-soluble jelly. In anxious patients, or those in whom intervention (e.g. dilatation) is required, insert a small plastic cannula into a peripheral vein and through it inject slowly 1–2 mg of midazolam until the patient's eyelids just begin to droop. Remember that it takes 2 minutes for the full effect of midazolam to develop.

FIBREOPTIC ENDOSCOPY

Lay the patient on the left side with hips and knees flexed. Place a plastic hollow gag between the teeth. Ensure that the patient's head is in the midline and that the chin is lowered on to the chest. Pass the endoscope tip through the plastic gag, over the tongue to the posterior pharyngeal wall. Depress the tip control slightly so that the instrument tip passes down towards the cricopharyngeal sphincter. Do not overflex the tip or it will be directed anteriorly and enter the larynx. Visualize the larynx and pass the endoscope just behind it.

Ask the patient to swallow. Do not resist the slight extrusion of the endoscope as the larynx rises but maintain gentle pressure so that it will advance as the larynx descends and the cricopharyngeal sphincter relaxes. Advance the endoscope under vision, insufflating air gently to open up the passage. Aspirate any fluid. Spray water across the lens if it becomes obscured. If there is no hold-up, pass the tip through the stomach into the duodenum then withdraw it slowly, noting the features. Remove biopsy specimens and take cytology brushings from any ulcers, tumours or other lesions.

If you encounter a stricture note its distance from the incisor teeth. If the instrument passes through, determine the length of the stricture. Always remove biopsy specimens and cytology brushings from within the stricture. If the stricture appears benign, gently dilate it to 12 mm if the patient is symptomatic. Dilatation of malignant strictures is not indicated as any benefit is short-lasting and the risk of perforation is high (6–8%). Get biopsies and confirm the diagnosis prior to intervention. If nutritional support is required, you can pass a feeding nasogastric tube under fluoroscopic control.

Oesophagitis is usually from gastro-oesophageal reflux, but is not necessarily associated with hiatal hernia. Confirm the diagnosis by taking mucosal scrapings. Sliding hiatal hernia produces a loculus of stomach above the constriction of the crura with a raised gastro-oesophageal mucosal junction. To determine the level of the hiatus, ask the patient to sniff, and note the level at which the crura momentarily narrow the lumen. A rolling hernia is visible only from within the stomach by inverting the endoscope tip. Frank ulceration is unusual except from severe reflux. In Barrett's oesophagus the lower gullet is lined with modified gastric mucosa and ulceration may develop in the columnar-lined segment; take 4-quadrant biopsies of the columnar segment at 2-cm intervals. In patients with dysplasia use 'jumbo' forceps to take biopsies. In most Western countries most cancers are adenocarcinomas, associated with Barrett's oesophagus. Take multiple biopsies and cytological brushings. Strictures develop from peptic oesophagitis, rarely from Barrett's oesophagus and cancer. Achalasia (failure to relax) of the cardia, Schatzki's ring, Zenker's diverticulum (pharyngeal pouch), caustic strictures, webs or strictures are also seen, as are mega-oesophagus in South American Chagas' disease, and pulsion diverticula. Learn the differing appearances by practice, from atlases and from a CD-ROM.

Fragile strictures do not always require endoscopic dilatation. The safest oesophageal dilator is soft, solid food, provided that each bolus contains only aggregated small particles. Dilatation with fixed maximum diameter balloons (Fig. 13.1) may require only a single session, but do not persist unduly in the face of difficulty or discomfort. It is not necessary to intubate all strictures that cannot be resected. Intubation produces a rigid channel through which food must fall by gravity; expanding metal stents (Fig. 13.2) may be inserted at endoscopy, by radiological screening or by a combination of both methods.

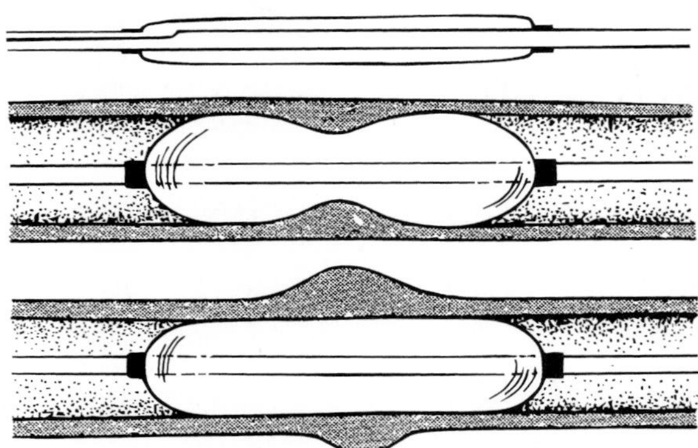

Fig. 13.1 Balloon dilatation. At the top is a balloon collapsed on its introductory catheter. There is a radio-opaque marker at each end of the balloon. In the middle drawing, the balloon is partly inflated within a stricture that has produced a waist. At the bottom, the waist has disappeared as the balloon is fully inflated.

Swallowed articles impact at the sites of narrowing. Smooth objects usually pass into the stomach. Most foreign bodies may be removed using a variety of methods in conjunction with fibreoptic endoscopes and an overtube under local anaesthesia with sedation.

Oesophageal varices develop in portal venous hypertension (see Ch. 25).They thrombose when injected with ethanolamine oleate; alternatively constricting bands can be applied with a special device.

OESOPHAGEAL EXPOSURE

NECK (Fig. 13.3)

The cervical oesophagus may be approached from either side. Operations for the removal of pharyngeal pouch, cricopharyngeal myotomy, are usually carried out from the left side. For oesophageal anastomosis following resection either side can be used. The right-sided approach minimizes risk of damage to the thoracic duct, although this is a rare complication for exposure of the oesophagus and usually occurs as a complication of biopsy of lymph nodes. Mobilize the posterior wall of the oesophagus with blunt dissection. Staying on the muscle wall of the oesophagus come anteriorly and over the front, separating the trachea and recurrent laryngeal nerve anteriorly.

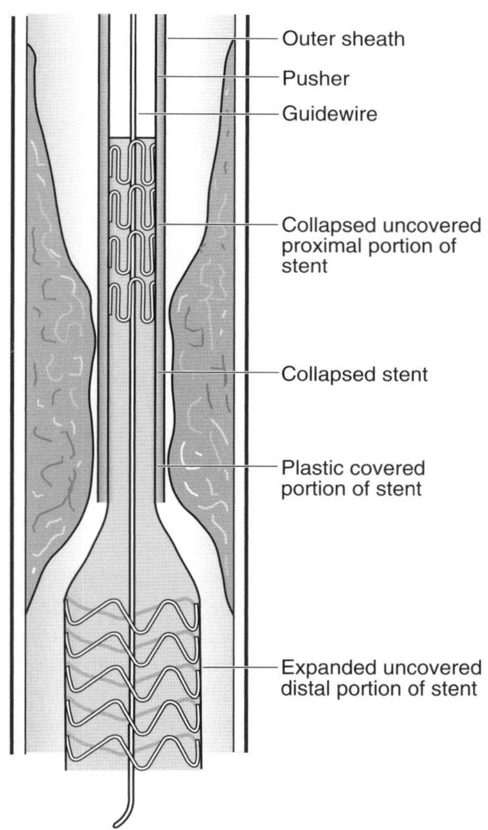

Fig. 13.2 Wall stent: self-expanding metal stent being deployed under fluoroscopic control.

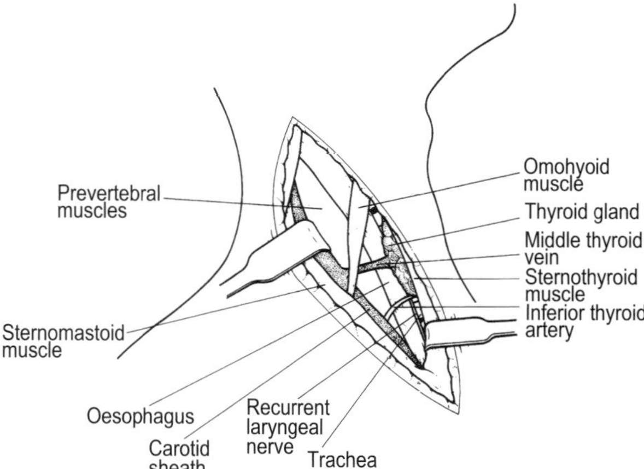

Fig. 13.3 Exposure of the cervical oesophagus on the right side. Sternomastoid muscle and the carotid sheath are drawn laterally. The space between these structures and the midline column of the pharynx and oesophagus, larynx, trachea and thyroid gland is crossed by the omohyoid muscle, middle thyroid vein and the inferior thyroid artery.

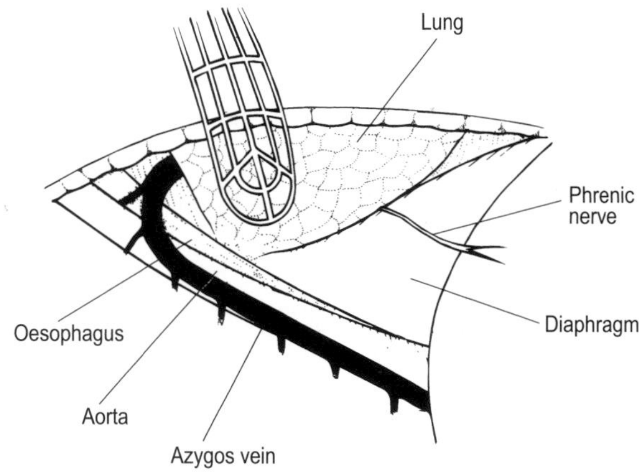

Fig. 13.4 Diagram of approach to the oesophagus through the right pleural space. The right lung is retracted anteriorly.

RIGHT POSTEROLATERAL THORACOTOMY (Fig. 13.4)

The patient lies on the left side. Carry out right posterolateral thoracotomy at the level of the fifth or sixth rib (see Ch. 36). Draw down the collapsed right lung to reveal the mediastinal pleura and the azygos vein arching over the lung root. Incise the mediastinal pleura, mobilize, doubly ligate and divide the azygos vein to reveal the oesophagus running posterior to the trachea and lung root.

LEFT THORACOTOMY (Fig. 13.5)

The lower thoracic oesophagus may be approached by left thoracotomy at the level of the seventh or eighth rib (see Ch. 36).

LEFT THORACOABDOMINAL APPROACH (Fig. 13.6)

The lower thoracic oesophagus and upper stomach are best approached using a combined thoracoabdominal approach (see Ch. 14). The patient lies on the right side, left leg

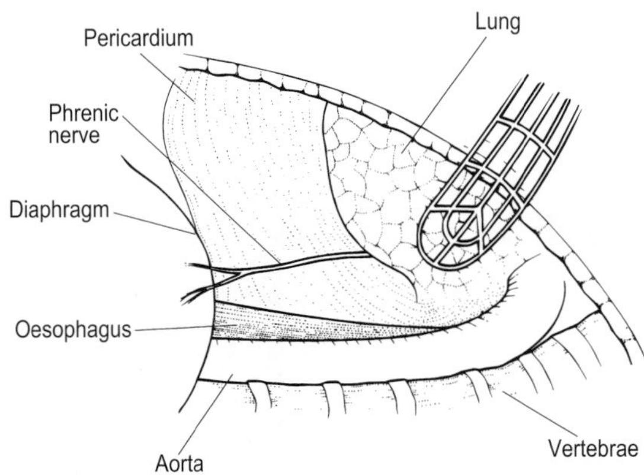

Fig. 13.5 Diagram of approach to the lower oesophagus through the left pleural space. The left lung is retracted anteriorly.

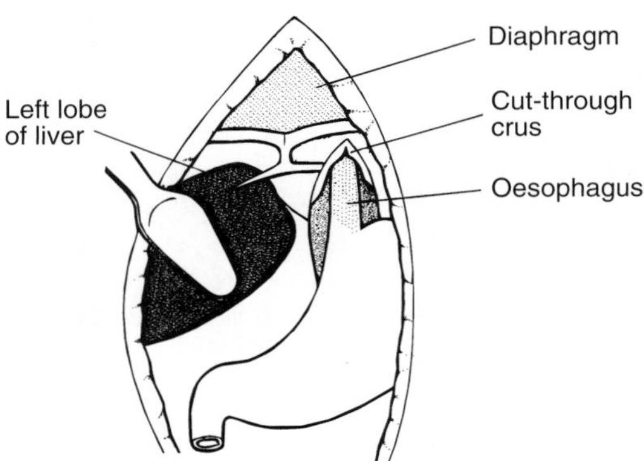

Fig. 13.7 Transabdominal approach to the lower oesophagus. The left lobe of the liver is folded to the right. If necessary, the diaphragmatic crus can be incised anteriorly.

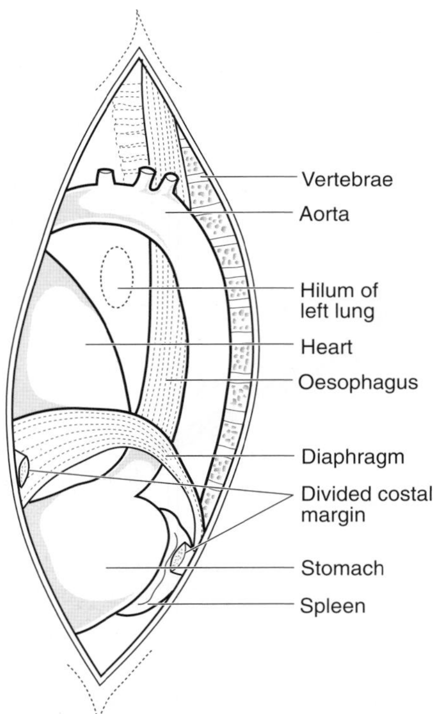

Fig. 13.6 Left thoracoabdominal approach. The diaphragm is divided circumferentially to enable the incision to open. It does not extend to the hiatus. The lung is elevated anteriorly.

extended, right leg flexed at hip and knee, both arms flexed with forearms before the face as though performing the hornpipe dance, with the shoulders at 30° from the vertical. Start the incision 2.5 cm under the right costal margin in the midclavicular line, carry it obliquely upwards and to the left to cross the costal margin along the line of the seventh or eighth rib, extending to the posterior angle of the chosen rib and up behind the scapula. Deepen the incision to enter the thorax along the line of the rib, cutting and removing 1 cm of the costal margin. Incise the diaphragm peripherally parallel to the chest wall far enough in to enable the chest to be opened but not as far as the hiatus. This method spares the phrenic nerve.

ABDOMINAL (Fig. 13.7)

The lower oesophagus is approachable through the abdomen and oesophageal hiatus via a roof-top or bilateral subcostal incision if the costal angle is narrow, through an upper midline incision extending to the costal margin. Draw down the stomach to reveal the lower oesophagus at the hiatus after incising the overlying peritoneum and fascia.

TRANSHIATAL APPROACH

This encompasses both the abdominal and cervical approaches described above.

LAPAROSCOPIC

With the patient supine induce a pneumoperitoneum and insert a 10-mm cannula in the midline. Retract the liver to approach and expose the abdominal oesophagus.

OPERATIVE CONSIDERATIONS

The oesophagus has no serous coat except on the anterior wall of the abdominal segment. A considerable part of the oesophageal wall is composed of longitudinal muscle. Longitudinally placed sutures thus have a tendency to cut out. The powerful longitudinal muscle produces shortening of the transected oesophagus when it contracts. Unless this is allowed for, the most carefully placed sutures may be torn out. A relaxed oesophagus has a large lumen but tone in the circular muscle contracts the lumen. Unless it is stretched by inserting a Foley catheter and inflating it, stitches placed closely are widely separated on stretching and permit leakage.

The blood supply to the oesophagus is tenuous when it is mobilized, especially at the lower end. The healthy oesophagus is easily damaged but disease may make it exceptionally fragile. A diseased or partially obstructed oesophagus is contaminated. Prophylactic antibiotics must be given to cover the operation. Although oral feeding may be stopped temporarily following oesophageal surgery, swallowed saliva must still pass through. Intrathoracic oesophageal leakage produces posterior mediastinitis and if the pleura is damaged a pleural collection develops. The best hope for the patient's survival if major leakage occurs is rapid clinical recognition with early reoperative repair and drainage. Minor leaks may be treated conservatively. Place chest drains in all opened chest cavities. Following transhiatal resection even if the pleura is not opened a chest drain in the posterior mediastinum will prevent haematoma collection. Place a feeding jejunostomy at operation in all cases for postoperative nutrition and do not start oral intake until the anastomosis is checked by contrast swallow at 5 days.

Never intubate the oesophagus unnecessarily or pass a rigid tube when a flexible one will suffice. Never carry out extensive oesophageal mobilization before forming an anastomosis and if the oesophagus retracts after division do not damage it by grabbing it with an instrument. Enquire about the level of anaesthesia since the longitudinal muscle is one of the last to relax. If the longitudinal muscle relaxes the oesophagus will reappear so stay sutures can be inserted. Never leave the oesophagus anastomosed under tension; ensure there will be no traction, even when the oesophagus fully contracts. Never attempt an oesophageal anastomosis with poor access, view, or when you are tired. Avoid using small forceps to grasp the oesophagus. Improve the view or change tactics. Never perform an oesophageal anastomosis when tired. Take a short break if necessary. Never use small forceps to grasp the oesophagus, as they cause damage; prefer those with a large surface area, taking a firm, but gentle grip.

Anastomosis

The tenuous blood supply of the oesophagus makes it rarely possible to excise a segment, mobilize the cut ends and carry out an end-to-end union, except in neonates. The stomach, with its rich blood supply and extensibility, is the favoured oesophageal substitute; jejunum is usually used for anastomosis to the lower one-third of the oesophagus only. Right or left colon or, preferably the transverse and left colon based on the ascending left colic artery, all placed isoperistaltically, will reach the floor of the mouth. Prefer the oesophageal bed as the route, otherwise the substernal or subcutaneous routes can be used for neck anastomoses, with sutures or staples.

Sutured anastomosis

The oesophagus and conduit, which may be stomach, jejunum or colon, must be united without tension and twist. The anastomosis depends mainly upon the submucous and mucous coats so divide the muscle coat to produce a mucosal tube 1 cm long. The hole in the conduit must match the slightly stretched oesophageal lumen. Use fine, 3/0 absorbable sutures, monofilament or braided, and continuous or interrupted stitches. If you use interrupted stitches, tie those uniting the posterior walls within the lumen, tie those uniting the anterior walls on the outer walls (Fig. 13.8). Insert further sutures to close any gaps.

Stapled anastomosis

Insert a purse-string suture using 2/0 Prolene with an over-and-over suture encompassing the mucosal/submucosal layer (Fig. 13.9). Select the largest size staple head that easily fits the lumen, usually 25 mm. Detach the anvil from the spindle, introduce it into the lower oesophagus and tighten and tie the purse-string suture onto the stem. If you are using stomach, create a temporary anterior gastrotomy and insert the spindle of the stapler into the fundus at least 2 cm from any suture or staple line. 'Open' the instrument so that its sharp point comes through the stomach (Fig. 13.9). If the jejunum or colon are joined end-to-side, insert the stapler without the anvil head through the cut end; this will be closed later. Protrude the stem through the antimesenteric wall at a suitable point. Attach the anvil onto its spindle

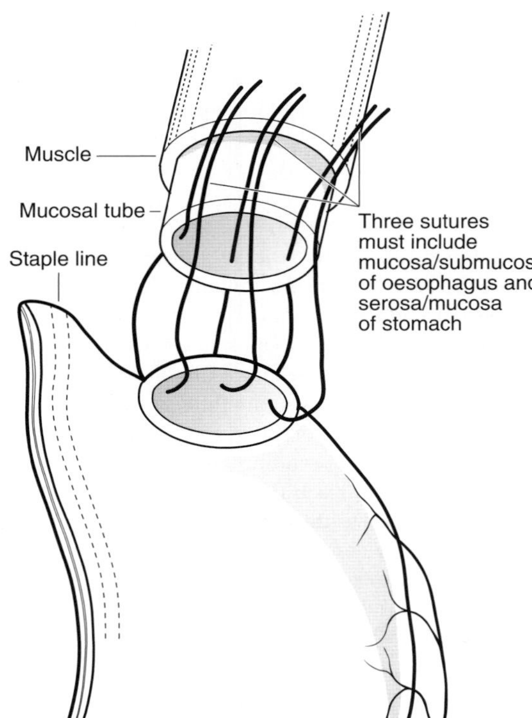

Fig. 13.8 Oesophageal anastomosis. The first three sutures are placed on the posterior wall to enable triangulation.

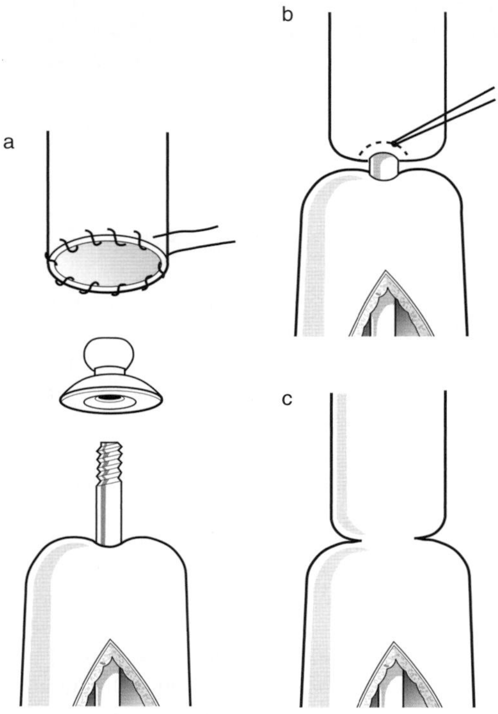

Fig. 13.9 A stapled oesophageal anastomosis: (a) the stapler shaft has been pushed through a hole in the stomach and the anvil is attached so that it can be introduced into the oesophagus; (b) the purse-string suture is tightened; (c) the device is actuated, producing an anastomosis.

to the instrument and close the anvil down onto the cartridge. Check that there is no twisting, nothing interposed or protruding. Release the safety catch and fully compress the handles to activate the stapler. Slightly separate the jaws, gently rotate and withdraw the device. Remove the anvil head and check that the toroidal ('doughnut'-shaped) oesophageal and viscus cuffs are complete before placing them in fixative solution for histology. Check the anastomosis with a finger and have the aspiration tube passed if necessary. Close the opening through which you passed the instrument and recheck the completed anastomosis.

TRAUMA, SPONTANEOUS AND POSTOPERATIVE LEAKS

Swallowed foreign body, stab or missile wounds may immediately rupture the oesophagus, but crush injuries such as those sustained in road traffic accidents may cause necrosis with late rupture. Boerhaave's tear of the lower oesophagus is caused by retching; a mucosal tear only is Mallory–Weiss syndrome. Iatrogenic rupture may follow endoscopy, dilatation of stricture or achalasia, removal of a foreign body, or follow an operation on the oesophagus including cardiomyotomy, vagotomy and resection or bypass.

Small cervical leaks following instrumental damage usually seal if the patient is fed parenterally for a few days. Treat conservatively tears in the thoracic oesophagus that are detected early, produced at endoscopy or instrumentation, associated with minimal contamination and are contained in the mediastinum. Intrathoracic leaks have a high mortality rate if not treated promptly. The worst results occur if the diagnosis is overlooked and the patient is fed.

CORROSIVE BURNS

Corrosives swallowed accidentally or in suicide attempts during acute depression burn the mouth, pharynx and larynx, and oesophagus into the stomach; inhalation causes hoarseness, stridor and dyspnoea. Immediately remove 'button' batteries swallowed by children which release caustics. The mucosa is damaged or destroyed but may regenerate within 14 days but wound contraction may cause strictures. If deeper layers are damaged or rupture, septic mediastinitis ensues. Order plain X-rays of the chest and abdomen. Contrast fluids are too painful but an expert may gently pass an endoscope. Stop oral intake, start intravenous fluids and antibiotics. If perforation has occurred expert emergency exploration is necessary.

GASTRO-OESOPHAGEAL REFLUX DISEASE

The continence of the gastro-oesophageal junction is maintained by a combination of anatomical and physiological factors and loss of function of the lower oesophageal function allows gastro-oesophageal reflux disease (GORD) of irritant gastroduodenal contents producing oesophagitis. Hiatal hernia is variably associated with GORD. Clinical assessment, endoscopy and 24-hour lower oesophageal pH recording are valuable to detect the pre-malignant complication of Barrett's oesophageal mucosal cells.

Consider an antireflux operation such as Nissen's fundoplication, or a modification of it, only if measures such as weight loss, stopping smoking, reducing alcohol and fatty foods, combined with treatment with antacids, H_2-receptor antagonists or proton-pump inhibitors, have failed. Persistent regurgitation is the best indication for operation, and in severe dysplasia or neoplasia in Barrett's oesophagitis, oesophagectomy may be indicated.

TRANSABDOMINAL FLOPPY NISSEN FUNDOPLICATION (Fig. 13.10)

Do not operate on an overweight patient until he or she has lost as much weight as possible. Never operate until you have fully confirmed the diagnosis and excluded other conditions of the upper gastrointestinal tract.

Have the head of the table elevated, use an upper midline incision with an on-table mechanical retractor lifting the sternum and fold the left lobe of the liver to the right (Fig. 13.11).

Action

First mobilize the stomach and divide most of the short gastric vessels that tether the stomach to the spleen, which

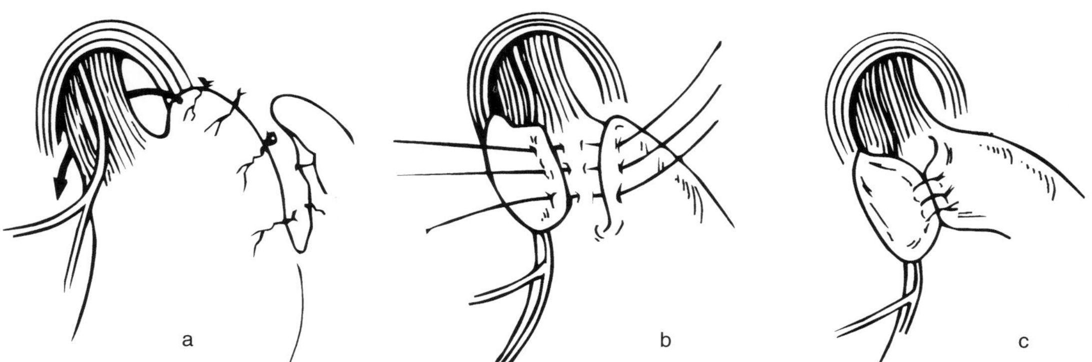

Fig. 13.10 Transabdominal Nissen fundoplication: free the oesophagus in the hiatus, while preserving the vagi and branches; isolate, doubly ligate and divide the upper short gastric vessels; (a) gently fold the freed fundus behind the lower oesophagus to emerge on its right side; (b) insert three or four non-absorbable sutures to pick up the fold, the lower oesophagus and the anterior wall of the stomach to the left of the oesophagus; include the submucosa but not the mucosa; avoid piercing or damaging the vagi; (c) gently tie the sutures; you should be able to insert a finger beneath the cuff so formed and rotate the cuff to the left in order to insert two or three sutures fixing the lower edge of the oesophagogastric junction.

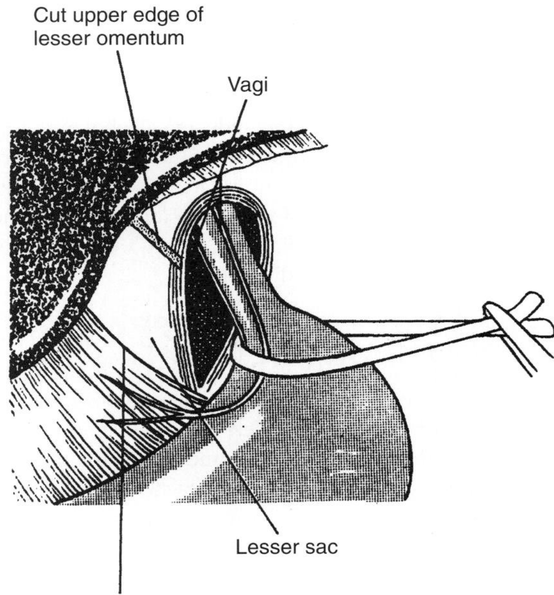

Fig. 13.11 Abdominal approach to the repair of hiatal hernia. The hernial sac has been excised to define the margins of the hiatus, and the upper edge of the lesser omentum has been detached from the diaphragm. Either an anterior or posterior repair may now be performed.

may be in two layers. Expose the lower oesophagus, crural margins, identifying and preserving the anterior and posterior vagal trunks. Divide the upper portion of the gastrohepatic omentum, to display the right margin of the hiatus, preserving the hepatic branches of the vagus nerve and an accessory hepatic artery. Trim the sac from the lower oesophagus.

Posterior repair

1 Ask the anaesthetist to pass a soft-tipped 50F Maloney tapered mercury dilator into the stomach. Displace the gullet forwards and stitch the margins of the hiatus together behind it using 2–4 non-absorbable sutures. Leave a space between the hiatus and the stented oesophagus that will admit a finger, avoiding overtightening. Excise the fat pad in front of the cardia, preserving the anterior vagus nerve. Gently fold the gastric fundus behind the lower oesophagus to emerge above the lesser curvature behind or in front of the posterior vagus nerve.

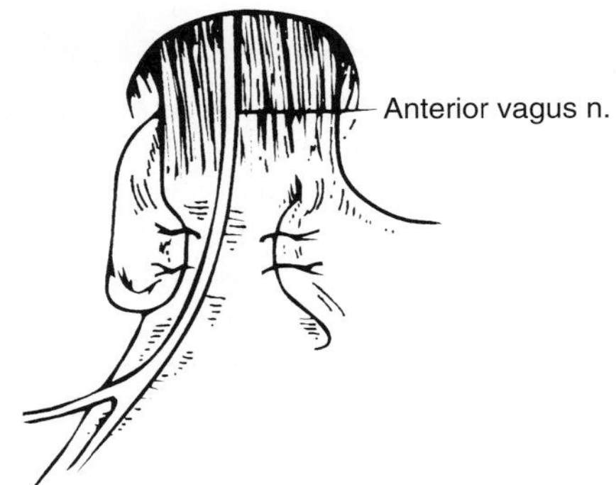

Fig. 13.12 Partial fundoplication, leaving 90° of the oesophageal circumference bare.

2 Insert a non-absorbable suture, such as braided polyamide, picking up the upper anterior wall of the stomach on the left of the oesophagus, the lower oesophagus immediately above the cardia and the part of the stomach that has been folded behind and to the right of the oesophagus. Each stitch is deep enough to incorporate the submucosa but not to pierce the mucosa. Tighten the stitch so that the two folds of stomach are brought together in front of the oesophagus. Check that a finger can be passed easily between the wrap and the oesophagus which contains the 56F dilator. The wrap must be really floppy to avoid postoperative dysphagia and gas bloat. Insert a second stitch 1 cm above the first one. Make the fundoplication not more than 1 cm long anteriorly, or risk dysphagia and gas bloat. Have the mercury dilator withdrawn but leave the nasogastric tube.

PARTIAL FUNDOPLICATION

To reduce the risk of dysphagia and 'gas bloat', have the wrap encircling only 270° of the lower oesophagus, not more than 3 cm long, around the lower oesophagus. Two or three stitches pick up the oesophagus and the left upper stomach, leaving the anterior 90° of oesophagus bare (Fig. 13.12). In the Toupet operation the hiatus is not repaired. Instead, the completed fundoplication is stitched to the crura on both sides.

LAPAROSCOPIC FUNDOPLICATION

(See Ch. 15.)

The operation is exactly the same in principle as the 'floppy' Nissen. However, the technique is different because of the different access to the organs and because laparoscopic instruments have a different set of disadvantages from those encountered during a conventional approach. Do not attempt laparoscopic fundoplication unless you are fully competent in the full range of laparoscopic skills.

ACHALASIA OF THE CARDIA

Achalasia (Greek *a* = not + *chaleein* = to relax), in which the lower segment of the oesophagus fails to relax ahead of a peristaltic wave, is probably part of a generalized condition of neuromuscular origin associated with abnormal vagal motor input and myenteric ganglionic degeneration. There is gradual dilatation of the oesophagus, retention of contents, risk of retained food aspiration and pulmonary fibrosis, so do not delay effective treatment with forceful balloon dilatation or surgical myotomy, which can be performed as an open operation or laparoscopically. The aim of cardiomyotomy is to weaken the lower oesophageal sphincter sufficiently to allow food to pass but not to allow gastro-oesophageal reflux by performing a limited myotomy (Fig. 13.13).

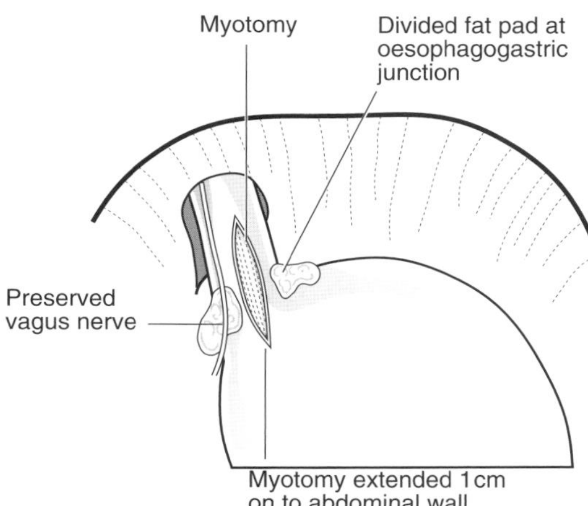

Fig. 13.13 Myotomy for achalasia. The defect can be covered with the gastric fundus to reduce reflux.

PHARYNGEAL POUCH

This pulsion diverticulum of Zenker is a mucosal herniation between the transverse and oblique fibres of the inferior pharyngeal constrictor muscle, thought to result from incoordination or achalasia of the cricopharyngeal sphincter. Recommend operation if the patient has dysphagia or regurgitation with the likelihood of aspiration pneumonia. It is now usually treated by transoral stapling in which a linear cutting device both divides cricopharyngeus and opens the diverticulum into the oesophagus. Reserve operation for failures of this technique.

FURTHER READING

Adam A, Mason RC, Owen WJ 2000 Practical management of oesophageal disease. Isis Medical Media, Oxford

Akiyama H 1990 Surgery for cancer of the esophagus. Williams & Wilkins, Baltimore, pp 73–80

Mason R 1996 Palliation of malignant dysphagia, alternatives to surgery. Annals of the Royal College of Surgeons of England 78:457–462

14

Oesophageal cancer

H. Udagawa, H. Akiyama, R. M. Kirk

CONTENTS

INTRODUCTION

The epidemiology of squamous oesophageal carcinoma is the most varied of any tumour, so that in certain geographical regions there is a very high incidence and in other areas it is rare. It is also well known that squamous cell carcinoma of the oesophagus very often shows multicentric occurrence, including associated head and neck tumours. These suggest that environmental factors are important and many such factors have been postulated.

The tumour spreads circumferentially and longitudinally within the mucosa (intraepithelial spread), and spreads also in the submucosa and the muscle layer continuously or sometimes apart from the main tumour (intramural metastasis). It invades the trachea, bronchi, lungs, thoracic duct, recurrent laryngeal nerves, pericardium and aorta. This tumour notoriously spreads to the lymph nodes, not just locally but also at a considerable distance. Because of its insidious development, many patients present with advanced disease, complaining of dysphagia, weight loss, substernal or back pain, aspiration pneumonia or hoarseness. Supraclavicular lymph nodes may be palpable on presentation. The prognosis at this stage is very poor.

Confirm the diagnosis by endoscopy with biopsy. Take a number of biopsy specimens and record the levels at which they are taken. If the cytological brushings and biopsy specimens are reported to be normal but you suspect carcinoma, repeat the examination, and go on repeating it until you are absolutely sure that you are not missing a cancer. Of the available imaging methods, the most valuable are double-contrast barium swallow, abdominal and cervical ultrasonography, computed tomography (CT), endoscopic ultrasonography and magnetic resonance imaging. The last three methods show the tumour size, invasion of contiguous structures and extent of lymph node involvement. Preoperative staging can now be attempted, using the TNM classification of the International Union against Cancer. Carry out a careful assessment of the patient to exclude or confirm the presence of incidental disease, particularly that of the cardiovascular and respiratory systems.

Recent advances in the field of chemoradiotherapy are rapidly changing the therapeutic scheme of this disease. Although surgery remains the standard measure of treatment for lesions where R0 resection is possible, an increasing number of patients, particularly those with advanced disease, are treated with chemoradiation as the first mode of treatment.

Because oesophageal carcinoma is so often advanced at the time of diagnosis, some surgeons feel that treatment should be palliative. This deprives the patients who might be cured of the opportunity to benefit from a radical approach. Our experience of over 20 years of extensive lymph node dissection proves that even patients with 'distant' lymph node metastases still have a chance of being cured by surgery. With the recent advance of non-surgical treatments, some T4 tumours have also become candidates for radical operation after neoadjuvant therapy.

We shall describe only the principles of these complex operations to allow you as an assistant to follow the steps.

RESECTION OF CARCINOMA OF THE LOWER OESOPHAGUS

Open the left upper abdomen obliquely along the line of the sixth or seventh intercostal space, starting in the midline halfway between the umbilicus and the tip of the xiphisternum and extending to the left costal margin (Fig. 14.1). Palpate the liver and the pelvis to detect distant spread. Determine the fixity of the cardia and feel for extensive lymph node involvement that would make resection useless. If resection seems feasible, cut across the costal margin and elongate the skin incision toward the posterior axillary line along the aimed intercostals space. In very advanced cases, laparoscopic observation of the abdominal cavity may prove peritoneal dissemination and avoid useless laparotomy. Cut the diaphragm radially 10–15 cm towards the right crus. Even in very advanced cases with direct tumour invasion to the crural muscle, you can get the safe surgical margin with circular resection of the muscle around the hiatus. It is usually unnecessary to cut through the diaphragm. Our routine operation for carcinoma of abdominal oesophagus and the cardia is resection of the lower thoracic oesophagus together with a cuff of the gastric cardia or entire stomach followed by jejunal interposition or Roux-en-Y reconstruction performed through the left thoracoabdominal approach (Fig. 14.2). During closure, insert an underwater-sealed drain into the left pleural cavity through a separate stab incision near the costophrenic angle in the posterior axillary line.

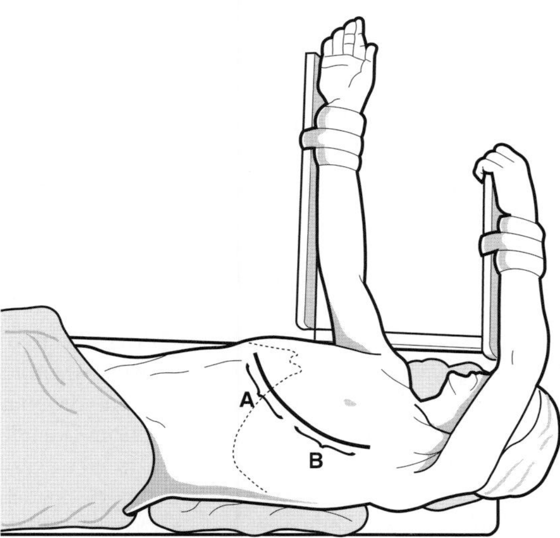

Fig. 14.1 Left thoracoabdominal approach to the lower oesophagus. Line A is for initial abdominal exploration. When the tumour is resectable, the incision is extended (line B). (Modified with permission from Akiyama H 1990 Surgery for cancer of the esophagus. Williams & Wilkins, Baltimore.)

OPERATIONS FOR THORACIC OESOPHAGEAL CARCINOMA

The two-step operation of Ivor Lewis is the classic method for dealing with mid-oesophageal carcinoma. Newer and more radical techniques are also applied these days. They include the extensive (three-field) lymph node dissection promoted by Akiyama and other Japanese surgeons. The operative mortality is satisfactorily low and the 5-year survival rate exceeds 50% for those who undergo a curative (R0) resection.

RADICAL CURATIVE SURGERY: EXTENSIVE LYMPH NODE DISSECTION (AKIYAMA)

Japanese surgeons have been performing extensive lymph node dissection for about 20 years, and it has also been done recently by some surgeons in North America and Europe. This extensive operation has been developed on the basis of investigation of the extent of lymphatic tumour spread, and careful attention to detail in planning and performing the operation has made it feasible. We do not take an inflexible attitude towards the extent of either oesophageal or lymph node excision but try to match the operation to the site and extent of tumour growth and to the likelihood of invasion and spread to the lymph nodes. Reliable preoperative assessment of the tumour by endoscopy, conventional ultrasound of the neck and abdomen, endoscopic ultrasound and CT is mandatory.

Access is through a right thoracotomy in the fourth intercostal space. The extensive resection of the oesophagus and dissection of the lymph nodes has been worked out by extensive studies, so that the procedure demands special expertise.

Through an upper median abdominal incision the stomach is mobilized; the line of resection of the oesopha-

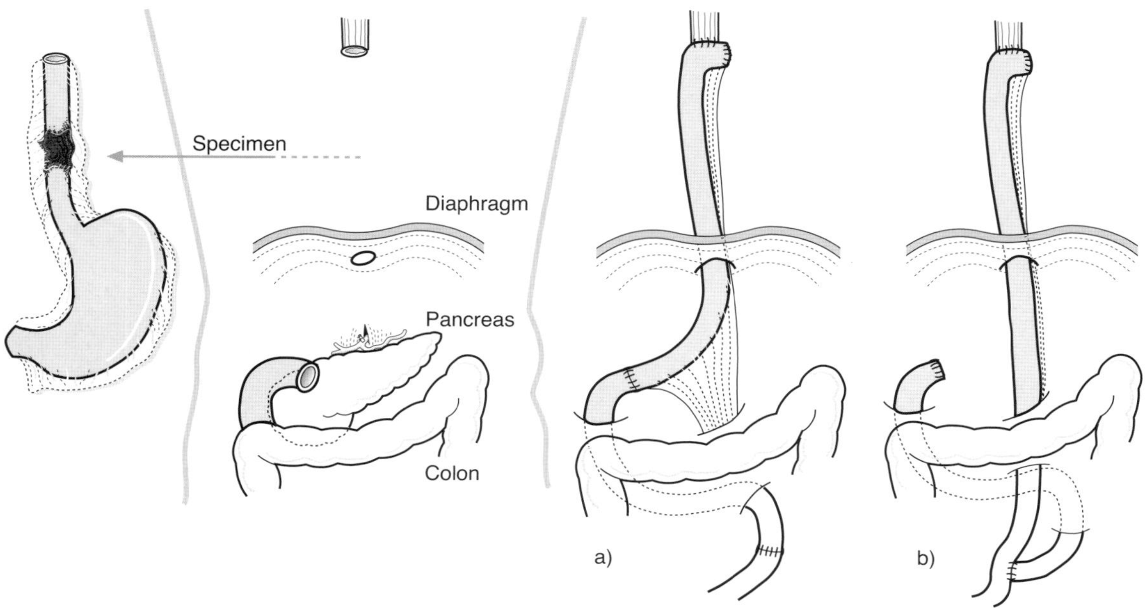

Fig. 14.2 Diagram of resection of lower oesophagus and stomach for cancer and reconstruction. On the left is the resected specimen. In the middle is the defect following resection. On the right are two possible methods of reconstruction. (a) A segment of jejunum has been taken out of circuit, retaining its blood supply, and interposed between the oesophagus and the distal stomach or duodenum. (b) A Roux loop of jejunum is taken up to the oesophagus. The distal stomach or duodenum is closed.

gus includes the gastric lesser curve and associated lymph nodes.

The cervical oesophagus is approached on the left side and transected so that the mobilized stomach is drawn up through the chest so that the fundus can be united to it (Fig. 14.3).

OTHER PROCEDURES

Palliative resection of the oesophagus may be achieved by combined transhiatal abdominal and cervical approaches. It should be restricted to high-risk patients in whom standard thoracotomy is impossible or dysphagic patients with resectable oesophageal carcinoma who have distant nodes or organ metastases but have a reasonable life expectancy.

If resection is not possible, the stomach can be mobilized and drawn up subcutaneously to the neck for bypass of an obstructed upper oesophagus.

The right or left colon can be taken out of circuit and used as an oesophageal replacement.

ADJUVANT TREATMENT

Although squamous carcinoma, and indeed adenocarcinoma, responds to external beam therapy, the effect of such adjuvant treatment on the prognosis is questionable. Brachytherapy (intracavity irradiation with caesium-137 or iridium-192) offers certain advantages, notably that the radiation is concentrated on the tumour. Endoscopic Nd-YAG laser therapy is valuable for palliation of dysphagia but it often has to be repeated to alleviate dysphagia and to maintain patency. Photodynamic therapy involves giving sensitizing drugs, usually haematoporphyrin derivatives or phthalylcyanates, which are retained by tumour cells.

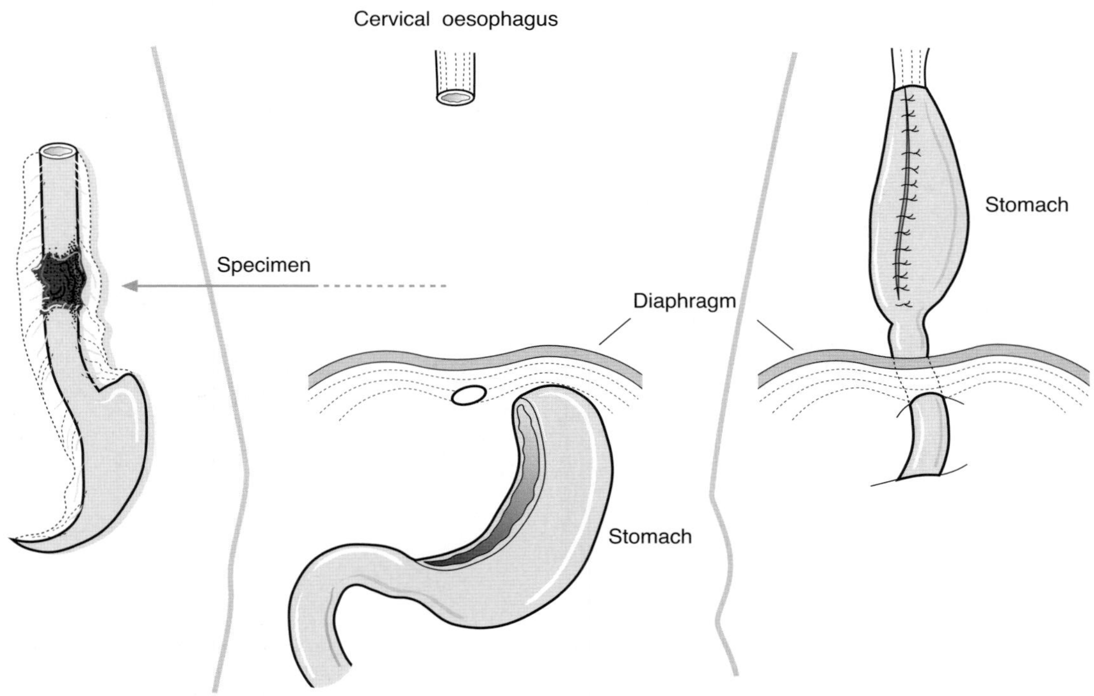

Fig. 14.3 Diagram of resection for thoracic oesophageal carcinoma. On the left is the specimen including the gastro-oesophageal junction and part of the gastric lesser curve. In the middle is the defect left following resection. On the right is the stomach, closed on the lesser curve, mobilized and drawn up through the mediastinum to be united to the cervical oesophagus.

FURTHER READING

Akiyama H 1980 Surgery for carcinoma of the esophagus. In: Current problems in surgery. Year Book Publishers, Chicago

Akiyama H 1990 Surgery for cancer of the esophagus. Williams & Wilkins, Baltimore

Akiyama H, Udagawa H 1999 Surgical management of esophageal cancer: The Japanese experience. In: Daly JM, Hennessy TPJ et al (eds) Management of upper gastrointestinal cancer. Saunders, London, pp 200–225

Akiyama H, Udagawa H 2002 Total gastrectomy and Roux-en-Y reconstruction. In: Pearson FG, Cooper JD et al (eds) Esophageal surgery, 2nd edn. Churchill Livingstone, New York, pp 871–879

Akiyama H, Tsurumaru M, Udagawa H et al 1997 Esophageal cancer. In: Current problems in surgery. Mosby, St Louis

Udagawa H, Akiyama H 2001 Surgical treatment of esophageal cancer: Tokyo experience of the three-field technique. Diseases of the Esophagus 14:110–114

15

Laparoscopic Nissen fundoplication

A. Darzi, P. A. Paraskeva

DESCRIPTION OF OPERATION

Gastro-oesophageal reflux disease (GORD; GERD, gastro-esophageal, in the USA), which often results from irreversible injury to the lower oesophageal sphincter, is not always responsive to medical therapy or recurs after stopping treatment. Persistent heartburn and regurgitation may be complicated by nocturnal choking, aspiration pneumonia, oesophageal stricture and oesophageal mucosal changes and ulceration described in 1950 by the London surgeon Norman Barrett (1903–1979). The description is for you as an assistant since you require adequate training before performing the procedure.

Confirm reflux with 24-hour pH monitoring. If manometric studies reveal ineffective lower oesophageal sphincter and oesophageal body peristalsis, some form of antireflux procedure is necessary. The motility disorders are often secondary to the reflux and will not respond to prokinetic or prolonged acid-reduction medication. Perform gastroscopy, barium swallow X-ray, 24-hour pH monitoring and oesophageal manometry.

Gain informed consent including possible conversion to open surgery and warning of 'gas bloat' syndrome, recurrence of symptoms, and other options.

Perform laparoscopic fundoplication under general anaesthesia with endotracheal intubation. A 'loose' Nissen, partial fundoplication such as the Toupet, a Hill procedure or Belsey mark IV are suitable. Laparoscopic Nissen fundoplication produces results comparable with open fundoplication (see Ch. 13) but benefits from the minimally invasive approach.

As a rule place the patient supine while you stand on the right side. Your assistant stands on the patient's left. The second assistant, who will hold the liver retractor and the camera, stands next to you on the patient's right.

Access

Create a pneumoperitoneum using a Veress needle or by an open Hassan entry.

Action

The technique is comparable with that of open operation (Fig. 15.1). The gastric fundus is brought posterior to the oesophagus but anterior to the posterior vagus nerve.

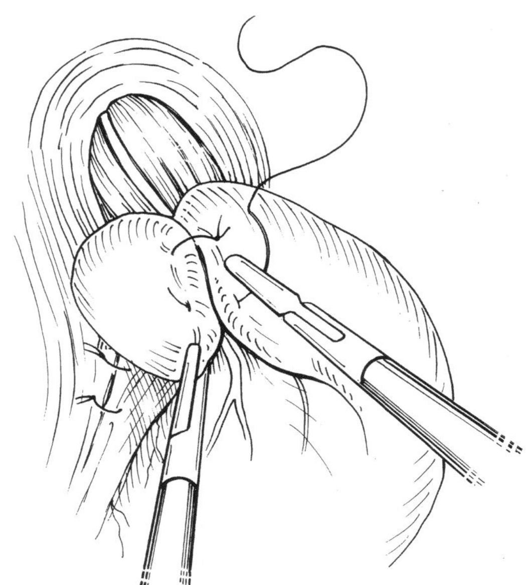

Fig. 15.1 The completed laparoscopic Nissen fundoplication.

16

Stomach and duodenum

M. C. Winslet

CONTENTS

ENDOSCOPY

Diagnostic endoscopy using flexible fibreoptic endoscopes has become so easy that even inexperienced clinicians can safely pass the instrument and interpret most abnormalities. Certainly all gastrointestinal operators should be familiar with the use of the endoscope. Endoscopy does not compete with radiology but is complementary to it. Consider endoscopy whenever there is any possibility of a lesion lying within its scope. It often provides authoritative diagnosis because of the facility to remove guided biopsy specimens or cytological brushings. It is no longer ethical practice to operate on a patient for suspected oesophagogastroduodenal disease without carrying out endoscopy when this is available, even when the diagnosis seems certain. Occasionally, diagnoses made by radiology and other means prove to be fallacious, or other, unsuspected, lesions are discovered in addition to or instead of the expected one. Conversely, many patients are spared operations because an expected condition is excluded. The examination is mandatory before operations for gastrointestinal bleeding. Even when the exact site of bleeding is not seen, it is often possible to exclude suspected lesions. In the duodenum the ampulla of Vater can be cannulated for radiological and cytological diagnosis. Therapeutic uses include dilatation of strictures by several methods, snaring polyps, sphincterotomy performed on the ampulla of Vater and stones extracted, insertion of stents to overcome strictures of the bile and pancreatic ducts.

Prepare

Learn on the slim end-viewing instrument. Other types offer wider suction and biopsy channels through which larger forceps can be passed for biopsy, grasping foreign bodies, or snaring polyps. The very flexible ends of end-viewing endoscopes make them very versatile, but side-viewing instruments are of value in special circumstances, notably when cannulating the ampulla of Vater (Fig. 16.1). Make sure that the instrument, light source, suction apparatus, biopsy forceps and air insufflation pump all work satisfactorily and that the instrument has been sterilized according to the manufacturer's recommendations.

Obtain written, informed consent from the patient, highlighting the indications for the procedure and the potential complications. Before starting, inspect any barium meal radiographs to assess potential difficulties and pinpoint areas requiring special attention.

Except in emergency the patient takes no food or fluids for 6 hours. In an emergency it is prudent to have an anaesthetist in attendance.

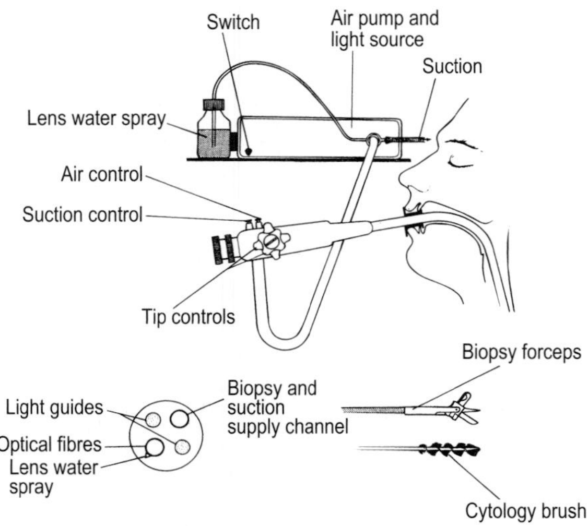

Fig. 16.1 Flexible fibreoptic endoscopy.

Apply protective gloves and spectacles before starting the procedure. Ensure that the patient has no dentures. Anaesthetize the pharynx with an aerosol spray of 4% lidocaine. For simple diagnostic endoscopy, adequate sedation can usually be obtained by giving diazepam (Valium) 10 mg or midazolam (Hypnovel) 2.5 mg through an indwelling cannula over a period of 1–2 minutes just before passing the instrument, giving further increments if necessary. If the procedure becomes painful call for senior advice. Apply a pulse oximeter monitor and be prepared to administer oxygen – elderly or infirm patients are at risk of hypoxia. If peristaltic activity is excessive, give hyoscine butylbromide (Buscopan) 20–40 mg through the indwelling cannula.

Insert a plastic mouthpiece between the patient's teeth or gums through which the instrument will slide. Smear the endoscope shaft with water-soluble lubricant, and smear the lens with silicone liquid to prevent the adherence of secretions and mucus. With the patient laid on the left side, the head is steadied and maintained in neck flexion by an assistant.

Access

1 Slightly flex the tip of the instrument. Pass it through the mouthpiece, over the tongue, keeping the flexed tip strictly in the midline pointing towards the cricopharyngeal sphincter. As the tip reaches the sphincter there is a hold-up. Ask the patient to swallow. The tip will be slightly extruded, and do not resist this, but suddenly the obstruction disappears as the sphincter relaxes and the instrument can be smoothly passed into the stomach after unflexing the tip. Do not use force or advance the instrument blindly.

2 Look down the instrument and concentrate on safely passing the instrument through the oesophagus and stomach and into the duodenum, noting incidentally if there is any abnormality. Insufflate the minimum of air to open up the passage. Hold the eyepiece with the left hand, adjusting the tip controls with the left thumb. Hold the shaft of the endoscope with the right hand close to the patient's mouth, advancing, withdrawing and rotating it as necessary. When the gastric angulus is passed, flex the tip to identify the pylorus. Advance the tip, keeping the pylorus in the centre of the field until the tip slips through.

3 The side-viewing endoscope has a rounded tip which makes it easier to negotiate the pharynx. If there is any doubt about the free passage, always examine the patient first with an end-viewing endoscope. Become familiar with the tip control and angle of view before passing it. When it has passed into the stomach, rotate it to bring into view the relatively smooth, straight lesser curve which ends at the arch of the angulus, below which can be seen the pylorus in the distance. Angle the instrument up towards the roof of the antrum while advancing the instrument. The view of the pylorus is lost momentarily as the tip slips through into the duodenum. Paradoxically, if the shaft is slightly withdrawn, the instrument is straightened and the tip advances further into the duodenum. Rotate the shaft to bring the medial duodenal wall into view and, as the instrument enters the second part of the duodenum, the ampulla of Vater is usually seen as a nipple, often with a hooded mucosal fold above it.

Assess

1 Withdraw the end-viewing instrument in a spiral fashion to bring into view the whole circumference of the duodenum and stomach. Withdraw the side-viewing endoscope whilst rotating it 180° either side to view the whole circumference. Do not overinflate the stomach and duodenum with air. In the duodenum and distal stomach, keep the endoscope still and watch the peristaltic waves form and pass distally, to estimate the suppleness of the walls and exclude rigidity from

infiltration or disease. With the tip of the end-viewing instrument lying in the body of the stomach, flex it fully while gently advancing the shaft to bring the fundus and cardia into view. Flex the side-viewing instrument to produce the same view. From just above the cardia the end-viewing instrument displays the pinchcock action of the diaphragmatic crura at each inspiration. If gastric mucosa is seen above this, there is a sliding hiatal hernia. The gastric mucosa is pink and shiny; at the crenated transition to the thinner and more opaque oesophageal squamous mucosa, the colour becomes paler and sometimes slightly bluish. Islands of pink gastric mucosa may be seen above the line of transition.

2 If the view disappears, withdraw the instrument and insufflate a little air. If the lens is obscured, clean it with the water jet or wipe it against the mucosa to free it of adherent mucus.

3 Look out for inflammation, atrophy, hypertrophy, ulcers, tears, diverticula, polyps, varices, tumours. Remove biopsy specimens under vision from any suspicious sites, including tumours, the edges of ulcers, irregularities of the mucosa and suspected inflammation. Take specimens from different places, preferably from each quadrant of an ulcer. If lymphoma is a possibility, take multiple deep biopsies, since the disease often spreads in the submucosa. Place the specimens in carefully labelled separate pots containing formol saline fixative for histological examination. Cytological diagnosis is extremely helpful. Pass the brush through the biopsy channel and rotate it against the suspicious area. Agitate the brush in a separate jar of fixative; this will be subsequently centrifuged and the cells stained and examined.

4 Lay a heavily sedated patient on the left side, slightly face-down, under the care of a trained nurse to be watched during recovery. Do not allow any fluids or foods to be given until the patient is fully recovered and until the effect of pharyngeal anaesthesia has worn off, usually 4 hours.

ACCESS IN THE UPPER ABDOMEN

Improve your access to the gastric cardia by tilting the whole patient slightly head-up. Kocher's duodenal mobilization (Fig. 16.2) raises the head of the pancreas contained within

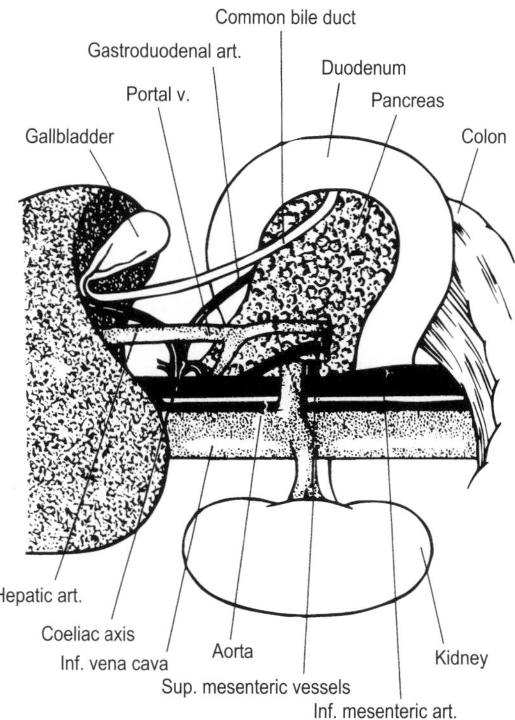

Fig. 16.2 Kocher's duodenal mobilization, as seen from the right side of the patient.

the duodenal loop into its embryological midline position, restrained by the structures in the free edge of the lesser omentum above, the superior mesenteric vessels below, and the body and tail of the pancreas to the left.

The head and neck of the pancreas and duodenum can be palpated between fingers and thumb as can the lower end of the common bile duct, and ampulla. Duodenotomy at the level of the ampulla allows inspection of the interior for tumours, stones, biopsy, excision of ampullary neoplasms, sphincterotomy, sphincteroplasty, and cannulation or instrumentation of the bile and pancreatic ducts. Mobilization is essential for a number of procedures.

SUTURING AND STAPLING THE STOMACH AND DUODENUM

Strong, reliably absorbed synthetic materials that elicit minimal inflammatory reaction are available, allowing finer thread to be used but they are severely weakened by crushing, abrasion and rough handling, especially when tying knots. Braided materials are flexible but use smooth monofilaments which have no interstices for bacteria in the presence of infection.

Innumerable papers have been written about the best ways of suturing stomach and intestine. Should we use interrupted or continuous, one layer or two, simple through-and-through or complex stitches, including or excluding the mucosa, inverted or edge-to-edge? There is but a single common factor and that is the care with which sutures are inserted and tied. The one layer that must always be included in the stitches, as shown by Halsted, is the submucosa.

As with sutures, ligatures (bindings) are applied using the finest possible materials, although silk and linen are still popular because of their excellent handling properties.

Reliable stapling instruments for joining bowel are valuable but they are not as versatile as sutures so as a trainee, first take every opportunity to master the accurate placement of sutures. There are two overriding indications for using stapling instruments: when access for suturing is difficult or when speed is essential, perhaps during a major operation.

GASTROTOMY AND GASTRODUODENOTOMY

Gastric, gastroduodenal and duodenal incision allows the interior of the bowel to be examined to confirm, biopsy or treat a suspected lesion such as an ulcer, tumour or source of bleeding. Gastrotomy allows access from below to the lower oesophagus. Strictures are often dilated more safely from below than from above. As a rule, open the stomach on the anterior wall midway between the greater and lesser curves. For the purpose of diagnosis, start with a small incision, 3–4 cm long, the proximal end of which is 5–6 cm from the pylorus allowing you to examine it while it is intact, though the incision can be extended distally through the pyloric ring onto the anterior wall of the duodenal bulb. To view the interior, first aspirate all the contents. Retractors may be placed to hold open the stomach so that it can be examined by adjusting the theatre light to shine through the opening. The stomach can be manoeuvred manually to bring different parts of the interior into view and evaginated through the incision. Close a gastrotomy in one or two layers, leaving a longitudinal suture line using a single edge-to-edge row of sutures.

OPERATIVE GASTROSTOMY

Gastrostomy offers a valuable method of feeding patients who are unable to swallow because of oesophageal obstruction, bulbar palsy and other causes. In Stamm's method a tube passes through the abdominal wall, through a stab hole in the middle of the anterior gastric wall. Two or three purse-string sutures (Fig. 16.3), invert the stoma like an inkwell. Several stitches draw the stoma up against the anterior abdominal wall where it seals, preventing intraperitoneal leakage. Open gastrostomy has been partly replaced by percutaneous endoscopic gastrostomy (PEG).

PERFORATED PEPTIC ULCER

Record the patient's age, blood pressure and the presence or absence of serious associated disease such as cardiac, respiratory or renal failure. Fully resuscitate the patient before performing the operation. Patients seen within 8 hours, in whom a confident diagnosis is made, and who are haemodynamically stable, may be treated conservatively. Ensure that the tip of an 18F nasogastric tube is accurately placed in the most dependent part of the stomach. Proceed to operation at once if the patient develops pyrexia, tachycardia, pain, distension or increasing intraperitoneal gas on X-rays. A few patients develop intraperitoneal abscesses if there has been significant leakage and soiling. Nasogastric suction, parenteral feeding, systemic antibiotics and chest physiotherapy are instituted, and operation is resorted to only if the patient fails to improve or deteriorates.

Perforated gastric ulcer carries a higher mortality than perforated duodenal ulcer, because the patients are, on average, older and less 'fit' generally. Most gastric ulcer perforations are successfully managed by simple suture after

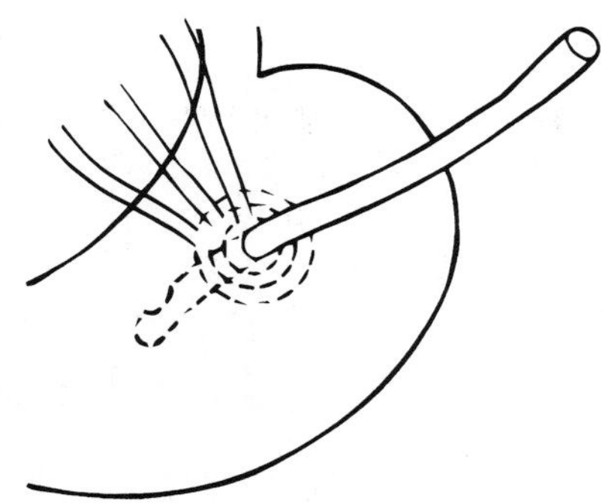

Fig. 16.3 Stamm gastrostomy.

excising a specimen from the edge for histology. Sometimes they are difficult to close and demand gastrectomy including the ulcer. Perforated gastric carcinoma may be amenable to the same operation as would be carried out electively.

The diagnosis has been confirmed through the laparoscope and followed by repair using sutures, staples or a plug. This may become an accepted method of diagnosis and treatment.

Action

1 Use a midline or right paramedian incision from the xiphisternum to the umbilicus, 10–12 cm long. Remove all instruments from the field with the exception of a retractor for your assistant and the sucker tube for yourself. Aspirate any free fluid after collecting a specimen for laboratory examination. Gastric juice is usually bile-stained. Examine the duodenal bulb and the stomach, especially along the lesser curve. If necessary, open the lesser sac of omentum through the lesser or gastrocolic omenta to view the posterior gastric wall. Remember that multiple perforations can occur. Always locally excise or remove a biopsy specimen from the edge of a gastric ulcer.

2 If you cannot find the perforation after a diligent search, explore the whole abdomen, if necessary extending the incision downwards. Examine in particular the gallbladder and sigmoid colon. If you are still puzzled, consider the possibility of Boerhaave's syndrome (spontaneous rupture of distal oesophagus). If you are a surgeon in training and find yourself in difficulty either because of failure to discover the cause, or indecision about the best course of action, or because the required procedure is beyond your capabilities, do not hesitate to contact your chief for advice and assistance.

> **KEY POINTS Treat the emergency condition – that is why you operated**
>
> - Your function at this emergency operation is to perform the simplest procedure that will correct the catastrophe.
> - If you do more than this, will you be able to justify it to yourself and others if the patient succumbs?

3 Place two or three parallel sutures of 3/0 synthetic absorbable material on eyeless needles through all coats, passing in 1 cm proximal to the ulcer edge and emerging 1 cm distal to the ulcer (Fig. 16.4). Do not pick up the opposite wall as this will obstruct the lumen. When all the sutures are in place, mobilize a tongue of omentum, place it over the perforation and tie the sutures just tightly enough to hold it in place.

4 Insert further sutures to reinforce the obturating action of the omentum to ensure that it is adequately sealed. Even when closure seems secure, do not hesitate to suture omentum over it. Aspirate any free fluid from above and below the liver, from within the lesser sac, the right paracolic gutter and from the pelvis. Re-examine the closure and aspirate collection areas before closing. Do not insert a drain if the perforation was sutured without delay, if the closure is secure and peritoneal toilet was adequate.

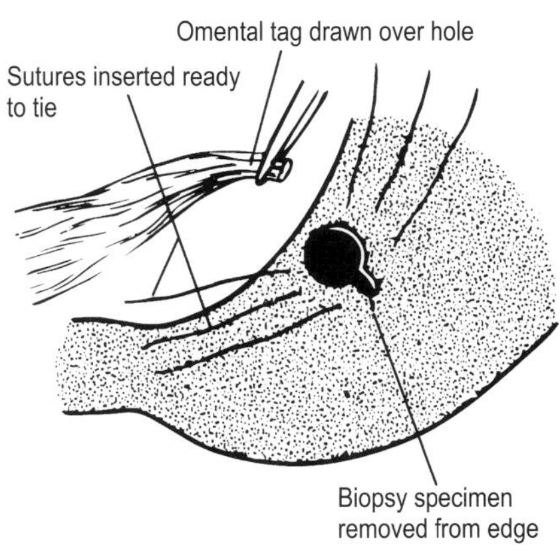

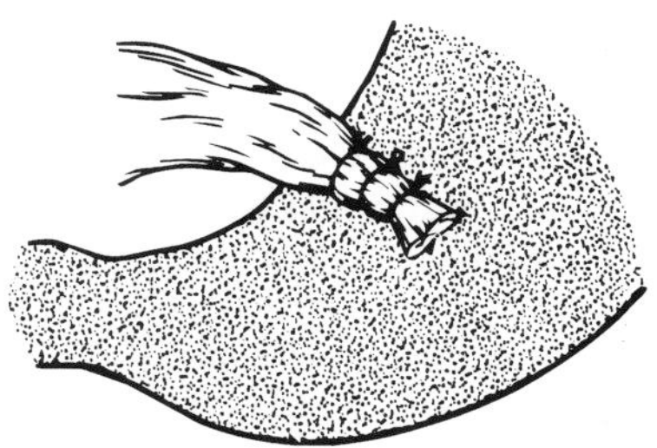

Fig. 16.4 Suture of a perforated peptic ulcer.

ELECTIVE SURGERY FOR PEPTIC ULCER

Medical treatment has become the mainstay with potent antacids, atropine-like drugs, liquorice extracts, mucosal-coating substances, histamine H_2-receptor-blocking drugs and H^+,K^+-ATPase inhibitors. The elimination of *Helicobacter pylori*, using so-called triple therapy of a proton-pump inhibitor combined with two antibiotics such as clarithromycin and metronidazole, reduces the relapse rate. Proximal gastric vagotomy, known also as highly selective vagotomy, is now rarely performed. Benign gastric ulcer was treated more aggressively, partial gastrectomy being advised if a 6–8-week course of medical treatment failed to heal the ulcer. Suspect Zollinger–Ellison syndrome associated with hypergastrinaemia, usually from G-cell hyperplasia or gastrin-secreting tumour in the pancreas, if peptic ulcers are multiple, or occur in unusual sites.

VAGOTOMY

The various types of vagotomy are now seldom used in the elective treatment of peptic ulceration, because of the success of medical treatment with antibiotics and potent antacids. Proximal gastric, or highly selective vagotomy is preferable to truncal vagotomy and 'drainage' because side-effects such as dumping and diarrhoea are fewer in incidence and less in severity.

Per-hiatal truncal vagotomy was formerly indicated for the management of uncomplicated duodenal ulcer when the full range of medical treatment had been tried and failed to control the symptoms. It is normally accompanied by pyloroplasty or gastroenterostomy to improve the rate of gastric emptying, so-called drainage procedures. Use a midline incision 20 cm long, skirting the umbilicus. Make sure there is a nasogastric tube in place, as a guide to the line of the gullet at the oesophageal hiatus, where you open the peritoneum and phreno-oesophageal ligament to reveal, mobilize and transect the anterior then the posterior vagal trunks (Fig. 16.5). Carry out the selected adjunctive procedure of pyloroplasty or gastroenterostomy.

Proximal gastric vagotomy aims to denervate only the acid-secreting proximal part of the stomach (Fig. 16.6) leaving the alkali-secreting antrum, with its muscular pumping action, still innervated. Use an upper midline or paramedian incision, skirting the umbilicus, 20 cm long. Separate the anterior and posterior nerves of Latarjet from the gastric lesser curve, extending from the hiatus to the gastric angulus. An adjunctive operation to improve gastric emptying is usually unnecessary.

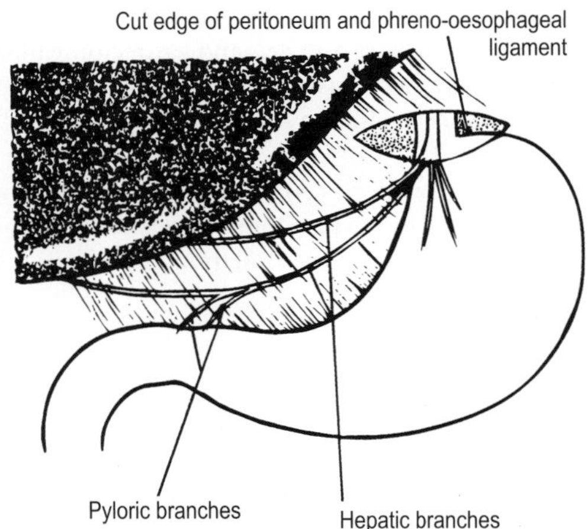

Fig. 16.5 Truncal vagotomy. Exposure of the anterior nerve; the distribution of the nerve is indicated.

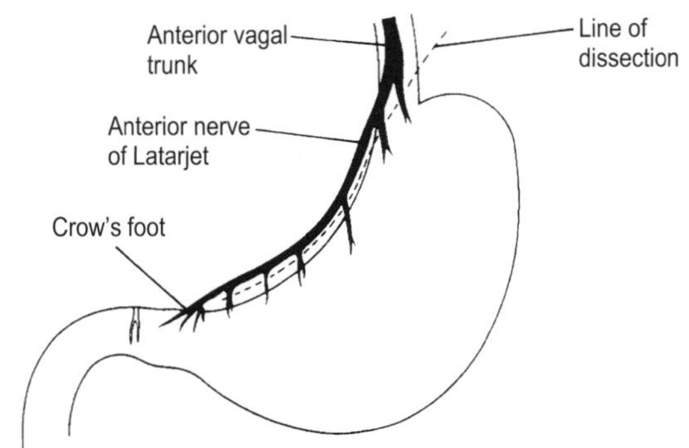

Fig. 16.6 Proximal gastric vagotomy. The anterior nerve of Latarjet, showing line of separation by dissection. The posterior nerve runs parallel to the anterior nerve.

PYLOROPLASTY

Re-formation of the pylorus has the effect of increasing the size of the lumen and also destroys the pyloric sphincteric metering function. It can be used to overcome stricture of the pylorus and also to improve gastric emptying following

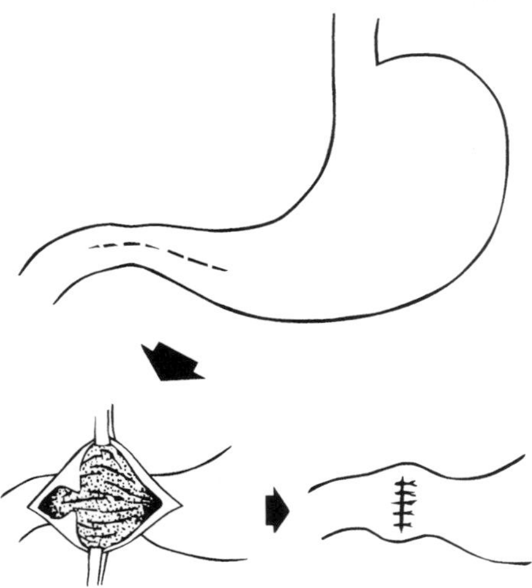

Fig. 16.7 Heineke–Mikulicz pyloroplasty; make a longitudinal incision, open it and close the defect as a transverse suture line.

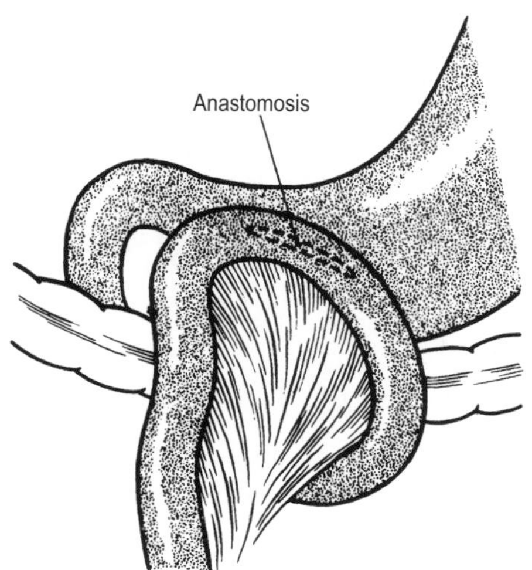

Fig. 16.8 Juxtapyloric anterior gastroenterostomy

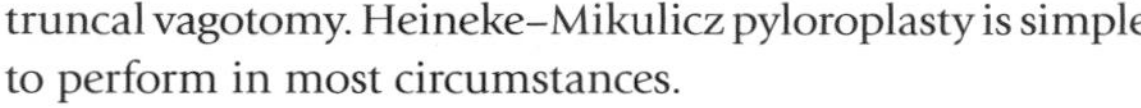

truncal vagotomy. Heineke–Mikulicz pyloroplasty is simple to perform in most circumstances.

Make a longitudinal incision through all coats starting on the anterior wall of the duodenal bulb, carried through the pylorus and on to the anterior gastric antral wall (Fig. 16.7). Gently apply tissue forceps to the middle of the upper and lower cut edges and draw them apart, allowing the proximal and distal limits of the incision to come together, transforming the longitudinal cut into a transverse slit, producing a shorter but wider passage. Close the incision.

GASTROENTEROSTOMY

Gastroenterostomy, originally applied to the relief of pyloric obstruction from distal gastric carcinoma, offers an important relief when gastrectomy cannot be carried out because the growth is locally too extensive or has already metastasized. Gastroenterostomy also relieves benign pyloric stenosis from duodenal ulceration and improves gastric emptying following truncal vagotomy. An advantage is that it can be disconnected if the patient develops subsequent postprandial symptoms (Fig. 16.8).

Through a right upper paramedian or midline incision 15 cm long explore the abdomen. If the patient proves to have extensive and inoperable carcinoma with no evidence of impending distal obstruction, carry out limited exploration only, but take a biopsy specimen.

Action

1. Pick up a longitudinal fold of anterior gastric wall and grasp it with one of Lane's twin clamps. Choose a fold as close to the pylorus as possible if this is for benign pyloric obstruction or accompanies vagotomy for ulcer. Choose a fold as high as possible if this is to bypass an unresectable distal gastric carcinoma.

2. Lift up the greater omentum and transverse colon to identify the duodenojejunal junction. Draw the first loop of jejunum up over the colon and greater omentum to the stomach, with the short but not taut afferent loop against the proximal part of the clamped gastric fold and the efferent loop against the distal end of the fold. Place the second twin clamp along the apposed bowel, avoiding the mesentery, to occlude the lumen but not the blood supply. Lock the clamps together and unite the adjacent gastric and jejunal walls with a running seromuscular stitch on an eyeless needle. Leave the ends long so that the stitch can be continued to encircle the anastomosis.

3. Open the stomach and jejunum parallel to the seromuscular stitch and 0.5 cm from it on each side, for 4–6 cm if this is for benign disease and for as long as possible if it is to bypass malignant obstruction. Apply fresh drapes to isolate the area and keep separate

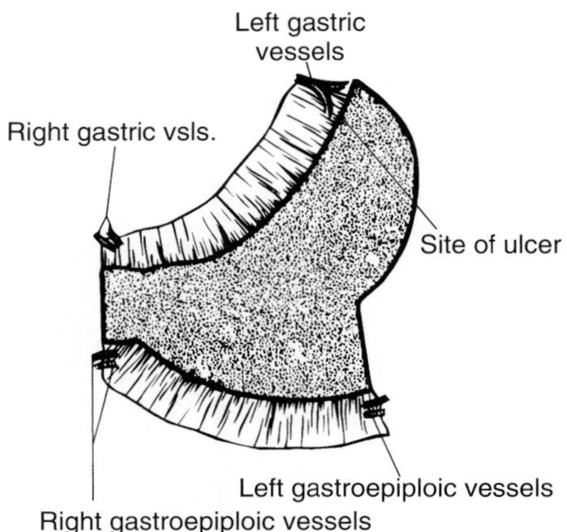

Fig. 16.9 Billroth I partial gastrectomy. The removed specimen.

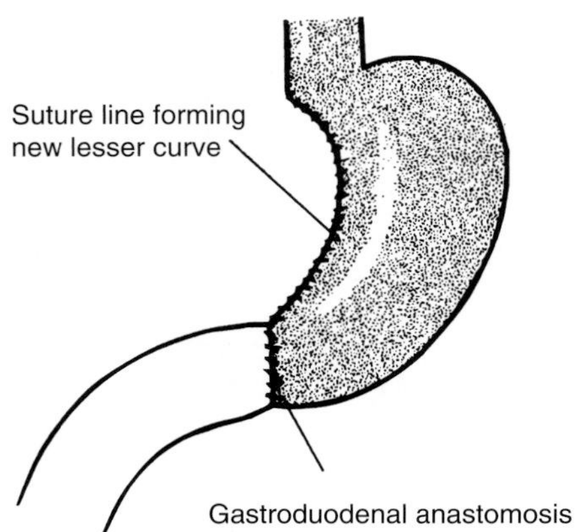

Fig. 16.10 Billroth I partial gastrectomy. The gastroduodenal anastomosis is complete, after re-forming the lesser curve of the stomach.

instruments during the next part of the operation when the potentially infected interior of the bowel will be exposed.

4 Unite the adjacent gastric and jejunal walls with a running all-coats stitch. Carry the stitch round the corner on to the anterior wall to complete the anastomosis. As the anterior gastric and jejunal walls are brought together, invert the edges. A Connell mattress stitch may be used as an alternative to the simple over-and-over stitch but take care that the blood vessels are picked up and tied along the edges since the Connell stitch is not haemostatic. Remove the twin clamps, discard and take sterile replacements for the soiled towels, instruments and gloves. Carry the seromuscular stitch round the end on to the anterior wall and complete it to encircle the anastomosis, burying the all-coats stitch. The anastomosis can be fashioned using a linear cutting staple device as an alternative to sutures.

5 Before closing make sure the anastomosis is patent, that there is no tension on the loop of jejunum and draw the transverse colon and greater omentum to the right so there is no weight of bowel to drag on the anastomosis.

BILLROTH I PARTIAL GASTRECTOMY

Billroth I gastrectomy was originally used to resect distal gastric carcinoma in 1881 but is now rarely used. The distal stomach is resected (Fig. 16.9) and the proximal remnant united to the duodenum (Fig. 16.10).

POLYA PARTIAL GASTRECTOMY

The most frequent indication for gastrectomy is distal gastric carcinoma. Prefer it to Billroth I gastrectomy because it allows the creation of a stoma the full width of the stomach and so is unlikely to obstruct if the tumour recurs. Since the duodenum is closed, this isolates it from distal spread as may occur if gastroduodenal anastomosis is used. The preferred method of resecting distal gastric carcinoma is by radical subtotal gastrectomy with Polya or Roux-en-Y reconstruction.

Assess

1 Explore the whole abdomen through a midline incision skirting the umbilicus, extending downwards from the xiphoid process for 20 cm. Ligate and divide the ligamentum teres and divide the falciform ligament.

2 If the operation is for carcinoma, start in the pelvis and lower abdomen, para-aortic region and root of the mesentery, proceeding to the liver before touching the stomach in order to avoid carrying malignant cells around the peritoneal cavity.

3 Carefully examine the stomach and duodenum to confirm the diagnosis and assess the strategy of the operation. If necessary, open the lesser omentum or gastrocolic omentum to examine the posterior wall of

the stomach and contents of the lesser sac, including the glands around the coeliac axis and along the superior border of the pancreas.

Resect

Benign disease

1 Make a hole in an avascular area of the gastrocolic omentum to the left of the gastroepiploic vascular arch. Identify the posterior gastric wall and separate it from the pancreas and transverse mesocolon.

2 Clamp in sections, divide and ligate the gastrocolic omentum, extending on the left up to and including the main left gastroepiploic vessels and the first one or two short gastric vessels. Avoid damaging the spleen directly or by exerting heavy traction on the stomach. To the right, divide and ligate the main right gastroepiploic vessels as they lie near the inferior border of the pylorus. The separation of this vascular tissue can be accomplished rapidly using a stapling device which places two clips across the tissue and cuts between them in a single action. Identify to avoid damaging the middle colic vessels, which lie within 1 cm of the right gastroepiploic vessels. Clamp, divide and ligate the right gastric vessels after identifying and isolating them as they run to the left in the lesser omentum just above the duodenal bulb and pylorus. Divide the lesser omentum proximally, if possible preserving an accessory hepatic artery if one is present.

3 Free the first 1–2 cm of duodenum after applying fine artery forceps on the small vessels posteriorly, dividing and ligating them with fine ligatures. Divide with a linear stapler or Payr's clamp across the duodenum just beyond the pylorus. Place a second clamp just proximal to this to occlude the stomach. If there is insufficient room for this, apply a non-crushing clamp across the distal stomach. Transect the duodenum just above the distal Payr clamp, ensuring that no gastric mucosa remains attached to the duodenum. Cover the cut distal stomach with a swab. Dissect the duodenum free for 2–3 cm so that it can be safely closed, applying fine forceps and ligatures to the vessels, keeping close to the duodenal wall. The common bile duct lies near the posterior and superior parts of the proximal duodenum and may be drawn out of its normal relationship by scar tissue. The gastroduodenal artery runs close to the medial wall of the duodenum.

4 Close the duodenal stump as a rule using a linear stapling device. This places a double row of staples across the duodenum. Apply it just distal to the pylorus in place of the Payr's crushing clamp and place a proximal clamp across the distal stomach. Activate the stapling device to staple and seal the duodenum and transect this with a scalpel applied closely to the upper edge of the stapler. Alternatively, close the distal stomach and duodenal stump with a mechanical stapler which inserts two double staggered rows of staples and simultaneously cuts and divides the tissues between the rows (Autosuture GIA). It is wise to invaginate or reinforce the everted staple line with a layer of sutures.

5 Alternatively close the duodenal stump with sutures. First use a running over-and-over spiral stitch that encircles the clamp and the enclosed crushed duodenum. Gently ease out the clamp, tightening the stitches seriatim as it is withdrawn. Tie the stitch. Insert a second invaginating seromuscular suture to cover the first stitch line or insert a purse-string suture and invaginate the first suture line as it is tightened and tied. If possible, insert a third stitch that picks up and draws together the ligated right gastric and right gastroepiploic vessel stumps, the anterior duodenal wall and the peritoneum over the head of the pancreas. Exert a little tension on the left gastric vessels by elevating the pyloric end of the stomach. Identify the artery by feeling for the pulsations. Isolate the vessels from the lesser curve of the stomach, doubly clamp, divide and ligate them.

6 Select the line for the transection of the stomach. When Polya gastrectomy was the standard operation for duodenal ulcer, a two-thirds gastrectomy was usually carried out. Ask the anaesthetist to withdraw the nasogastric tube until the tip lies above the line of transection.

Malignant disease

Radical subtotal gastrectomy is described later, but non-radical partial gastrectomy is appropriate in frail patients and in those who have a resectable carcinoma but already have metastatic deposits in the liver or elsewhere which make radical resection impossible. It may not be possible to be sure that the distal resection is clear of growth but always ensure that the proximal line of resection is well clear of growth. Aim at a minimum of 5 cm apparently tumour-free margin. If the resection line cuts through tumour, the anastomotic line may break down during recovery from the operation. If it does not do so, recurrent tumour at the anastomosis may soon obstruct the lumen. It is useless to carry the line of resection widely beyond the stomach, so adopt the same technique as for resection for benign disease. Plan to provide a full-width gastroenterostomy to guard against recurrent tumour causing obstruction.

Unite

1 Place one of the twin gastroenterostomy clamps across the stomach 2 cm above the proposed line of transection, from greater to lesser curve. Place a long non-crushing clamp across the stomach 3 cm distal to the twin clamp and parallel to it. The stomach will be transected just above this clamp. Fold the distal part of the stomach upwards. Reach down and identify the duodenojejunal junction. Draw up to the stomach the first loop of jejunum, with afferent loop to the lesser curve, with no slack but not tight. The efferent loop is placed at the greater curve. Place the second of the twin clamps across this loop of bowel, occluding only the lumen and not the mesentery. Marry and lock the clamps together. Run a continuous seromuscular stitch to unite the adjacent gastric and jejunal walls.

2 Incise the full width of the posterior gastric wall 0.5 cm above the clamp, taking care at this time to leave the anterior wall intact. Make a parallel incision in the jejunum, 0.5 cm from the seromuscular suture line. Join the adjacent gastric and jejunal edges with an all-coats stitch on an eyeless needle. Now cut through the anterior wall of the stomach 1 cm distal to the clamp and remove the specimen of distal stomach. Continue the all-coats stitch round on to the anterior wall and along it to completely encircle the anastomosis.

3 Remove the clamps, discard and take sterile replacements of the towels, gloves and instruments. Complete the seromuscular suture line on to the anterior wall to encircle the anastomosis (Fig. 16.11).

4 Before closing, check the anastomosis, the main vascular ligatures, mesocolon and middle colic vessels, the spleen, the duodenal closure and aspirate any blood from under the cupolas of the diaphragm and the subhepatic space. Draw the greater omentum, transverse colon and mesocolon through to the right so there is no weight of colon resting on the anastomosis.

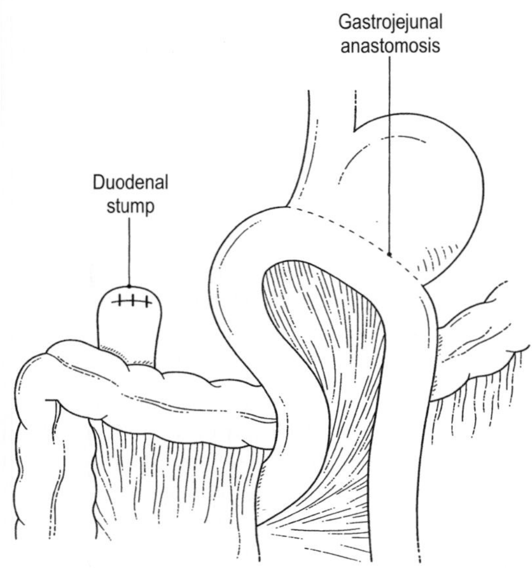

Fig. 16.11 Polya partial gastrectomy. The full-width antecolic gastrojejunal anastomosis, with afferent loop joined to lesser curve, is complete. The duodenal stump is closed.

Technical points

The inside of the stomach and bowel are infected with microorganisms. While fashioning anastomoses, isolate the interior of the bowel from the peritoneal cavity and wound edges by using separate towels, instruments and gloves. When the bowel is repaired, discard and replace them with sterile gloves, towels and instruments.

The gastroenterostomy can be accomplished using stapling devices.

GASTRODUODENAL BLEEDING

Bleeding is the most life-threatening complication of peptic ulcer and demands management by experienced clinicians, endoscopists and surgeons acting as a team, who achieve the best survival. Remember that more than 80% of gastrointestinal bleeding stops spontaneously, but also remember that you do not know which 80%.

Erosive bleeding sometimes complicates bleeding elsewhere, sepsis, burns, head injury and major trauma. Drugs such as steroids and non-steroidal anti-inflammatory drugs (NSAIDs) can cause erosive and ulcer bleeding as can alcoholic acute gastritis, and retching from this and Mallory–Weiss tears around the cardia. For this reason take a careful history, asking specific questions about drugs.

Assess the patient's general condition so that you can carry out appropriate resuscitation. Check the blood haemoglobin and haematocrit, and exclude clotting deficiencies if suspected. In appropriate circumstances have blood cross-matched. Routinely give intravenous omeprazole or an equivalent proton-pump inhibitor. Do not make a once-and-for-all assessment but carefully monitor the patient thereafter. Remember that mortality is highest among the over-60s, those with massive haemorrhage and shock, and those with serious associated disease.

Carry out endoscopy as soon as possible to determine the cause, site, state and number of lesions. Look for continuing bleeding and the presence of visible vessels which indicate that the bleeding is likely to continue or recur. Even if you cannot identify the source you can usually exonerate particular areas, for example excluding oesophageal varices. Experts have a range of methods of haemostasis deliverable through the endoscope.

Relative indications for operation when other methods of control have failed are continuing bleeding which fails to respond to other measures, bleeding that recurs, patient more than 60 years old, gastric ulcer bleeding and cardiovascular disease patients, who do not withstand hypotension well. This makes it dangerous to defer operation if bleeding is serious and not controllable.

Always have an endoscope available in the operating theatre, even when the diagnosis seems certain and be willing to perform endoscopy in case of doubt when anaesthesia is induced, if only to exclude possible causes, including multiple sites. Although exploratory laparotomy allows access to the abdomen, the exterior of the gut is exposed, not the interior, where the cause lies.

Bleeding duodenal ulcer is preferably treated at present by pyloroplasty or duodenotomy, and suture of the bleeding vessels. Vagotomy is now usually omitted in favour of postoperative medical treatment of the ulcer.

GASTRIC CARCINOMA

At present, the best hope of cure is early diagnosis and radical resection. Gastric carcinoma is usually resistant to radiation therapy, but responses to chemotherapy are improving. In Japan a high proportion of early cancers are detected by screening or open-access endoscopy and are successfully treated by surgery. Endoscopy with cytology and biopsy is the best method of screening and diagnosis. It is valuable in detecting early gastric cancer. The ability to determine the extent of the tumour before operation saves many patients from fruitless exploratory laparotomy. Careful, mainly Japanese studies demonstrate the sequential spread of cancer from various sites in the stomach to the lymph nodes. Local nodes within 3 cm of the primary tumour are designated N_1, the next nodes to be affected are N_2, the third tier is N_3 and distant spread is N_4. En bloc resection of the tumour with the N_1 nodes is designated a D_1 resection, with the N_1 and N_2 nodes a D_2 resection. D_2 resection is the standard procedure. On occasion a D_3 resection may be performed, incorporating the N_3 nodes.

Removal of the primary tumour is valuable even when the growth has spread beyond the limits of radical resection. When resection is impracticable, try to relieve existing or impending obstruction.

D_2 RADICAL ABDOMINAL SUBTOTAL AND TOTAL GASTRECTOMY

Radical resection for localized carcinoma of the distal stomach (subtotal) resembles radical total gastrectomy except that a fringe of proximal stomach is retained, which should be 5 cm clear of detectable tumour; this allows gastrojejunostomy to be accomplished through the abdomen. It is carried out on patients who have no evident involvement of the peritoneum distant from the tumour or of N_3 and N_4 nodes. Any local invasion of contiguous structures must be resectable with the stomach, such as proximal duodenum, a segment of small bowel, transverse colon, pancreas, liver lobe or parietal wall.

If radical resection cannot encompass all the detectable growth, carry out a more modest palliative resection if possible. Ensure that the resection margin is well clear of growth, because a resection that does not protect the patient against stomal recurrence and obstruction is not worth carrying out. If there are extensive metastases, even palliative resection is probably inappropriate. Bypass existing or impending pyloric obstruction with proximal gastroenterostomy.

Assess

Through a long vertical midline incision skirting the umbilicus, or a paramedian incision, first note any ascites and peritoneal deposits. Do not immediately palpate the stomach but start your complete exploration from the pelvis and work towards the stomach to avoid dispersing malignant cells. Now draw the omentum caudally to examine the upper compartment. Feel both lobes of the liver and adjacent diaphragm and the other structures. This part of the examination cannot be exact – repeat it as the dissection allows. If you are seriously in doubt whether to proceed, incise the lesser omentum in an avascular area near the liver and examine the coeliac axis and emerging arteries and assess the spread across the lesser sac and also perform Kocher's manoeuvre in order to palpate the head of pancreas.

Resect

The sequence of involvement of lymph node tiers is dependent on the site of the tumour (Fig. 16.12). Total gastrectomy includes the gastric fundus and cardia.

Unite

Following subtotal gastrectomy draw up a loop of proximal jejunum in exactly the same manner as following Polya gastrectomy for benign disease. The anastomosis can be made using sutures or a combined linear stapling and cutting device. Alternatively, use a Roux-en-Y method of reconstruction, which spares some patients the discomfort of bilious vomiting.

Following total gastrectomy, oesophagojejunostomy is preferably performed using a Roux-en-Y jejunal loop (see Ch. 17). Transect the jejunum close to the ligament of Treitz and divide sufficient primary vascular arcades to allow the distal portion to be taken up to the oesophagus. Transect the bowel beyond the duodenojejunal junction and join the cut proximal end into the side of the Roux loop 50 cm downstream. If you will create a sutured oesophagojejunal anastomosis, close the end of the jejunum in two layers, or staple it. Lead the loop up to the oesophagus posterior to the transverse mesocolon avoiding tension or twisting. Insert a posterior running suture line of Lembert stitches joining the posterior wall of the oesophagus to the posterior wall of the Roux loop about 5 cm from the closed end. Now transect the oesophagus below the suture line and remove the specimen.

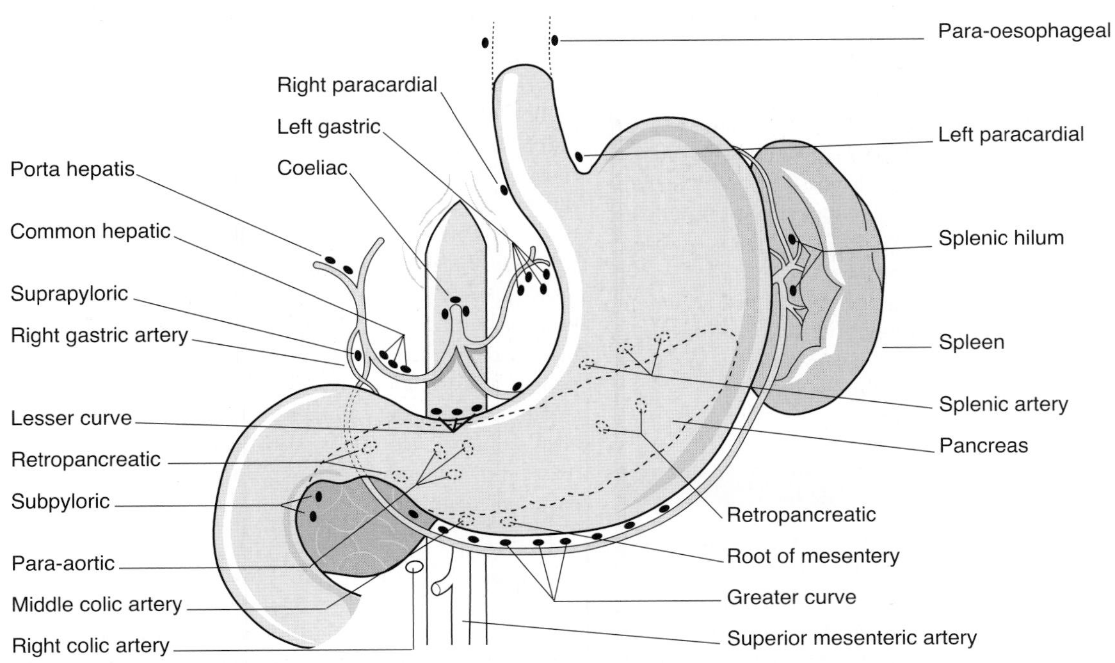

Fig. 16.12 The lymph nodes likely to be involved by gastric carcinoma.

RADICAL THORACOABDOMINAL TOTAL GASTRECTOMY

Never embark upon this operation without first obtaining a tissue diagnosis with endoscopic biopsy or cytology or frozen-section histology at operation. Never embark upon it without making every effort by preoperative and operative assessment to exclude metastatic tumour. As a rule, this is a radical operation undertaken for carcinoma of the proximal stomach or cardia which can apparently be totally encompassed by this major resection of the stomach, lower oesophagus, omenta, spleen, body and tail of the pancreas, with all the primary lymph nodes and the next tier, completing a D_2 resection.

Accomplish it through a left thoracoabdominal incision (Fig. 16.13). The specimen is shown in Figure 16.14 and the union is shown in Figure 16.15. It can be carried out through an upper midline abdominal incision only if the upper stomach is free of growth and in that case it is merely an extension of radical partial gastrectomy to include the upper fringe of stomach in the resection. Transabdominal total gastrectomy is usually contraindicated, except in very thin patients, if the growth extends proximally to within 2–3 cm of the gastro-oesophageal junction since at least a 3-cm segment of apparently uninvolved lower oesophagus should be resected.

ZOLLINGER–ELLISON SYNDROME

The classic syndrome consists of severe, intractable, sometimes multiple peptic ulcer developing as a rule in expected sites but sometimes distally in the duodenum and proximal jejunum, associated with gastric acid hypersecretion of marked degree. The syndrome is caused by a gastrin-

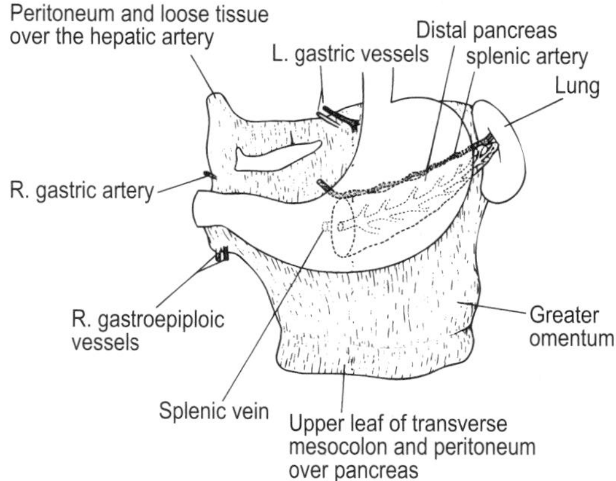

Fig. 16.14 Radical total gastrectomy. The resected specimen.

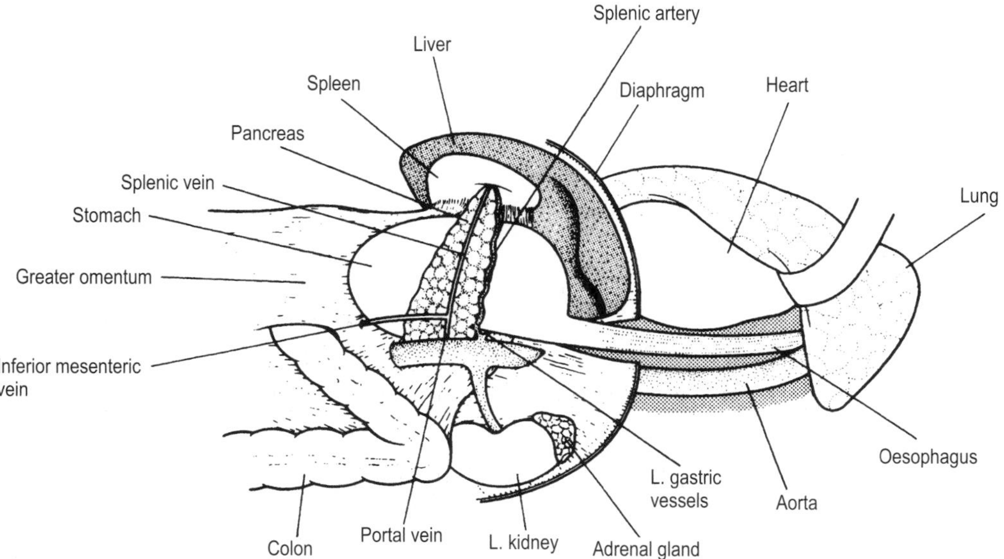

Fig. 16.13 Through a left thoracoabdominal incision the diaphragm has been incised. The spleen, splenic vessels and body and tail of the pancreas have been elevated, together with the greater curve of the stomach.

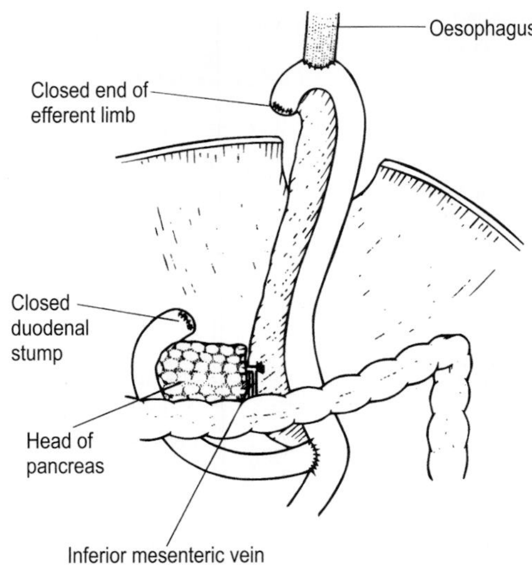

Fig. 16.15 Radical total gastrectomy. The oesophagojejunal anastomosis is complete, using a Roux loop of jejunum taken behind the mesocolon. The duodenal bulb is closed, and duodenal loop is joined end-to-side to the jejunum.

secreting tumour of the pancreatic islets which may be benign or malignant, or there may be hyperplasia without tumour formation (see Ch. 24). The serum gastrin is raised and appears to act as a trophic hormone acting on gastric parietal cells which undergo hyperplasia. It is part of a multiple endocrine neoplastic (MEN) syndrome in a quarter of cases, the parathyroid glands being particularly frequently involved.

FURTHER READING

Akiyama H 1979 Thoracoabdominal approach for carcinoma of the cardia of the stomach. American Journal of Surgery 137:345–349

Allum WH, Griffin SM, Watson A et al on behalf of the Association of Upper Gastrointestinal Surgeons of Great Britain and Ireland, the British Society of Gastroenterology, and the British Association of Surgical Oncology 2002 Guidelines for the management of oesophageal and gastric cancer. Gut 50(Suppl V):v1–v23

So JBY, Yam A, Cheah WK et al 2000 Risk factors related to operative mortality and morbidity in patients undergoing emergency gastrectomy. British Journal of Surgery 87:1702–1707

17

Small bowel

R. C. N. Williamson, L. R. Jiao

CONTENTS

EXAMINATION OF THE SMALL BOWEL

Diverticula

Meckel's diverticulum is considered below. Acquired diverticula may affect the duodenum, jejunum and to a lesser extent the ileum, and are frequently multiple. Do not remove incidental diverticula, but excise localized groups if they are causing symptoms, such as pain or bleeding.

Inflammation

Crohn's disease may affect any part of the alimentary canal but especially the terminal ileum. Affected segments of bowel are inflamed, thickened, narrowed, often covered with fibrinous exudate, with thickened mesentery encroaching on the circumference of the bowel; adjacent lymph nodes are enlarged; tuberculous and yersinial infection can produce similar changes. Coeliac disease particularly affects the jejunum, indicated by dilated subserous and mesenteric lymphatics, thinning and pigmentation of the bowel wall and splenic atrophy and confirmed by full-thickness biopsy. Small-bowel ulcers and strictures may occur spontaneously or follow either radiotherapy, transient strangulation in an external hernia or the ingestion of potassium tablets.

Infarction

Check the viability of the small bowel after reducing a strangulated hernia or untwisting of a volvulus. Excise frankly necrotic or perforated loops. If the viability is in doubt, return it to the abdomen and wait for 5 minutes (timed by the clock). The return of a shiny, pink appearance, pulsation of the mesenteric vessels (or bleeding if pricked) and peristalsis across the affected segment indicate viability. If you are still in doubt, resect. Carefully invaginate constriction rings with interrupted seromuscular sutures.

Tumours

Serosal deposits occur in carcinomatosis peritonei and may cause kinking and obstruction of the small bowel, requiring side-to-side bypass. Primary neoplasms are less common. Benign tumours include adenoma, leiomyoma, lipoma and Peutz–Jeghers hamartomas; they can cause intussusception. Carcinoid tumours favour the ileum, but may be multiple and metastasizing; they are hard with a yellowish cut surface. Malignant tumours comprise adenocarcinoma, lymphoma and leiomyosarcoma in that order of prevalence. Excise primary neoplasms or, if irresectable, bypass and biopsy them. Biopsy of duodenal lesions can be performed with fibreoptic endoscopy, and enteroscopy is also available.

INTESTINAL ANASTOMOSIS

Intestinal anastomoses heal rapidly but leakage of intestinal contents into the peritoneal cavity is potentially lethal. Most of the intestinal canal is contaminated with bacteria, especially towards the distal end. Take appropriate precautions against disseminating faecal organisms (Ch. 7) before dividing and re-suturing the bowel; clamps are usually indicated to prevent faecal spillage. Postoperative abscess formation is likely to impair anastomotic healing.

Ensure that the bowel ends are pink and bleeding freely, and leave the mesentery attached to the bowel right up to the point of intestinal transection. Excise bruised or dusky ends.

Tension, usually resulting from inadequate mobilization, stretches the mesenteric vessels and distracts the bowel ends. Avoid twisting of the mesentery and as a rule repair mesenteric/mesocolic defects after completing an intestinal anastomosis to prevent postoperative internal herniation; but take care not to injure the supplying vessels.

Distended loops of bowel are heavy, difficult to handle, thin-walled, somewhat ischaemic, with impaired healing. Decompress it by milking contents upwards into the reach of the nasogastric tube or by enterotomy and insertion of a sucker.

Hand-suturing techniques

Bowel is traditionally united in two layers, using absorbable suture material such as polyglactin 910 for the inner, all-coats layers and an outer stitch, named after its inventor in 1826, the Parisian surgeon Antoine Lembert (1802–1851), to join the seromuscular layers. One-layered anastomosis can sometimes be achieved. The best suture material, type of stitch, number of layers and best methods of fashioning a suture are disputed; they are less important than achieving accurate and tension-free coaptation of two healthy mucosal surfaces. As an assistant, follow the method of your present chief; as you pass through rotations you thus experience a number of methods from which to select for yourself.

If you anticipate impaired healing, as in Crohn's disease, consider using an inner layer of continuous polyglactin 910 (Vicryl) and an outer layer of interrupted silk to provide added security. Non-absorbable sutures are usually indicated when joining small bowel or colon to the oesophagus, pancreas or rectum; suitable materials include silk (2/0 or 3/0), polypropylene (Prolene), monofilament nylon and stainless-steel wire.

Whichever type of suture and suture material you employ, take care to achieve the correct degree of tension when pulling through and tying the stitch. Insert each stitch separately and invert the bowel edges as you tighten the suture. Once the bowel edge is inverted, prevent the suture material from slipping by getting your assistant to follow up. Alternatively, follow up yourself, using the taut suture as a means of steadying the bowel against the thrust of the needle. The objective is a snug, water-tight anastomosis. Excessive tension risks strangulating the bowel incorporated in the stitch and perhaps causing subsequent leakage.

Do not place the sutures so close to the edge of the bowel that they might tear out, or so deep that they turn in an enormous cuff of tissue and narrow the bowel; usually 3–5 mm is about the correct depth of 'bite'. Be sure that the all-coats suture does in fact incorporate all coats of the bowel wall. The muscularis tends to retract and may escape being sutured, especially posteriorly. The best way to master these important technical points is to assist at, and then perform under supervision, a number of intestinal anastomoses.

The seromuscular stitch unites the adjacent bowel walls outside the all-coats stitch. Sometimes the posterior seromuscular layer is inserted before opening the gut, as in side-to-side anastomoses. After the all-coats stitches have been inserted, carry the seromuscular sutures round the ends of the anastomosis and across the front wall, ultimately encircling the anastomosis so that the all-coats stitches can no longer be seen. For end-to-end anastomoses in small and large intestine it may be simpler to complete the all-coats layer before placing any Lembert sutures. Thereafter, the seromuscular layer can be inserted all the way round by rotating the bowel.

The all-coats stitch is accepted as the paramount stitch for holding bowel edges, since it catches the strong submucosa. There are many ways of inserting these stitches; three popular methods are described here:

- *Continuous over-and-over suture.* Approximate the two edges of cut bowel. Starting at one end, insert a corner stitch from outside to in, then over the adjacent edges of bowel and out through the other corner. Tie the suture and clip the short end. Pass the stitch back through the nearest bowel wall, over the contiguous cut edges and back through the full thickness of both walls. Continue over-and-over stitches to the opposite corner (Fig. 17.1a). After the last stitch is inserted right into the corner, take it back through the nearest corner leaving a loop on the mucosa so that the stitch emerges from the outer wall of the bowel (Fig. 17.1b). Now sew the front walls together by passing the stitch over and over, from out to in and then from in to out (Fig. 17.1c). Continue until the anastomosis has been encircled and

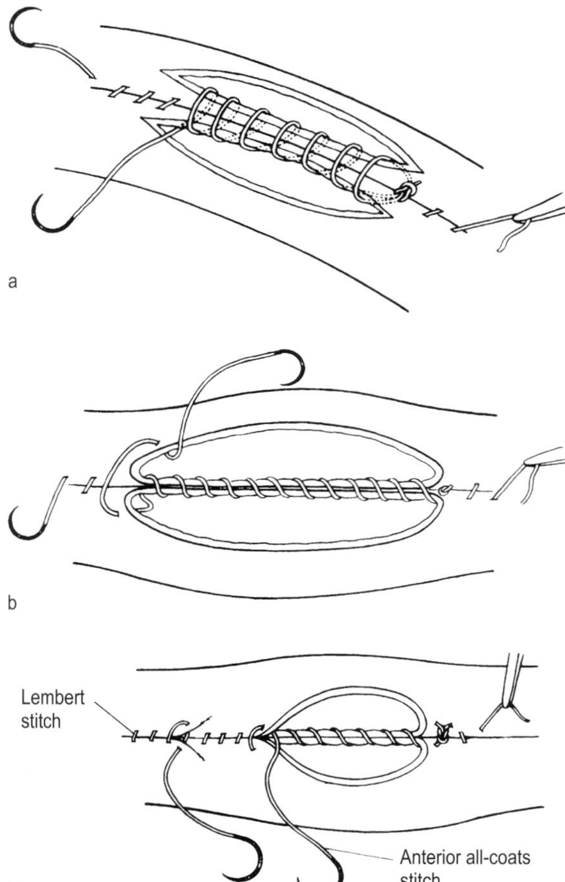

Fig. 17.1 Continuous over-and-over stitch. (a) The all-coats stitch is being inserted in a continuous over-and-over fashion. Care is taken to include mucosa and muscularis in each bite. (b) The all-coats stitch is continued round the corner. A single loop-on-the-mucosa stitch starts the return over-and-over stitch. (c) The anterior all-coats stitch is continued, then the anterior seromuscular stitch completes the anastomosis.

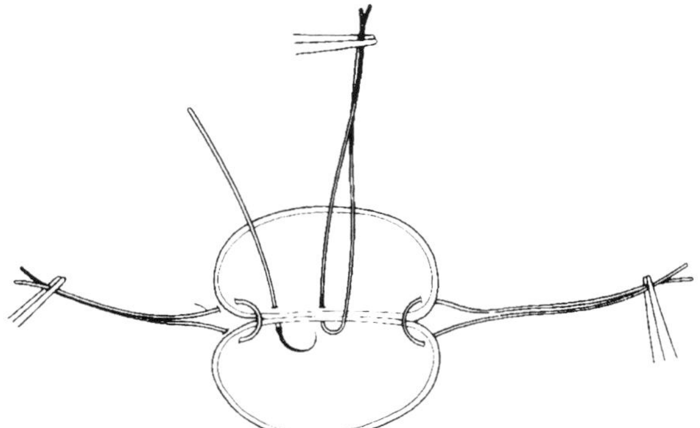

Fig. 17.2 End-to-end anastomosis using interrupted sutures. The two corner stitches are tied with the knots on the outside, but for the remainder of the posterior wall the knots are placed on the inside. If access is restricted, each suture is inserted and held in a clip before any one is tied (as shown).

the edges inverted, then tie off the ends of suture material. This over-and-over stitch is haemostatic.

- *Continuous over-and-over plus Connell suture.* Commence in the middle of the posterior wall by placing a stitch between the adjacent cut edges of bowel and tying it on the luminal surface. Now continue towards one corner with over-and-over stitches. At the corner the needle passes from in to out on the nearside cut surface, then crosses to the far edge and is passed in and out to leave a loop on the mucosa. The needle returns to the near edge and another loop-on-the-mucosa stitch (named after the American surgeon Gregory Connell born 1875, who popularized it) is inserted. They turn the corner neatly. Once you are round the corner, leave this stitch and return to the middle of the posterior wall. Use a new length of suture material, unless there is a needle at each end of the original length. Insert and tie a stitch close to the site of the original ligature, tie the two short ends of suture material and proceed towards the opposite corner, using Connell sutures to negotiate the corner again. Either continue with Connell stitches along the anterior wall from each end or return to over-and-over stitches once you are round the corners. Tie off the ends of suture material in the middle of the anterior wall. The Connell stitch is not fully haemostatic, so secure all bleeding points.
- *Interrupted suture.* Insert a stitch from out to in and in to out at each corner. If the anastomosis is easily accessible, tie each stitch at this stage. Clip the ends of suture material and get your assistant to hold the clips to exert traction on the posterior cut edges of bowel (Fig. 17.2). Insert a row of posterior sutures 2–3 mm apart, tying the knots on the luminal surface. If the anastomosis is relatively inaccessible, avoid tying any sutures until the entire posterior row has been inserted. Then approximate the bowel ends and tie the sutures snugly and in

order, proceeding from one corner to the next. Now place an anterior row of interrupted sutures. It is easier to tie the knots on the outside at this stage, and inversion does not appear to be essential. Indeed, some surgeons practise edge-to-edge or eversion techniques routinely for intestinal anastomosis, preferring not to turn in a ridge of tissue that might obstruct the lumen.

Mechanical stapling techniques

Stapling machines are now available to carry out most types of gastrointestinal anastomosis. Disposable and angled instruments are available for use in particular circumstances, and the metal staples come in different lengths to accommodate the different tissue thicknesses encountered. For end-to-end anastomosis (e.g. colorectal, oesophagojejunal) the stapling gun (Fig. 17.3a) is introduced into the intestinal lumen downstream, brought out through the distal cut end of bowel and then insinuated into the proximal cut end.

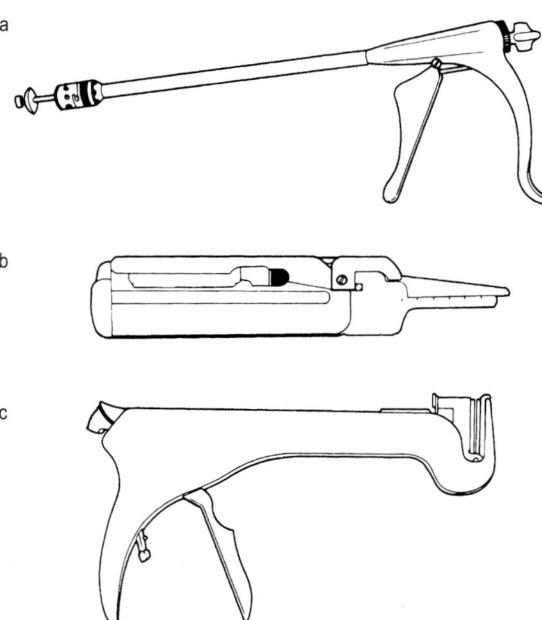

Fig. 17.3 Autosuture instruments used for gastrointestinal anastomosis: (a) model EEA is for end-to-side anastomosis; (b) model GIA is for side-to-side anastomosis; (c) model TA30 is for closing off the end of the bowel.

Choose the largest anvil that will fit comfortably into the proximal lumen. Tightly snug the proximal and distal gut around the central rod using purse-string sutures, and then approximate the anvil to the cartridge by closing the instrument. When the gun is fired, a circular double row of stainless-steel staples is inserted and at the same time a complete 5-mm rim of each bowel end (the 'doughnut') is resected. Withdraw the machine and check the 'doughnuts' to confirm that they are complete and that the anastomosis is perfect.

For side-to-side anastomosis use a different instrument, resembling a pair of scissors (Fig. 17.3b). One 'blade' is inserted into each of the two intestinal segments to be united, and the blades are closed. Firing the gun advances a knife, which divides the adjacent surfaces of bowel between two parallel rows of staples.

Yet another set of instruments has been designed to place a double row of staples across the end of a segment of intestine or stomach (Fig. 17.3c). The staple line can be 30, 55 or 90 mm long. After firing the staples, leave the instrument attached and use it as an anvil on which to transect the gut. Some surgeons prefer to bury the staple line with a continuous Lembert suture.

KEY POINTS Stapled anastomosis

- Using a mechanical stapler does not guarantee a perfect result. It is just as important to prepare healthy bowel ends and avoid tension as it is in hand-sewn anastomoses, and a different set of technical details has to be learnt.
- Sutures are more versatile than staples. As a trainee, take every opportunity to practise perfect stitching.

Stapling machines reduce the time involved in fashioning an anastomosis and facilitate certain operations that can be difficult to complete by hand, such as oesophageal transection, oesophagogastrectomy (Fig. 17.4) or low anterior resection of the rectum. The introduction of disposable stapling guns obviates the need for careful maintenance of the reusable instrument and may reduce the substantial costs involved in mechanical stapling. On the other hand, there are many situations where the stapler is inappropriate such as choledochojejunostomy, or unnecessary as in most small-bowel anastomoses.

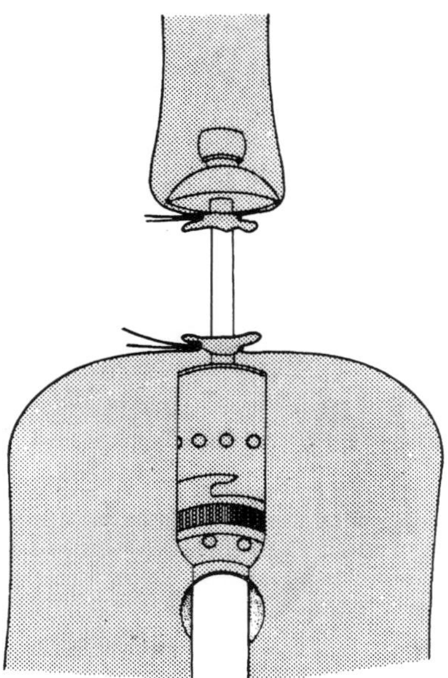

Fig. 17.4 Oesophagogastric anastomosis, using the EEA stapling gun inserted through a small gastrotomy. After tying each purse-string suture around the central rod, the anvil is approximated to the cartridge and the staples are discharged.

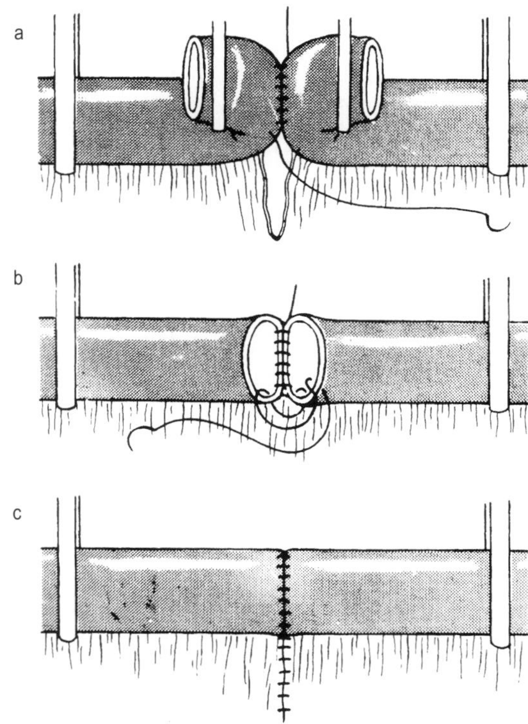

Fig. 17.5 End-to-end intestinal anastomosis: (a) and (b) two layers of stitches being inserted; (c) the completed anastomosis with the mesentery repaired.

Types of anastomosis

End-to-end anastomosis

This is the simplest way of restoring intestinal continuity after partial enterectomy and/or colectomy. After removal of the resected specimen, clean and approximate the bowel ends. The anastomosis is usually created in two layers, using a continuous absorbable suture (e.g. 2/0 or 3/0 Vicryl) swaged on to an eyeless needle (Fig. 17.5).

Insert the all-coats stitch, using one of the techniques described above or a variant that you have been shown. Remove the intestinal clamps and check that the anastomosis is airtight and watertight by gently squeezing intestinal contents across it. Now insert the circumferential seromuscular stitch, taking care not to turn in too thick a cuff of tissue. Make sure the thumb and forefinger can invaginate bowel wall on each side through the anastomosis. Some surgeons prefer to unite the bowel ends with a posterior layer of Lembert sutures before embarking on the all-coats stitch, but we resort to this manoeuvre with end-to-end anastomosis only if we anticipate subsequent difficulty in placing the posterior seromuscular layer. Lastly, unite the cut edges of mesentery and/or mesocolon on each aspect with interrupted Vicryl sutures, taking care to avoid damaging the vessels.

Oblique anastomosis

When the ends of bowel are disproportionate in size, they may be matched by incising the antimesenteric border of the narrow bowel longitudinally.

This manoeuvre is useful in joining obstructed bowel to collapsed bowel or ileum to colon. In neonates with congenital intestinal atresia, the lumen of the distal bowel is particularly narrow and this type of 'end-to-back' anastomosis is necessitated. The mesentery of the proximal bowel is also disproportionately big and should be shortened with a few gathering stitches before being united to the distal cut edge of mesentery. When two segments of narrow intestine must be united, they may both be opened along their antimesenteric borders, which are then joined

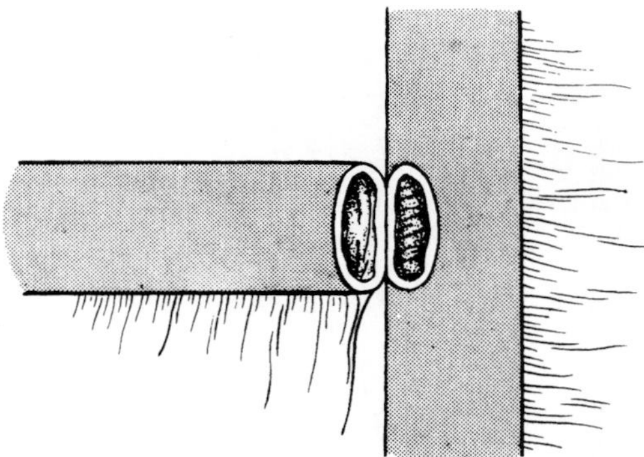

Fig. 17.6 End-to-side anastomosis.

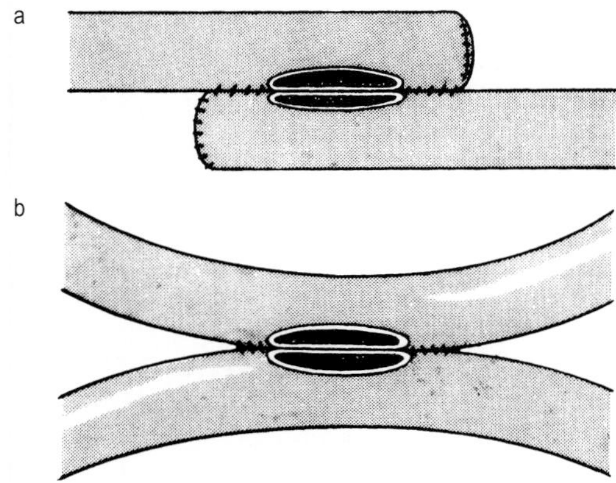

Fig. 17.7 Side-to-side anastomoses: (a) after transection of the bowel, with closure of each end; (b) two segments are joined without dividing the bowel.

back-to-back. The mesenteries are now on opposite sides of the anastomosis and cannot always be neatly approximated. Poth has described an elegant variant of this technique, in which the end of the larger segment is sutured to the end-to-lateral aspect of the smaller segment of bowel.

End-to-side anastomosis

This is most commonly used when creating a Roux-en-Y anastomosis. Approximate the cut end to the side of bowel to which it will be joined and insert a posterior seromuscular suture (Fig. 17.6).

Incise the antimesenteric border of the side of bowel to accommodate the cut end. Insert the all-coats stitch as before, remove the clamps and complete the seromuscular stitch. Lastly, join the cut edge of mesentery to the side of the intact mesentery.

Side-to-side anastomosis

This can be used to joint two loops of bowel without resection, or to unite intestine to stomach, bile duct, etc. (Fig. 17.7).

It may also be employed as an alternative to end-to-end anastomosis after intestinal resection, in which case the cut ends of bowel should first be closed and invaginated. The advantages of the side-to-side anastomosis are that the segments of bowel to be united have no interruption to their blood supply at all and that the incisions can be made exactly congruous. The disadvantages are that there are more suture lines involved and that there may be some degree of stasis and bacterial overgrowth.

Lay the segments to be joined side by side in contact for 8–10 cm and insert a posterior seromuscular stitch. Incise the antimesenteric borders for about 5 cm and insert an all-coats stitch. Remove the clamps and complete the anterior seromuscular layer of stitches. When side-to-side anastomosis follows bowel resection, suture the cut edge of mesentery to the adjacent intact mesentery on each side of the anastomosis.

ENTERECTOMY (SMALL-BOWEL RESECTION)

Resection is often indicated for congenital lesions of the small bowel such as atresia and duplication; traumatic perforation; critical ischaemia from mesenteric trauma, strangulation or arteriosclerosis; Crohn's disease or other cause of stricture; tumours of the bowel or its mesentery. Resection is sometimes indicated for fistula, diverticulitis, intussusception and a symptomatic blind loop. Small portions of the duodenum and ileum are removed during partial gastrectomy and right hemicolectomy respectively.

Avoid unnecessary resection in *Crohn's disease*: it is indolent, it tends to relapse, and to recur anywhere in the intestinal tract (>50%), but especially at and just proximal to the anastomosis. It is unpredictable with little agreement about the factors predisposing to recurrence. Most patients eventually require resection because of subacute obstruction, fistula or abscess. Bypass is obsolete: the defunctioned segment is unlikely to heal, bacterial overgrowth of the blind loop may aggravate diarrhoea and there is a long-term risk of carcinoma. For 'burnt-out' stenotic areas of bowel, strictureplasty (see later) is an alternative to resection.

When operating for *radiation enteropathy* establish the extent both of the original cancer and of the radiation damage. Try to avoid bypass or exclusion; the leakage rate is probably no lower than after resection and anastomosis, and the defunctioned bowel may bleed and develop fistulas. Prefer wide resection ensuring that at least one side of the anastomosis is healthy, and non-irradiated.

Prepare

In the presence of obstruction ensure adequate resuscitation, nasogastric intubation and intravenous rehydration. In the absence of obstruction, pass a nasogastric tube after induction of anaesthesia. Nutritional status may be impaired in Crohn's disease, cancer, radiation enteropathy or enterocutaneous fistula. In the absence of obstruction or fistula give supplemental enteric feeds, otherwise arrange preoperative parenteral nutrition.

Healthy ileum has a resident bacterial flora; in obstruction the entire small bowel may be colonized. Cover all intestinal resections with prophylactic antibiotics, such as a cephalosporin plus metronidazole given preoperatively in a single intravenous injection.

Access

We usually employ a midline incision that skirts the umbilicus and can be extended in either direction as necessary. Take care – the small bowel quite often adheres to the back of a previous laparotomy incision.

Assess

Expose and examine the entire small bowel. Continue by examining the stomach, large bowel and remaining abdominal viscera (Ch. 7). If a loop of small bowel has been strangulated in an external hernia, for example, release it and check its viability after a minimum of 5 minutes.

Healthy small intestine has great functional reserve and adaptability to tissue loss by compensatory villous hyperplasia but do not gratuitously sacrifice healthy bowel, particularly specialized terminal ileum. Except for primary malignant tumours do not excise a deep wedge of mesentery, which requires excessive bowel removal. In Crohn's disease do not remove more than a few centimetres of gut on either side of the affected segment, but include any fistulas or sinuses; microscopic inflammation of the bowel at the resection margin does not appear to increase subsequent anastomotic recurrence. Conventional right hemicolectomy is unnecessary for small-bowel Crohn's disease; undertake conservative ileocaecal resection.

Sometimes a partial resection of small bowel can be performed, leaving the mesentery intact. Appropriate conditions include Richter's hernia, Meckel's diverticulum and small tumours arising on the antimesenteric border.

Action

Isolate the diseased loop of bowel from the other abdominal contents by means of large, moist packs or a special towel. Hold up the bowel and examine the mesentery against the light to note the vascular pattern.

Standard resection

1 Determine the proximal and distal sites for dividing the bowel, and select the line of vascular section in between; keep fairly close to the bowel wall, except when resecting a neoplasm (Fig. 17.8). Incise the peritoneum along this line on each aspect of the mesentery. This manoeuvre is most easily accomplished by inserting one blade

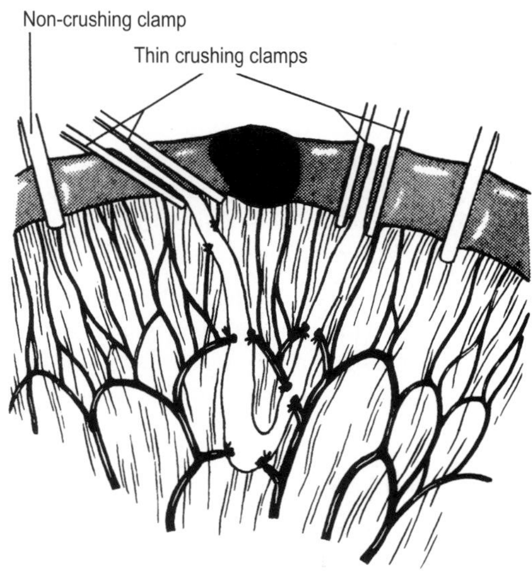

Fig. 17.8 Resection of a small-bowel tumour. A deeper wedge of mesentery is included than in operations for benign disease. As before, the narrower segment of bowel (on the left) is transected obliquely, removing more of the mesenteric border with the specimen.

of a pair of fine, curved scissors beneath the peritoneum and cutting superficially to expose the mesenteric vessels.

2 Using small artery forceps, create a small mesenteric window close to the bowel wall at each point chosen for intestinal transection. Starting at one end, insinuate a curved artery forceps through this window and back through the mesentery, denuded of peritoneum, 1–2 cm away, thus isolating a small leash of mesentery with its contained vessels. Either doubly ligate this leash in continuity and divide between ligatures, or divide between artery forceps, ligating the mesentery beneath each pair of forceps. Proceeding in this manner, divide the mesentery right up to the bowel wall at the further end of the line of peritoneal incision. Take care in placing and tying each ligature; if the knot slips, there can be troublesome haemorrhage. We use polyglactin 910 (Vicryl) or silk ties, 2/0 or 3/0 according to the thickness of the mesentery.

3 Apply four intestinal clamps. The first two clamps are crushing clamps (Payr's, Lang Stevenson's or Pringle's). They should be applied obliquely at the points of intended intestinal transection, so that slightly more of the antimesenteric border is resected than of the mesenteric border; the obliquity reduces the risk of a tight anastomosis. Now apply a non-crushing clamp about 5 cm outside each crushing clamp, having milked the intervening bowel free of contents.

4 Place a clean gauze swab beneath the clamps at each end to catch spills, and divide the bowel with a knife flush against the outer aspect of each crushing clamp. Place the specimen and the soiled knife in a separate dish, which is then removed.

5 Cleanse each bowel end, using small swabs or pledgets of gauze soaked in cetrimide. Then remove the protective gauze swab and proceed to intestinal anastomosis. In an attempt to limit contamination, some surgeons divide the intestine between two pairs of light crushing clamps (i.e. six clamps in all) and insert the posterior seromuscular layer of sutures before removing the outer clamps and excising the narrow rim of crushed tissue (Fig. 17.8). Now perform a two-layer, end-to-end anastomosis.

Partial resection

1 Locally excise a diverticulum on the antimesenteric border. Clamp and cut it off at the neck, then close the defect in two layers as a transverse linear slit. Try to avoid narrowing the intestinal lumen during this procedure.

2 A diamond-shaped area of the antimesenteric border may be included in the resection of a localized tumour or wide-mouthed Meckel's diverticulum. Apply two light crushing clamps (Lang Stevenson's or Pringle's) across the antimesenteric border, meeting in a 'V' (Fig. 17.9). Incise the bowel flush with the outer aspect of each clamp, and close the wall in two layers, leaving a transverse suture line.

3 A similar defect results if the antimesenteric lesion is excised through a longitudinal ellipse. Approximate the ends of the ellipse, pull apart the sides and close transversely as before.

Checklist

Before closing check the anastomosis, bowel colour, closure of mesenteric defects and perfection of haemostasis. Recheck the swab count, replace intestine and the greater omentum in their normal anatomical positions. Suck out the peritoneal cavity. Place a fine-bore suction drain to the region of the anastomosis.

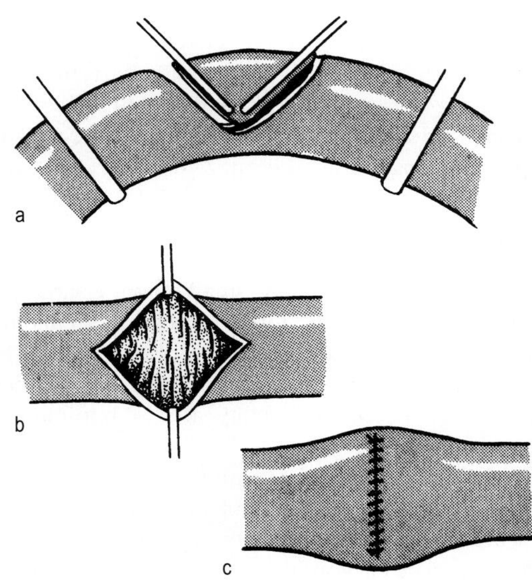

Fig. 17.9 Partial resection of small bowel: (a) a wedge of antimesenteric bowel is removed; (b) the defect is opened out transversely; (c) closure across the long axis of the bowel prevents narrowing.

? **DIFFICULTY**

1. *Is the bowel obstructed?* Decompress obstructed jejunum by milking its contents upwards until they can be aspirated through the nasogastric tube. Decompress obstructed ileum by inserting a sucker tube, either into the end of the proximal bowel after releasing the clamps or via a separate enterotomy. Do this without allowing bowel contents to spill.
2. In the presence of obstruction there may be marked disparity between the diameters of the bowel ends. In practice, moderate incongruities can be overcome by adjusting the size of bite, while suturing proximal to distal bowel. The diameter of the distal bowel can be increased by transecting it more obliquely, sparing the mesenteric border, and by opening it along the antimesenteric border. If there is gross disparity, consider oblique or side-to-side anastomosis.
3. Resection and anastomosis can usually be completed outside the abdomen. Sometimes this is not possible, in which case you may not be able to apply all the clamps described above. Try and retain the non-crushing clamps placed at a distance from the anastomosis, if possible. In difficult circumstances, concentrate on completing the all-coats suture without defect, if necessary using interrupted sutures. You may subsequently be able to insert seromuscular sutures around all or most of the circumference.
4. *A haematoma develops in the mesentery or in the submucosa at the point of intestinal transection.* Compression of the area with a swab usually stops the bleeding. Alternatively, gently close swab-holding forceps or non-crushing clamps across the bleeding point and wait for a few minutes. If the bleeding is not fully controlled, incise the peritoneum, find the bleeding point, pick it up with fine artery forceps and ligate it. Check the colour of the bowel to confirm that the blood supply is not prejudiced.
5. *One or other intestinal end becomes dusky during the anastomosis.* Allow time to declare the issue. Non-viable bowel will not heal, so if you are in any doubt excise a few more centimetres and make a fresh start. Leave the mesentery attached to the bowel as close as possible to the point of transection, and check for visible pulsations in the edge of the mesentery.

Aftercare

Anticipate a period of postoperative paralytic ileus during which maintain the patient on intravenous fluids. Leave the nasogastric tube on open drainage, aspirated regularly for the first 24–48 hours. Allow water 30 ml/hour by mouth. The tube can usually be removed when bowel sounds return, the volume of aspirate drops below the volume of fluid taken by mouth and there is passage of flatus. Peristalsis returns to the small bowel before the stomach and colon regain their motility.

Remove the drain when the fluid loss diminishes, generally at 2–3 days.

If restoration of oral feeding is very delayed, consider instituting a period of parenteral nutrition.

Complications

Wound infection is a potential risk of any procedure involving an intestinal anastomosis. Good surgical technique in limiting contamination from bowel contents certainly reduces the incidence. If wound sepsis develops, remove sufficient sutures to allow the pus to drain, irrigate the wound, obtain bacteriological cultures and, in severe cases, institute appropriate antibiotic therapy. Once the infection is controlled, the wound usually heals without the need for secondary suture. Wound dehiscence is considered in Chapter 7.

As with any abdominal operation there is a risk of chest infection resulting from atelectasis. Institute vigorous physiotherapy to avert the need for antibiotics.

Occasionally a collection of infected material develops within the abdominal cavity. Abscess sites may be subphrenic, subhepatic, pelvic or adjacent to the anastomosis.

The patient develops fever and leucocytosis. Ultrasound scan localizes the collection and allows percutaneous drainage in many cases (Ch. 11).

A leaking anastomosis often presents with pain, fever, tachycardia and erythema of the wound or drain site before intestinal contents begin to discharge. The management of an established small-bowel fistula is described at the end of this chapter.

It is occasionally necessary to undertake massive resection of the small bowel, for example when volvulus complicates an obstruction.[1] Repeated enterectomies in Crohn's disease can similarly remove a substantial percentage of the small intestine. Increased frequency of bowel actions may follow loss of a third to a half of the small bowel, and more extensive resections produce short-bowel syndrome.[2] During the initial phase of recovery and adaptation, anticipate and replace losses of fluid and electrolytes, notably potassium. Give codeine or loperamide to control diarrhoea. The body compensates better for proximal than distal enterectomy. After an extensive ileal resection regular injections of vitamin B_{12} may be needed indefinitely; colestyramine may diminish the irritative diarrhoea that results from bile-acid malabsorption. Consider nutritional support by the enteral or parenteral routes in severe short-bowel syndrome. Cimetidine or, rarely, vagotomy may be needed for gastric acid hypersecretion.

REFERENCES

1. Hill GL 1985 Massive enterectomy: indications and management. World Journal of Surgery 9:833–841
2. Bristol JB, Williamson RCN 1985 Postoperative adaptation of the small intestine. World Journal of Surgery 9:825–832

ENTERIC BYPASS

Appraise

Small-bowel loops may become obstructed as a result of carcinomatosis peritonei or a particularly dense set of adhesions, sometimes deep in the pelvis. Irradiated small bowel may fistulate into other organs, such as the bladder or vagina. In these unfavourable circumstances it is often better just to bypass the affected segment of intestine (Fig. 17.10) rather than embark on a difficult and hazardous disentanglement. In radiation enteritis choose overtly normal bowel for the anastomosis, since healing is likely to be impaired.

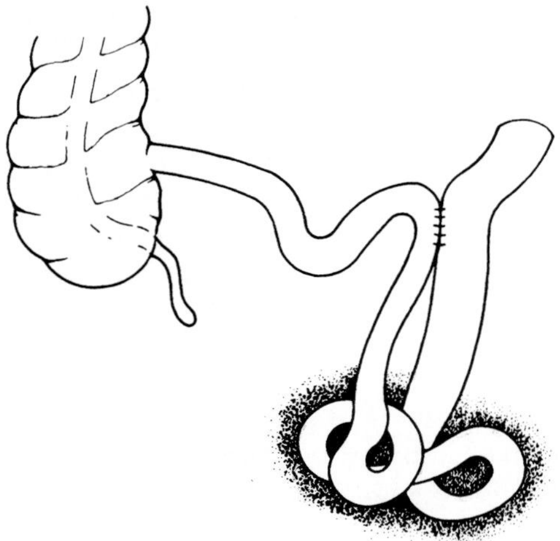

Fig. 17.10 Bypass procedure for small-bowel obstruction resulting from irresectable pelvic cancer. A side-to-side anastomosis is fashioned between a (proximal) distended loop of bowel and a (distal) collapsed loop.

Resection is almost always a better option than simple defunction in Crohn's disease of the small bowel. For irresectable carcinoma of the caecum, however, side-to-side bypass is indicated between the terminal ileum and the transverse colon – ileotransversostomy.

Subtotal jejunoileal bypass has been recommended for intractable morbid obesity. Patients lose weight because of malabsorption, diarrhoea and impaired appetite. The operation provides a metabolic insult to the body, and there are many potential long-term complications. The alternative procedure of gastric reduction causes fewer metabolic upsets and is generally preferred nowadays.

Bypass of the distal one-third of the small intestine is rarely indicated for certain types of hyperlipidaemia. The ileum is divided, the distal end is closed and the proximal end is reimplanted into the caecum. The operation reduces the levels of cholesterol and triglyceride in the blood.

Action

Bypass of an irresectable lesion

1 A midline incision is usually appropriate. Aim to anastomose healthy bowel on either side of the diseased

segment. Side-to-side anastomosis avoids the risk of closed-loop obstruction developing in a sequestered loop of bowel.

2 Occasionally if there are multiple sites of actual or imminent obstruction, two or more side-to-side anastomoses between adjacent loops may cause less of a short circuit than one enormous bypass.

3 Approximate a distended loop of proximal intestine to a collapsed loop of distal small bowel (Fig. 17.10) or transverse colon. Pack off the remaining viscera. Consider decompression of the obstructed loops.

4 Carry out a two-layer, side-to-side anastomosis, as previously described. Take care with the anastomosis and subsequent wound closure, since healing may be impaired, but do not prolong the operation unnecessarily if the patient has advanced disease.

Aftercare and complications

The principles of management are as for enterectomy. Short-bowel syndrome is inevitable after subtotal (about 90%) jejunoileal bypass, although adaptation can still be anticipated.

STRICTUREPLASTY

Appraise

This technique is virtually confined to patients with Crohn's disease causing a single or a few strictures in the small intestine.[1] It can avoid the need for resection and may therefore be appropriate for patients with disease at several sites or those with recurrent disease and a limited length of residual small bowel.

Florid inflammatory change or bowel containing several strictures within a relatively short segment is better treated by local resection. Sometimes you may combine one or more strictureplasties with resection to reduce the total length of bowel excised.

Assess

The tightness of the stricture(s) can be assessed by making a small enterotomy and passing a balloon catheter. Moderate strictures of 20–25 mm diameter may be treated by balloon dilatation, but tight strictures of less than 20 mm diameter require either strictureplasty or resection.

Action

1 Carry a longitudinal full-thickness incision across the stenotic area and for 1 cm into the 'normal' bowel on either side.

2 Close the bowel transversely, using either one or two layers of 3/0 Vicryl sutures. Test that the anastomosis is airtight and watertight.

3 This modification of the Heineke–Mikulicz pyloroplasty is suitable for short stenoses. For longer strictures perform resection and anastomosis.

Complications

Wound infections are uncommon.

Anastomotic leakage may occur, particularly if tight strictures distal to the strictureplasty are not treated.

As strictureplasty is a relatively recent innovation, long-term follow-up is limited. Several studies have reported excellent symptomatic improvement following operation, however. Moreover, perioperative complication rates are comparable to standard surgical treatment, with low rates of recurrent stricture. Recurrent stricture can sometimes occur at a later date.

It is of concern that small bowel adenocarcinoma has been reported at the site of a previous strictureplasty, so bear this possibility in mind if there is a sudden clinical deterioration.[2]

REFERENCES

1. Andrews HA, Keighley MRB, Alexander-Williams J et al 1991 Strategy for management of distal ileal Crohn's disease. British Journal of Surgery 78:679–682
2. Jaskowiak NT, Michelassi F 2001 Adenocarcinoma at a strictureplasty site in Crohn's disease: report of a case. Diseases of the Colon and Rectum 44:284–287

THE ROUX LOOP

Appraise

A defunctioned segment of jejunum provides a convenient conduit for connecting various upper abdominal organs to the remaining small bowel. The technique was originally described by the Swiss surgeon César Roux in 1907 for oesophageal bypass.

KEY POINT The versatile Roux loop

- The method has proved invaluable in gastric, biliary and pancreatic surgery.[1] It can be used to bypass or replace the stomach, the distal bile duct and to drain the pancreatic duct or pseudocyst.

Roux-en-Y anastomosis has two advantages over an intact loop: it can stretch further and it is empty of intestinal contents, thus preventing contamination of the organ to be drained such as the bile duct. Active peristalsis down the loop encourages this drainage.[2]

Probably the commonest indications for Roux-en-Y anastomosis are biliary drainage in irresectable carcinoma of the pancreatic head and reconstruction after total gastrectomy (Fig. 17.11) or oesophagogastrectomy. Conversion to a Roux loop may cure duodenogastric reflux after partial gastrectomy, provided the loop is 40–50 cm long. Allison has shown that with meticulous attention to technique it is possible to bring a Roux loop up to the neck to replace the oesophagus.[1]

Although Roux-en-Y anastomosis is the most versatile technique, other types of jejunal loop are sometimes indicated. Intact loops are used for cholecystoenterostomy, gastroenterostomy and Polya (Billroth II) reconstruction after partial gastrectomy. Isolated loops may be interposed between the stomach and duodenum in an isoperistaltic or antiperistaltic direction for different facets of the postgastrectomy syndrome. A reversed loop can be used further downstream in certain cases of intractable diarrhoea.

Action

1 Select a loop of proximal small bowel, beginning 10–15 cm distal to the ligament of Treitz. Hold up the jejunum and transilluminate its mesentery to display the precise blood supply, which varies from patient to patient. The number of vessels requiring division depends on the length of conduit required.

2 Starting at the point chosen for intestinal transection, incise the peritoneal leaves of the mesentery in a vertical direction (Fig. 17.12). Divide at least one vascular arcade and the smaller branches that lie between the arcade vessels and the bowel. Ligate these vessels neatly

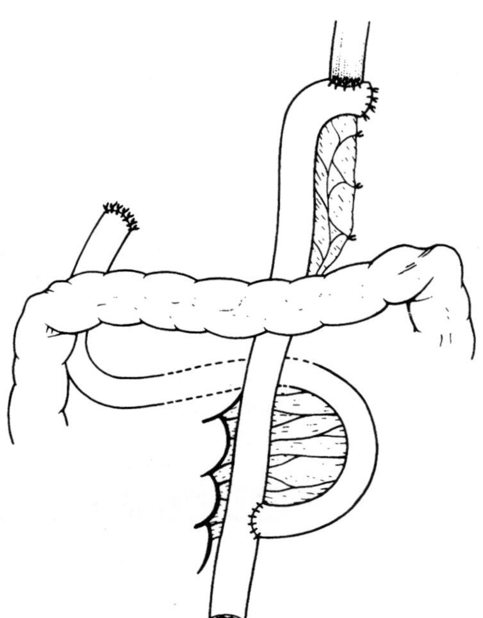

Fig. 17.11 One indication for a Roux loop: Roux-en-Y anastomosis between the oesophagus and jejunum after total gastrectomy.

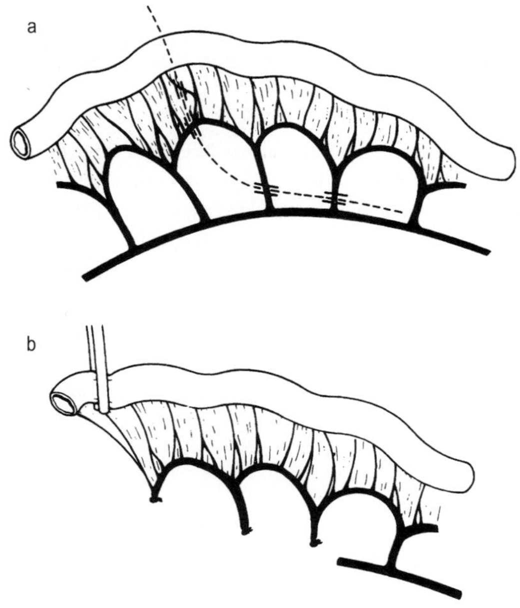

Fig. 17.12 Creation of a long Roux loop: (a) three arcade vessels have been divided; (b) the bowel is transected at a point previously selected and the loop is mobilized.

in continuity and avoid using artery forceps, which can bunch up the tissues and prevent mobilization of the loop. Now divide the bowel between clamps.

3 If a longer loop is required, sacrifice two or three main jejunal vessels, preserving an intact blood supply to the extremity of the bowel via the arcades (Fig. 17.12). The peritoneum may require further incision to facilitate elongation of the loop without tension. Individual ligation of the arteries and veins is recommended, using fine silk sutures. Check the viability of the bowel at the tip of the loop, and sacrifice the end if it is dusky.

4 Straighten out the efferent limb and take it up by the shortest route for anastomosis to the oesophagus, stomach, bile duct, common hepatic duct or pancreatic duct. It is often easier to close the end of the limb and fashion a new subterminal opening of the correct diameter. Make a window in the base of the transverse mesocolon, to the right of the duodenojejunal flexure, for passage of the Roux loop. At the end of the operation suture the margins of this defect to the Roux loop to prevent internal herniation.

5 Restore intestinal continuity by uniting the short afferent limb to the base of the long efferent limb, using an end-to-side anastomosis. Ensure that the efferent limb is at least 30 cm long and that the afferent loop is joined to its left-hand side.

REFERENCES

1. Allison PR, da Silva LT 1953 The Roux loop. British Journal of Surgery 41:173–180
2. Kirk RM 1985 Roux-en-Y. World Journal of Surgery 9:938–944

ENTEROTOMY

Appraise

Probably the commonest reason for making an incision into the lumen of the small bowel is to decompress the intestine proximal to the site of an obstruction. The enterotomy should be made halfway between the ligament of Treitz and the site of obstruction, so that the sucker can be inserted both proximally and distally to reach all the distended loops. It is usually possible to avoid enterotomy in a high obstruction by advancing the nasogastric tube through the duodenum and squeezing luminal contents upwards until they can be aspirated. In other circumstances the decompressing sucker can be inserted through the proximal cut end of bowel, if enterectomy is planned, or through the caecum and ileocaecal valve after appendicectomy.

Sometimes enterotomy is needed to extract a foreign body, for example in gallstone ileus or bolus obstruction. After partial gastrectomy, the absence of the antropyloric mill means that whole orange segments or pith, for example, are inadequately broken up and may impact further down the gut. Benign mucosal or submucosal tumours may be explored and removed through an enterotomy incision.

Traumatic enterotomy can result from blunt or penetrating abdominal injuries. After a closed injury there is typically a rosette of exposed mucosa on the antimesenteric border of the upper jejunum. After knife or gunshot injuries, look for entry and exit wounds; holes in the small bowel nearly always come in multiples of two.

Occasionally, operative enteroscopy may be indicated for unexplained bleeding localized to the small bowel. A flexible colonoscope can be introduced through a mid-enterotomy and threaded up and down the gut.

Action

Decompression enterotomy

1 The objective is to empty the small bowel without contaminating the peritoneal cavity. Pack off the area and apply non-crushing clamps on either side of the site chosen for enterotomy. Insert an absorbable purse-string stitch, make a small nick through the wall of the bowel and introduce a Savage decompressor, which consists of a long trocar and cannula connected to the sucker tubing (Fig. 17.13).

2 Pass the sucker up and down the bowel, removing first one clamp and then the other. The assistant feeds the distended loops of gut over the end of the sucker, while you control the force of suction by placing a finger over a side-port on the decompressing cannula. Sometimes the bowel appears to be only partly deflated, because of interstitial oedema.

3 After emptying the bowel, remove the sucker, tighten and tie the purse-string and discard the contaminated packs. Place a second purse-string suture or Lembert sutures to bury the wound.

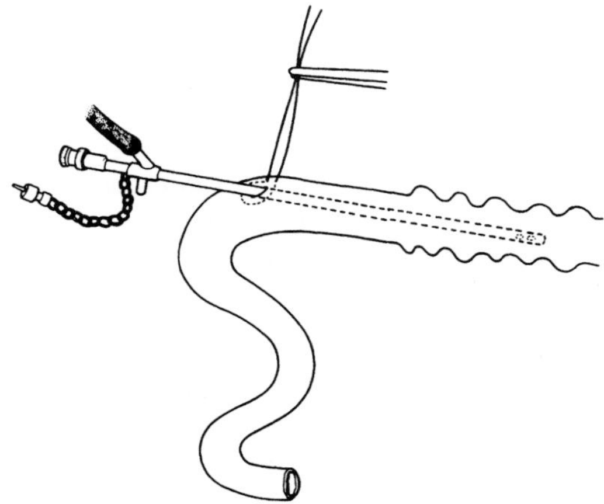

Fig. 17.13 Decompression enterotomy. After insertion of the Savage decompressor, the trocar is withdrawn and the cannula is gently passed along the distended loops of bowel in either direction. Suction tubing is attached to the side-arm of the decompressor.

Extraction enterotomy

1 It may be possible to knead a foreign body, especially a bolus of food, onwards into the caecum. If so, it will pass spontaneously per rectum. Do not persist with this manoeuvre if it is difficult.

2 Before opening the bowel, pack off the area carefully. Try and manipulate an impacted foreign body upwards for a few centimetres, away from the inflamed segment in which it was lodged.

3 Apply non-crushing clamps across the intestine on either side of the enterotomy site. Open the bowel longitudinally over the foreign body or tumour and gently extract or resect the lesion. Close the bowel transversely in two layers to prevent stenosis.

4 In gallstone ileus examine the right upper quadrant of the abdomen. Consider whether it is appropriate to proceed to cholecystectomy, choledochotomy and possible closure of the biliary–enteric fistula. Since the patient is often elderly and unfit, concentrate on relieving the intestinal obstruction. Examine the rest of the small bowel to exclude a second gallstone.

Traumatic enterotomy

1 Excise devitalized tissue and close the intestinal wound(s) in two layers. Explore an associated haematoma in the mesentery and ligate any bleeding points. Check the viability of the bowel thereafter, and if in doubt resect the damaged segment with end-to-end anastomosis.

2 Examine the other abdominal viscera for concomitant injuries (see Ch. 7).

ENTEROSTOMY

Appraise

A feeding jejunostomy permits enteral nutrition in patients who are unable to take sufficient food by mouth.[1] The development of parenteral nutrition has limited its use to certain circumstances, for example the preoperative hyperalimentation of malnourished patients with cancer of the stomach or oesophagus. Better still, it may be possible to pass a fine transnasal feeding tube through the malignant stricture under endoscopic control.

A feeding tube should always be placed as high as possible in the jejunum. Nevertheless it can be difficult to introduce enough calories and nitrogen by this route without causing troublesome diarrhoea. Some surgeons use feeding jejunostomy routinely after major oesophagogastric resections. Others reserve it for postoperative complications such as fistula, or serious upper gastrointestinal conditions such as corrosive oesophagogastritis or pancreatic abscess.

The ideal feeding jejunostomy is easily inserted, if necessary under local anaesthesia, and seals off immediately it is removed. It neither obstructs the bowel nor permits the escape of intestinal contents. We favour the use of a T-tube for this purpose.

A feeding jejunostomy tube can be placed at laparotomy either transnasally or via an enterostomy. Insert a fine-bore nasojejunal tube peroperatively and milk it down into jejunum. The sophisticated Frecka tube contains three separate lumens – to allow gastric aspiration, pressure measurement and jejunal feeding; it includes a clever device for insertion. It is sometimes possible to avoid laparotomy for insertion of a feeding jejunostomy by radiological puncture of the jejunum and initial placement of a guidewire, using a Seldinger technique similar to that for Hickman line insertion.

A terminal ileostomy replaces the anus after total colectomy for multiple neoplasia, ulcerative proctocolitis or Crohn's colitis. The ileostomy may be temporary, if subsequent ileorectal anastomosis is planned, or permanent after panproctocolectomy. Improvements in stoma care make ileostomy less of a burden to patients, many of whom are young. It is desirable and usually possible to select and mark the site for ileostomy preoperatively. Choose a point just below waist level and 5 cm to the right of the midline, unless there is a previous scar in this region. It is important to create a spout that will discharge its irritative contents well clear of the skin.

Other types of ileostomy are sometimes fashioned. Increasingly, defunctioning loop ileostomies are being used as forms of faecal diversion. Historically this stoma was used to defunction distal bowel affected by inflammatory bowel disease or to cover a precarious anastomosis in the right colon. With the advent of ultralow anterior resection, however, its use has spread. In comparison with transverse colostomy, it produces predictable volumes of relatively inoffensive faecal effluent and it is a truly defunctioning stoma to which an appliance can easily be attached. For these reasons, it has become the temporary stoma of choice. Split ileostomy, with separated stomas, completely defunctions the distal bowel and has been advocated in selected cases of colitis. Split enterostomy has also been advocated to protect a lower enteric anastomosis created in the presence of peritonitis. The distal cut end is either exteriorized as a mucous fistula or oversewn and fixed to the parietal peritoneum to facilitate later retrieval. Kock's continent ileostomy consists of an ileal reservoir discharging by a short conduit to a flush stoma; a nipple valve is created to preserve continence, and the patient empties the reservoir regularly with a soft catheter. Lastly, a 'wet' ileostomy together with an ileal conduit provides one of the commoner methods for achieving urinary diversion.

Action

Feeding jejunostomy

1 Expose the upper jejunum through a small left upper paramedian or transverse incision. Trace the bowel proximally to the duodenojejunal flexure. Select a loop a few centimetres distal to this point, so that it will easily reach the anterior abdominal wall.

2 Insert a Vicryl purse-string suture on the antimesenteric border of the bowel. Make a tiny enterotomy in the centre of the purse-string and introduce a T-tube (14F) into the lumen of the bowel (Fig. 17.14). Tighten the purse-string snugly around the tube.

3 An alternative method employs a Foley catheter subsequently inflated with 5–10 ml of water. After tightening the purse-string, the catheter and its point of entry into the bowel are buried with Lembert sutures. This is a Witzel jejunostomy.

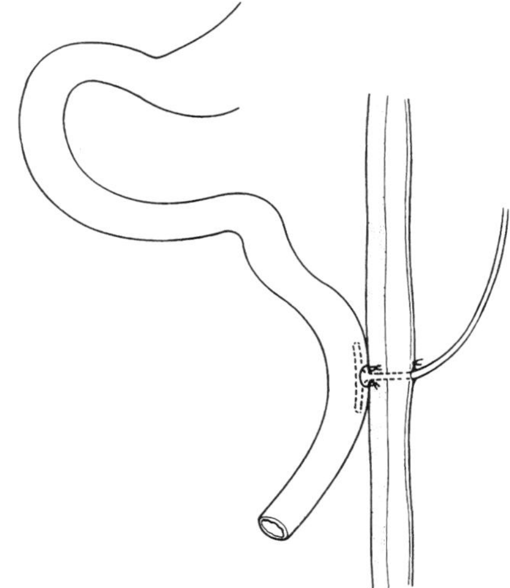

Fig. 17.14 Feeding jejunostomy. The T-tube is brought out through the abdominal wall, and the jejunum is stitched to the peritoneum around the margins of the stab incision.

4 Whichever tube is used, introduce it first through a stab incision in the abdominal wall and then into the jejunum. Traction on the tube approximates the intestine to the underside of the abdominal wall. Suture the bowel to the parietal peritoneum.

Terminal ileostomy

> **KEY POINT A durable ileostomy**
>
> - Permanent ileostomies are prone to complications such as retraction, prolapse and parastomal hernia that require operative correction. Take extra care when fashioning an ileostomy to reduce the incidence of these problems

1 Excise a circular disc of skin and subcutaneous fat, 3 cm in diameter, at the site chosen and marked preoperatively. Make a cruciate incision in the exposed anterior

rectus sheath, split the fibres of the rectus muscle and open the posterior sheath and peritoneum. The defect should comfortably accommodate two fingers.

2 The terminal ileum will previously have been clamped and transected. Now exteriorize 6–8 cm of bowel with its mesentery intact, through the circular opening in the abdominal wall, leaving its end securely clamped. Make sure that the mesentery is neither twisted nor tight and that the tip of the ileum remains pink.

3 Some surgeons close the lateral space between the ileostomy and the abdominal wall, using a running Vicryl suture (Fig. 17.15). Others tunnel the ileum extraperitoneally. We prefer transperitoneal ileostomy, leaving the lateral space widely open. In this case, however, it is important to suture the seromuscular layer of the bowel to the margins of the defect at peritoneal level.

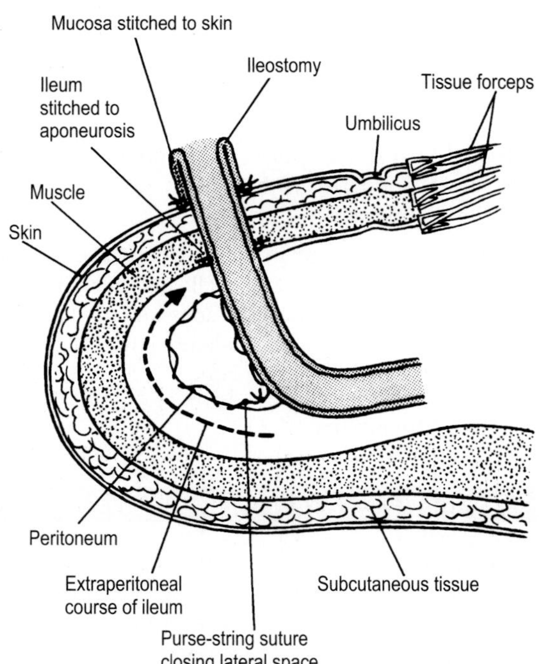

Fig. 17.15 Terminal ileostomy. Two methods of closing the lateral space are shown: a purse-string suture or taking the ileum along an extraperitoneal track. Alternatively, the lateral space can be left widely open. Tissue forceps on each layer of the wound edge prevent retraction of the layers while the ileostomy is being fashioned.

Take great care not to enter the lumen of the ileum when inserting these stitches.

4 After closing the main abdominal incision, remove the clamp and trim the crushed portion of ileum. Now suture the edge of the ileum directly to the skin, using Vicryl mounted on an atraumatic taper-pointed needle. After inserting three or four evenly spaced sutures, the bowel begins to evert spontaneously; if not, use Babcock's forceps to encourage eversion. Complete the circumferential sutures, producing a spout, which should project about 3 cm from the abdominal wall.

5 Carefully clean and dry the skin around the ileostomy and apply an ileostomy bag at once.

Loop ileostomy

1 Excise a disc of skin and fat and deliver a loop of ileum on to the abdominal wall.

2 Open the bowel, not at the apex of the loop as for a loop colostomy (Ch. 19), but close to skin level.

3 Suture the mucosa of the distal bowel to the skin. Use Babcock's forceps to evert the mucosa of the proximal bowel before suture.

4 The completed loop ileostomy looks very like a standard end ileostomy. As for loop colostomy, insert a plastic rod to prevent the bowel slipping back in, and fit a suitable appliance, with flange and clip-on bag, to the skin over the stoma.

Aftercare

Feeding jejunostomy

Keep the tube patent by introducing 5–10 ml of sterile water hourly. When bowel sounds return, increase the amount of water before switching to half-strength and then full-strength liquid feed. Consult the dietitian about the patient's individual nutritional needs. Give codeine or loperamide to control diarrhoea. When oral feeding is resumed, spigot the tube for 24–48 hours before removal.

Ileostomy

Increase oral fluids when the stoma commences to discharge. The effluent will be very loose at first but will gradually thicken as the ileum adapts. Give bulking agents or antidiarrhoeal drugs as needed. Consult the stomatherapist directly, if he has not already seen the patient before operation. Make sure that the patient is competent and confident at managing the stoma before he leaves hospital.

REFERENCE

1. Hesp WLEM, Lubbers EJC, de Boer HHM et al 1988 Hendriks T enterostomy as an adjunct to treatment of intra-abdominal sepsis. British Journal of Surgery 75:693–696

MISCELLANEOUS CONDITIONS

MECKEL'S DIVERTICULUM

Potential complications include bleeding, infection, peptic ulceration, perforation, intestinal obstruction or fistulation to the umbilicus. Usually this remnant of the allantois gives no trouble at all, however, throughout the patient's life.

Incidental Meckelian diverticulectomy has been advocated by some surgeons because of the supposed lower morbidity and mortality rates before complications arise. Others have argued that the low risk of complications arising from a Meckel's diverticulum does not justify prophylactic resection. A retrospective analysis[1] found that the conditional probabilities of producing surgical morbidity and mortality in the adult population were far higher when resecting incidental diverticula.

> **KEY POINT Removal of Meckel's diverticulum**
>
> - Do not carry out incidental Meckelian diverticulectomy in adults.

The first step in Meckelian diverticulectomy is to divide the small vessel that crosses the ileum to supply it. Depending on the size of its mouth, the diverticulum can simply be transected across the neck using a linear stapler or excised with a portion of the antimesenteric border of the bowel. Local resection of the ileum with end-to-end anastomosis may be preferable in a complicated case.

INTUSSUSCEPTION

In infants

Ileocolic intussusception usually presents in a child of a few months old with abdominal colic and rectal passage of blood and mucus. Besides confirming the diagnosis, barium enema may reduce the intussusception totally or subtotally. On examination under anaesthetic, if not before, a mass can be felt in the central or upper abdomen with an 'empty' right iliac fossa.

Open the abdomen through a right Lanz incision and find the sausage-shaped mass. Starting at the apex, squeeze the intussusceptum back along the intussuscipiens as though extracting toothpaste from the bottom of the tube. Do not remove the bowel from the abdominal cavity during this manoeuvre.

The final portion of the intussusception is the most difficult to reduce. Deliver the affected segment from the abdomen and gently compress it with a moist swab, before resuming the squeeze. Make certain that reduction is complete before replacing the bowel. No fixation is required, except in the rare event of a recurrent intussusception.

If the bowel is clearly gangrenous or the intussusception cannot be reduced, proceed to resection. Usually an end-to-end ileoileostomy can be performed.

In adults

Intussusception is rare and is nearly always associated with an underlying lesion in the bowel wall such as a benign tumour or Meckel's diverticulum.

Reduce the intussusception as far as possible, then proceed to local resection of the affected segment of bowel with end-to-end anastomosis.

INTESTINAL ISCHAEMIA

The small intestine is supplied by the superior mesenteric, midgut, vessels. Thrombosis may occur on arteriosclerotic plaques at the origin of the superior mesenteric artery, especially if the patient is shocked. The superior mesenteric artery is an uncommon site for peripheral embolism in patients with cardiac arrhythmia or a recent myocardial infarction. Venous gangrene may result if the superior mesenteric or portal veins suddenly undergo thrombosis, for example in extreme dehydration or disseminated intravascular coagulation. Lastly, non-occlusive mesenteric infarction may occur secondary to microcirculatory damage in critically ill patients. With the advent of ever-improving intensive care units, a greater proportion of patients have mesenteric ischaemia secondary to this cause. Although the diagnosis may be difficult to make, suspect it if unexplained acidosis develops in a postoperative or critically ill patient.

Patients with severe mesenteric vascular insufficiency are extremely ill with evidence of peritonitis and shock. Early operation is needed to prevent death.[2] At laparotomy, the bowel appears ischaemic or frankly infarcted without evidence of strangulation.

Examine the whole intestinal tract and feel for pulsation in all accessible gut arteries. Examine the aorta and its main divisions to determine the extent of atherosclerosis. If the main intestinal vessels and their arcades are patent, the circulation is probably occluded at capillary level.

Resect obviously necrotic bowel. Recovery is unlikely if the entire midgut is infarcted following occlusion of the main superior mesenteric vessels. If an extensive segment is affected, be as conservative as possible to avoid severe short-bowel syndrome. Multiple patches of ischaemia can be oversewn or locally resected.

Early cases of arterial embolus or acute in-situ thrombosis may be amenable to revascularization. It is much easier to mobilize the caecum and identify the ileocolic artery than to expose the origin of the superior mesenteric artery itself. Control the vessel with tapes and perform a longitudinal arteriotomy. Pass a Fogarty catheter proximally into the superior mesenteric artery and aorta to dislodge the clot, and try to establish free flow. Rapid injection of heparin saline up the vessel may achieve the same effect. If the bowel regains its normal colour, close the arteriotomy with a venous patch. Otherwise consider side-to-side anastomosis between the ileocolic and right common iliac arteries.

Following direct arterial surgery, or in any case in which bowel of doubtful viability has been left in the abdomen, plan to repeat the laparotomy after 24 hours. Further resection of bowel may be clearly indicated at this time.

KEY POINT Mesenteric ischaemia: urgency of management

- Regardless of aetiology, the prognosis of patients with mesenteric ischaemia is dependent upon rapid diagnosis and institution of treatment. Conservative management may be sufficient in selected cases; more often laparotomy is required and can be life-saving.

SMALL-BOWEL FISTULA

The spontaneous discharge of bowel contents on to the abdominal wall is a rare event. The vast majority of external fistulas arise either from a leaking anastomosis or from operative injury to the intestine. Besides impaired healing, radiation enteritis, multiple adhesions, diffuse carcinoma and Crohn's disease predispose to fistula formation.[3]

Do not rush to reoperate once there is an established small-bowel fistula. Correct fluid and electrolyte depletion. Switch to total parenteral nutrition both to maintain health and to reduce the amount of intestinal contents discharged. Consult a stomatherapist on how best to protect the wound and abdominal wall from the effluent, using adhesive seals and collecting bags as appropriate. Consider constant suction through a catheter placed in the fistula if the discharge is particularly profuse.

Obtain an early fistulogram to delineate the leak. A side hole may well close if there is no distal obstruction, but a complete anastomotic dehiscence is almost certain to require reoperation once the patient's general condition allows.

If the patient is toxic, early drainage of an associated abscess may improve the patient's general health and sometimes allow the fistula to heal. If you encounter a complete dehiscence at this time, it is probably better to exteriorize the bowel ends rather than attempt a repeat anastomosis under unpromising circumstances. This counsel may not be appropriate for a high jejunal fistula, however.

Do not ordinarily undertake a definitive operation to close a small-bowel fistula if you are an inexperienced surgeon. As a rule resect the damaged portion of bowel. Take care to divide any adhesions that could partially obstruct the distal gut and lead to recurrence of the fistula. Continue nutritional support during the postoperative healing phase.

REFERENCES

1. Peoples J 1995 Incidental Meckel's diverticulectomy in adults. Surgery 118:649–652
2. Bradbury A 1995 Mesenteric ischaemia: a multidisciplinary approach. British Journal of Surgery 82:1446–1459
3. Frileux P, Parc Y 1999 External fistulas of the small bowel. In: Taylor TV, Watson A, Williamson RCN (eds) Upper digestive surgery. Oesophagus, stomach and small intestine. Saunders, London, pp 741–763

LAPAROSCOPIC APPROACH TO THE SMALL BOWEL

Appraise

Diagnostic laparoscopy can be performed with little morbidity and can obviate additional complications arising from laparotomy. In addition to this diagnostic role, laparoscopic surgical techniques can now be applied to a variety of therapeutic procedures that traditionally were performed in an open fashion.

> **KEY POINT Laparoscopy: risk of small-bowel injury**
>
> - In patients in whom previous laparotomy has been carried out and in those with distended loops of bowel, prefer the open method of trocar placement to avoid inadvertent puncture of the small bowel.

With regard to diagnosis, laparoscopy is useful in patients with peritonitis or possible small-bowel ischaemia, any therapeutic procedures being carried out either laparoscopically or via the open route. The small bowel can be examined in detail via the laparoscope. Use a standard infra-umbilical port and a 30°-angled endoscope. Identify the ligament of Treitz initially. Thereafter, by alternately using two atraumatic graspers, expose the entire length of the small bowel to the caecum, dividing any intervening adhesions with scissors. Inspect both the serosal surface and the mesentery.

The clinical diagnosis of small-bowel ischaemia is notoriously difficult to make. Laparoscopic examination of the bowel is helpful, therefore, and other diagnostic aids such as fluorescein and Doppler examinations, which assess perfusion and viability of the bowel, can be adapted for use via the laparoscope. If you are in doubt about the viability of the bowel, make a small incision in order to deliver the suspect segment for closer inspection. Diagnostic laparoscopy is safe and can be performed with minimal risk and a negligible mortality rate. It is perhaps most useful in critically ill patients in whom you wish to avoid unnecessary laparotomy.

Small-bowel resection can be performed entirely laparoscopically or with laparoscopic assistance (Ch. 8). Determine the segment for resection, dissect the mesentery and devascularize it using clips, sutures or linear cutting staplers that have been designed to fit through a laparoscopic port. Perform subsequent anastomosis intraperitoneally or, as is more conventional, by standard extracorporeal anastomosis after delivering the bowel to the exterior through a small abdominal incision. Intraperitoneal resection and anastomosis is possible, using either stapling devices or laparoscopic suturing.

The placement of a feeding jejunostomy can be achieved via the percutaneous route using a laparoscope to anchor the bowel to the anterior abdominal wall. Sutures, clips or T-fasteners, with a metal bar attached to a nylon suture, can be used to secure the bowel. Once attached, the bowel is cannulated using an 18G needle and a guidewire. When performed by experienced laparoscopic surgeons, this technique is safe, effective and perhaps superior to open jejunostomy. Complications can still arise, however, and as with open jejunostomy catheters may become dislodged. Leaks seldom occur as the bowel is flush to the abdominal wall, and catheter replacement can usually be carried out without resorting to laparotomy.

Laparoscopic creation of stomas for faecal diversion can be performed using a variety of organs as conduits; loop ileostomy, loop sigmoid colostomy and end colostomy have all been described. Studies have reported a high success rate, in excess of 95%, and a low morbidity rate.

Laparoscopic management of acute small-bowel obstruction is theoretically attractive, but experience is limited.[1] Adhesions and distended loops of bowel make trocar placement more hazardous, therefore prefer open trocar placement. If obstruction is due to a single adhesion, as is often the case, this can easily be identified and divided. If adhesions are more extensive, adhesiolysis and relief of obstruction are more difficult. The procedure demands painstaking care, whether performed by the open or the laparoscopic route. Several studies have shown that laparoscopy is both effective and safe in patients with small-bowel obstruction. One study in particular[2] reported that laparoscopy was effective in a high proportion of patients and that hospital stay was reduced; early unplanned reoperation was increased in patients managed laparoscopically, reinforcing the fact that experience is limited in this field.

REFERENCES

1. Navez B 1998 Laparoscopic approach in acute small bowel obstruction. A review of 68 patients. Hepatogastroenterology 45:2146–2150
2. Wullstein C, Gross E 2003 Laparoscopic compared with conventional treatment of acute adhesive small bowel obstruction. British Journal of Surgery 90: 1147–1151

SMALL-BOWEL OBSTRUCTION

See Chapter 7.

FURTHER READING

Duh Q 1993 Laparoscopic procedures for small bowel disease. Baillièrés Clinical Gastroenterology 7:833–850

Durdey P 1996 Small intestine. In: Keen G, Farndon J (eds) Operative surgery and management, 3rd edn. Butterworth-Heinemann, London, pp 210–225

Galland RB, Spencer J 1990 Radiation enteritis. Edward Arnold, London

Hyman NH, Fazio VW 1991 Crohn's disease of the small bowel. Comprehensive Therapy 17:38–42

Irwin ST, Krukowski ZH, Matheson NA 1990 Single layer anastomosis in the upper gastrointestinal tract. British Journal of Surgery 77:643–644

Mackey WC, Dineen P 1983 A fifty year experience with Meckel's diverticulum. Surgery, Gynecology and Obstetrics 156:56–64

Marston JAP 1986 Vascular disease of the gut: pathophysiology, recognition and management. Edward Arnold, London

McConnell DB, Turkey DD 1999. Injuries to the small intestine. In: Taylor TV, Watson A, Williamson RCN (eds) Upper digestive surgery. Oesophagus, stomach and small intestine. Saunders, London, pp 732–740

Michelassi F 1998 Strictureplasty for Crohn's disease: techniques and long-term results. World Journal of Surgery 22:359–363

Murray J 1998 Controversies in Crohn's disease. Baillière's Clinical Gastroenterology 12:133–155

Newman T 1998 The changing face of mesenteric infarction. American Surgeon 64:611–616

O'Toole G 1999 Defunctioning loop ileostomy: a prospective audit. Journal of the American College of Surgeons 188:6–9

Ottinger L 1990 Mesenteric ischaemia. In: Williamson RCN, Cooper MJ (eds) Emergency abdominal surgery. Churchill Livingstone, Edinburgh, pp 242–257

Richelsen B 1998 Long term follow up of patients who underwent jejunoileal bypass for morbid obesity. European Journal of Surgery 164:281–286

Studley JGN, Williamson RCN 1999 Malignant tumours of the small bowel. In: Taylor TV, Watson A, Williamson RCN (eds) Upper digestive surgery. Oesophagus, stomach and small intestine. Saunders, London, pp 949–962

Thodiyil PA, El-Masry NS, Peake H et al 2004 T-tube jejunostomy feeding after pancreatic surgery: a safe adjunct. Asian Journal of Surgery 27:80–84

Thomas WEG 1990 Complications of small bowel diverticula. In: Williamson RCN, Cooper MJ (eds) Emergency abdominal surgery. Churchill Livingstone, Edinburgh, pp 191–208

Williams JG, Wong WD, Rothenberger DA et al 1991 Recurrence of Crohn's disease after resection. British Journal of Surgery 78:10–19

Williams NS, Nasmyth DG, Jones D et al 1986 De-functioning stomas: a prospective controlled trial comparing loop ileostomy with loop transverse colostomy. British Journal of Surgery 73:566–570

Williamson RCN 1991 Small intestine. In: O'Higgins NJ, Chisholm GD, Williamson RCN (eds) Surgical management, 2nd edn. Butterworth-Heinemann, Oxford, pp 562–593

18

Colonoscopy

R. J. Leicester

CONTENTS

INTRODUCTION

Colonoscopy has revolutionized the diagnosis and treatment of colonic disease, allowing accurate mucosal visualization, biopsy and therapeutic polypectomy. Technological advances in instrumentation allow rapid and safe examination of the whole colon, provided the endoscopist has been adequately trained in the technique.

Use diagnostic colonoscopy to evaluate an abnormal or equivocal barium enema, particularly where diverticular disease or colonic spasm may often obscure a small mucosal lesion. In elderly patients, who often tolerate barium enema badly, colonoscopy should be the first-line investigation for unexplained rectal bleeding or anaemia and is the investigation of choice for all patients with a positive faecal occult blood test. Colonoscopy is the most accurate diagnostic tool for differential diagnosis and assessment of extent in inflammatory bowel disease, but should be avoided in acute disease, where technetium-labelled white cell scanning is a safer alternative.

Therapeutic colonoscopy has changed the surgical management of colorectal polyps, facilitating removal of all pedunculated and most sessile adenomatous lesions, thus providing an opportunity for colorectal cancer prevention. Diathermy coagulation or laser therapy of vascular abnormalities such as angiodysplasia may pre-empt laparotomy in acute colonic haemorrhage or cure anaemia due to chronic blood loss. Relief of obstruction in colorectal cancer, either as an initial procedure prior to surgical resection or as long-term palliation, may be achieved using either laser vaporization or stent insertion.

Following polypectomy or curative resection for colorectal cancer, carry out regular follow-up colonoscopy, initially after 3 years and thereafter 5-yearly if no new polyps are detected. Commence screening of high-risk groups (e.g. polyposis coli) from age 15 years (if gene-positive) and continue approximately 2-yearly until the age of 40 years. Hereditary non-polyposis coli families should undergo 1–2-yearly surveillance, commencing at least 10 years younger than the index case. If facilities exist, then screen subjects with a strong family history of colorectal cancer (i.e. one first-degree relative with onset before 40 years of age, or more than one first-degree relative of any age) in the hope of reducing the incidence of colorectal cancer by removing adenomatous lesions.

Carry out emergency colonoscopy in cases of acute, severe rectal bleeding after anorectal and upper gastrointestinal causes have been excluded by rigid proctosigmoidoscopy and gastroscopy. Bleeding usually ceases in up to 80% of patients, allowing colonoscopy within 24–48 hours, after bowel preparation. Even in the presence of active bleeding, while small mucosal lesions may be overlooked, you can obtain valuable clues as to the segment of colon from which the haemorrhage is arising, or note blood emerging through the ileocaecal valve, indicating a small-bowel lesion. When a diagnosis has not been reached and emergency laparotomy becomes necessary, you may perform colonoscopy under general anaesthetic with the peritoneal cavity exposed, following on-table lavage with saline or water introduced via a Foley catheter through a caecostomy.

PROCEDURE

Prepare

Accurate, rapid examination depends upon effective bowel preparation. Advise patients to discontinue any iron preparation or stool-bulking agents 1 week prior to endoscopy, and change to a low-residue diet. Twenty-four hours before examination, restrict oral intake to clear fluids such as coffee or tea without milk, concentrated meat extract and glucose drinks. Give a purgative such as sodium picosulfate 12–18 hours before colonoscopy and repeat it 4 hours before examination. Alternatively, give balanced electrolyte solutions combined with polyethylene glycol, which have been shown to produce rapid preparation without the need for dietary restriction. Give oral metoclopramide 10 mg prior to ingestion of the 3–4 litres of solution, which enhances gastric emptying and reduces nausea and vomiting.

Obtain from all patients written, informed consent for the procedure. Give reassurance about the examination to allay fears, allowing minimal levels of sedation to be used.

Colonoscopy is usually performed under intravenous sedation with the addition of an analgesic. Do not give excessive sedation or analgesia, to avoid circulatory or respiratory depression. Additionally, it will dull appreciation of severe pain, which should occur only when a poor technique is used, causing dangerous overstretching of the bowel. For similar reasons do not perform colonoscopy under general anaesthesia, apart from as an intraoperative procedure in cases of acute colonic haemorrhage. Elderly patients in particular can suffer significant hypotension following pethidine, and this, combined with the synergistic effect of opiates and benzodiazepines, can also cause significant falls in oxygen saturation. In order to avoid these complications, use only small doses of analgesic and hypnotic such as intravenous pethidine 50 mg or pentazocine 30 mg plus midazolam 2.5–5 mg. Monitor all patients by pulse oximetry, during and after the procedure, and give added inspired oxygen as appropriate. Always have available antidotes to benzodiazepines (flumazenil) and opiates (naloxone), together with full cardiorespiratory resuscitation equipment and trained staff to use it in case of emergency. Occasionally an antispasmodic, either intravenous hyoscine butylbromide (Buscopan) or intraluminal peppermint oil suspension, may be employed.

As a rule, examine the patient in the left lateral position or, alternatively, supine. Use a tipping trolley in case of cardiorespiratory problems. Have available at least two trained assistants: one to observe the patient's vital signs and the other to assist with the accessories for biopsy or snare polypectomy. Videoendoscopes are an essential tool to ensure accurate and safe polypectomy and also to maintain the interest of the assistants.

Check all equipment prior to intubation. The colonoscope must have been adequately cleaned and disinfected. The light source, endoscope angulation controls, air–water insufflation and suction facilities must be in full working order. Check the diathermy equipment for correct, safe operation. Ensure that all accessories such as biopsy forceps and polypectomy snares operate correctly.

Access

Modern colonoscopes are sophisticated precision instruments designed to enhance intubation of the colon in the most efficient manner. As well as a wide-angled lens to allow a greater field of vision, a graduated torque characteristic assists variability in the stiffness of the instrument. During intubation, the instrument may be pushed forward or pulled back (Fig. 18.1). Change of direction may be achieved by angulation of the distal end, up/down or left/right. Change of direction may also be achieved by up/down deflection, combined with rotation. Keeping the distal section of the instrument as straight as possible, restoring this to a neutral position as soon as possible after angulation around an acute bend, helps to prevent loop formation. Avoid maximum up/down and left/right angulation, as this results in a J-shape and rotation of the end of the instrument rather than change of direction. Advancement may also be achieved by the straightening of a loop using torque and withdrawal or by suction causing a concertina effect of the bowel over the endoscope.

Colonoscopy is made easier if the anatomy of the colon is properly understood. The rectum is fixed in a retroperitoneal position and consists of alternating mucosal folds forming the valves of Houston. The sigmoid colon is freely mobile on its mesentery and of variable length and configuration. The descending colon and splenic flexure are

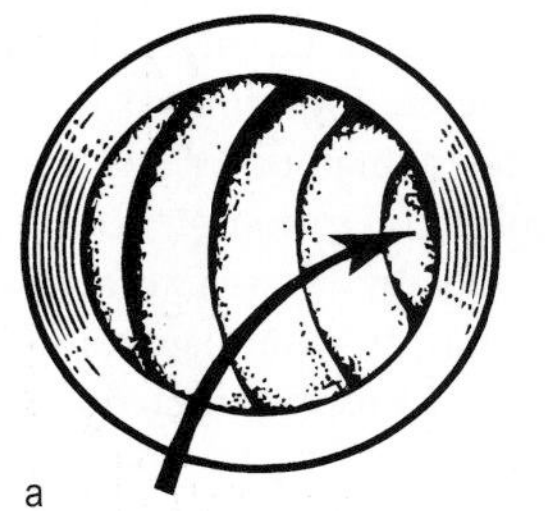

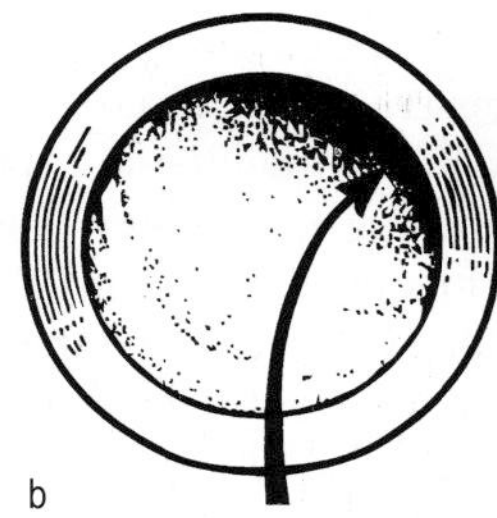

Fig. 18.1 Steer towards the concavity of the folds (a) and away from the bright light reflex (b).

relatively fixed by their peritoneal attachments. At the splenic flexure, the direction of the colon is forwards and downwards to the transverse colon which, like the sigmoid, is of variable length and freely mobile on the transverse mesocolon. The bowel becomes fixed again at the hepatic flexure and the direction passes forwards and downwards into the ascending colon and caecum, which are usually fixed by peritoneal attachments, though less consistently than the descending colon. It is the mobile and variable-length sigmoid and transverse colon that cause the most difficulty through looping of the instrument.

The aim of colonoscopy is to achieve intubation from the anus to caecum with the minimum possible length of instrument. Characteristically, the colonoscope, when straight and without loop formation, should be in a roughly U-shaped configuration with 70–80 cm of instrument inserted to the caecal pole. Significantly greater insertion length indicates the presence of a loop.

19

Colon

C. R. G. Cohen, C. J. Vaizey

CONTENTS

EXAMINATION OF THE LARGE BOWEL

Preoperative assessment

In addition to a full history carry out a complete examination including the abdomen, and palpation and sigmoidoscopy of the anus and rectum. Carry out further investigations as necessary.

- *Fibreoptic sigmoidoscopy,* a simple outpatient procedure, can be undertaken after one or two phosphate enemas, revealing polyps or a carcinoma in the proximal sigmoid or descending colon.
- *Colonoscopy* (Ch. 18) is the investigation of choice for the large bowel although it is not without risks, especially in the elderly, those with co-morbidity, with diverticular disease or if polyp removal is carried out. Biopsies can be obtained from tumours and inflammatory bowel disease in the proximal colon. Pedunculated polyps can be removed by colonoscopic snaring, and more advanced procedures such as endoscopic mucosal resection and stenting are now available in many centres. Colonoscopy is often useful in cases of gastrointestinal bleeding and can be safely carried out at the acute admission.
- *CT colography and virtual colonoscopy* offers a sensitive alternative to colonoscopy.
- *Double contrast barium enema* is less sensitive than colonoscopy but still has a valuable place.
- *Other examinations.* These include: mucosal biopsy in inflammatory bowel disease to help in the differentiation of ulcerative colitis, Crohn's disease and infective colitis; stool microscopy and culture to differentiate bacterial and parasitic infection from inflammatory bowel disease; straight X-ray of the abdomen in suspected large-bowel obstruction or perforation. Serial abdominal films are important in evaluating the progress of acute colitis and the onset of toxic megacolon. Imaging scans are of value in elucidating abdominal masses, abscesses and possible metastases. Ultrasonography is more readily available than CT scanning, but diagnostic accuracy is operator-dependent. Angiography can help in the evaluation of severe gastrointestinal haemorrhage and localizes haemangiomatous malformations.

Avoid performing elective operations to establish colonic or rectal disease; diagnostic laparotomy allows access to the exterior of the bowel; disease is mainly confined to the interior.

ELECTIVE OPERATIONS

CARCINOMA

Prepare

Plan elective surgery carefully. Always get informed consent for removal of any adjacent organs that may be affected by the disease process. Always have X-ray films and results of other investigations available for study in the operating theatre. Ensure you have the right equipment and assistance available. Always have an endoscope available to re-examine the bowel lumen if necessary during the procedure. Re-examine the abdomen and rectum when the patient is asleep and relaxed.

Assess

Examine the contents of the whole abdomen, and the whole of the colon from the appendix to the anus. Small adenomatous polyps cannot be felt. Synchronous carcinomas occur in 4% of patients. Avoid handling the carcinoma; cover it with a swab soaked in dilute aqueous povidone-iodine (Betadine) solution. Feel for enlarged lymph nodes in the mesentery and in the para-aortic regions. Look and feel for liver metastases. Look for peritoneal metastases.

Estimate the resectability and curability of the tumour. Palpate and visualize the liver to exclude metastases or biopsy them to confirm the diagnosis. If a tumour is locally resectable but fixed to other organs such as bladder, uterus, another piece of large or small intestine, the duodenum, stomach, gallbladder, liver or kidney, or to the abdominal wall, it may still be curable, so be prepared to resect it en bloc with part or all of the adjacent organ or abdominal wall. If the carcinoma is resectable but metastases are present, be willing to modify surgical treatment, but tumour resection provides better palliation than a bypass procedure. After subsequent investigation you may then plan to perform partial hepatectomy or an ablation technique in 3–4 months' time.

Treat potentially curable carcinoma of the right colon by one-stage right hemicolectomy, taking the ileocolic and middle colic vessels at their origin from the superior mesenteric vessels. If metastases are present perform a less extensive resection without wide mesenteric clearance.

Treat carcinoma of the transverse colon by extended right hemicolectomy or transverse colectomy, taking the hepatic and/or splenic flexure if the lesion is situated proximally or distally in the transverse colon. With a lesion at the splenic flexure and distal diverticular disease, you may need to perform an extended left hemicolectomy; swing the right colon down on the right side of the abdomen and perform an anastomosis to the rectum. Alternatively, perform an extended colectomy and ileosigmoid anastomosis.

Treat carcinoma of the descending and sigmoid colon by left hemicolectomy, taking the inferior mesenteric artery at its origin from the aorta and the inferior mesenteric vein at the same level.

Treat most cases of carcinoma of the rectum by anterior resection using either a sutured, stapled or per-anal anastomosis. Abdominoperineal excision of the rectum is required in only 15–20% of cases when it is impossible to obtain a 2–5-cm distal clearance of the tumour. Dissection in the pelvis is essential to ensure removal of the lymphovascular bundle (mesorectum) without breaching the fascial plane in which it is contained. Identify and preserve the hypogastric nerve plexus, if it is uninvolved with tumour. This avoids ejaculatory, erectile and urinary complications. A discussion of the merits and problems with so-called 'total mesorectal excision' is beyond the scope of this chapter; suffice to say that in expert hands it provides very low local recurrence rates with an acceptable incidence of complications.

For rectal carcinoma with metastases, carry out anterior resection if you can perform this safely without the need to perform a defunctioning colostomy, since many of these patients deteriorate and never have the colostomy closed. For low rectal carcinoma with local extension to the side walls of the pelvis or involved internal iliac nodes, select a palliative abdominoperineal excision of the rectum or a Hartmann's operation.

DIVERTICULAR DISEASE

Diverticular disease is very common and found incidentally, especially in the sigmoid colon, in elderly patients. Symptomatic disease is usually produced by muscle hypertrophy, thickening and shortening of the sigmoid colon. Even in elective resection the disease may be associated with marked pericolic inflammation and oedema with pericolic abscess formation in the mesentery.

Fewer operations are now undertaken than formerly, except for fit patients with severe attacks of lower left-sided and suprapubic pain with marked diverticular disease on a barium enema X-ray, muscle hypertrophy and narrowing of the colonic lumen unresponsive to dietary change and antispasmodic drugs. The barium enema findings and pathology do not always correlate, and patients often wait too long before being offered surgical treatment. Definite indications for surgical treatment include males under 50 years with symptomatic disease such as frequent acute attacks with fever, mass, and radiologically demonstrable pericolic abscess, or urinary infections suggesting bladder or ureteric adhesion signalling impending fistula formation, or recurrent bleeding, since statistically over 80% eventually come to surgery, many with complications.

Avoid operation in patients with irritable bowel syndrome and few diverticula; their symptoms will persist.

Operative treatment is always by resection and anastomosis. If there is acute on chronic inflammation at the time of surgery or the anastomosis is difficult, then be prepared to perform a defunctioning ileostomy as a temporary measure. It is unnecessary to remove all the proximal diverticula. Resect all hypertrophied sections of bowel, usually including the whole of the sigmoid colon, with anastomosis between the middle or upper descending colon and the upper third of the rectum below the sacral promontory.

ULCERATIVE COLITIS

Offer elective operation to patients with persistent or recurrent attacks of diarrhoea with the passage of blood, anaemia, weight loss and general ill-health who do not respond to treatment with corticosteroids and salazines. The majority of these patients have total or extensive colitis. Patients with purely distal disease, such as sigmoid or left-colon, do not usually require operation. Try to operate on patients who have several severe attacks of acute colitis during remission.

Total colitis of 10 or more years' duration may result in dysplastic epithelial changes and eventual carcinoma, even in the absence of any symptoms. Carefully monitor them with colonoscopy and mucosal biopsy. Operate if they develop moderate or severe dysplasia. Operate on patients with total colitis and strictures or filling defects on barium enema X-ray or colonoscopy. Steroid therapy does not contraindicate surgery as it makes no difference to the outcome, but administer steroid cover during and after the operation.

In quiescent total colitis, the colon is slightly thickened, shortened and greyish white in colour. Even at elective operation, part of the colon may appear much more actively inflamed with thickening, oedema and marked hyperaemia. The paracolic and mesenteric nodes may be considerably enlarged.

The most straightforward procedure is a proctocolectomy with a conventional ileostomy. If operation is performed early in the course of the disease when the rectum is still distensible and there is no dysplasia in rectal biopsies, consider performing a colectomy and ileorectal anastomosis. To spare patients from permanent conventional ileostomy, perform a conservative proctocolectomy leaving the anal sphincters and create an ileoanal reservoir. If the patient is incontinent as a result of previous sphincter damage, you may construct an ileostomy with a reservoir (Kock) to avoid the patient having to wear an appliance. If you are inexperienced in these operations, carry out a colectomy and ileostomy, retaining the whole rectum.

CROHN'S DISEASE

This can develop anywhere within the gastrointestinal tract and is primarily treated medically. Undertake surgical treatment if medical treatment fails to control the disease, or for complications such as stenosis causing obstructive symptoms, abscesses or internal or external fistula formation. Surgery is not curative, so make sure you treat the patients and their symptoms, not appearances on radiological imaging.

The whole or part of the colon may be involved in Crohn's disease. Carefully exclude disease in the stomach, duodenum and the whole of the small bowel. Measure and record the length of the small bowel and the sites and extent of the disease. These patients often require multiple operations and may end up with 'short-bowel syndrome' unless surgery is carefully planned.

When the disease affects the terminal ileum and/or caecum and ascending colon, carry out ileal resection with removal of the caecum or right colon as necessary. In a primary operation, remove 5–10 cm of macroscopically normal ileum proximal to the lesion. If there is a chronic abscess cavity in the right iliac fossa, extend the right hemicolectomy so that the anastomosis lies in the upper abdomen away from the abscess cavity.

If the whole colon is severely involved and requires resection, perform a colectomy and ileorectal anastomosis or a total proctocolectomy and conventional ileostomy. Distal disease involving only the rectum may require an abdominoperineal excision with an end colostomy.

POLYPS AND POLYPOSIS

When you discover rectal polyps on routine sigmoidoscopy, remove one or more for histology. If the polyp proves to be an adenoma, carry out a colonoscopy to search for and treat proximal polyps. Sessile villous adenomas usually occur in the rectum and can be removed by endoanal local excision. Transanal endoscopic microsurgery is available in specialist centres. If several large polyps are present in a patient with carcinoma, extend the resection to include these. In a patient with one or more carcinomas and several large polyps, consider colectomy and ileorectal anastomosis.

Perform anterior resection with coloanal anastomosis or a modified Soave procedure on circumferential villous tumours extending above 10 cm from the anal vent. Familial adenomatous polyposis demands operation to avoid inevitable malignant change. Options include colectomy and ileorectal anastomosis, or proctocolectomy and ileoanal pouch reconstruction. Following ileorectal anastomosis the rectum still carries the potential for malignant change, so plan to perform follow-up sigmoidoscopy every 6 months. Fulgurate rectal polyps if they are over 5 mm in diameter.

URGENT OPERATIONS

Urgent operations on the colon or rectum are carried out for obstruction, perforation, acute fulminating inflammatory bowel disease and acute haemorrhage. You are operating in an emergency to achieve a specific, urgent goal. Do not lightly undertake procedures that prejudice the patient's recovery. Improve the patient's condition before operation by replacing blood, fluid and electrolyte loss. Counteract major sepsis with antibiotics such as a cephalosporin, together with metronidazole.

Severe bleeding, major abdominal sepsis or perforation demand operation as soon as the patient's condition allows. Large-bowel obstruction and inflammatory bowel disease rarely require emergency surgery. Whenever possible avoid operating in haste at night, when you are tired, the patient is ill-prepared and your assistance and equipment are inadequate.

OBSTRUCTION

Define the level of obstruction with a CT scan or water-soluble contrast enema. If the patient is medically unfit for operative surgery, the stenosing tumour may be suitable for radiological insertion of a stent to open up the lumen, allowing the patient to be optimized for elective surgery.

If you need to carry out an urgent resection, make sure it is as radical as would be achieved at an elective operation at the same site, provided cure is possible. If there are metastases, carry out palliative resection. It is rare to find a proximal tumour that is not resectable. Avoid the alternative procedure of a bypass operation if possible as this may relieve the obstruction but it will not stop bleeding from the tumour and consequent anaemia nor will it stop the pain or complications from the mass invading other structures. If a left-sided tumour is unresectable, create a proximal defunctioning colostomy.

Perform a right hemicolectomy for carcinoma of the right colon causing acute intestinal obstruction. In the past, left-sided obstruction was treated by a staged procedure. Initially a proximal defunctioning stoma was created to relieve the obstruction; subsequently the tumour was resected and, when it was safely healed, the stoma was closed. More commonly, carcinoma of the sigmoid or descending colon is resected by a one-stage colectomy with ileosigmoid or ileorectal anastomosis.

Treat carcinoma of the rectosigmoid junction or rectum by resection, peroperative irrigation of the obstructed colon and primary anastomosis with or without a defunctioning ileostomy. Alternatively, perform a Hartmann's procedure (see later).

Acute obstructive diverticular disease is rare but is often complicated by paracolic abscess formation. The most commonly performed operation is immediate resection with a Hartmann's procedure. However, if the infection is localized and would be completely removed by resection, it should be safe to carry out a resection and anastomosis with or without a defunctioning ileostomy.

PERFORATION

Perforation of a carcinoma or diverticular disease demands resection and anastomosis with a covering colostomy or, in the presence of major faecal contamination, a Hartmann's procedure. If you detect a significant abscess using CT, drain it percutaneously.

If initially localized abdominal signs become more generalized, or if the infection fails to settle despite adequate conservative therapy, operate. A minority of patients operated on for localized diverticulitis are amenable to primary resection and primary anastomosis. Generalized peritonitis secondary to a free perforation is more commonly associated with purulent peritonitis than with faecal peritonitis. Resection and primary anastomosis is possible in the majority of cases without faecal contamination but do not carry this out in the presence of faecal peritonitis.

Primary anastomosis is popular because patients require one operation rather than two, whereas following a Hartmann's operation many patients are left with a permanent stoma, either because of unwillingness or unfitness to have further surgery – and reversal operation after Hartmann's resection can be very difficult.

Aim to resect the perforated segment, even in the acutely ill patient, minimizing the risk of continued contamination, since it is difficult, at operation, to differentiate a perforated carcinoma from diverticulitis.

ACUTE INFLAMMATORY OR ISCHAEMIC BOWEL DISEASE

Treat acute fulminating colitis, with or without toxic megacolon, by colectomy and ileostomy with a mucous fistula. Do not excise the rectum. It is much safer to make a mucous fistula than to close the rectal stump. In order to avoid creating a second stoma, close the stump directly under the wound so that if it breaks down it will not contaminate the peritoneal cavity.

Excise a segment of acute ischaemic colitis and create a proximal and distal colostomy. Always leave the rectum and sigmoid colon as these usually recover sufficiently for an anastomosis to be carried out later.

ACUTE MASSIVE HAEMORRHAGE

Determine if possible the site of bleeding by sigmoidoscopy, colonoscopy, upper gastrointestinal endoscopy and angiography. Remember that 50% of patients with episodes of haemorrhage and diverticular disease have another cause for the bleeding.

If the site can be accurately determined it may be possible to stop the bleeding by interventional radiologically controlled embolization. If you cannot determine the site and origin of colonic bleeding preoperatively, organize on-table colonoscopy and possible enteroscopy.

SURGERY OF THE LARGE BOWEL

Morbidity and mortality following colonic surgery is higher than following resections of the small bowel. The colonic blood supply is tenuous and easily damaged, and tissue perfusion is often decreased postoperatively, resulting in a degree of ischaemic colitis. Infection is common, resulting in abscess formation with potentiation of collagenase activity. Collagen undergoes lysis and may result in anastomotic dehiscence.

Prepare

1 Ensure that this is the correct, 'consented' patient, equipment and assistance are adequate, and imaging results are available at operation.

2 Most surgeons use bowel preparation before elective operations although there is no clear-cut evidence to support it. Certainly there is no need to clear the colon for a right hemicolectomy. Sodium picosulfate and magnesium citrate provide a stimulant preparation, polyethylene glycol is a mechanical preparation. Give adequate fluids for 24 hours preoperatively. Intravenous fluids may be required in elderly patients. If necessary order enemas in the absence of a bowel preparation to reduce the presence of hard stools distal to the anastomosis.

3 Oral antibiotics are of little value; give peroperative prophylactic antibiotics at induction of anaesthesia. A cephalosporin and metronidazole or beta-lactamase inhibitor/broad-spectrum penicillin (Augmentin) are popular. Give a further dose of antibiotics if the operation is prolonged more than 2 hours, or if there is significant intraoperative contamination. Routine use of more than one dose of prophylactic antibiotics does not appear to reduce the risk of infection but gross faecal contamination may demand continued therapeutic antibiotics for several days postoperation.

4 Catheterize the patient after induction of anaesthesia and monitor urinary output during and after surgery.

Action

1 Clamp the bowel to be resected with Parker–Kerr clamps or use a cross-stapling technique. Place no clamps on the ends to be sutured but use non-crushing clamps away from the bowel ends to avoid contamination. Clean the ends of the bowel to be sutured with moistened swabs wetted in 1:2000 aqueous chlorhexidine solution or aqueous 10% povidone-iodine (Betadine) solution.

2 Divide the colon at right-angles to the mesentery. If there is disparity in size between the ends as in right hemicolectomy or ileorectal anastomosis, slit up the antimesenteric border of the ileum or narrower colon

until the two ends approximate in size. Alternatively carry out an end-to-side or side-to-side anastomosis. Ensure there is no twist in the bowel.

3 Suture the bowel in a one-layer interrupted or continuous seromuscular fashion with an appropriate suture such as 3/0 PDS (polydioxanone), or 4/0 Ethibond (polybutylate-coated polyester). Invert the edges to prevent mucosal protrusion, without producing an obstructing anastomotic cuff. Alternatively, carry out a stapled anastomosis. Undertake rectal anastomosis using a circular stapling device such as the EEA stapler, using a 28- or 31-mm diameter device, particularly when forming an anastomosis low in the pelvis, when suturing is technically difficult.

4 Avoid contamination during the operation. If the colon is loaded, place a non-crushing clamp across the bowel 10 cm from the end before this is swabbed out and cleaned. If possible, screen the anastomosis from the peritoneal cavity and contents while it is being constructed. When it is complete, discard and replace the towels, gloves and instruments before closing the abdomen.

5 Colonic anastomosis are traditionally drained but probably unnecessary, except for a very low pelvic anastomosis.

RIGHT HEMICOLECTOMY

Perform this operation for carcinoma of the caecum and ascending colon and for the occasional benign tumour of the right colon. Undertake it for a perforated caecal diverticulum, so-called solitary ulcer of the caecum and carry out a limited resection for carcinoma of the appendix or a carcinoid tumour at the base of the appendix. If possible avoid performing an ileocolic bypass even for an extensive carcinoma; a palliative resection gives better results.

Treat benign disease of the terminal ileum, particularly Crohn's disease, by resecting an appropriate amount of ileum together with the caecum and 2–3 cm of the right colon. When Crohn's disease is associated with abscess formation in the right iliac fossa, extend the operation so that the anastomosis lies in the upper abdomen away from the abscess with the intention of protecting it from post-operative fistula formation.

Never make a small-bowel anastomosis close to the ileocaecal valve. Preferably remove the caecum and a small part of the ascending colon, and carry out an ileocolic anastomosis. In the presence of obstructing lesions of the colon, the caecum may be ischaemic. You must include the region in any resection, either in the form of an extended right hemicolectomy or even a colectomy with ileorectal anastomosis.

Action (Fig. 19.1)

1 Handle the tumour as little as possible. If the serosa and surrounding fat are infiltrated by carcinoma, cover it with a swab soaked in aqueous 10% povidone-iodine solution. Leave the omentum adherent to the right colon. Draw the caecum and ascending colon medially. Cut through the parietal peritoneum lateral to the colon from the caecum to the hepatic flexure. If the carcinoma infiltrates the lateral abdominal wall, excise a large disc of peritoneum and underlying muscle with the specimen.

2 Dissect the right colon from the posterior abdominal wall. Identify and preserve the right ureter, gonadal vessels and duodenum. Mobilize the hepatic flexure and divide any ileal bands so that the whole of the right colon can be lifted from the abdomen. You are elevating the bowel on its embryological mesentery, containing its blood vessels, lymphatics, nerves and contained fat. Keep meticulously in the correct plane between the mesentery and posterior wall peritoneum.

3 Transilluminate the mesentery to identify the vessels. Clamp and divide the ileocolic artery and vein close to the superior mesenteric vessels. Divide the right colic vessels and the right branch of the middle colic vessels close to their origin.

4 The extent of the resection depends to some degree on the size and site of the tumour but normally includes approximately 25 cm of terminal ileum to the middle third of the transverse colon. Remove the right half of the greater omentum with the specimen. If the tumour is situated near the hepatic flexure remove the right side of the gastroepiploic arch of vessels to obtain a wider clearance. Place a Parker–Kerr clamp or cross-staples across the ileum and transverse colon at the site of division. If the patient is obstructed or the colon is unprepared, place towels around the bowel at the time of division. Divide the bowel and remove the specimen. Hold the ends of the ileum and colon to be anastomosed in Babcock's forceps and clean them with mounted swabs wetted with aqueous 10% povidone-iodine solution.

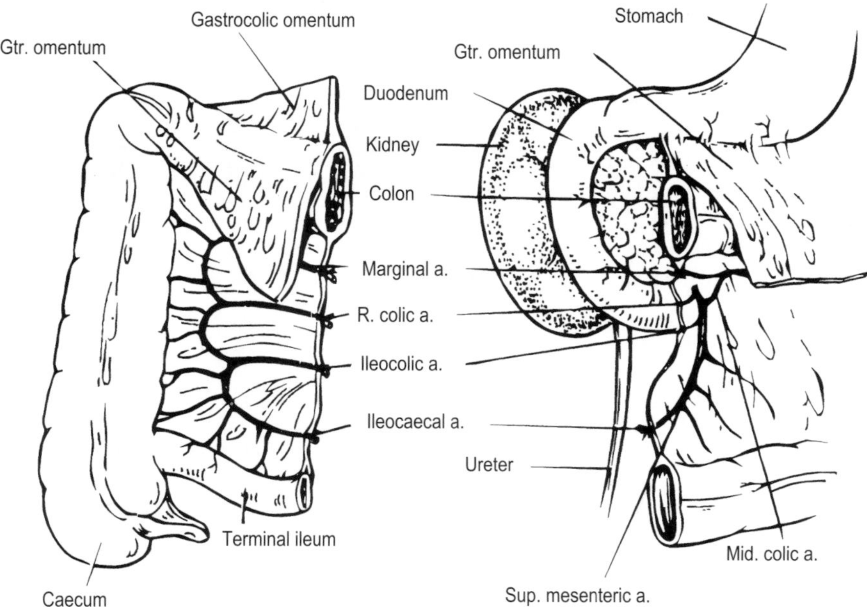

Fig. 19.1 Radical right hemicolectomy. The resected specimen is on the left and comprises the right half of the colon, the terminal ileum and the mesentery with vessels and nodes. Also included are the right halves of the gastrocolic and greater omenta. The ileocolic artery and vein are divided at their origins from the superior mesenteric vessels. The right branch of the middle colic artery is divided. The duodenum, pancreas and right kidney and ureter have been identified and protected from damage.

5 Anastomose the terminal ileum end-to-end to the transverse colon, if necessary widening the ileum with an antimesenteric slit. Mark the anastomosis with haemostatic clips if desired. Alternatively, divide the colon using a linear cutter stapling device and perform an end-to-side anastomosis, or construct a functional end-to-end anastomosis using the same linear cutter stapling device. Suture the cut edges of the mesentery with a polyglactin 910 (Vicryl) suture. Cover the anastomosis with the remaining omentum.

6 Make sure the bowel on each side of the anastomosis is viable and check that the anastomosis lies freely without twist or tension.

7 Examine the raw surfaces, particularly in the right flank, and stop any bleeding. Remove any blood collected above the right lobe of the liver and in the pelvis.

Technical points

1 If the resection is for a benign condition such as Crohn's disease or a caecal diverticulum, it need not be extensive. The vessels can be divided in the middle of the mesentery rather than at their origin.

2 If the carcinoma is locally invasive but can be excised radically, widen the scope of the operation to include abdominal wall or part of the involved organs.

3 If the carcinoma is situated at the hepatic flexure or in the right side of the transverse colon, mobilize the splenic flexure as well. Divide the middle colic vessels close to their origin and anastomose the terminal ileum to the descending or sigmoid colon. If there are multiple metastases carry out a limited segmental resection rather than a bypass procedure.

LEFT HEMICOLECTOMY

Undertake left hemicolectomy for carcinoma of the left and sigmoid colon, and for diverticular disease. If the operation is for an obstructed neoplasm, carry out an extended colectomy with an ileosigmoid or ileorectal anastomosis. Alternatively, carry out a resection with on-table irrigation of the obstructed proximal colon and create a primary anastomosis. Try to avoid a Hartmann's operation as patients are frequently left with their stoma and reversal can be a major undertaking.

In diverticular disease, resect the sigmoid colon and as much of the ascending colon as is necessary. Leave isolated diverticula in the upper descending and transverse colon, providing the bowel wall is not thickened. Anastomose the proximal bowel to the upper third of the rectum below the sacral promontory and not to the sigmoid colon. In any left hemicolectomy, the splenic flexure and the left half of the transverse colon must be mobilized.

Assess

1 Have the catheterized patient in the lithotomy Trendelenburg (Lloyd-Davies) position. Stand on the patient's right side. Make a long midline incision. You require access to the spleen when you mobilize the splenic flexure of colon, and in the pelvis when you construct the anastomosis. If the operation is for a carcinoma, carefully palpate the liver bimanually, examine the colon and the whole of the small bowel, palpate the mesenteric and para-aortic nodes and the whole of the peritoneal cavity and pelvis.

2 Gently palpate the carcinoma to assess its mobility but touch it as little as possible. If the serosal surface is involved, cover it with a swab soaked in 10% aqueous povidone-iodine solution. If you are performing partial colectomy for a benign condition, assess the diseased and normal colon to decide the extent of resection.

3 Determine on radical resection of a carcinoma if possible. Tie the inferior mesenteric artery at its origin from the aorta and the inferior mesenteric vein below the inferior border of the pancreas. If the patient is very elderly and clearly unfit, and the blood supply to the colon is tenuous because of severe atheroma, undertake a less radical procedure, retaining the origin of the inferior mesenteric artery, and ligate the left colonic artery and sigmoid branches as appropriate. If the resection is for a benign condition, or a palliative resection for carcinoma, then the bowel resection need not be so wide and you may ligate and divide the vessels close to the bowel wall.

RADICAL RESECTION OF THE LEFT COLON

Action (Fig. 19.2)

1 Exteriorize the small bowel to the right side and cover it with a moist pack. Never pack the small bowel into the wound as it severely restricts access. Divide the congenital adhesions that bind the sigmoid colon to the abdominal wall in the left iliac fossa and then divide the adhesions between the descending colon and the lateral peritoneum. This is most efficiently achieved by following the plane of zygosis (Greek *zygon* = yoke; true conjunction of posterior peritoneum and visceral peritoneum) or white line. Do not divide the peritoneum

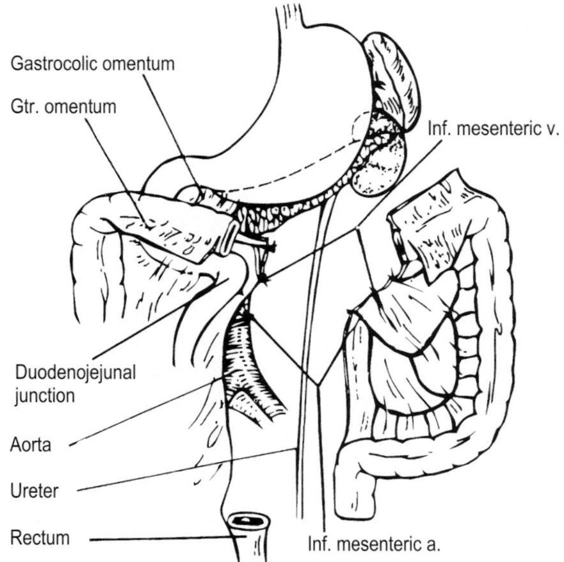

Fig. 19.2 Radical left hemicolectomy. The resected specimen is on the right and comprises the left half of colon, the mesocolon and the left halves of the gastrocolic and greater omenta. The left division of the middle colic artery and the origin of the inferior mesenteric artery have been ligated and divided. The duodenojejunal junction, left ureter and kidney, pancreas and spleen have been protected from damage.

but stay on the mesenteric side of the white line to ensure that you remain in the correct plane.

2 Rotate the patient to the right side and then mobilize the splenic flexure by dividing the phrenocolic ligament. Ligate the few vessels in it. Avoid damaging the spleen and the tail of the pancreas. If the carcinoma is distal you may preserve the greater omentum by dividing the adhesions between the omentum and the colon as far proximally as the middle of the transverse colon and dividing the peritoneum along the end of the lesser sac. If the tumour is situated near the flexure, excise the left half of the greater omentum with the tumour by dividing the left side of the gastroepiploic arch and removing the lesser and greater omentum with the specimen.

3 Elevate the left colon on its mesentery and dissect it free from the duodenojejunal flexure, the left ureter and gonadal vessels. Incise the peritoneum overlying the aorta and mobilize the inferior mesenteric artery to its origin. Ligate and divide the artery and then identify the inferior mesenteric vein lying laterally and clamp, ligate and divide it a little below the lower border of the pancreas.

4 Mobilize the sigmoid colon if the anastomosis is to be made to the upper third of the rectum. Do not divide the sigmoid higher than about 10 cm above the rectum or you will endanger its blood supply. Divide the mesentery and marginal vessels to the edge of the colon at the site chosen for resection in the transverse colon and rectum or sigmoid colon.

5 Place a non-crushing right-angled clamp across the rectum at the site of resection. Then irrigate the rectum by means of a catheter passed through the anus with povidone-iodine solution or a 1:2000 aqueous chlorhexidine solution, until it is perfectly clean.

? DIFFICULTY

1. If the abdominal wall is involved with carcinoma, excise part of the wall with the tumour and repair the defect at the end of the procedure. If small bowel is involved, be prepared to resect one loop or more as necessary and anastomose the cut ends. Be willing to excise a portion of the bladder fundus. If other organs are involved, such as the left ureter or uterus, deal with them appropriately.
2. Never fail to call for assistance and advice if you are not experienced enough to deal with unfamiliar techniques.
3. If the tumour is situated in the left half of the transverse colon or at the splenic flexure, excise most of the transverse colon and unite the hepatic flexure or ascending colon to the lower descending or sigmoid colon. Alternatively, perform an extended right hemicolectomy with an ileo-descending anastomosis.

6 While the rectal irrigation is being carried out, prepare the proximal colon for division. Place a non-crushing clamp across the bowel well proximal to the intended site of division. Cross-staple or use a Parker–Kerr clamp just distal to the intended site of division. Divide the colon, hold the proximal end in Babcock's forceps and swab the bowel out with Betadine solution or 1:2000 aqueous chlorhexidine solution.

7 Divide the rectum or sigmoid colon below the right-angled clamp and remove the specimen consisting of the left half of the colon, the inferior mesenteric artery and vein and the whole of the mesentery. If you need to mobilize the transverse colon or hepatic flexure to ensure a tension-free anastomosis, do this before dividing the colon.

Unite

Unite the bowel ends with one layer of seromuscular-inverting sutures according to your preferred technique. Beware of using the EEA stapler at the top of the rectum. Introducing it around the rectal valves may tear the rectum. If you employ this technique, either resect more of the rectum or anastomose the colon end-to-side to the rectum. Suture the cut edge of the transverse mesocolon to the cut edge of the peritoneum overlying the aorta.

CARCINOMA OF THE RECTUM

Assess all patients before operation by sigmoidoscopy, rectal biopsy and a colonoscopy or CT colography to evaluate the proximal colon. Assess low tumours and those placed anteriorly, with magnetic resonance imaging, to assess tumour stage. Consider preoperative radiotherapy particularly for T_3 and T_4 lesions. A few patients with small early carcinomas (assessed by transrectal ultrasound) are suitable for a per-anal local excision.

ANTERIOR RESECTION OF THE RECTUM

Assess

1 With the catheterized, anaesthetized patient in the lithotomy Trendelenburg (Lloyd-Davies) position, carry out an examination under anaesthetic to assess the fixity of low tumours (below the peritoneal reflection). Standing on the patient's right, make a long midline incision, as the splenic flexure will require mobilization and the rectal anastomosis may be deep within the pelvis.

2 Palpate and visualize the liver to establish if there are metastases. Note any local or distant peritoneal metastases. Examine the omentum. Palpate any nodes in the mesentery and note any para-aortic nodes. Finally, palpate the tumour, note its size and position above or below the peritoneal reflection and decide whether it is mobile, adherent to other organs or fixed within the pelvis.

3 Do not be daunted to discover that a large rectal carcinoma lies in a small male pelvis. Determine not to compromise on the standard of radical resection by breaching the planes of direction. Take time and proceed in an ever-deepening circumferential manner. As you mobilize the rectum, dissection becomes progressively easier.

Action (Fig. 19.3)

1 Mobilize the left side of the colon from the peritoneum by dividing the congenital adhesions from the sigmoid colon to the splenic flexure. Fully mobilize the splenic flexure and the left half of the transverse colon, preserving the omentum unless there are metastases present in it. Avoid damage to the spleen.

2 Mobilize the left colon on to its embryological mesentery – make sure you do not wander from the correct tissue plane; pull it to the right on its mesentery and separate and preserve the left ureter and gonadal vessels.

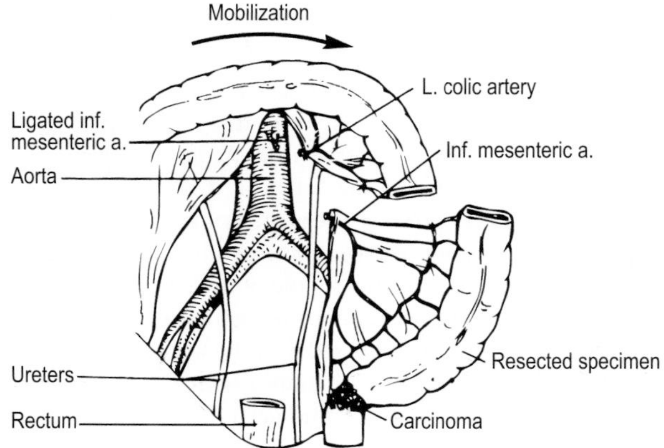

Fig. 19.3 Anterior resection of the rectum: the resected specimen is on the right and consists of the upper rectum, the sigmoid and part of the descending colon, together with the sigmoid mesocolon. The inferior mesenteric artery has been ligated and divided on the aorta and the inferior mesenteric vein at the upper border of the pancreas. The splenic flexure has been mobilized. Both ureters have been identified and preserved.

Take care not to damage the duodenojejunal flexure or the tail of the pancreas.

3 To enter the 'mesorectal plane' lift the sigmoid loop vertically. Observe the arc of the inferior mesenteric artery as it leaves the aorta and enters the mesorectum. Divide the peritoneum on the right side just beneath the arc of the artery, follow it back up to its origin and down into the loose areolar tissue that denotes the beginning of the mesorectal plane. Push away the tissue deep to this arcing peritoneal incision, which contains the pelvic nerve plexus. Both branches of this plexus should be apparent as they divide around the rectum at the level of the sacral promontory.

4 Make a similar incision in the peritoneum of the left side to produce a window with artery above and nerves below from the origin of the inferior artery to the start of the mesorectal plane. Clamp, divide and ligate the inferior mesenteric artery at its origin from the aorta, but if the patient is old and arteriosclerotic, preserve the left colic artery. Divide the inferior mesenteric vein at a slightly higher level, close to the lower border of the pancreas. Select a suitable area to transect the descending colon and divide the mesentery up to this point.

Bowel transection at this stage facilitates the rectal dissection because the specimen can be pulled anteriorly while leaving the descending colon and small bowel packed up and out of the way in the upper abdomen. The extent of rectal mobilization depends upon the level of the tumour. If it is retroperitoneal, you must completely mobilize the rectum and its mesorectum.

5 Move to the left of the patient. Pull the rectum forwards and dissect anteriorly to the sacral promontory and presacral fascia, as far down as the tip of the coccyx and the pelvic floor muscles. This is best done by holding a St Mark's lipped retractor in your left hand to pull the rectum forwards while carrying out sharp dissection with scissors or diathermy. Take care to visualize and preserve the presacral nerves.

6 As the posterior dissection deepens, divide the peritoneum over each side of the pelvis, close to the lateral wall. Eventually join the incisions anteriorly in the midline. The ideal site for this anterior division is about 1 cm above the most dependent part of the peritoneum. This usually corresponds to the bulge in the peritoneum overlying the seminal vesicles.

7 Hold the seminal vesicles forwards with a St Mark's lipped retractor and dissect between the vesicles and the rectum to uncover the rectovesical fascia described by the Parisian anatomist and surgeon Charles Denonvilliers (1808–1872). Incise this transversely and dissect down between the fascia and the rectum as far distally as necessary, and down behind the prostate to the pelvic floor. In a female, dissect distally between the rectum and vagina as far down as necessary, even to the pelvic floor.

8 By traction on the rectum to one side and then the other side of the pelvis, identify the tissue described as the 'lateral ligaments'. This can be cauterized and divided without the need for formal clipping and dividing. Avoid tenting up and damaging the third sacral nerve root at this point.

9 Straighten out the rectum and draw the tumour upwards. Choose a suitable site for division of the rectum. If possible allow a 5-cm clearance below the lower edge of the carcinoma. If the tumour is low down, this degree of clearance may be impossible to achieve in a restorative procedure. Be willing to compromise but without jeopardizing a curative procedure. Obtain at least a 2-cm clearance. For lesions of the upper rectum, the mesorectum is present at the site selected for division of the rectum. Divide this perpendicularly to the rectal wall, taking care not to 'cone down' on to the rectum, getting so close that you risk leaving mesorectum containing tumour deposits. Apply a transverse stapler or right-angled clamp to the rectum at the site selected for division. Remember, if you intend using a stapled anastomosis, that the stapler removes an extra 8 mm of rectum.

10 Irrigate the rectum through the anus with povidone-iodine solution or 1:2000 aqueous chlorhexidine solution. If only a small cuff of sphincter and rectum remains, simply swab it out. If you have not already divided it, select the site for division of the descending colon, place a Parker–Kerr clamp at right angles across the bowel and transect above it, holding the upper end of the colon with Babcock's forceps so that it can be swabbed out. Divide the rectum below the stapler or clamp with a long-handled knife. Remove the specimen containing the rectal carcinoma, the complete mesentery and nodes up to the origin of the inferior mesenteric artery.

Unite

The anastomosis can be carried out in one of two ways, depending upon the level of anastomosis, the ease of access to the pelvis and the obesity of the patient.

Sutured anastomosis (Fig. 19.4)

Suture the bowel in one layer to produce an end-to-end inverted anastomosis. Insert vertical mattress sutures into the posterior layer and hold each suture with artery forceps until they have all been inserted. Now 'rail-road' the descending colon down to the rectum. The sutures are all held taut while the descending colon is pushed down until its posterior edge is in contact with the rectum, sometimes also called the 'parachute' technique. Tie the sutures with the knots within the lumen. Hold the two most lateral sutures and cut the others. Suture the anterior layer using interrupted seromuscular-inverting stitches, inserting them all before they are tied. Place a haemostatic clip on each side of the anastomosis to mark it radiologically.

Stapled anastomosis (Fig. 19.5)

If the anastomosis is too low to suture conventionally or if you prefer the technique, unite the bowel with the EEA circular stapling device. Carry out the operation exactly as described until the ends of the bowel have been prepared

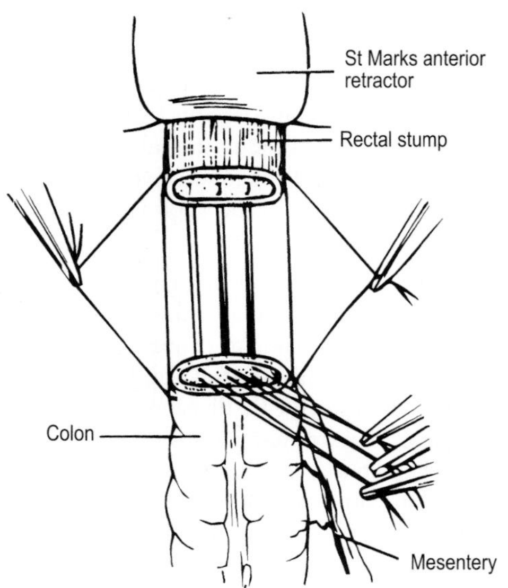

Fig. 19.4 Anterior resection of the rectum with sutured anastomosis. One-layer anastomosis, showing the insertion of sutures in preparation for the descending colon to be 'railroaded' down to the rectum.

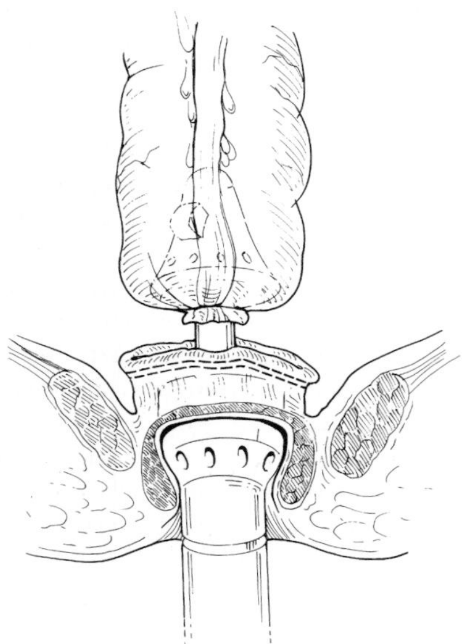

Fig. 19.5 Anterior resection of the rectum with stapled anastomosis, showing insertion of the circular stapling device through the anus with stapled rectal stump with the descending colon tied over the anvil.

for anastomosis. Now insert the sizing heads into the colon to see if the stapling gun should be 25, 28 or 31 mm in diameter. For the colon it is best to select a 28- or 31-mm gun. Remember that the stapler removes an extra 8 mm of rectum and this can be taken into account when estimating the distal clearance below the tumour.

Introduce the EEA gun through the anus and open it. Allow the spike of the gun to pass through the posterior aspect of the stapled rectal stump in the middle and just behind the staple line. Insert a purse-string suture into the end of the descending colon. Manipulate the end of the descending colon over the top of the anvil and tie the purse-string suture as tightly as possible. Connect the anvil and secured descending colon into the cartridge.

Have the assistant operating the gun approximate the anvil to the cartridge while you make sure that the gun is pushed firmly upwards and that the descending colon is pulled up tightly over the anvil. Ensure that no appendices epiploicae and no part of the vagina are trapped between the ends of the bowel to be stapled. Rotate the descending colon 90° to the left so that the mesentery lies to the right side. Fire the staple gun to construct the anastomosis. Open the gun to separate the anvil from the cartridge, twist it to make sure the anastomosis is lying free, and then gently rock it and pull it free from the anus.

Check the integrity of the stapled anastomosis. Examine the 'doughnuts' of colon and rectum removed from the gun. They should be complete. Identify the distal doughnut and send it for histological examination. Feel the anastomosis digitally with a finger through the anus. Pass a 1-cm sigmoidoscope to examine the anastomosis. Place fluid in the pelvis and gently blow air into the colon through the sigmoidoscope. If no bubbles appear and the doughnuts are complete, the anastomosis is satisfactory.

Whichever method of anastomosis you used, make certain that there is no bleeding, particularly in the region of the splenic flexure and spleen, no tension on the anastomosis, with the whole colon viable and the descending colon lying in the sacral hollow. Following a low anastomosis, do not close the mesentery. Drain the pelvis, preferably using a sump suction drain inserted through a stab wound in the left iliac fossa, and replace and arrange the small bowel and cover it with omentum before closing the abdomen.

HARTMANN'S OPERATION

This was described by the Berlin anatomist Robert Hartmann (1831–1893). After carrying out an anterior resection of the rectum or rectosigmoid it may be inadvisable to proceed with an anastomosis if the procedure is palliative and the anastomosis would demand the addition of a defunctioning colostomy, or there is residual carcinoma in the lateral pelvic wall or internal iliac nodes.

Close the distal rectum. If the rectum is cut off low down and the end is difficult to suture, leave it open and insert a drain through the anus into the pelvis. Close the peritoneum over the rectal stump if possible. Bring out an end colostomy as described later (following abdominoperineal excision of the rectum).

ABDOMINOPERINEAL EXCISION OF THE RECTUM

This operation may be performed by one surgical team carrying out the abdominal part of the operation and then the perineal part, or by a synchronous combined approach with two teams. The catheterized patient is in the lithotomy Trendelenburg position with the sacrum overhanging the end of the table.

The abdominal team resects the rectum from above through a lower midline incision (Fig. 19.6), entering the mesorectal plane in the same manner as for anterior resection of the rectum, to meet the perineal operator. After dividing the sigmoid colon, construct a left iliac terminal colostomy at a preoperatively identified site.

The perineal operator excises the anus and rectum, including in the female the posterior vaginal wall, in the male preserving the urethra and prostate gland, to meet the abdominal operator.

As a rule the abdominal operator can close the pelvic peritoneum.

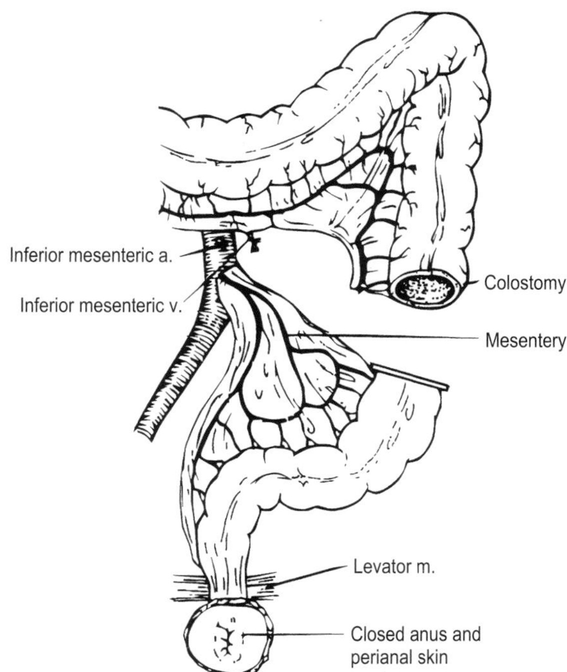

Fig. 19.6 Abdominoperineal excision of the rectum. The excised specimen consists of the rectum, anus, perianal skin and sigmoid colon and mesocolon. The inferior mesenteric artery is divided at its origin from the aorta and the inferior mesenteric vein is divided at a similar level.

TRANSVERSE COLOSTOMY

KEY POINT Carefully assess the options

- Transverse colostomy is a particularly unpleasant stoma so try to avoid it if at all possible.

Try to avoid the need for transverse colostomy since it is an unpleasant stoma, reserving it for the rare cases of distal obstruction in patients unfit to have an urgent resection carried out, or if you are too inexperienced to do this. It can be performed under a local anaesthetic in a severely ill patient. Site it in the right upper quadrant of the abdomen, midway between the umbilicus and the costal margin as far to the right in the transverse colon as possible to minimize the risk of prolapse. The next stage of the operation may require you to take down the splenic flexure and mobilize the distal transverse colon.

Make a transverse incision 5 cm long centred on the upper right rectus muscle between the umbilicus and the costal margin so that an appliance can be fitted without encroaching upon either. Divide the anterior and posterior rectus sheath, and split the rectus muscle. Through this locate the transverse colon, which you can recognize by the presence of omentum, and the lack of appendices epiploicae.

The abdomen may be already open when you make a decision to perform a colostomy. When a midline or left paramedian incision has been used, make a transverse incision as described above but only 6–7 cm long. If a right upper paramedian incision was used, bring the colostomy through the upper end of the incision, provided it is clear of the costal margin. If it is undertaken through a laparotomy to relieve a distal obstruction, examine the relevant structures and feel the obstructing mass in the distal colon. It may be impossible to determine if this is due to carcinoma or diverticular disease. Palpate the liver for metastases and the rest of the colon and the peritoneal cavity to determine if there are other metastases.

Action (Fig. 19.7a)

1 Draw the right side of the transverse colon and omentum out of the wound. Manipulate it so that a loop of proximal transverse colon lies in the wound without tension. Separate the omentum from the colon and turn it upwards to expose the mesentery. Pull the loop upwards through the incision and make a hole through the mesentery close to the bowel wall at the apex of the loop with a pair of long artery forceps, taking care not to damage the blood supply. Pass a piece of narrow rubber tubing or a catheter under the mesentery. Pull the loop right out through the incision with the rubber tubing, making certain that the loop is not twisted and that the proximal opening is to the right and the distal opening to the left.

2 Pass a plastic colostomy device through the mesentery to form a bridge for the colostomy. Open the end of the colostomy device to keep it in place. Do not insert any internal sutures. If the colostomy is made to relieve obstruction, open it immediately by cutting across the apex of the bowel through half the circumference. Turn back the edges of the opened colon and suture the whole thickness of the colon to the edge of the skin incision with interrupted 2/0 Vicryl sutures mounted on a cutting needle.

3 Insert a finger into each loop of the colostomy to make sure it is not too narrow and that the finger passes straight into the underlying colon. Fix a suitable disposable appliance over the loop colostomy rod. Plan to remove the device forming the bridge in about 7 days.

Closure

1 Do not close the colostomy until at least 6 weeks after it has been formed. This allows the oedema to settle down and makes the operation safer and easier. Before closure ensure that any distal anastomosis is satisfactory following the definitive operation, as shown on sigmoidoscopy and/or Gastrografin enema X-ray. Prepare the proximal bowel as for colonic resection and anastomosis. Make an incision in the skin close to the mucocutaneous junction.

2 Insert six 2/0 silk stay sutures into the mucocutaneous junction, each held in an artery forceps so that traction may be applied while dissecting (Fig. 19.7b). Deepen the incision to reveal the colon and the external rectus sheath. Dissect the colonic loops from the abdominal wall until the whole of the loop is freed and can easily

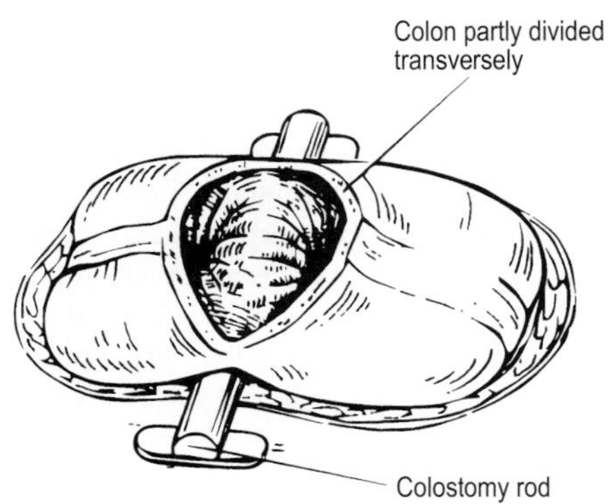

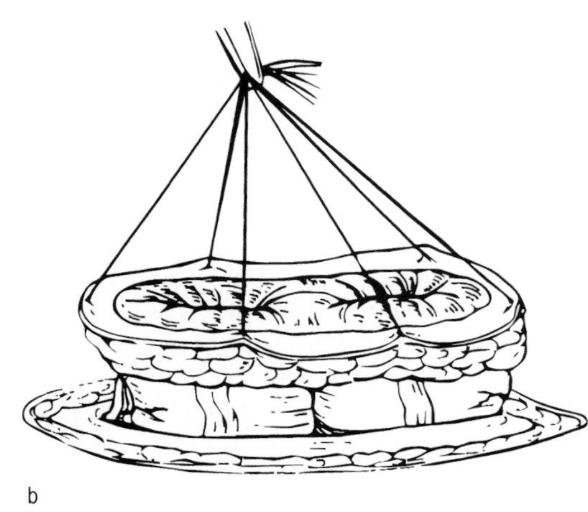

Fig. 19.7 (a) Transverse colostomy: bring a loop of colon through the wound and keep it in place with a colostomy device or simple glass rod. Open the colostomy by a transverse incision. (b) Closure of colostomy: insert stay sutures to help mobilization.

be drawn out from the abdominal cavity. Excise the mucocutaneous junction.

3 Close the colostomy transversely using a single layer of seromuscular sutures. Replace the re-sutured colostomy in the peritoneal cavity, place the omentum over it and manipulate it so that it lies away from the abdominal incision. Close the abdominal wound in one layer with a continuous or interrupted nylon suture. If the patient is obese, drain the subcutaneous space with a slip of corrugated latex sheet brought out through the end of the wound, or through a separate stab wound. Close the skin.

SIGMOID END COLOSTOMY

Use this when you require to fashion a permanent colostomy because of sphincter damage, in some cases of constipation, prolapse and solitary ulcer when no other definitive operation is possible. If no previous surgery has been undertaken, you do not need to perform a laparotomy. Consider performing the operation using the laparoscope.

COLECTOMY FOR INFLAMMATORY BOWEL DISEASE

Acute fulminating colitis, with or without toxic megacolon, usually occurs in idiopathic ulcerative colitis but may occur in Crohn's colitis. The operation of choice is colectomy and ileostomy. Emergency proctocolectomy carries a higher mortality and morbidity, and there is no opportunity to carry out a secondary ileorectal anastomosis. Manage these patients jointly with a senior gastroenterologist. Surgical treatment is usually indicated if the patient's condition does not improve within 72 hours, the patient does not improve in 24 hours and still has more than six bowel actions containing blood each day, or has a fever of more than 38°C and a tachycardia over 100 beats/min. If there is toxic dilatation or evidence of perforation, carry out an emergency operation.

ELECTIVE COLECTOMY AND ILEORECTAL ANASTOMOSIS

This may be indicated for ulcerative colitis provided there is no carcinoma or severe dysplasia, Crohn's disease provided the rectum is relatively disease free, or familial adenomatous polyposis provided there is no rectal carcinoma. After completing the colectomy perform an ileorectal anastomosis. Widen the narrow ileal lumen with a longitudinal slit to accommodate the wider rectum and use a single layer of seromuscular stitches or EE stapler.

ELECTIVE TOTAL PROCTOCOLECTOMY

Either excise the rectum conservatively using a close rectal dissection to conserve the pelvic floor and protect the pelvic autonomic nerves, or take care as for 'mesorectal excision' of the rectum for cancer to ensure these structures are preserved. Create the ileostomy at the preoperatively marked site.

In patients with ulcerative colitis or familial adenomatous polyposis who wish to avoid a permanent conventional ileostomy but are not suitable for an ileorectal anastomosis, two alternative procedures can be carried out. Restorative proctocolectomy entails creating a reservoir in the terminal ileum by folding and anastomosing before uniting it to the rectum (Fig. 19.8). An alternative is to create an ileostomy with a reservoir and an intussuscepted nipple valve to produce a continent ileostomy.

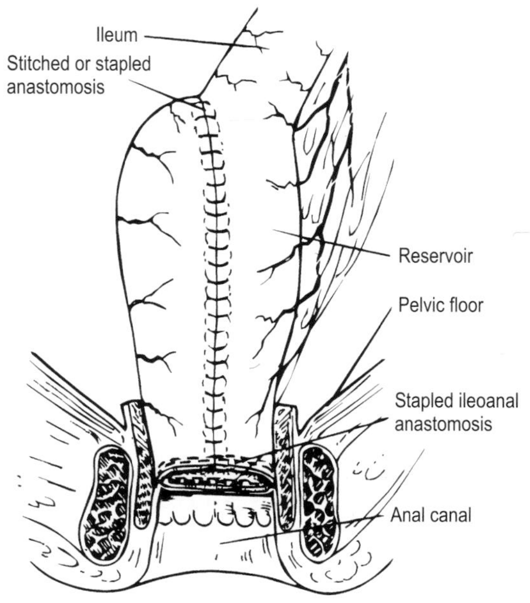

Fig. 19.8 Ileoanal reservoir. Depicted is a 'J' configuration reservoir, stapled to the anal canal 1–2 cm above the dentate line.

DUHAMEL OPERATION

Described by the Parisian surgeon Bernard Duhamel in 1956, this is the most satisfactory procedure for treating adult Hirschsprung's disease; for children see Ch. 43. Excise the thickened dilated colon, leaving, closing, mobilizing forward and washing out the rectal stump of about 10 cm. Bring the cut proximal colon behind the rectal stump. Open the stump posteriorly and through the abdomen and per-anally, unite the colon and rectum with sutures and staples.

SOAVE OPERATION

It is a useful procedure for revision of a failed pelvic anastomosis and can be modified for treating large villous tumours, irradiation proctitis, rectovaginal and rectoprostatic fistulas and haemangiomas of the rectum. Excise diseased bowel, leaving 10-cm rectum but denude this of mucosa. Draw down the proximal colon within the denuded tube of rectum, uniting the colon to the dentate line.

FURTHER READING

Keighley MRB, Williams NS 1999 Surgery of the anus, rectum and colon, 2nd edn. Saunders, London
Nicholls RJ, Dozois RR 1997 Surgery of the colon and rectum. Churchill Livingstone, Edinburgh
Phillips RKS 1998 Colorectal surgery: a companion to specialist surgical practice. Saunders, London

20

Laparoscopic colorectal surgery

A. Darzi, T. Rockall, P. A. Paraskeva

CONTENTS

PREOPERATIVE CONSIDERATIONS

Advocates cite numerous potential advantages: less pain, faster patient recovery with less postoperative disability, shorter hospitalization, earlier return to work, better quality of life, with better cosmetic results. Technical capability is comparable to that of the open technique. Laparoscopic colectomy is technically demanding and may be difficult.

Potential advantages are claimed for sigmoid resection, abdominoperineal resection, Hartmann's procedure, and assisted right hemicolectomy. Restorative proctocolectomy and completely intracorporeal right hemicolectomy require advanced technical skill.

Conditions amenable to a laparoscopic approach include carcinoma, benign neoplasms, diverticular disease, inflammatory bowel disease, rectal prolapse, idiopathic constipation, volvulus and stomas for diversion.

RIGHT-SIDED COLECTOMY

The same routine is followed as in the open technique. The colectomy can be performed with a laparoscopic-assisted technique by making a small incision to allow the bowel to be delivered to the surface of the mid-abdominal wall. If the procedure is performed for carcinoma, shield the incision with a wound protector to avoid contamination by malignant cells. Transect the bowel, usually with staples, and perform the anastomosis, either by functional end-to-end anastomosis using a stapling device or by suturing.

LEFT COLECTOMY

The specimen can be removed. Perform an intracorporeal stapled anastomosis via the anus using a triple-staple technique.

Alternatively, use the laparoscopically assisted colectomy techniques. Make the planned incision for specimen removal and draw the mobilized colon into the wound. Isolate, ligate and divide the vessels. Dissect the transection sites clean of fat and accomplish standard stapler transection. Anastomosis can be performed intraperitoneally, but it is easier to use a double-stapling technique.

RECTOPEXY

Laparoscopic surgery can be especially effective in benign disease such as rectal prolapse. Mobilize the rectum while identifying the ureters and preserving the lateral stalks. Clear the sacrum of overlying tissues on the sacral promontory. Sew the lateral stalks to the clean site on the sacrum; this pulls and holds the rectum up in the pelvis. Insert two sutures as a rule through each lateral stalk. In time, the rectum will adhere, preventing further prolapse. Some authors use a mesh to fix the rectum to the sacrum.

HAND-ASSISTED LAPAROSCOPIC COLORECTAL SURGERY

This is a newly developed technique involving the insertion of a hand or forearm through a mini-laparotomy incision, while maintaining pneumoperitoneum. The hand can be used as in an open procedure to palpate organs or tumour, reflect organs atraumatically, retract structures, identify vessels, dissect bluntly along a tissue plane and provide finger pressure to bleeding points while proximal control is achieved (Fig. 20.1).

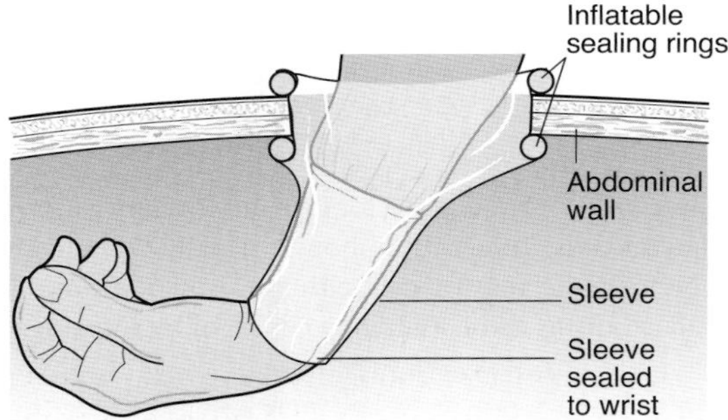

Fig. 20.1 Hand assisted laparoscopic surgery. A special ring fits within an incision, which can be sealed. From it, a sleeve extends which is sealed to the operator's wrist, thus maintaining the pneumoperitoneum.

FURTHER READING

Darzi A, Lewis C, Menzies-Gow N et al 1995 Laparoscopic abdominal perineal excision of the rectum. Surgical Endoscopy 9:414–417

Guillou PJ, Darzi A, Monson JRT 1993 Laparoscopic assisted colectomy for colorectal cancer. Surgical Oncology 2:43–49

Monson JRT, Darzi A, Carey PD et al 1992 Prospective evaluation of laparoscopic assisted colectomy in an unselected group of patients. Lancet 340:831–833

Monson JRT, Hill ADK, Darzi A 1995 Laparoscopic colonic surgery. British Journal of Surgery 82:150–157

Paraskeva PA, Purkayastha S, Darzi A 2004 Laparoscopy for malignancy. Current status. Seminars in Laparoscopic Surgery 11:27

Puttick M, Gould SW, Darzi A 1999 Early experience with a new device for hand assisted laparoscopic colorectal surgery. British Journal of Surgery 86 (Suppl 1): 94 (abstract)

21

Anorectum

C. R. G. Cohen, C. J. Vaizey

CONTENTS

Invariably perform a full rectal examination, including inspection, palpation, sigmoidoscopy and proctoscopy, before carrying out any procedure. In appropriate circumstances exclude serious diseases, such as neoplastic or inflammatory bowel disease with colonoscopy or computed tomography (CT) colography. Most operations can be performed with the patient in the lithotomy position. The prone (Latin *pronus* = bent forward) jack-knife position has the advantage of superior visibility and access for your assistant.

ANATOMY

The anal canal extends from the anorectal junction superiorly to the anus below and is approximately 3–4 cm long in men and 2–3 cm long in women. There is a line of anal valves midway along the canal, loosely called the 'dentate line' (Fig. 21.1). Fusion between the embryonic hindgut and the proctoderm occurs higher, between the anal valves and the anorectal junction with a mixture of columnar and squamous epithelium. The internal sphincter is the expanded, 2 mm thick, distal portion of the smooth circular muscle of the large intestine and is grey/white in colour. Outside this, with a palpable gutter between them, is the near-centimetre thick external sphincter, with brown, striated muscle, supplied by the pudendal nerve. The skin over the outer margin of the external anal sphincter muscle is paler than that over the muscle and towards the anal canal – a useful demarcation when siting the skin incision to operate on the external anal sphincter. The levator ani and puborectalis muscles hold the anal canal in its correct position in relationship to the bony pelvis; this is with the top of the anal canal on the line joining the tip of the coccyx to the inferior aspect of the symphysis pubis. They also maintain the correct angle between the rectum and anal canal at less than 90°.

There are three spaces around the anal canal which are important in the spread of sepsis and in certain operations:

- The *intersphincteric space* lies between the two sphincters and contains the terminal fibres of the longitudinal muscle of the large intestine and also the anal intermuscular glands, approximately 12 in number, arranged around the anal canal; their ducts pass through the internal sphincter and open into the anal crypts.
- The *ischiorectal fossa* lies lateral to the external sphincter and contains fat. Abscesses may occur here as the result of horizontal spreading infection across the external sphincter.
- The *supralevator space* lies between the levator ani and the rectum, and is also important in the spread of infection.

Prepare

Familiarize yourself with the small range of essential instruments for examination of the patient, such as the proctoscope and the rigid sigmoidoscope. In awake patients with anal sphincter spasm, use a small paediatric sigmoidoscope. Operating proctoscopes of the Eisenhammer, Parks and

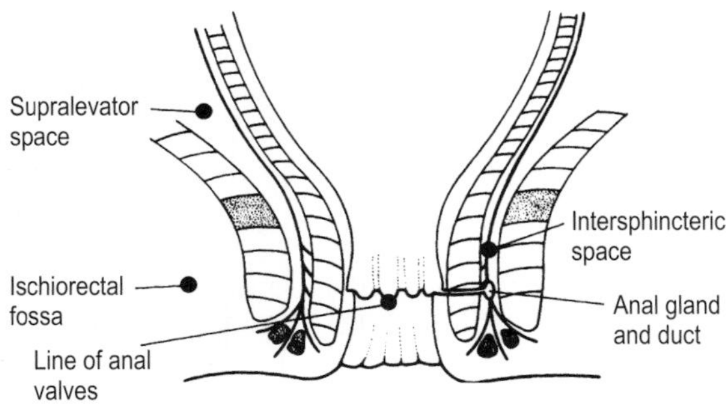

Fig. 21.1 Diagram to show the essential anatomy of the anal canal.

Sims type are essential for operations on and within the anal canal. Use fine scissors, fine forceps (toothed and non-toothed), a light needle-holder, Emett's forceps and a small no. 15 scalpel blade for intra-anal work. Alternatively, diathermy dissection creates a virtually bloodless field. For fistula surgery have a set of Lockhart–Mummery fistula probes together with a set of Anel's lacrimal probes.

Most patients require no preparation, or two glycerine suppositories, to ensure that the rectum is empty before anal surgery. If for any reason the bowels need to be confined postoperatively, then carry out a full bowel preparation to empty the whole large intestine. Minor operations can be performed under local infiltration anaesthesia; larger procedures demand regional or general anaesthesia. For outpatient procedures use the left lateral position, or alternatively the knee–elbow position. For anal operations most British surgeons favour the lithotomy position, although the prone jack-knife position can also be used. If you prefer to shave the area before starting an anal operation, carry it out in the operating theatre immediately beforehand, where there is good illumination.

HAEMORRHOIDS

Minimally symptomatic haemorrhoids may not require treatment if you have excluded a primary cause. Small internal haemorrhoids can be treated by injection sclerotherapy. Prolapsing haemorrhoids may be ligated with rubber-bands. Large prolapsing haemorrhoids, which are usually accompanied by a significant external component, are best treated by haemorrhoidectomy. With the advent of day-case diathermy haemorrhoidectomy, which gives a satisfactory result, we are willing to offer surgical treatment more readily than in the past. As a rule, avoid treating haemorrhoids if the patient also has Crohn's disease.

INJECTION SCLEROTHERAPY

This is an outpatient procedure and does not require any anaesthesia. It is most conveniently carried out following a full rectal examination if no further investigation is required. Leave the patient in the left lateral position.

Pass the full-length proctoscope and withdraw it slowly to identify the junction – the area where the anal canal begins to close around the instrument. Place a ball of cotton wool into the lower rectum with Emett's forceps to keep the walls apart. Since you will not usually remove it, warn the patient that it will pass out with the next motion.

Identify the position of the right anterior, left lateral and right posterior haemorrhoids. Fill a 10-ml Gabriel pattern syringe with 5% phenol in arachis oil with 0.5% menthol (oily phenol BP). Through the full-length proctoscope, insert the needle into the submucosa at the anorectal junction at the identified positions of the haemorrhoids in turn. Inject 3–5 ml of 5% phenol in arachis oil into the submucosa at each site, to produce a swelling with a pearly appearance of the mucosa in which the vessels are clearly seen. Move the needle slightly during injection to avoid giving an intravascular injection. Delay removing the needle for a few seconds following the injection, to lessen the escape of the solution. If necessary, press on the injection site with cotton wool to minimize leakage. Warn the patient to avoid attempts at defecation for 24 hours.

KEY POINT Injection sclerotherapy caution

- Avoid injecting the solution too superficially. This produces a watery bleb, which may ulcerate and subsequently cause haemorrhage. Avoid injecting the solution too deeply. This produces an oleogranuloma with subsequent features of an extrarectal swelling. Too deep anterior injection in male patients causes perineal pain and sometimes haematuria from prostatitis. This is a serious problem. Halt the injection immediately. If you suspect that the needle has entered the urinary tract, administer antibiotics. Do not hesitate to admit the patient, since septicaemia is common and may be severe.

RUBBER-BAND LIGATION

This is also an outpatient procedure and does not require anaesthesia. There are several different designs of band applicator; the simplest is illustrated in Figure 21.2. The suction bander is relatively expensive but is convenient and easy to use. Have available a pair of grasping forceps such as Patterson's biopsy forceps. There are two conceptually different strategies. One is to band, or inject, above the haemorrhoid in order to 'hitch' it back into its normal place. The other is to destroy the haemorrhoid itself; this will be described here but the hitch can be achieved by grasping the redundant mucosa proximal to the haemorrhoid and banding that instead.

Load two elastic bands on to the band applicator. Pass the full-length proctoscope and withdraw it slowly to identify the anorectal junction. Position the end of the proctoscope midway between the anorectal junction and the dentate line. Pass the tips of the grasping forceps through the ring of the band applicator, within the lumen of the proctoscope, and take hold of the selected haemorrhoid, or above it if you are employing the 'hitch-up' approach. Pull the haemorrhoid through the ring of the band applicator while pushing the band applicator upwards. If the patient experiences little additional discomfort when asked, 'fire' the band on to the haemorrhoid. If the manoeuvre causes increased discomfort, reposition the grip on the haemorrhoid slightly higher and retest before applying the band. Any number of haemorrhoids can be banded on each occasion. Repeat banding when necessary but delay it for 6–8 weeks.

Warn the patient to avoid attempts at defecation for 24 hours and to take a mild analgesic if the procedure causes discomfort.

If the procedure produces severe pain it may be because you applied the band too low on to sensitive epithelium. Try the effect of analgesics. If they do not control the pain, remove the bands in the operating theatre under general anaesthesia, using an operating proctoscope. Pain developing slowly in 1–2 days may be from ischaemia. Analgesics relieve the pain. Give metronidazole tablets 200 mg three times daily, which may help reduce inflammation. Advise the patient that the haemorrhoid and the band should drop off after 5–10 days and may be accompanied by a small amount of bleeding. Warn the patient that secondary haemorrhage occurs in approximately 2% any time up to 3 weeks after the application. Tell the patient to report to hospital if this is severe, since it may require transfusion and operative control of the bleeding. Monitor the temperature; if the patient develops severe fever, suspect HIV infection and admit the patient for treatment with intravenous antibiotics.

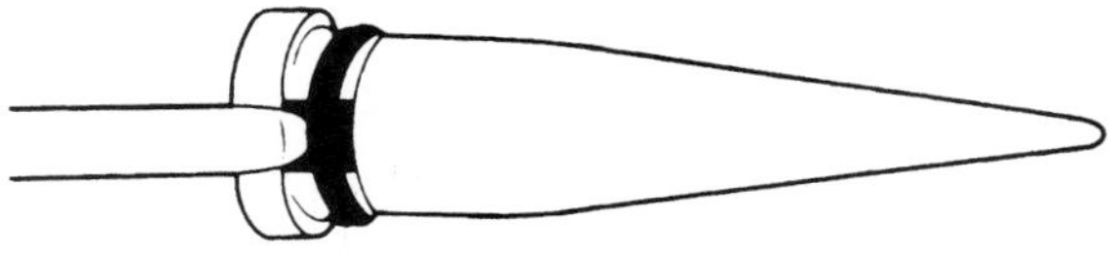

Fig. 21.2 A simple instrument with which to perform elastic-band ligation of haemorrhoids.

HAEMORRHOIDECTOMY

There are several methods of performing a haemorrhoidectomy. We shall describe the diathermy technique, which has evolved out of the ligation and excision technique of Milligan and Morgan. Haemorrhoidectomy should be a curative procedure. Perform it carefully and thoroughly. Closed haemorrhoidectomy is a limited removal of anoderm with immediate suturing. Randomized trials have failed to show any advantage. Stapled haemorrhoidectomy is painful from impinging of the staples on the skin.

Start lactulose, a non-absorbed disaccharide which produces an osmotic bowel action, 30 ml twice daily 2 days preoperatively. This reduces postoperative pain. Give oral metronidazole 400 mg three times a day for 5 days, which significantly reduces postoperative pain. Place the anaesthetized patient in the lithotomy position with some head-down tilt. Avoid caudal anaesthetic as it may provoke retention of urine.

Plan the operation by inserting the Eisenhammer retractor and establish which haemorrhoids need to be removed; also estimate the state and size of the skin bridges (Fig. 21.3). Determine whether a three-quadrant haemorrhoidectomy will be sufficient, if there is one additional haemorrhoid that needs removal, or if the situation is more complex than this. If there is one additional haemorrhoid you may leave it and be prepared to return on another occasion if it proves troublesome, or fillet it out by undermining the skin bridge, or divide the skin bridge above the dentate line, reflect it out of the anus, and trim the haemorrhoid with the back of a pair of scissors. Now excise any redundant mucosa and stitch the trimmed flap back into position with 2/0 synthetic absorbable sutures of Vicryl. If the haemorrhoids are even more extensive and circumferential, you may perform a standard three-quadrant haemorrhoid-

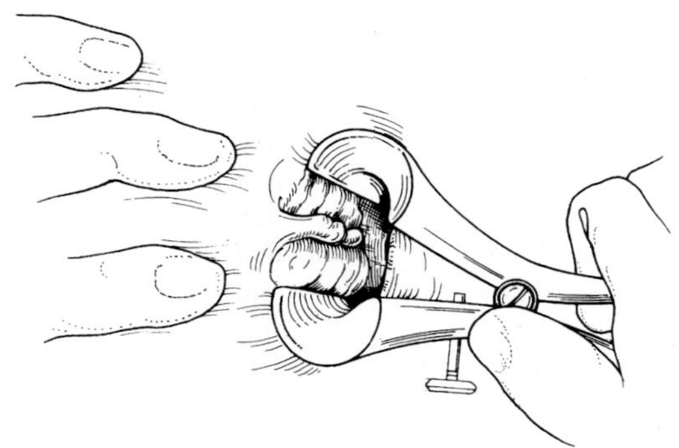

Fig. 21.3 Plan the operation by inserting the Eisenhammer retractor, establish the site and size of the haemorrhoids and identify the skin bridges to preserve them.

ectomy and return on another occasion to deal with any residual haemorrhoids. If you are experienced in the technique, consider performing the circumferential Whitehead haemorrhoidectomy described in 1882; he described the excision of a tubular segment of the anal canal, with mucosal–cutaneous re-anastomosis. Use polyglactin 910 (Vicryl). Beware of the difficulty, avoiding Whitehead deformity – mucosal ectropion (Greek *ek* = out + *trepein* = to turn) – and later stenosis.

Action

1 Inject bupivacaine (Marcaine) 0.25% with adrenaline (epinephrine) 1 : 200 000 into each skin bridge and into the external component of each haemorrhoid to be excised. Wait, and gently massage away excess fluid from the injection with a moistened gauze.

2 Commence with the left lateral haemorrhoid. Place the Eisenhammer retractor in the anal canal and open it sufficiently to put the internal sphincter under tension. This demonstrates the plane of the dissection. Group the external component and excise it with electrocautery, using cutting diathermy on skin and coagulating diathermy for all other dissection. Do not linger in one area with cutting diathermy or the skin develops indolent burn marks.

3 Now extend the haemorrhoidal dissection up the anal canal, separating the haemorrhoid from the underlying internal sphincter. Narrow the pedicle as you dissect up towards the apex, otherwise you risk encroaching on the skin bridge. When you have encompassed the internal component of the haemorrhoid, simply transect the pedicle with diathermy. Repeat the procedure on the right anterior haemorrhoid and then the right posterior haemorrhoid. Ensure complete haemostasis and check each wound and apex. Inspect the skin bridges and perform any further procedure as necessary. Do not apply any anal canal dressing. Insert a diclofenac (Voltarol) suppository into the anus.

Aftercare

Remember that bleeding comes from what remains inside the patient, not from what has been removed. Allow the patient home after recovery from the anaesthetic. Warn that there is likely to be an early increase in pain 3–5 days postoperatively. Control pain with non-steroidal anti-inflammatory drugs (NSAIDs). Manage the bowels with lactulose 30 ml orally twice daily until defecation is comfortable. Try the effect of creating a reversible chemical sphincterotomy with 0.2% glyceryl trinitrate (GTN) applied locally three times daily. Review the patient in the outpatient clinic within 10–12 days.

FISSURE

Most ulcers at the anal margin are simple fissures in ano, possibly associated with a sentinel skin tag and/or hypertrophied anal papilla or anal polyp. Exclude excoriation in association with pruritus ani, Crohn's disease, primary chancre of syphilis, herpes simplex, leukaemia and tumours.

Treat superficial fissures with 0.2% GTN (glyceryl trinitrate) cream twice a day or 2% diltiazem ointment, a calcium-channel-blocking drug, also twice daily. GTN can cause headaches; occasionally diltiazem causes local irritation. Botulinum toxin injection is an alternative therapy. Anal dilatation is no longer an acceptable treatment. Reserve operation for failures, usually associated with sentinel tag, an anal polyp, exposure of the sphincter and undermining of the edges (Fig. 21.4). The standard procedure is a lateral (partial internal) sphincterotomy.

LATERAL SPHINCTEROTOMY

Introduced by Eisenhammer in 1951, this can be carried out as a 'day-case' procedure and is very successful, curing more than 95% of patients. To avoid exacerbating the pain, avoid preoperative preparation. Warn the patient of a 1 in

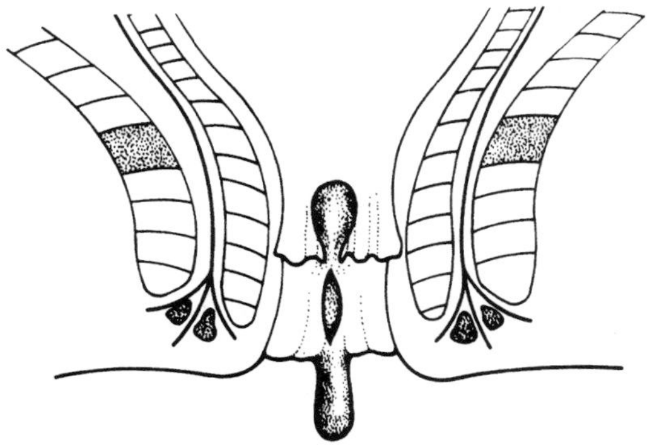

Fig. 21.4 A fissure with a sentinel skin tag, an anal polyp and undermining of the edges of the ulcer.

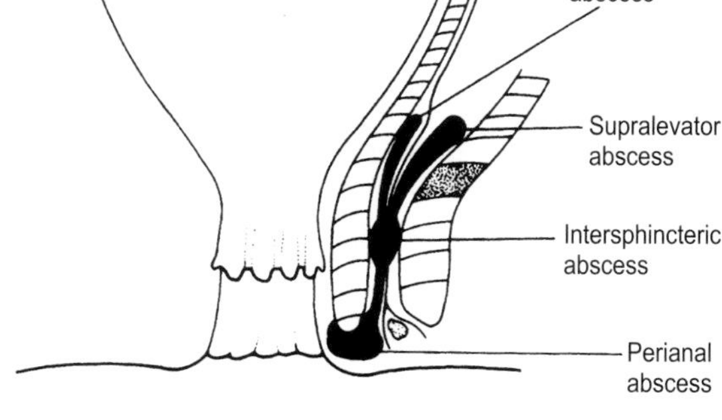

Fig. 21.5 Spread of intersphincteric abscess. Vertical spread upwards and downwards from a primary intersphincteric abscess.

20 chance of permanent flatus incontinence and a 1 in 200 chance of faecal leakage.

Action

1 Place the patient in the lithotomy position, with general or regional anaesthesia. Pass an Eisenhammer bivalve operating proctoscope. Examine the fissure to exclude induration suggestive of an underlying intersphincteric abscess. Remove hypertrophied anal papillae or a fibrous anal polyp, sending them for histopathological examination. Remove a sentinel skin tag. Rotate the operating proctoscope to demonstrate the left lateral aspect of the anal canal. Palpate the lower border of the internal sphincter muscle. Replace the Eisenhammer retractor with a Parks' retractor, which permits outward traction, making the internal sphincter more obvious.

2 Make a small incision 1 cm long in line with the lower border of the internal sphincter. Insert scissors into the submucosa, gently separating the epithelial lining of the anal canal from the internal sphincter, and also into the intersphincteric space to separate the internal and external sphincters. If you make a hole in the mucosa open it completely to avoid the risk of sepsis. Clamp the isolated area of internal sphincter with artery forceps for 30 seconds. This markedly reduces haemorrhage.

3 With one blade of the scissors on each side of it, divide the internal sphincter muscle up to the level of the top of the fissure. Do not extend the division above the upper end of the fissure or the anal valves. Press on the area for 2–3 minutes to stop the bleeding. The wounds do not normally need to be closed. Do not apply a dressing unless there is excessive bleeding that will be controlled by pressure from it. The dressing exacerbates postoperative pain. Apply a perineal pad and pants.

4 Prescribe a bulk laxative such as sterculia (Normacol) 10 ml once or twice a day. Bruising under the perianal skin signifies a haematoma, but it requires no treatment.

ANAL ABSCESS AND FISTULA

Most abscesses and fistulas in the anal region arise from a primary infection in the anal intersphincteric glands. Furthermore, they represent different phases of the same disease process. An acute-phase abscess develops when free drainage of pus is prevented by closure of either the internal or external opening of the fistula, or both, which is the chronic phase. Other causes of sepsis in the perianal region include pilonidal infection, hidradenitis suppurativa, Crohn's disease, tuberculosis and intrapelvic sepsis draining downwards across the levator ani.

Once established, an intersphincteric abscess may spread vertically downwards to form a perianal abscess or upwards to form either an intermuscular abscess or supralevator abscess, depending upon which side of the longitudinal muscle spread occurs (Fig. 21.5). Horizontal spread medially across the internal sphincter may result in drainage into the anal canal, but spread laterally across the external sphincter may produce an ischiorectal abscess. Finally, circumferential spread of infection may occur from one intersphincteric space to the other, from one ischiorectal fossa to the other and from one supralevator space to the other.

Once an abscess has formed, surgical drainage must be instituted; antibiotics have no part to play in the primary management. As the tissues are inflamed and oedematous, do the minimum to promote resolution of the infection. More tissue can be divided later to resolve the condition. Send a specimen of pus to the laboratory for culture. The presence of intestinal organisms suggests the presence of a fistula.

Avoid preoperative preparation of the bowel as it causes unnecessary pain. Place the anaesthetized patient in the lithotomy position and now shave the operation area.

Perianal abscess

Recognize the abscess as a swelling at the anal margin. Make a radial incision and excise overhanging edges. Allow pus to drain and send a sample to the laboratory. Gently examine the wound to see if there is a fistula. Insert a gauze dressing soaked in normal saline solution and surrounded by Surgicel. Do not pack the wound tightly.

Intermuscular abscess

Recognize the abscess as an indurated swelling, sometimes mobile within the lower rectal wall. As this is an upward extension of an intersphincteric abscess, manage it similarly, but the upper limit of division of the internal sphincter and/or circular muscle of the rectum is higher. Control bleeding from the divided edges of the rectal wall. Insert a gauze dressing soaked in normal saline to the upper limit of the wound. Do not pack the wound tightly.

Supralevator abscess

Recognize this as a fixed indurated swelling palpable above the anorectal junction. Drain it and insert a gauze dressing soaked in normal saline.

Ischiorectal abscess

Recognize this as a brawny inflamed swelling in the ischiorectal fossa which often spreads circumferentially from one side to the other, so carefully examine the patient under anaesthesia to determine if this has occurred. Recognize the abscess by feeling the induration inferior to the levator ani muscle and employ a circumanal incision to establish drainage. Excise the skin edges to create an adequate opening and send a specimen of pus to the laboratory. Never use a probe; gently explore with your finger to avoid spreading infection and then gently insert a gauze dressing soaked in normal saline surrounded by Surgicel to the upper limit of the wound. Do not pack the wound tightly.

Remove the dressing on the second postoperative day while the patient lies in the bath, having been given an intramuscular injection of pethidine 100 mg or papaveretum 7–15 mg. Initiate a routine of twice-daily baths, irrigation of the wound and the insertion of a tuck-in gauze dressing soaked in physiological saline or 1:40 sodium hypochlorite solution. If the patient has evidence of persistent local or systemic sepsis, administer systemic antibiotics guided by the culture report. Metronidazole is effective against anaerobic organisms.

Assess the patient for the possible presence of a fistula detected at the time of abscess drainage, or a history of recurrent abscesses, or palpable induration of the perianal area, anal canal and lower rectum, or the presence of gut organism in the pus. If so, plan to re-examine the patient under anaesthesia and carry out the appropriate treatment.

FISTULA

A fistula is an abnormal communication between two epithelial-lined surfaces. Therefore, in the context of fistula in ano, there should be an external opening on the perianal skin, an internal opening into the anal canal and a track between the two. There may be no external opening, or it may be healed over. Likewise there may be no internal opening as the sepsis arises in the area of the intersphincteric gland, which is the primary site of infection. It may not drain across the internal sphincter into the anal canal. Finally, the track may follow a very complicated path. The presence of infection is characterized by the physical sign of induration, detected by palpation with a lubricated, covered finger.

SUPERFICIAL FISTULA

Place the anaesthetized patient in the lithotomy position. Always perform sigmoidoscopy, looking especially for inflammatory bowel disease. Palpate the perianal skin, anal canal and lower rectum to detect induration. This is confined to the distal anal canal and localized to one area, as superficial fistulas are really fissures covered with skin and lower anal canal epithelium.

Insert a bivalve operating proctoscope and pass a fine probe along the track. Lay open the fistula using a no. 15 bladed knife or electrocautery. Curette the granulation tissue and send a specimen for histopathology. If there is no induration deep to the internal sphincter, fashion the external skin wound so that it becomes pear-shaped and perform a lateral sphincterotomy (see above). Insert a gauze dressing soaked in normal saline solution and surrounded by Surgicel to the upper limit of the wound.

INTERSPHINCTERIC FISTULA

An intersphincteric fistula results when the sepsis is inside the striated muscle of the pelvic floor and the anal canal. It may be necessary to totally divide the internal sphincter and the muscle of the lower rectum, to lay open the fistula and create an adequate external wound to allow drainage.

TRANS-SPHINCTERIC FISTULA

The primary track passes across the external sphincter from the intersphincteric space to the ischiorectal fossa. The infection may also have drained across the internal sphincter into the anal canal, where you find the internal opening of the fistula, which is usually at the level of the anal valves (Fig. 21.6), but there may be no internal opening. The external opening(s) are usually laterally placed and indurated, The infection may spread circumferentially and other secondary tracks may also develop. Laying open the fistula requires expertise to avoid causing incontinence. It is often safer to drain the track by inserting a length of fine silicone tubing (1 mm diameter) or no. 1 braided suture material (seton). Once all the septic areas have been drained, fashion the wound so that drainage can continue and the wound can heal from its depths. You almost certainly need to trim the skin and fat. In a suprasphincteric fistula, the primary track crosses the striated muscle above all the muscles of continence.

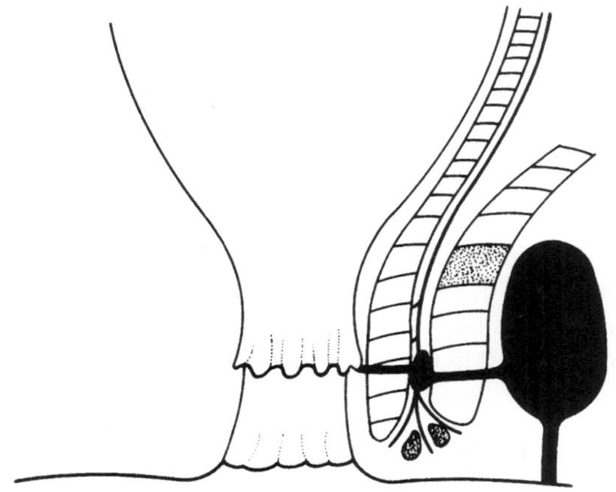

Fig. 21.6 Trans-sphincteric fistula.

EXTRASPHINCTERIC FISTULA

This arises from an upward extension of infection from the ischiorectal fossa. Create a defunctioning loop colostomy as a preliminary to closing the opening in the rectum and treat the fistula along the lines indicated above. Manage a fistula arising from pelvic sepsis from, for example, acute appendicitis, Crohn's disease or diverticular disease, and not, therefore, of anal gland origin, by treating the primary disease.

POSTOPERATIVE

Remove the dressing on the second or third postoperative day after giving an intramuscular injection of pethidine 100 mg or papaveretum 7–15 mg. Carry out the first dressing in the operating theatre under general anaesthesia if the wound is very extensive. Initiate a routine of twice-daily baths, irrigation of the wound and insertion of gauze soaked in physiological saline. Inspect the wound at regular intervals until healing is complete. Encourage the bowel movements to coincide with these dressing times by giving laxatives. If they do not coincide, arrange bath–irrigation–dressing routines as necessary.

If there is voluminous discharge of pus, review the wound in the operating theatre under general anaesthesia after 10–14 days. In patients with large wounds, this may need to be repeated. Lay open any residual tracks and curette away the granulation tissue. Administer antimicrobial agents such as erythromycin 250 mg 8-hourly and metronidazole 400 mg 8-hourly for up to 28 days, to assist in the elimination of the sepsis.

A seton does not complicate the postoperative routine. A tight seton is designed to cut through the fistula track slowly, in the hope of reducing the separation of muscle ends. Apply it firmly but not tightly. Replace it at monthly intervals. Allow the wound to heal around it; this may take 3 months. Then, under general anaesthesia, remove the seton and curette its track free of granulation tissue. Spontaneous healing occurs in approximately 40% of patients. If healing does not occur, lay open the residual track. The advantage of this staged division of the external sphincter is that healing occurs around the 'scaffolding' of the external sphincter. When it is subsequently divided – and this is not always necessary – its ends separate only slightly. This produces a better functional result than if it were divided at the outset.

Failure to heal may be from inadequate or inappropriate drainage of intersphincteric abscess of origin, or of secondary tracks, or of the primary track, demanding the skills of an experienced surgeon.

PILONIDAL SINUS

Pilonidal sinus detected as a chance finding during routine examination probably does not require treatment. Operate only if it is painful or infected, producing a pilonidal abscess. After shaving the skin on the anaesthetized patient, excise the skin over the septic area, curette out the granulation tissue and embedded hairs. Detect and open any side tracks and overhanging edges, stop bleeding and dress the wound with saline-soaked gauze. Initiate a twice-daily routine of bath, irrigation and dressing. Keep the wound edges shaved. Cauterize any excess granulation tissue with silver nitrate. Complications include haemorrhage, delayed healing and recurrence. If necessary, repeat the operative procedure to get healing.

Alternative techniques include laying open a simple pilonidal sinus and marsupializing it (Latin *marsupium* = pouch; create a pouch with an open mouth) to keep it open until the interior has filled up. In Bascom's operation excise each pit with a no. 11 bladed knife. Drain the cavity through a laterally placed incision. Various rotation flaps can be used; all are intended to avoid having a midline suture line.

RECTAL PROLAPSE

The symptom of prolapse (i.e. tissue slipping through the anus) may result from causes other than complete rectal prolapse. Distinguish haemorrhoids, anal polyps, mucosal prolapse and rectal adenomas. Treatment consists of control of the prolapse, re-education of the bowel habit and improvement, if necessary, of sphincter function.

First control the prolapse. While an internally intussuscepted rectum lies in the lower third of the rectum (the first phase of prolapse), sphincter function is inhibited, as it will be as a complete prolapse passes through the anal sphincter and keeps it open. Many operations have been described to achieve control. Complete rectal prolapse can be treated by abdominal rectopexy in which the rectum is mobilized, drawn up and suspended from the intervertebral disc just distal to the sacral promontory. Alternatively, Delorme's procedure performed from the perineum consists of fully reproducing the prolapse, circumferentially incising the mucosa and dissecting it down to the apex, then up the internal surface of the prolapse; now unite the internal and external mucosal edges while plicating the denuded, redundant rectal wall.

FAECAL INCONTINENCE

Determine the cause of faecal incontinence. If the anal sphincter is normal consider causes such as faecal impaction or irritable bowel. If the anal sphincter is abnormal consider the possibility of a congenital abnormality, complete rectal prolapse (see above), a lower motor neurone lesion, disruption of the sphincter ring due to trauma (including surgical and obstetric trauma) or muscle atrophy.

Operative treatment may be employed for the correction of some congenital abnormalities and complete rectal prolapse. Simple disruption of the external sphincter may be repaired by overlapping the mobilized edges of the tear. Severe incontinence may need to be treated with the implantation of an artificial, inflatable bowel sphincter. Sacral nerve stimulation is an alternative approach which is gaining in popularity.

MISCELLANEOUS

Hidradenitis

Hidradenitis (Greek *hidros* = sweat + *aden* = gland + *itis* = inflammation) suppurativa (Latin = pus-forming) is a septic process that involves the apocrine (Greek *apo* = off + *krinein* = to separate; the secretion is a breakdown product of the cell) sweat glands. It occurs in the perineum as well as the axillae. It does not communicate with the anal canal. Drain each abscess and allow defects to heal by second intention.

Anal manifestations of Crohn's disease

Anal manifestations of Crohn's disease occur in approximately 50% of patients affected with Crohn's disease. The perianal area has a bluish discoloration and there may be oedematous skin tags. Ulceration, which can be extensive, may involve the perianal skin, anal margin and anal canal. Sepsis may occur in the form of either an abscess or a fistula. Remove a small biopsy specimen of a skin tag, or granulation tissue together with a rectal mucosal biopsy for histopathological examination. Drain any abscess in the usual way, taking care not to divide any muscle, and fully investigate the patient.

Condylomata acuminata

Condylomata acuminata (warts) result from human papillomavirus (HPV) infection of the squamous epithelium. Papilliferous lesions may develop on the perianal skin, within the anal canal and on the genitalia. Exclude other forms of sexually transmitted disease and attempt to trace contacts. Treat scattered lesions by applying 25% podophyllin in compound benzoin tincture. Treat more extensive lesions by operation – a technique of scissors excision.

Anal tumours

Anal tumours may be divided into two groups, although opinions differ as to the anatomical level of division.

For the purposes of this chapter anal canal tumours arise from the dentate line and above. Anal margin tumours arise below the dentate line and include condylomata acuminata, kerato-acanthoma, apocrine gland tumours, premalignant Bowen's disease and Paget's disease which are benign, and squamous and basal cell carcinomas.

Anal canal tumours are almost always malignant and include squamous cell carcinoma, basaloid carcinoma, adenocarcinoma and malignant melanoma. Carcinoma may be amenable to radiotherapy or chemotherapy but failure may demand abdominoperineal resection.

Rectal adenomas

Rectal adenomas of the rectum may be classified on a histopathological basis into tubular, tubulovillous and villous, clinically similar in their behaviour with no invasion across the muscularis mucosae. They may be pedunculated or sessile. Multiple small adenomatous polyps in the rectum suggest the diagnosis of familial adenomatous polyposis. Exclude other lesions, benign or malignant, in the large intestine. Order a colonoscopy.

Totally remove lesions less than 5 mm across, by twisting with a pair of Patterson biopsy forceps. Employ diathermy snare excision for those that are pedunculated. Submucosally excise those that are sessile, non-circumferential and confined to the lower two-thirds of the rectum, using a bivalve operating proctoscope. Employ anterior resection for sessile non-circumferential tumours with the lower border in the upper third of the rectum, and circumferential tumours with the lower border in the upper two-thirds of the rectum.

FURTHER READING

Beck DE, Wexner SD 1998 Fundamentals of anorectal surgery, 2nd edn. Saunders, Philadelphia

Fielding LP, Goldberg SM 1993 Rob and Smith's operative surgery, 5th edn. Butterworth-Heinemann, Oxford

Keighley MRB, Williams NS 1999 Surgery of the anus, rectum and colon, 2nd edn. Saunders, London

Nicholls RJ, Dozois RR 1997 Surgery of the colon and rectum. Churchill Livingstone, Edinburgh

Phillips RKS 1998 Colorectal surgery: a companion to specialist surgical practice. Saunders, London

22

Open biliary operations

R. C. N. Williamson, L. R. Jiao

CONTENTS

INTRODUCTION

This chapter concentrates on open operations for gallstones, since until lately these have been by far the most common indication for 'open' biliary surgery. Introduced as recently as 1987, laparoscopic cholecystectomy has rapidly been taken up by many centres throughout the world. At present almost all elective cholecystectomies are carried out by the laparoscopic route (Ch. 23), but open operation is still commonly performed in some developing countries and also in difficult or complicated circumstances when it cannot be completed with a laparoscopic approach. Always ensure that the patient is positioned on the operating table so that the upper abdomen overlies a radiolucent tunnel. Alert the radiographer and theatre staff in advance that an operative cholangiogram may be required.

Give a single routine antibiotic prophylactic dose shortly before operation with a broad-spectrum agent excreted in bile, such as a cephalosporin, which should be continued if the bile is obviously infected. Carry out thromboprophylaxis routinely unless there is a specific contraindication. We use subcutaneous low-dose heparin and below-knee compression stockings.

OPEN CHOLECYSTECTOMY

Whether symptomatic or 'silent', gallstones are the major indication for cholecystectomy, the second most common intra-abdominal operation in Western countries after appendicectomy. It is occasionally indicated for acalculous cholecystitis, gallbladder carcinoma or cholecystoses (cholesterosis, adenomyosis), or during the course of partial hepatectomy or pancreatoduodenectomy. As a rule, remove a diseased gallbladder encountered incidentally at operation provided there is adequate access and an additional procedure would not be inappropriate.

Prefer open to laparoscopic cholecystectomy for the Mirizzi syndrome in which gallstones within the cystic duct or Hartmann's pouch externally compress the common hepatic duct (CHD), causing symptoms of obstructive jaundice, or if you do not clearly understand the anatomy or you are inexperienced in dealing with a problem such as bleeding. Extracorporeal shock-wave lithotripsy, percutaneous cholecystolithotomy and dissolution therapy with cheno- or ursodeoxycholic acid are occasionally used but the diseased gallbladder remains and may form more stones. Consider open operation following previous upper abdominal operations, acute cholecystitis, cirrhosis, pregnancy, cholecystoenteric fistula or suspected gallbladder carcinoma.

Acute cholecystitis generally settles with rehydration and antibiotics, allowing operation to be delayed. Operate if there is persistent fever, local tenderness or evidence of spreading peritonism because of the risk of gangrene or perforation. About 10% of patients with acute cholecystitis have acalculous disease, carrying particular risk of perforation.

Following acute cholecystitis or biliary colic and confirmation of the diagnosis by ultrasonography or contrast radiology, we operate on the next elective operating list, avoiding recurrent attacks or complications, such as acute pancreatitis. The operation may be more difficult but often inflammatory oedema assists dissection of the gallbladder. Laparoscopic cholecystectomy is safe but expect a higher rate of conversion to open operation.

Transient jaundice is compatible with stones confined to the gallbladder. Continuing jaundice suggests obstruction of the bile duct and requires further investigation, including an 'invasive' cholangiogram (either percutaneous transhepatic or endoscopic retrograde).

Learn the common anatomical variations, since half the population have some anatomical variation in the arterial supply of the gallbladder or the disposition of the bile ducts.

Access

Choose between a right upper paramedian, an oblique subcostal (Kocher's) or a transverse incision, according to your experience and the shape of the patient's abdomen. In a paramedian incision it is simpler to split the fibres of rectus abdominis than to mobilize and retract the muscle belly; no harm ensues from denervation of the medial portion of the rectus. Start the incision at the costal margin 5 cm from the midline and run down to just below the umbilicus. Kocher's oblique subcostal incision extends parallel to the costal margin for about 15 cm; if you take it further to the right, isolate and preserve the ninth thoracic nerve. Divide the muscles with diathermy in the line of the skin incision. A transverse incision provides a better cosmetic scar at the expense of slightly limited access. 'Mini-cholecystectomy' through a short (5 cm) transverse incision with careful retraction gives an excellent cosmetic result but has probably been superseded by laparoscopic cholecystectomy.

Assess

1 Examine the gallbladder to see if it is inflamed, thickened or contains stones. With the patient supine, stones sink to the neck of the gallbladder. If the organ is hard and adherent to the liver, consider the possibility of carcinoma. Gallstone symptoms can mimic those of other diseases so explore the abdomen, looking in particular for hiatal hernia, peptic ulcer, diverticular disease of the colon and diseases of the liver, pancreas and appendix.

2 Examine the common bile duct. It should not exceed 6–8 mm in diameter. Insert your left index finger through the epiploic foramen of Winslow, feeling the duct between finger and thumb. Is it thickened, does it contain stones? Feel the lower duct after splitting the peritoneum in the floor of the foramen with the edge of a finger.

3 Examine the head of pancreas between finger and thumb, again passing your left index finger through the epiploic foramen and down behind the gland. Normal pancreas has a softish nodular feel, but with experience you will learn to detect the induration that denotes chronic inflammation or neoplasia.

Action

1 Place your hand over the liver and gently manipulate the right lobe downwards into the wound. Ask the anaesthetist to empty the stomach by aspirating the nasogastric tube. Divide any omental adhesions to the undersurface of the gallbladder. Place one pack in the subhepatic space to retract the intestines and another just covering the duodenal bulb.

2 Decide whether to commence gallbladder dissection at the fundus or in the region of the cystic duct. We generally prefer to display the structures in Calot's triangle (Fig. 22.1) and to ligate and divide the cystic artery

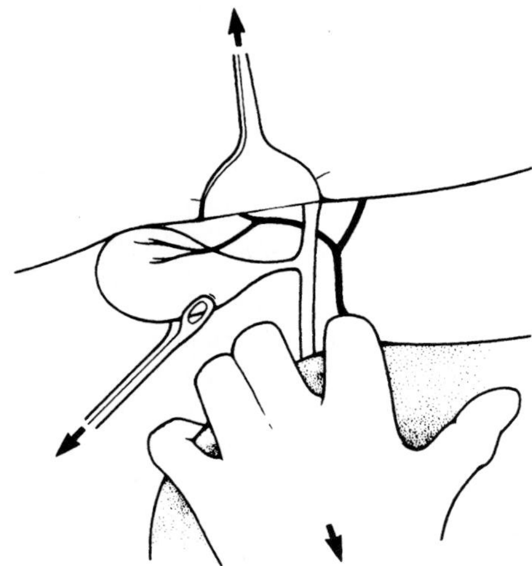

Fig. 22.1 Cholecystectomy. Traction in three directions displays Calot's triangle, which is bounded by the cystic duct, common hepatic duct and inferior border of the liver. The triangle has been extended by mobilization of the neck of the gallbladder. The cystic artery normally arises from the right hepatic artery within Calot's triangle.

before proceeding to the fundus and working back towards the cystic duct. If chronic inflammation is severe, it is safer to start at the fundus; some surgeons advocate this approach routinely.

3 Cholecystectomy may be performed with you standing on the right- or left-hand side of the operating table. Try both positions on different occasions and see which you find more comfortable.

4 If the gallbladder is very distended, aspirate it before proceeding. The empty gallbladder is easier to grasp for dissection and less likely to contaminate the peritoneal cavity if accidentally entered. Pack off the fundus and insert an Ochsner trocar, which is connected to the sucker tubing. Alternatively, use a syringe and wide-bore needle. Afterwards, seal the defect by grasping it with tissue-holding forceps.

'Duct-first' technique

1 The first assistant's left hand draws the duodenal bulb downwards, while a retractor draws the liver upwards. Grasp the neck of the gallbladder with sponge-holding forceps and draw it to the patient's right. This three-way traction provides good exposure (Fig. 22.1).

2 Incise the peritoneum over the neck of the gallbladder and continue for a short distance along its superior border. Using blunt dissection, gently open the space between the gallbladder and the liver at this point and expose the cystic artery. Follow the vessel on to the gallbladder wall and confirm that it is the cystic artery and not the right hepatic artery. Ligate the vessel twice in continuity and divide it between the ligatures.

3 Prior division of the cystic artery helps to straighten out the cystic duct. Now expose the duct by a combination of sharp and blunt dissection, and trace it to its junction with the common hepatic duct to form the bile duct. It is vital to display this three-way junction before dividing the cystic duct.

4 Perform an operative cholangiogram via the cystic duct if required (see next section). Take a swab of the bile for bacteriological culture on opening the duct. While awaiting the X-ray films (this is avoided if you can perform the cholangiogram with real-time fluoroscopic images), proceed to dissect the gallbladder from its liver bed. Leave the cholangiogram catheter in situ but complete the division of the cystic duct, grasping its gallbladder end with Moynihan's cholecystectomy forceps.

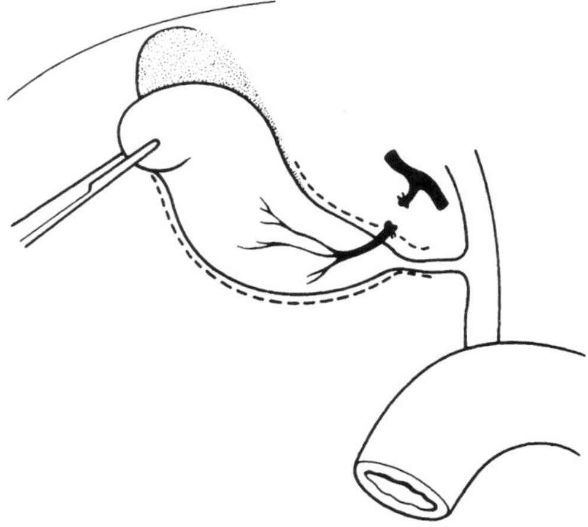

Fig. 22.2 Cholecystectomy: separation of the fundus of the gallbladder from the liver. The lines of peritoneal division are shown. The fundal dissection may be carried out after ligation and division of the cystic artery (as shown) or as the first stage of cholecystectomy.

Incise the peritoneum along the anterior and posterior aspects of the gallbladder, proceeding either towards or away from the fundus. Traction on the fundus assists the dissection (Fig. 22.2).

Numerous small vessels and occasionally accessory bile ducts traverse the areolar tissue between the liver and the gallbladder. Diathermy coagulation is effective to secure these vessels, but it may be simpler to ligate leashes of tissue on the hepatic side and then divide them with scissors. Remove the gallbladder, preserving it for subsequent gross and histological examination. Routinely open the gallbladder, inspect its contents and submit any suspicious nodule or ulcer to urgent frozen-section examination to exclude carcinoma.

5 If the cholangiogram pictures are technically satisfactory, withdraw the catheter and ligate the cystic duct close to the origin of the bile duct. Try and avoid leaving too long a cystic duct stump but do not struggle to place the ligature exactly flush with the bile duct. Avoid tenting or narrowing the bile duct while tying the ligature. We use an absorbable suture material for the ligature, such as 2/0 or 3/0 polyglactin 910 (Vicryl). If the cystic duct is large, use a transfixion suture.

6 Use diathermy to stop any residual oozing from the liver bed. Often the application of a surgical pack to

the gallbladder fossa, with or without the aid of a haemostatic agent such as Surgicel for a few minutes, will stop most bleeding. If you observe a leak of bile from a small cholecystohepatic duct, close the duct with a Vicryl stitch. Do not attempt to close the raw area of liver with sutures. Remove the packs and aspirate any blood.

'Fundus-first' technique

1 Grasp the fundus of the gallbladder with tissue-holding forceps. Incise the peritoneum between the fundus and the liver, using frequent diathermy to secure the many fine vessels. Larger vessels can be ligated on the hepatic side and divided. Extend the peritoneal incision along the anterior and posterior aspects of the gallbladder (Fig. 22.2). Open up the plane between the liver and the gallbladder, and proceed towards the neck of the organ, staying close to the gallbladder. Identify the cystic artery. Ligate and divide the artery close to the gallbladder wall.

2 The advantage of the 'fundus-first' technique is that it brings you directly on to the cystic duct from the safe side and lessens the risk of bile duct injury. Trace the cystic duct to its junction with the common hepatic duct. Perform a cholangiogram. Ligate and divide the cystic duct and remove the gallbladder.

3 Secure haemostasis in the liver bed. Remove the packs.

KEY POINT The golden rule: display the ductal anatomy

- Usually straightforward, cholecystectomy can sometimes, unpredictably, be a major technical challenge. Under such circumstances take great care to avert future disaster. The golden rule is never to cut any major structure, whether duct or artery, until you have displayed the crucial anatomy – notably the entry of the cystic duct into the bile duct. Always call for help from a senior surgeon if you are in trouble.

? DIFFICULTY

1. *Is the gallbladder stuck to the duodenum or transverse colon and obscured by inflammatory adhesions?* The organ can usually be freed by gentle digital dissection, but remember that calculi may have fistulated into the adherent viscus.
2. *Can you not identify the cystic artery or the three-way union of ducts?* Perhaps the tissues are fibrotic or bleed too easily. The liver may be enlarged and stiff; the gallbladder may be inaccessible because the costal margin is low or the patient obese. Do not proceed until you have improved the view. Enlarge the incision if necessary. Have the light adjusted. Use the sucker. Place and employ your assistants usefully, or summon further assistance.
3. *Can you still not safely progress?* Adopt the 'fundus-first' technique. Seek senior help. If the dissection is very difficult, consider an alternative procedure, either cholecystostomy or subtotal cholecystectomy.
4. *Are you proceeding with the dissection, but the anatomy is anomalous or confusing?* In these circumstances do not divide any structure until you have fully displayed the anatomy, and you understand it. Remember the common variations, summon a textbook of surgical anatomy or seek assistance from a senior surgeon. If you can confidently identify the cystic duct, perform cholangiography in order to clarify the remaining ductal anatomy.
5. *Do you suspect damage to the common hepatic duct or the bile duct?* If the possibility exists, you must declare the issue and not just hope for the best. Enlist the help of the most experienced surgeon available and discuss the case with a regional hepatopancreatobiliary centre. Cholangiography may be helpful. Repair partial division of the main duct immediately using fine absorbable sutures, and place a T-tube across the anastomosis through a

separate stab incision. It is often better, following complete transection, and particularly resection of a length, of duct, to perform a hepaticojejunostomy repair using a Roux loop of jejunum. Anastomosis can be difficult with a normal bile duct. Do not undertake this procedure unless you are fully trained to do it; otherwise, discuss the problem with a hepatopancreatobiliary specialist. Resolve to make accurate notes, with drawings to display the exact situation.

6. *Severe bleeding?* Do not panic and apply haemostats blindly or use inappropriate diathermy; the situation is almost certainly recoverable. Control the bleeding by local pressure. Arrange for blood to be available and for arterial sutures, tapes and bulldog clamps. Summon further advice and assistance if necessary.
   a. If the bleeding is arterial, compress the free edge of the lesser omentum between finger and thumb or apply a non-crushing intestinal clamp just tightly enough to control bleeding (Pringle's manoeuvre; Fig. 22.3). Dissect out and control the hepatic artery, which normally lies on the left-hand side of and below the bile duct. Remember that accessory hepatic arteries arising from the left gastric or superior mesenteric arteries are not controlled by occluding the main hepatic artery. Expose the damaged vessel. If it is large, repair it with arterial sutures; if it is small, ligate each end. You may find that you have pulled the cystic artery off the right hepatic artery. If so, suture the defect in the parent vessel. In the absence of jaundice or hypotension, ligature of the right hepatic or even the common hepatic artery, although best avoided, does not lead to infarction of the liver.
   b. If the bleeding is venous, control it by compression for 5 minutes timed by the clock, then explore, evaluate and repair the damage as necessary.

7. *Can the gallbladder not be separated from the liver?* Suspect carcinoma, and consider frozen-section examination if the diagnosis is equivocal. Resect carcinoma of the gallbladder if you are able to achieve a curative resection. This usually necessitates resection of the gallbladder bed and the nodes at the porta hepatis. This decision is often guided by the depth of tumour invasion into the gallbladder wall on histology. Although some surgeons favour partial hepatectomy, any attempted resection is best performed by a fully trained hepatobiliary surgeon. If severe but benign fibrosis makes it extremely difficult to develop a safe plane of dissection, be willing to leave the back wall of the gallbladder attached to the liver and destroy the exposed mucosa with diathermy current.

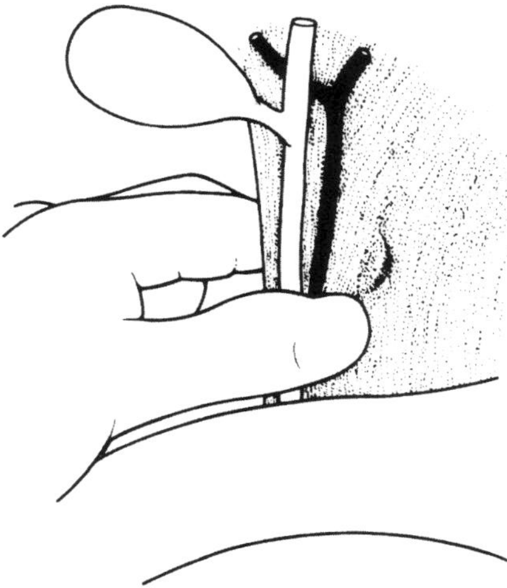

Fig. 22.3 Pringle's manoeuvre. Digital compression of the hepatic artery within the free edge of the lesser omentum controls haemorrhage from branches of the vessel beyond that point.

Closure

Have you reviewed the clinical and radiological criteria for continuing to exploration of the bile duct (see below) and examined the gallbladder bed, the common duct and the ligatures on the cystic duct and cystic artery?

Place a tube drain or fine-bore suction drain to the subhepatic pouch if you are concerned about possible biliary leak from the gallbladder bed on the liver, or if the area is oozing and there is the possibility of haematoma formation.

Close the abdominal wall in layers as for a standard laparotomy incision (see Ch. 7).

Aftercare

The nasogastric tube can usually be removed at 12–24 hours and the drain at 48 hours. In straightforward cases introduce a light diet at 24–36 hours and discharge patients at 3–8 days.

A small amount of bile may drain at first from the raw surface of the liver but ceases spontaneously within a few days. Regard a larger leak of more than 100 ml bile per day or a persistent fistula as a complication and manage it accordingly.

> **KEY POINT Initial management of a postoperative bile leak**
>
> - In the setting of postoperative biliary ascites and sepsis, first control the bile leak and treat the sepsis. This can often be achieved by positioning a percutaneous drain. Before contemplating reoperation and repair you must carry out imaging of the bile ducts, either from above by percutaneous transhepatic cholangiography or HIDA (hepatobiliary iminodiacetic acid) scan, or from below by endoscopic retrograde cholangiography, and often both.

Complications

Copious bile drainage through the wound or drain site suggests unrecognized injury to the bile duct or a slipped ligature on the cystic duct. Under these circumstances a retained calculus in the bile duct may be associated with persistence of the biliary fistula. Damage to the main duct is often accompanied by jaundice. Confirm the diagnosis by cholangiography, obtained either by transhepatic needling or by retrograde cannulation of the ampulla. Endoscopic retrograde cholangiopancreatography (ERCP) is extremely valuable for both diagnosis and treatment of postoperative bile leak. The only action needed may be decompression of the bile duct with the insertion of a temporary stent to control a leak from either the cystic duct or a small tear in the bile duct. Reoperation is needed if the leak continues. A small defect in the bile duct may be amenable to repair over a T-tube, after ensuring that there are no ductal calculi, but a larger defect or complete transection requires Roux-en-Y hepaticojejunostomy (see later).

Wound infection is uncommon unless the bile duct is explored or there is severe acute cholecystitis.

Subhepatic abscess occasionally results from an undrained collection of blood or bile; management is considered in Chapter 11. True subphrenic abscess is rare, likewise septicaemia.

The mortality rate of cholecystectomy is well under 1%. Most deaths occur in the elderly, those with gangrene or perforation of the gallbladder or those with concomitant ductal stones. Most postcholecystectomy symptoms result from unrecognized intercurrent disease.

OPERATIVE CHOLANGIOGRAPHY

Cholangiography is an integral part of cholecystectomy. Carry it out at an early stage unless preoperative visualization of the ducts by, for example, retrograde cholangiography has been excellent and they are normal. This policy of routine cholangiography has been challenged in the laparoscopic era (Ch. 23) but, as most cases performed with open operation are likely to represent the more difficult cases, we still believe that this traditional teaching holds true during open cholecystectomy.

EXPLORATION OF THE BILE DUCT

Absolute indications for exploration of the bile duct at laparotomy are stones unequivocally shown on a preoperative or operative cholangiogram, stones that can be palpated within the bile duct and stones causing obstructive jaundice. Preoperatively detected stones should usually be treated by ERCP and stone extraction unless the patient is to be subjected to open operation anyway. The detection of duct stones during laparoscopic cholangiography is usually not an indication to convert to an open procedure as in most cases the duct can be cleared by laparoscopic duct exploration or postoperative ERCP. In the latter case, a transcystic duct drain can be left in situ to provide adequate drainage until the ERCP is organized. This strategy may be appropriate in the elderly patient, although the mortality rate of open common bile duct exploration is low at 1%.

Endoscopic papillotomy may avoid the need for laparotomy in selected patients with bile duct stones, especially those without a gallbladder.

INTERNAL DRAINAGE FOR DUCTAL STONES

Some form of permanent drainage operation is indicated during exploration of the bile duct when multiple stones and biliary mud are encountered, or when papillary stenosis impedes the onward passage of contrast or instruments. Such patients are likely to have a history of jaundice and dilatation of the extrahepatic biliary tree.

Choledochoduodenostomy is a satisfactory alternative, especially in the elderly.

Transduodenal sphincteroplasty (Fig. 22.4) is intended to create a passage into the duodenum equal in size to the diameter of the bile duct, so that any remaining stones can enter the duodenum.

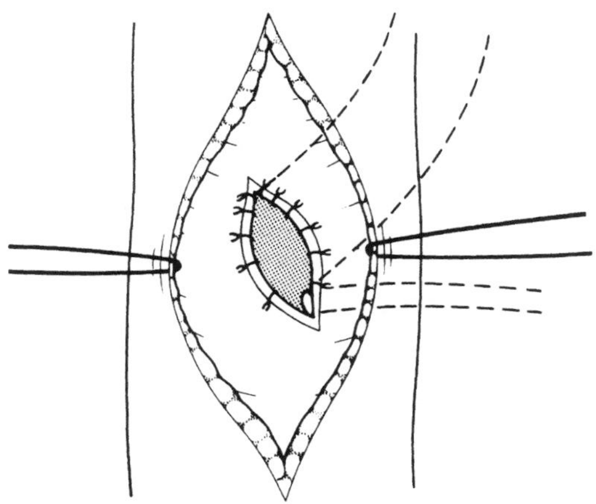

Fig. 22.4 Transduodenal sphincteroplasty. Approach the papilla through a longitudinal duodenotomy to incise it. Insert interrupted sutures to coapt the mucosa of the terminal bile duct and duodenum. The orifice of the major pancreatic duct is visible at the lower end of the sphincteroplasty.

Endoscopic papillotomy can also provide ductal drainage without the need for a major surgical operation.

ALTERNATIVES TO CHOLECYSTECTOMY

Cholecystostomy is a temporary expedient for draining an obstructed or infected gallbladder to the exterior when cholecystectomy unsafe. It can be performed under local anaesthesia.

Subtotal cholecystectomy may be a better option than cholecystostomy if you encounter difficulty in removing the entire gallbladder for stones because of oedema and fibrosis in Calot's triangle. Remove the gallbladder piecemeal, leaving part of the posterior wall in situ. It avoids the need for further surgery.

Percutaneous cholecystostomy may be a better option than open cholecystostomy in a patient with severe acute cholecystitis, especially the acalculous type, who is unfit for operation. Under ultrasound guidance a fine needle is inserted percutaneously into the gallbladder. A guidewire is passed through it and after withdrawing the needle, dilators are passed over the wire, followed by a catheter.

MISCELLANEOUS OPERATIONS

Hepaticojejunostomy may be performed for traumatic biliary stricture, almost always resulting from inadvertent damage at cholecystectomy. Excise the stricture and close off the lower cut end. Dissect at least 1 cm of the normal proximal duct and unite it to a Roux loop of jejunum (Fig. 22.5). If you anticipate recurrent stenosis, an extension of the Roux loop can be brought to the abdominal wall, fixed and marked with a radio-opaque marker ring. Subsequently a radiologist may puncture into the loop and insert radiology catheters, dilators and stents percutaneously.

Malignant stricture from cholangiocarcinoma, gallbladder cancer or metastases from breast, gastric or pancreatic cancer may be amenable to resection and Roux-loop reconstruction, resection into the hilum, or major hepatectomy. Irresectable blockage may be dilated and held open with a stent, or bypassed by resecting the tip of one lobe of the liver and joined to a Roux loop.

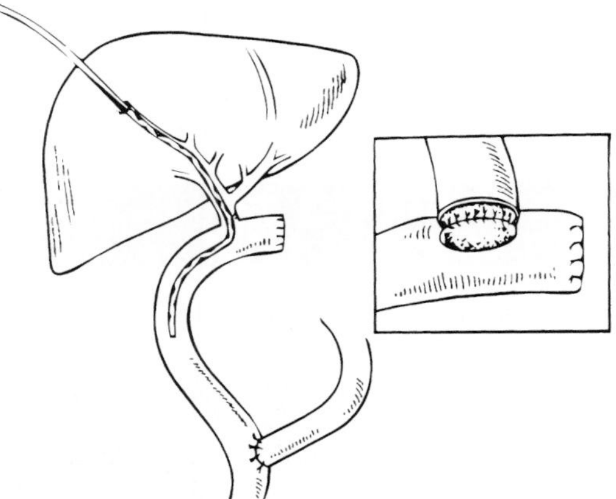

Fig. 22.5 Hepaticojejunostomy Roux-en-Y. A retrocolic jejunal conduit has been brought up for anastomosis to the upper common hepatic duct. A transhepatic splinting tube has been placed across the anastomosis. Side holes are created in those segments of the tube destined to lie within the liver and jejunum. An alternative ploy is to position the upper end of the tube within the intrahepatic biliary tree and bring the lower end out through the jejunum below the anastomosis. The insert shows a close-up of the biliary–enteric anastomosis after tying the posterior row of sutures (and with the tube omitted for the sake of clarity).

FURTHER READING

Adam A, Roddie ME 1991 Acute cholecystitis: radiological management. In: Williamson RCN, Thompson JN (eds) Gastrointestinal emergencies: part II. Baillière Tindall, London, pp 787–816

Blumgart LH, Fong Y 2000 Surgery of the liver and biliary tract, 3rd edn. Saunders, London

Williamson RCN 1988 Acalculous disease of the gallbladder. Gut 29:860–872

Williamson RCN, Abdulhadi ALY 1994 Recent advances in diagnosis and treatment of carcinoma of the gallbladder. In: Serio G, Huguet C, Williamson RCN (eds) Hepatobiliary and pancreatic tumours. Graffham Press, Edinburgh, pp 127–138

23

Laparoscopic biliary surgery

J. N. Thompson, S. G. Appleton

CONTENTS

KEY POINT Respond to circumstances

- In the face of these findings, convert to an open procedure sooner rather than later. This is not a failure of surgical technique but safe practice.

LAPAROSCOPIC CHOLECYSTECTOMY

This is now the treatment of choice for patients with symptomatic gallstones. Additional indications for the operation include selected patients with gallstones who have no symptoms but are at risk of severe complications and those who have no stones but suffer severe biliary symptoms. There are few absolute contraindications. Cirrhosis with portal hypertension is dangerous because of the substantial risk of uncontrollable bleeding during the operation, which may also precipitate hepatic failure. Sustained carbon dioxide pneumoperitoneum can cause significant cardiovascular changes in patients with ischaemic heart disease and significant hypercarbia in patients with respiratory disease. If carcinoma of the gallbladder is diagnosed preoperatively, avoid laparoscopic excision.

Contraindications to the laparoscopic technique may become apparent during the procedure, including discovery of an unexpected pathology; inability to identify the anatomy safely – usually because dense adhesions make safe dissection impossible; and uncontrollable bleeding and damage to adjacent structures or organs.

Some centres now perform laparoscopic cholecystectomy as a day-case procedure, although this requires appropriate facilities and good postoperative support. It has rendered virtually obsolete non-operative treatments of gallstones such as lithotripsy or dissolution therapy. Mini-cholecystectomy performed through a 5-cm right upper quadrant incision is an alternative to laparoscopic cholecystectomy and has comparable results. However, as with the laparoscopic procedure, special instruments and training are required.

Prepare

1 Obtain informed consent for laparoscopic cholecystectomy, having discussed the possibility of conversion to an open operation during the procedure, which varies from unit to unit but is of the order of 5%. Bleeding, infection and ductal injury may occur. If you perform cholangiography you find common duct stones in about 10% and you must be prepared to deal with them.

2 Institute thromboprophylaxis with subcutaneous heparin and compression stockings because the reverse Trendelenburg position, together with a positive-

pressure pneumoperitoneum, encourages the development of deep venous thrombosis.

3 General anaesthesia is required, with endotracheal intubation and muscle relaxation.

4 Biliary tract surgery rarely involves anaerobic microorganisms so you need prescribe only cefuroxime 1.5 mg intravenously as a single dose at the induction of anaesthesia. If there is leakage of bile during the operation, give a further two postoperative doses.

5 Place the patient supine on a radiolucent operating table that allows on-table cholangiography, with the upper abdomen and lower chest over the radiolucent section. Ensure there is room for the C-arm of the image intensifier both above and below the table.

6 Pass a nasogastric tube to deflate the stomach. This decreases aspiration associated with the pneumoperitoneum, reduces the risk of accidental perforation by a trocar and improves visibility during the procedure. Similarly, if you use a closed technique for inserting the initial trocar, pass a catheter to empty the urinary bladder and avoid accidental perforation.

7 Most surgeons stand on the patient's left with the first assistant opposite. Alternatively, the patient may be placed in the Lloyd-Davies position while you operate from the foot of the table between the patient's legs.

8 Prepare the skin of the abdomen from the nipples to the suprapubic region using 10% povidone-iodine in alcohol (Betadine) or other cleansing agent. Ensure the skin is prepared up to the posterior axillary line on the patient's right side, for the lateral port. Similarly, ensure that the drape at the top end extends above the level of the xiphisternum and that the right drape is placed as far lateral as possible.

9 Arrange the various leads and tubes that may be required before establishing the pneumoperitoneum; these include the gas tubing, diathermy lead, light source and irrigation–suction tubing. Secure them with clips or tape to the surgical drapes around the operating field, to minimize tangling.

Access

1 We use an 'open' laparoscopic technique to access the peritoneal cavity, insert the primary subumbilical cannula and establish a pneumoperitoneum. Use a Veress needle to establish a pneumoperitoneum in the closed technique, followed by blind insertion of the initial trocar and cannula (see Ch. 8). Insert all subsequent trocars under direct vision. Maintain an intra-abdominal pressure of 10–14 mmHg throughout the procedure.

2 A 30° laparoscope is better than a 0° scope for obtaining 'angled' views and for 'looking down' onto Calot's triangle (described by the French surgeon Jean François Calot, 1801–1844), bounded above by the liver, below by the cystic duct and medially by the common hepatic artery, although definitions vary.

3 Four ports are required initially: a 10-mm umbilical port for the camera; a 5-mm lateral port to retract the fundus of the gallbladder; a 5-mm right upper quadrant port placed in the midclavicular line to manipulate the neck of the gallbladder; a 10-mm cannula with a 5-mm reducer or a 5–12-mm disposable port in the epigastrium, just to the right of the midline and 2–5 cm below the xiphisternum. Introduce the epigastric port into the abdominal cavity through or just to the right of the ligamentum teres. It is the main port for dissecting instruments, diathermy, clip applicators, suction and irrigation. A large or floppy left lobe of the liver occasionally obstructs the view of Calot's triangle. Overcome this with a liver retractor placed through an additional 5-mm port in the left upper quadrant.

Assess

1 As in a laparotomy, the initial task is to examine the abdominal cavity. Carry out a systematic inspection of the contents of the four quadrants and pelvis. This is equivalent to the exploratory laparotomy in open biliary surgery. Note common disorders of a benign nature, for example colonic diverticular disease or pelvic adnexal disease in the female, but these do not preclude the performance of laparoscopic cholecystectomy. More serious findings, particularly if you suspect neoplasia, may necessitate conversion to open laparotomy or postponement of the surgical treatment pending further investigations and preparation of the patient.

2 Facilitate your assessment of the subhepatic region by tilting the operating table 25–35° head up and 10–15° sideways to the left; this encourages the abdominal contents to fall away from the area.

3 *Assess feasibility of laparoscopic cholecystectomy.* This is an assessment of the technical difficulty and safety of

gallbladder excision using the laparoscopic method. To a large extent, the decision is influenced by your experience of laparoscopic surgery. The situations that may be encountered are:

a. *Easy cases*. The patient is thin and the intraperitoneal fat is minimal. The gallbladder is floppy and non-adherent. When the gallbladder is lifted and retracted upwards by a grasping forceps, the cystic pedicle – the fold of peritoneum covering the cystic artery, duct and lymph node – is readily identified as a smooth triangular fold between the neck of the gallbladder, the inferior surface of the liver and the common bile duct. These patients are undoubtedly better served by laparoscopic than by open cholecystectomy.
b. *Feasible but more difficult cases*. These include obese patients in whom the cystic pedicle is fat-laden. A gallbladder containing a large stone load may be difficult to grasp and this can cause problems with retraction and exposure. The gallbladder may be distended by cholecystitis or because of a stone impacted in the neck. Difficulties may also be encountered due to adhesions from previous surgery. Provided you are experienced and prepared to proceed carefully, laparoscopic cholecystectomy can be accomplished with safety and a good outcome.
c. *Cases of uncertain feasibility – trial dissection*. This group includes patients with dense adhesions, those in whom the cystic pedicle cannot be visualized and patients with contracted fibrotic gallbladders where the neck or Hartmann's pouch appears to be adherent to the common bile duct. If you are experienced, it is reasonable to perform a careful trial dissection. The feasibility or otherwise of the operation becomes apparent as the dissection proceeds.

▶ KEY POINT Be willing to convert

- Trial dissection does not equate with a long or hazardous procedure. If you cannot clearly identify and expose the structures of the cystic pedicle in Calot's triangle, convert to an open procedure.

d. *Unsuitable cases*. These include patients with the following findings:
   i. Severe acute cholecystitis with gangrenous patches or a gross inflammatory phlegmon obscuring the structures of the porta hepatis.
   ii. Chronically inflamed gallbladder with the neck adherent to the common hepatic duct, indicative of the syndrome described in 1948 by the Argentinian surgeon Pablo Mirizzi. This was obstructive jaundice caused by compression of the common hepatic duct by a stone on the cystic duct or neck of the gallbladder; variations have subsequently been described.
   iii. Cirrhosis with established portal hypertension and large high-pressure varices surrounding the gallbladder and cystic pedicle.

In patients with severe acute cholecystitis that precludes safe dissection, a laparoscopic cholecystostomy may be performed, with interval cholecystectomy at a later date (see later). It is foolhardy to attempt laparoscopic cholecystectomy in patients in whom the gallbladder neck/Hartmann's pouch is densely adherent or fistulated into the common hepatic duct, since the risk of damage to the bile duct is considerable. These patients are best served by open operation (see Ch. 22).

4 If the gallbladder is not visible then use blunt-tipped grasping forceps or a probe in the lateral port to gently sweep away omentum, colon or small bowel. Alternatively, insert grasping forceps under the edge of the liver and gently lift it to expose the fundus of the gallbladder.

5 Grasp the fundus of the gallbladder with self-retaining toothed grasping forceps inserted through the lateral port. Gently push the gallbladder up over the liver towards the diaphragm as far as it will comfortably go and have your assistant hold it in this position. It is difficult to grasp a distended and tense gallbladder so decompress it with a Veress needle or a 16G Abbocath passed through the abdominal wall just below the costal margin in the midclavicular line. Aspirate gallbladder contents using a 20-ml syringe or suction tubing put in the barrel of a 10-ml syringe with the plunger removed. Send the bile to microbiology for culture and sensitivity. Withdraw the Veress needle or Abbocath and place the grasping forceps over the

puncture site in the gallbladder to limit further bile spillage.

6 If the gallbladder has been previously inflamed, it often has adhesions on its serosal surface; pull off flimsy adhesions with fine non-toothed grasping forceps, divide thicker, vascular adhesions with diathermy, close to the gallbladder wall. Avoid the hepatic flexure of the transverse colon laterally, and the duodenum medially, both of which may be closely adherent to the gallbladder.

Action

1 Start the dissection of Calot's triangle by holding the neck of the gallbladder with grasping forceps, fairly close to the origin of the cystic duct, if it is visible. This is probably the most important instrument in the initial dissection, as it allows the structures in the cystic pedicle to be exposed under tension and the gallbladder neck can be moved up and down so you can see both superior and inferior surfaces of Calot's triangle. Never embark on this dissection unless you know the anatomy intimately and make certain what the structure you intend to cut is before you cut it.

2 If there is a stone impacted in the neck of the gallbladder, massage it back into the body with forceps. If this fails, the grasping forceps may be positioned just behind the stone and still permit adequate movement of the gallbladder. Alternatively, replace the 5-mm port in the right upper quadrant with a 10-mm port and use heavy grasping forceps to hold the stone within the gallbladder.

3 Begin the dissection by using the diathermy hook or scissors to make a small hole in the peritoneum overlying the cystic duct close to the gallbladder neck to dissect Calot's triangle (Fig. 23.1) in one of three ways.

a. Grip the free edge of peritoneum just created with fine-tipped, straight or curved grasping forceps and peel the peritoneum medially to expose the structures of the cystic pedicle. Sometimes the peritoneum peels back easily to reveal the cystic duct and cystic artery but if you feel any resistance it is safer to proceed to one of the following methods.

b. With the diathermy hook divide the peritoneum on the undersurface of Calot's triangle, aiming posterolaterally towards the junction of gallbladder wall and liver. Remember to keep the peritoneum under tension using the grasping forceps on the neck of the gallbladder and to keep close to the gallbladder wall. When you reach the sulcus between the body of the gallbladder and the liver, continue dividing the peritoneum along the inferior border of gallbladder and liver for about 1–2 cm laterally. Move the neck of the gallbladder down and divide the peritoneum over Calot's triangle in a similar manner laterally towards the junction of gallbladder and liver, again taking care to keep close to the gallbladder wall. Continue the dissection for 1–2 cm laterally along the gallbladder–liver junction to open out Calot's triangle and improve the view.

c. Employ a similar approach as above but use dissecting scissors attached to diathermy instead of the hook. This technique demands careful attention to ensure that you know what is between the blades of the scissors before you cut.

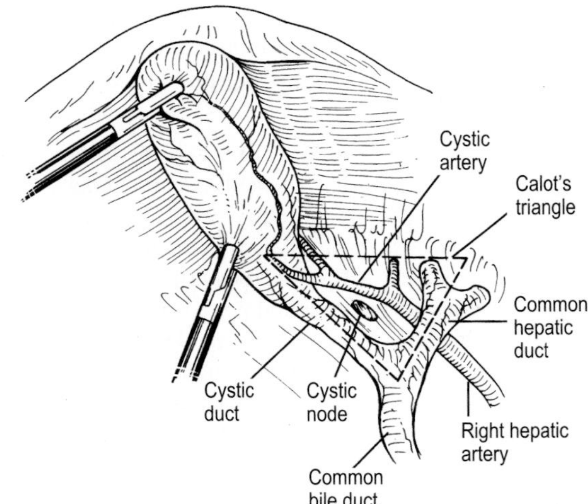

Fig. 23.1 Gallbladder retracted to show anatomy of Calot's triangle.

4 Aim to identify and clear the cystic duct and cystic artery so they may be clipped and divided safely. Frequently, this requires a disjointed dissection that alternates between the superior and inferior aspects of Calot's triangle, which is why the grasping forceps on the neck of the gallbladder is so important. The cystic duct and artery usually run parallel to each other. The

peritoneum overlying them will have been divided at right angles to these structures but create the window between them by inserting the tips of the scissors or dissecting forceps and opening them parallel to the duct and artery.

5 Diathermize any small bleeding vessels immediately; blood quickly obscures the view of Calot's triangle. It also absorbs the light from the camera, so darkening the view considerably. Remove clots with the suction/irrigation device. In difficult cases 'hydrodissection' of the tissues with the irrigation device may be helpful. Clear and skeletonize the cystic duct close to the neck of the gallbladder for 1–1.5 cm if possible. Ensure that the structure you think is cystic duct is entering the gallbladder and has no 'branches' or other connections. There is no advantage in dissecting out the junction of cystic duct and common hepatic duct; you are more likely to injure the bile duct if you attempt to identify the T-junction.

6 Sometimes the cystic artery can be seen to divide into its terminal anterior and posterior branches; this may occur more medially than anticipated and require distal clips on each of the branches before dividing the artery. To confirm a structure as an artery, observe it carefully and closely, to detect visible pulsation. To ensure it is the cystic artery that has been identified, and not the right hepatic artery, follow the vessel to the gallbladder wall.

7 When clipping either artery or duct, ensure that both tips of the clip applicator can be seen behind the structure being clipped in order to avoid inadvertently clipping important adjacent structures such as the common hepatic or common bile duct. When there is a short cystic duct avoid placing clips close to the junction with the common duct; instead, divide the neck of the gallbladder and use an Endoloop suture ligature.

Peroperative cholangiogram?

The necessity and indications for peroperative cholangiography during laparoscopic cholecystectomy are fiercely debated. Peroperative cholangiography may be performed routinely, selectively if there is a history of jaundice, dilated common bile duct or abnormal liver function tests, or rarely, following, for example, preoperative endoscopic retrograde cholangiography (ERCP). We use a selective approach and suggest that you should be familiar with the technique of laparoscopic cholangiography. You occasionally encounter aberrant or uncertain ductal anatomy and also it may be helpful to image the biliary ducts during operation. Cholangiography is usually performed via the cystic duct.

Gallbladder resection

1 Close the medial end of the cystic duct in one of three ways:

a. *Clips.* Use metal (titanium) clips or absorbable polydioxanone (Ethicon) clips to close the cystic duct stump. Apply these at right angles to the duct and check that they occlude the whole width of the duct. Failure to do this could result in a postoperative bile leak. Most surgeons use two clips on the medial cystic duct stump for added safety. Do not squeeze the clips too tightly – a particular hazard with reusable instruments – because they may 'cut through' the duct.

b. *Endoloop.* Apply a 2/0 polyglactin 910 (Vicryl) Endoloop once the cystic duct has been divided. This is particularly useful for a wide, oedematous or inflamed cystic duct where clips are liable to slip or cut through. Pass the Endoloop through the epigastric port. Pass the tips of dissecting forceps through the Endoloop and pick up the cystic duct stump. Apply enough tension on the cystic duct to slide the Endoloop down over it without tenting up the bile duct. Tighten the Endoloop securely around the cystic duct stump and then cut the ligature.

c. *Ligate in continuity.* Pass a length of 2/0 polyglactin 910 (Vicryl) thread behind the intact cystic duct. The duct can then be ligated in continuity using intra- or extracorporeal knotting techniques.

2 When the medial end of the cystic duct has been secured the duct can be divided using scissors. The gallbladder is now detached from the structures of the porta hepatis.

3 Gallbladder dissection from the liver can be relatively straightforward in a non-inflamed gallbladder, especially one attached to the liver by a mesentery. However, more often than not, the gallbladder is chronically inflamed, contracted, adherent or partially buried in the liver bed. Keep the gallbladder on the stretch using grasping forceps attached to the fundus and neck respectively. Divide the serosa along the upper and lower junctions of gallbladder and liver using scissors

or the hook attached to diathermy. Coagulate any obvious vessels before dividing the peritoneum.

4 Retract the gallbladder neck laterally, raising the neck of the gallbladder from the liver bed, revealing the loose fibrous tissue plane that separates the gallbladder wall from the liver parenchyma. Divide this fibrous tissue using a combination of blunt and sharp dissection with scissors and diathermy using scissors and/or hook. Stay close to the gallbladder wall; if you wander too close to the liver parenchyma, you cause bleeding; if so, push the gallbladder back into the fossa, compressing it for a few minutes, slowing or stopping the bleeding. Midway through the dissection, move the grasping forceps from the gallbladder neck to its undersurface – the liver aspect, allowing better control of dissection for the lateral half of the gallbladder. If you encounter the small cystohepatic bile duct of Luschka (German anatomist, 1820–1875) entering the gallbladder directly from the liver parenchyma, clip it to avoid postoperative bile leak.

5 Before the gallbladder is completely detached, push it up over the liver towards the diaphragm. This retracts the liver edge and exposes the gallbladder fossa, allowing you to thoroughly inspect and coagulate residual bleeding points. Pay particular attention to the cut peritoneum at the edge of the gallbladder fossa. Irrigating the gallbladder fossa with saline under pressure helps to identify bleeding points, which may occasionally need clipping. This manoeuvre also allows inspection of the cystic pedicle to check the clips on the cystic duct and artery.

6 Dissecting the fundus of the gallbladder can be difficult, particularly if the gallbladder is large or embedded in the liver. Techniques that may be helpful include:

a. Retract the fundus of the gallbladder medially and the undersurface laterally to reverse the usual position of the gallbladder.

b. Remove the grasping forceps from the fundus and place them on the undersurface of the gallbladder to push it upward over the liver edge. Frequently a combination of manoeuvres is required to detach the fundus completely.

7 Once detached, place the gallbladder out of the way on the superior surface of the liver. Use blunt-tipped grasping forceps or a probe to lift up the liver edge to allow a final inspection of the gallbladder fossa and cystic pedicle for any bleeding or bile leaks. Aspirate any remaining blood or clots from the subhepatic fossa, over the right lobe of the liver and the right paracolic gutter.

Extracting the gallbladder

1 The gallbladder may be removed via the epigastric or umbilical port sites.

2 We routinely place the gallbladder in a retrieval bag before removing it. In any case use a bag if the gallbladder has been perforated during the procedure or is very distended with bile or stones, or you risk perforation and spillage during extraction. A number of bags are available, some attached to introducing instruments. We use a Bert bag. Moisten a fabric bag with saline to ease its manipulation. Insert fine grasping forceps into the base of the bag and then twist it around the shaft of the forceps. Insert the bag and forceps through the epigastric port and place it on top of the liver. Unfurl the bag and have your assistant grab one edge of the open end with grasping forceps in the lateral port while you grab the other edge to open out the bag. Using the forceps in the right upper quadrant port, guide the gallbladder into the bag either fundus or cystic duct first. Grab the edges of the retrieval bag with alligator forceps and extract both the bag and gallbladder in the manner described below.

3 *Gallbladder removal through the epigastric port.* This is suitable for small, non-distended gallbladders. Insert a pair of heavy, self-grasping, toothed (alligator) forceps through the epigastric port. Bring the bag, or gallbladder, into view and grasp the edge, or the clipped cystic duct end. Under direct vision, gently withdraw the bag or gallbladder into the epigastric cannula as far as it will go. Slide the cannula and alligator forceps out of the abdominal cavity. Grasp the exteriorized edge of the bag or neck of the gallbladder, on the abdominal surface, with a pair of Kocher's forceps or a heavy arterial forceps to prevent retraction back into the abdominal cavity. Release the alligator forceps and, with a combination of gentle rotation and traction, extract the bag or gallbladder. If you have not used a bag, avoid excessive traction on the gallbladder as this may cause perforation with intraperitoneal spillage of bile and stones.

4 *Gallbladder removal through the umbilical port.* Remove the laparoscope from the umbilical port and replace it in

the epigastric port. Insert alligator forceps into the umbilical port and under direct vision follow them up to the liver. Grasp the bag or clipped cystic duct end of the gallbladder, and withdraw it through the umbilical port in the manner described above. We use the umbilical port since fascial closure is easier. If the intraperitoneal portion of the gallbladder is distended with bile, grasp the exteriorized neck between two clips. Cut between them to enter the lumen of the gallbladder and insert the suction device to aspirate the bile and allow extraction of the gallbladder. If the gallbladder has a large stone load that prevents extraction, open the exteriorized neck, aspirate the bile and insert a Desjardins or Spencer–Wells forceps into the gallbladder lumen to crush or extract the stones. You risk perforating the fundus of the gallbladder with resultant stone spillage and wound contamination, especially if you have not used a bag.

5 You may insert large forceps such as Spencer–Wells down the outside of the partially extracted bag or gallbladder. When you see the tips laparoscopically in the abdominal cavity, open the forceps. This may stretch the port site sufficiently to allow you to remove the gallbladder. To remove larger stones that are heavily calcified or impacted you may need to enlarge the trocar site by cutting it. Take care to suture-repair the defect in the linea alba to prevent subsequent herniation.

Checklist

Re-establish the pneumoperitoneum after extracting the gallbladder, and insert the laparoscope to make a final check for bleeding or bile leak. Check that there is no previously unnoticed damage to other organs, including the liver such as lacerations or tears, transverse colon and duodenum including diathermy burns, or small bowel, by trocar injuries.

? DIFFICULTY

1. Convert to an open operation if laparoscopic cholecystectomy proves to be too difficult, if bleeding cannot be controlled or if you damage any viscera.
2. If a thin-walled gallbladder is perforated during the procedure, bile and often also small stones spill into the peritoneal cavity. Insert the suction device into the perforation to aspirate the gallbladder to dryness before sucking out as much of the escaped bile as possible. Multiple small stones may be more easily aspirated using a 10-mm suction device. Prevent further escape of stones by closing the perforation with grasping forceps or metal clips. Try to locate and remove all stones from the peritoneal cavity. Larger stones may be placed in a retrieval bag with the gallbladder, for extraction.
3. *Retrograde (fundus-first) cholecystectomy.* This is a useful technique in experienced hands when the gallbladder is acutely inflamed or when dense adhesions distort Calot's triangle. When necessary, use it with caution and not as an alternative to conversion to open operation. Insert a retractor through the lateral port. Position it under the liver to the left of the gallbladder and lift up the liver edge. It is then possible to start the dissection at the fundus of the gallbladder and work down towards its neck. Mobilize the gallbladder fully. Retract the mobilized gallbladder laterally and in a caudal direction to open out Calot's triangle, which assists in identifying the anatomy. Since the cystic artery is patent, you may encounter heavier than usual bleeding during dissection of the gallbladder.
4. *Partial cholecystectomy.* In chronic fibrotic cholecystitis, when the gallbladder is very adherent to the liver, dissection of the gallbladder can produce significant bleeding and result in damage to the hepatic parenchyma. In these circumstances it is acceptable to perform an incomplete cholecystectomy. After dividing the cystic duct, open the gallbladder with scissors close to its junction with the liver. Aspirate the gallbladder to dryness and remove any stones with grasping forceps or suction. Cut along the gallbladder wall close to its junction with the liver and follow this all the way round, so leaving the back wall of the gallbladder in

situ. Coagulate the mucosal surface of the residual gallbladder with diathermy to prevent mucus production.

5. *Subtotal cholecystectomy.* If Calot's triangle is obliterated or considered hazardous to dissect, divide the gallbladder with scissors at the level of Hartmann's pouch. Extract stones and place them in a retrieval bag, and aspirate bile. It is usually possible at this stage to dissect out a short length of Hartmann's pouch/cystic duct, in order to ligate it with an Endoloop or oversew it. Dissect the body and fundus of the gallbladder from the liver in the usual way and place it in a bag for extraction.

Closure

1 *Drains.* Many surgeons do not use a subhepatic drain after routine laparoscopic cholecystectomy unless there is concern about bleeding or bile leakage. Routine drainage overnight has the advantage of detecting the occasional postoperative bile leak at an early stage, thus avoiding inappropriate early discharge from hospital. A suction or non-suction drain can be inserted through the lateral or right upper quadrant port and placed in the subhepatic space with grasping forceps inserted through the epigastric port. Secure the drain to the skin with a suture.

2 Remove the cannulas under vision and ensure there is no bleeding from the abdominal wall puncture sites. Deflate the pneumoperitoneum as much as possible to reduce referred pain to the shoulder after operation.

3 Close wounds greater than 1 cm in the linea alba under direct vision with 0 polyglactin 910 (Vicryl) or PDS to avoid subsequent hernia formation. Infiltrate the skin wounds with long-acting local anaesthetic such as bupivacaine, and approximate the edges using sutures, skin tapes or staples.

Postoperative

Remove the nasogastric tube at the end of the operation. Following reversal of muscle relaxation and extubation, insert an oropharyngeal airway. Administer oxygen by mask for the first 3 hours. Remove the drain, if inserted, on the day following operation if there is no bile in it and blood loss of less than 50 ml per 24 hours. The majority of patients are ready for discharge from hospital on the day following operation.

Complications

Bile leak

If a drain has been placed then this complication is usually recognized by the presence of bile in the drain bottle on the day following operation. In the absence of a drain the patient may be discharged from hospital only to return unwell 3–5 days following operation with pain and tenderness in the right upper quadrant of the abdomen and jaundice. Biliary leaks may arise from the cystic duct stump, divided cystohepatic duct of Luschka in the gallbladder bed, or injury to a major bile duct (see below). An ultrasound or CT scan helps determine the size and position of any intra-abdominal collections and they can also be drained under imaging control. If a significant bile leak continues after drainage, undertake early ERCP to demonstrate the site of the leak and determine if any significant bile duct injury has occurred. The majority of minor biliary leaks seal in time with external drainage alone; however, a temporary biliary stent inserted endoscopically decompresses the biliary system, hastening closure of the leak and shortening hospital stay.

Major bile duct injury

The incidence of bile duct injury was initially higher following laparoscopic cholecystectomy than following open operation, but the incidence is now comparable at 1 in 300–500 operations. Major bile duct injuries include complete transections and clipping the common duct. This is complex and best dealt with in a unit specializing in their treatment.

LAPAROSCOPIC EXPLORATION OF THE COMMON BILE DUCT

Stones in the common duct are discovered in up to 10% on peroperative cholangiography. Clearance of the ducts requires either laparoscopic or open exploration of the ducts at the time of surgery, or postoperative ERCP. The *transcystic duct approach* is the most commonly used for small ductal stones less than 8 mm diameter, performed under X-ray image intensification and/or direct visual guidance using a narrow flexible choledochoscope. *Laparoscopic choledochotomy* is technically more difficult.

LAPAROSCOPIC CHOLECYSTOSTOMY

Percutaneous cholecystostomy under ultrasound control is often used to decompress the gallbladder and relieve symptoms in poor-risk and elderly patients with acute cholecystitis. Laparoscopic cholecystostomy also has a role when you find acute inflammatory changes at operation.

> **KEY POINT Respond to the findings**
>
> - If you are a relatively inexperienced laparoscopist and discover at initial laparoscopy a distended and severely inflamed gallbladder with areas of patchy necrosis of its wall and vascular adhesions, proceed to laparoscopic cholecystostomy.

LAPAROSCOPIC CHOLECYSTOJEJUNOSTOMY

Laparoscopic diagnosis and staging of pancreatic malignancies is complementary to other imaging modalities and palliative biliary bypass may be performed at the time of the staging laparoscopy as an alternative to insertion of an endoscopic or percutaneous biliary stent (Fig. 23.2).

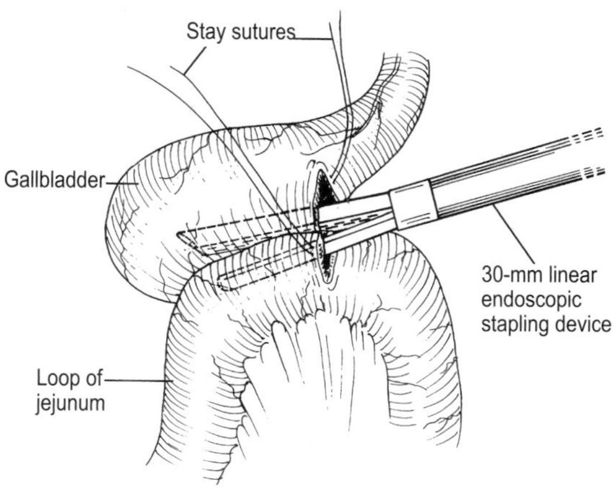

Fig. 23.2 Formation of cholecystojejunostomy using a 30-mm endoscopic linear stapler.

FURTHER READING

Cueto JG, Jacobs M, Gagner M 2002 Laparoscopic surgery. Higher Education, New York

MacFayden BV, Arrequi ME, Eubanks S et al (eds) 2003 Laparoscopic surgery of the abdomen. Springer-Verlag, Berlin

Nathanson L 2001 Gallstones. In: Garden OJ (ed.) Hepatobiliary and pancreatic surgery: a companion to specialist surgical practice, 2nd edn. Baillière Tindall, London

Scott-Conner CEH, Cuschieri A, Carter F (eds) 2000 Minimal access surgical anatomy. Lippincott Williams & Wilkins, Philadelphia

Internet websites

www.limit.ac.uk
www.websurg.com
www.laparoscopy.com
http://consensus.nih.gov/cons/090/090_intro.htm

24

Pancreas

R. C. N. Williamson, A. Shankar

CONTENTS

INTRODUCTION

Operations on the pancreas are some of the most challenging in abdominal surgery. It is inaccessibly retroperitoneal, intimately related to other organs, and following partial resection and union to a hollow viscus, leakage of powerful, digestive enzymes would cause severe tissue destruction. Disease of the head of the pancreas causing obstructive jaundice impairs many body functions.

For these reasons surgery of this organ is beyond the scope of junior surgeons and we shall display the principles only, so that you can assist intelligently, understand the procedures and improve your knowledge.

Pancreatic imaging is dramatically improved since the introduction of ultrasonography, spiral computed tomography (CT), endoscopic retrograde cholangiopancreatography (ERCP), endoscopic ultrasound, and other special processes.

Islets of pancreatic endocrine tissue are scattered throughout, described in 1869 by the Berlin physician and anatomist Paul Langerhans (1847–1888); major pancreatic resection can impair both endocrine and exocrine function sufficiency to cause diabetes and/or steatorrhoea.

We routinely employ a transverse ('gable') incision for pancreatic surgery, that is a curved bilateral subcostal incision. Cover pancreatic operations with broad-spectrum antibiotics, such as a cephalosporin. If there is any likelihood of operative cholangiography or pancreatography being required, place the patient on an operating table with X-ray tunnel.

EXPLORATION OF THE PANCREAS

First examine the duodenum, liver, spleen and bile duct, and mobilize the duodenal loop and pancreatic head by Kocher's manoeuvre (Fig. 24.1). See the pancreas and feel the head between finger and thumb. Expose the body and tail through the lesser sac, entered through the greater or lesser omentum. Divide the peritoneum along the inferior border, preserving the superior and inferior mesenteric veins. Expose the tail at the splenic hilum, if necessary dividing several short gastric arteries and the splenic flexure of the colon. Be willing to divide the peritoneum lateral to the spleen and lift the spleen and tail of pancreas forwards.

Normal pancreas is firm and nodular, chronic pancreatitis is sclerotic. Carcinoma may be hard, soft or cystic. If necessary open the duodenum to elucidate an ampullary mass.

Pancreatic biopsy carries a risk. Percutaneous wide-bore needle biopsy or narrow gauge cytology is guided by ultrasound or CT scans. Endoscopic retrograde cholangiopancreatography allows biopsy and cytology. Prefer biopsy of a liver, peritoneal or lymph node if present, otherwise take a direct biopsy, use a Tru-Cut needle, or fine needle cytology.

Operative pancreatography by cannulating the duct or through needle puncture can be performed if preoperative ERCP or magnetic resonance cholangiopancreatography

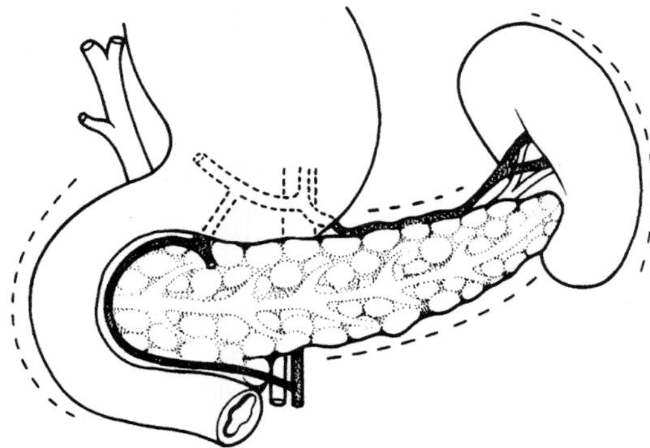

Fig. 24.1 Exposure of the pancreas. The lines of peritoneal incision are shown. The head of the pancreas and uncinate lobe are supplied by the superior and inferior pancreaticoduodenal arteries and the body and tail by the splenic artery.

(MRCP) were not performed or were unsuccessful. Elucidate pseudocysts and their ductal communication using cystography.

LAPAROTOMY FOR ACUTE PANCREATITIS

Diagnostic laparotomy is rarely required with the availability of abdominal CT but debridement of necrotizing pancreatitis after confirming infection with fine-needle aspiration may help, the alternative being percutaneous drainage inserted using local anaesthetic. Avoid laparotomy in the first week – it is too early for safe debridement and resection carries a formidable mortality. Pseudocysts, bleeding and abscesses are now often managed radiologically. Gallstone pancreatitis may improve after ERCP bile duct stone extraction. Ensure that the fluid depletion has been fully corrected by intravenous administration of colloid and crystalloid solutions before embarking on the operation. Anticipate hypoxaemia, monitor central venous pressure and urinary output. Give prophylactic broad-spectrum antibiotics.

Bloodstained free fluid is usually present in the abdominal cavity in acute pancreatitis. Whitish plaques of fat necrosis are visible on serosal surfaces, especially in the region of the pancreas. Lift up the greater omentum and transverse colon. There is oedema and blackish discoloration of the retroperitoneal tissues. The pancreas itself is swollen and may be haemorrhagic or even necrotic.

Examine the gallbladder and, if possible, the bile duct to determine if these organs are diseased. A more thorough examination is required if the patient has obstructive jaundice. In a case of infected pancreatic necrosis, extensively explore the retroperitoneal tissues to carry out a full assessment.

Diagnostic laparotomy

Do nothing unless there is a definite indication; attempted debridement at this stage can be disastrous. Consider placing a peritoneal dialysis catheter through a stab incision into the pelvis for postoperative peritoneal lavage. This treatment has not been shown to be of definite value but may be useful if the pancreatitis is complicated by renal failure. Wound dehiscence is common following laparotomy for acute pancreatitis. Take extra care in closing the linea alba or rectus sheath, and consider inserting tension sutures.

Infected pancreatic necrosis

Enter the lesser sac by dividing the greater omentum. The lesser sac is often obliterated by the inflammatory process and you quickly enter a large cavity containing pus and necrotic debris. Although the pancreas itself can undergo haemorrhagic infarction in a severe case of pancreatitis, more often the gland is viable and there is peripancreatic necrosis affecting the retroperitoneal fat.

Digitally explore the necrotic cavity and remove all dead tissue. Be gentle but thorough; the cavity may ramify extensively. Send samples of fluid and necrotic material for bacteriological examination.

Check the viability of the small and large intestine. Irrigate the large retroperitoneal cavity thoroughly with warm saline and secure haemostasis. You must now choose between closing the abdomen with generous drainage and leaving it open as a 'laparostomy', making no attempt to close the abdominal wall.

DRAINAGE OF PANCREATIC CYSTS

True cysts are congenital or neoplastic and are rare. Cysts complicating acute or chronic pancreatitis and pancreatic trauma are 'false' pseudocysts, in that they have no epithelial lining. Both types are best diagnosed by ultrasound and CT scanning of the upper abdomen. Drain a painful, expanding mass or one that fails to resolve or becomes infected. Employ percutaneous needle aspiration but after 4–5 weeks internal drainage is feasible, either cystgastrostomy for moderate-sized cysts or cystjejunostomy Roux-en-Y. Pseudocysts developing in association with chronic pancreatitis are generally contained within the pancreas and frequently communicate with the main ductal system. Always obtain a biopsy of the cyst wall at operation. Endoscopic techniques are now available for internal drainage of a pseudocyst, using endoscopic ultrasound guidance.

DRAINAGE OF THE PANCREATIC DUCT

Ductal drainage is preferable to resection for the relief of pain in chronic pancreatitis, since it preserves the remaining functioning tissue. The operation of choice is longitudinal pancreaticojejunostomy, which creates a long side-to-side anastomosis between the incised duct and a Roux loop of jejunum.

PRINCIPLES OF SURGERY FOR PANCREATIC CANCER

Ductal adenocarcinoma of the pancreas is common, difficult to treat and of unknown cause. Most tumours are irresectable by the time they are diagnosed, especially cancers of the body and tail, where early symptoms are scarce and non-specific, but distal pancreatectomy is feasible in a few (Fig. 24.2). Tumours within the head may present with obstructive jaundice while the tumour is still small and localized.

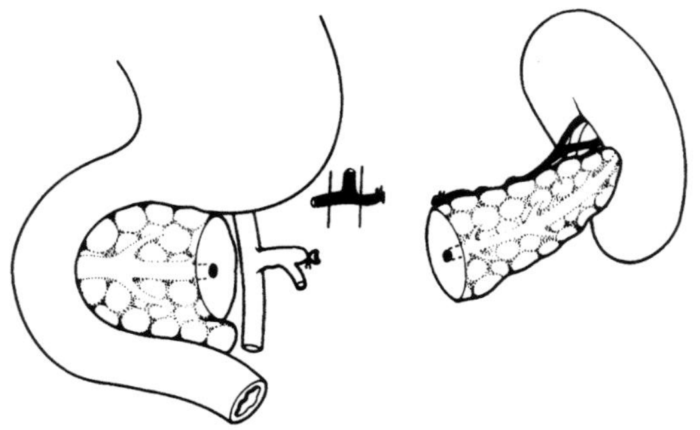

Fig. 24.2 Conventional distal pancreatectomy including splenectomy. Transection just to the right of the portal vein removes about 60% of the gland.

Some patients with cancer of the head of pancreas require laparotomy to confirm the diagnosis, determine the potential resectability of the tumour and allow a choice to be made between resection and bypass. Despite the scale of the operation required, carry out resection for potentially curable tumours in those of reasonable general health, since this policy offers the only chance of cure (Figs 24.3 and 24.4). In resection for chronic pancreatitis and cancer of the ampulla, lower part of the head and uncinate process, the whole stomach can be preserved – pylorus-preserving proximal pancreatoduodenectomy (PPPP).

Staging laparoscopy, possibly combined with laparoscopic ultrasound, allows detection of peritoneal deposits, small liver metastases and even portal venous invasion, but the additional information above that obtained from conventional imaging is controversial. Most patients with cancer of the body or tail of pancreas do not require laparotomy because the tumour either metastasizes or encases the superior mesenteric vessels at an early stage and is therefore seldom resectable. Moreover, jaundice and duodenal obstruction occur late if at all.

It is debatable whether non-operative stenting or surgical bypass is the better option for irresectable cancer of the

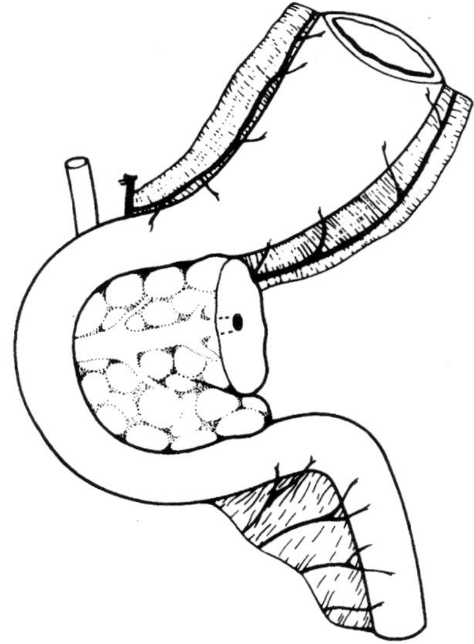

Fig. 24.3 Conventional pancreatoduodenectomy (Whipple's operation). The resection specimen is shown and includes the distal half of the stomach, the duodenal loop and duodenojejunal flexure, the terminal bile duct and the head and uncinate process of the pancreas.

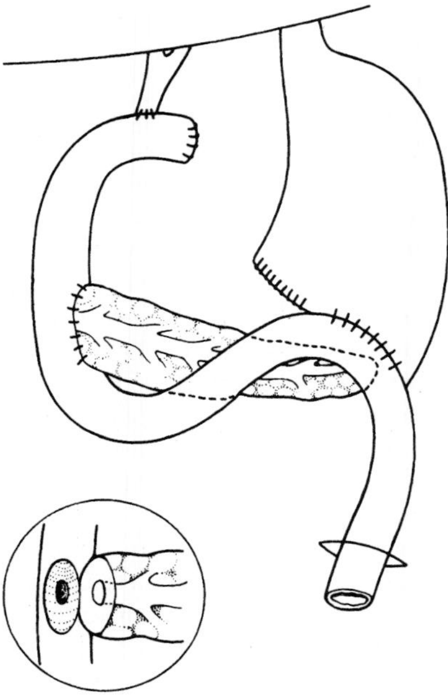

Fig. 24.4 Reconstruction after conventional pancreatoduodenectomy with an end-to-side pancreaticojejunostomy. To create the pancreatic anastomosis (inset), the pancreatic duct is sutured directly to the jejunal mucosa; the anastomosis can be splinted by a fine polythene tube.

pancreatic head. Stenting can be achieved by either the percutaneous transhepatic route or the endoscopic transpapillary route.

Patients with prolonged obstruction of the extrahepatic biliary tree tolerate major resectional procedures very poorly. Anticipate and counter coagulopathy, hepatorenal syndrome, sepsis, malnutrition and wound failure. Preoperative decompression of the obstructed biliary tree is controversial.

Action

The gallbladder is distended and there is such diffuse metastatic spread that the patient is unlikely to live very long

Patients with carcinomatosis are better served by nonoperative stenting. At operation relieve obstructive jaundice by the simple expedient of cholecystojejunostomy (see Ch. 22). For those with a better prognosis but irresectable tumours prefer to use the common hepatic duct for anastomosis; it prevents recurrence of jaundice from encroachment of tumour on the cystic duct.

The tumour is clearly irresectable but not as advanced as the above

The tumour is clearly irresectable but not as advanced as the above; alternatively, the gallbladder is collapsed or contains calculi. Do not use the gallbladder for anastomosis. Prefer choledochojejunostomy Roux-en-Y (see Ch. 22), dividing the bile duct above the 'leading edge' of tumour to limit upward spread. Cholecystectomy generally facilitates the operation and is certainly advisable if the gallbladder is obstructed.

The tumour could be resectable and there is no overt metastasis

Embark upon a trial dissection.

You have decided against resection

Obtain a positive tissue diagnosis by appropriate biopsy with frozen-section confirmation. Consider palliative procedures to relieve jaundice, vomiting and pain. Carry out biliary diversion as described above. Options for pain relief include coeliac plexus block; intraoperative nerve block involves injection of 15–20 ml of 50% alcohol on each side at the level of the diaphragmatic crura, or thoracoscopic division of the splanchnic nerves within the chest. Palliative resection is unjustified.

Once the patient recovers from operation and there is an unequivocal tissue diagnosis, consider the advisability of radiotherapy and/or chemotherapy.

TOTAL PANCREATECTOMY

Total pancreatectomy has sometimes been recommended for the routine management of resectable cancers on the grounds that it avoids the problems of multifocal origin of ductal carcinoma and potential leakage from the pancreaticojejunostomy. The counter-arguments are that it increases the risks of the procedure, conveys no actual survival advantage and renders the patient an obligate diabetic. Reserve the procedure for bulky tumours encroaching on the neck, for cancer in diabetics and for the occasional patient in whom frozen-section examination is positive during partial pancreatectomy. There is no evidence to suggest that total pancreatectomy for cancer provides any survival advantage, and in fact it may be associated with a worse outcome.

LAPAROTOMY FOR ISLET CELL TUMOUR

Insulinoma is the commonest islet cell tumour. It is usually solitary and benign. It presents with episodic hypoglycaemia and the diagnosis is confirmed by finding a low blood sugar and an inappropriately high serum insulin either spontaneously or after provocation by fasting. Most insulinomas are sufficiently vascular to be localized as a 'blush' on selective pancreatic arteriography. Local excision is sufficient.

Gastrinoma can arise in the pancreas, the duodenal wall or sometimes further afield. It presents with the Zollinger–Ellison syndrome of intractable peptic ulceration and diarrhoea. The best surgical treatment is to identify and resect all tumour tissue, but subtotal or even total gastrectomy is sometimes required. Some patients with islet cell tumour, especially gastrinoma, have coincident tumours of the parathyroid or pituitary gland as a part of *multiple endocrine neoplasia* (MEN I – multiple endocrine neoplasia type I).

Glucagonoma, somatostatinoma and other hormone-secreting tumours are rare entities, but a more common condition is the *non-functioning neuroendocrine tumour* of the pancreas.

FURTHER READING

Aldridge MC, Williamson RCN 1991 Distal pancreatectomy with and without splenectomy. British Journal of Surgery 78:976–979

British Society of Gastroenterology 1998 United Kingdom guidelines for the management of acute pancreatitis. United Kingdom guidelines for the management of acute pancreatitis. Gut 42 (Suppl 2):S1–S13

Buter A, Imrie CW, Carter CR et al 2002 Dynamic nature of early organ dysfunction determines the outcome in acute pancreatitis. British Journal of Surgery 89:298–302

Usatoff V, Brancatisano R, Williamson RC 2000 Operative treatment of pseudocysts in patients with chronic pancreatitis. British Journal of Surgery 87:1494–1499

25

Liver and portal venous system

S. Bhattacharya

CONTENTS

INTRODUCTION

The liver is considered by many surgeons to be a hallowed organ, and one that presents them with insurmountable problems. They fear massive haemorrhage after any violation of the capsule and dread the thought of attempting any elective procedure. These are unfounded myths: the liver is as amenable to surgery as any other organ, providing you respect certain principles. As a trainee learn the principles and perioperative care.

TRAUMA

The most frequent and frightening procedure you are called upon to perform on the liver is to arrest haemorrhage following trauma or spontaneous rupture of a tumour. Liver injuries can result from penetrating trauma such as stab or gunshot injuries, usually producing liver laceration, although high-velocity bullets may also cause significant contusion. Blunt trauma, often sustained in road traffic accidents, is usually associated with contusions and haematomas. Contusion carries a very high mortality rate, directly related to the severity and number of other affected organs.

Appraise

1 The patient may present with a typical history, in a shocked state. Maintain the patient's airway, breathing and circulation (ABC), following the principles of advanced trauma life support (ATLS). Now direct your attention to the internal bleeding. In case of doubt about intra-abdominal bleeding in a severely shocked patient, obtain an urgent contrast-enhanced computed tomography (CT) scan, to demonstrate liver parenchymal injury. Emergency portable abdominal ultrasound may also demonstrate a ruptured liver.

2 Treat penetrating injuries in general, and gunshot wounds in particular, by laparotomy. Treat conservatively only selected patients with stab injury who are haemodynamically stable and in whom there is no evidence of hollow viscus perforation.

3 Treat conservatively those patients with blunt trauma who are haemodynamically stable, even if there is demonstrable liver injury on CT or ultrasound scan. If the patient becomes haemodynamically unstable or develops signs of impending peritonitis, proceed to a laparotomy. Carry out urgent laparotomy on a shocked patient who fails to respond adequately despite aggressive initial fluid replacement.

EXPLORATION OF A DAMAGED LIVER

Have you booked an intensive care unit bed if needed postoperatively? Pass a bladder catheter to monitor urine flow and ensure adequate fluid volume replacement. Place a central venous line, wide-bore peripheral venous lines, and ideally an arterial catheter to monitor arterial pressure. Ensure there are at least 12 units of blood available, together with fresh-frozen plasma (FFP) and platelets to replace lost clotting products.

Access

A right subcostal incision 3 cm below the costal margin can be extended across as an inverted 'V', or vertically upwards. You may open the chest to control the supra-diaphragmatic inferior vena cava (IVC). If you discover the rupture at diagnostic laparotomy through a midline incision, extend it as necessary. If a lower abdominal incision is inappropriate, close it and re-site it.

Assess

There is usually much blood clot in the peritoneal cavity and probably some fresh bleeding. Remove clot with your hands and a sucker. Look systematically for damage to the liver, the gut from oesophagus to rectum, spleen, pancreas, anterior and posterior abdominal wall and the diaphragm. If necessary pack the abdominal cavity with sterile packs, removing them serially, inspecting each of the four quadrants in succession.

Action

1 If there is obvious damage to, and haemorrhage from, another intra-abdominal viscus such as the spleen, and that is the primary source of bleeding, surround the damaged area of the liver with large sterile packs and have an assistant apply gentle pressure to control the bleeding. Attend to the lesion in the other organ first, and then turn your attention to the liver. Remove blood and blood clot to gain adequate exposure of the bleeding area of the liver. Control the haemorrhage. Most patients do not require major surgical procedures. Attempt only the minimum surgery necessary to control haemorrhage. Avoid exploring and rough handling of sites of injury that are not bleeding at the time of exploration provided the blood pressure is normal. If the patient is hypotensive there is risk of reactionary haemorrhage when the patient becomes normotensive.

2 Explore the tear of the liver locally and remove any avascular tissue. If the laceration still bleeds and extends deeply into the liver parenchyma, gently explore the depth of the wound but avoid creating further damage. In contusion injuries major branches of liver vessels may be ruptured, producing large areas of devascularized tissue. Do not explore tears that are not bleeding, since you only encourage further bleeding. Identify bleeding points and apply fine haemostatic forceps. Ligate them with fine synthetic absorbable material. If there is vascular oozing from a large raw area of liver, cover it with one layer of absorbable haemostatic gauze and apply a pack. Fibrin sealants may help. Avoid deep mattress sutures to control such bleeding, since they may produce areas of devascularization which predisposes to subsequent infection.

? DIFFICULTY

Is there uncontrolled haemorrhage from torn liver? If haemorrhage is massive, attempt control by inserting a finger through the opening into the lesser sac behind the hepatic hilar structures and apply a Satinsky or other non-crushing clamp across them (Pringle manoeuvre). If this does not achieve control, pack gauze rolls around the liver; do not insert them into the depths of a liver laceration.

Aftercare

Admit the patient to an intensive care unit or high-dependency nursing area.

Maintain intravascular volume and normal clotting. Transfuse with blood and FFP as required. Maintain urine flow. If it falls below 30 ml/hour, first check that the circulating blood volume is adequate, with normal blood pressure and central venous pressure. Give a versatile antibiotic mixture such as a combination of cefuroxime and metronidazole. If gastrointestinal activity does not return within 2–3 days, institute intravenous nutrition. Sudden collapse suggests that the patient has developed further internal bleeding or septicaemia.

PRINCIPLES OF ELECTIVE SURGERY

Do not undertake an elective operation on the liver without complete preoperative investigation and a fairly certain working diagnosis. If you discover a lesion in the liver during a laparotomy, carefully consider the risks before trying to excise or biopsy it, or you may expose the patient to serious risks. Operation on a patient with impaired liver function can be very hazardous and carries a high morbidity and mortality.

Always obtain histological confirmation of the nature of any underlying parenchymal liver disease. First, correct any clotting or platelet abnormalities. The biopsy can be carried out percutaneously, by blind insertion, with CT or ultrasound direction, at peritoneoscopy, or at laparotomy. Use either a Tru-Cut or a Menghini needle. The needle track can be embolized by injecting Gelfoam suspension into the needle sheath as it is removed. If clotting cannot be corrected, an expert can obtain a transjugular biopsy using a special catheter introduced into an hepatic vein branch through a jugular vein puncture.

OPERATIVE LIVER BIOPSY

1 Check the patient's blood group but if a major procedure may be needed cross-match blood, platelets, and have available some FFP.

2 Take the liver biopsy early during laparotomy, otherwise histological changes may occur. Select an area of diseased liver or an edge that presents easily through the incision. Place two mattress stitches of 3/0 Vicryl or PDS on an atraumatic round-bodied needle to form a 'V', the apex of this pointing towards the hilum of the liver. Gently but firmly tie these stitches and remove the wedge of tissue between them. If the cut liver edges bleed, use diathermy or insert another stitch.

3 You may also use a Tru-Cut needle to take a liver biopsy. After removing the needle, check that you have an adequate core of tissue. Gently shake or tease the core of tissue into a pot of formalin, taking care not to crush it. The puncture site occasionally requires a figure-of-eight or Z-stitch with 4/0 Vicryl or PDS to obtain haemostasis.

INFECTIVE LESIONS AND CYSTS

Bacterial liver abscesses rarely require open surgical drainage; pus can be aspirated percutaneously through a large bore needle, under imaging guidance, with antibiotic cover. At laparotomy, first isolate the area with packs. Send contents for immediate examination and aerobic and anaerobic culture. Incise the abscess, suck out the contents, gently insert a finger to identify and breakdown all loculi. Wash out the cavity with physiological saline and insert a tube drain through a separate stab, preferably as a closed system. If possible, draw some omentum into the cavity. Now close the abdomen. Leave the drain until drainage ceases and the cavity is demonstrably collapsed on ultrasound, CT or a sinogram, then stop the antibiotics.

Amoebic abscess rarely requires surgical treatment. Positively confirm the diagnosis by identifying trophozoites in the aspirate, or by a positive serological test. Treatment is with metronidazole, 400–800 mg orally 8-hourly in an adult for at least 7 days. Resolution of the abscess can be monitored using regular ultrasound screening. If it becomes secondarily infected or is discovered at laparotomy then treat it like any other liver abscess.

Hydatid cyst is the likely diagnosis in patients who present with a liver mass and who live or have lived in an endemic area. Confirm it by the presence of eosinophilia, positive hydatid serology and classic ultrasound and CT appearances.

Past treatment was mainly surgical with cystectomy and omentoplasty, but percutaneous treatment, combined with antihelminthic drug therapy is safe and effective in selected patients with uncomplicated cysts. Administer an initial course of albendazole, followed by puncture of the cyst under imaging guidance, aspiration of the cyst contents, instillation of hypertonic saline and then re-aspiration – the acronym is PAIR.

If operation becomes necessary, give at least a 4-week cycle of albendazole tablets (10 mg/kg/day in divided doses for an adult) before and after surgery to prevent growth of any spilt protoscolices (Greek *protos* = first + *scolex* = a worm). At operation isolate the cyst from the rest of the peritoneal or chest contents with packs. If possible attach a metal funnel to the exposed cyst using liquid nitrogen before aspirating the cyst, filling it repeatedly with 20% saline solution to kill off any live scolisces (Greek *scolex* = worm; the head of the worm). Finally, empty it and then gently remove the yellow-grey cyst membrane containing the daughter cysts without spilling any. External drainage of the emptied cavity is controversial.

Massive polycystic disease of the liver is rare but can cause severe pain. In 50% there is associated polycystic renal disease.

NEOPLASMS

Liver neoplasms can be solid or cystic, benign or malignant, primary or secondary, single or multiple. Proven benign neoplasms may not require excision. Preoperative assessment of AFP and CEA levels may indicate if the lesion is a primary or secondary tumour. Ultrasound, CT and MR scans, angiograms and biopsy are valuable. Consider for laparotomy patients with malignant, suspected malignant or symptomatic benign disease. Correct any clotting abnormality before surgery. Give jaundiced patients vitamin K_1 injections. Assess the state and function of the unaffected liver. Administer intravenous prophylactic antibiotics with the premedication, such as a cephalosporin and metronidazole and plan to maintain this postoperatively for 3 days.

Wedge excision

After applying a gentle clamp across the hilar vessels. Incise the capsule and excise the tumour by dividing the liver by finger and thumb pinch technique. After achieving haemostasis, pack omentum against the raw surface and close the abdomen.

Right or left hepatectomy

The liver is divided into two anatomical lobes, each being supplied by its own branch of the hepatic artery, portal vein and hepatic duct. By ligating hepatic artery and portal vein branches supplying either lobe, it is possible to see the junction between them as a fairly sharp colour change. The liver is further divided into eight segments (Fig. 25.1). It is possible to divide the liver through the main plane separating the right and left lobes or remove segments of the liver. Left, right or extended right hepatectomy can be carried out depending on the location of the tumour and the desired clearance margin, which is ideally at least 1 cm.

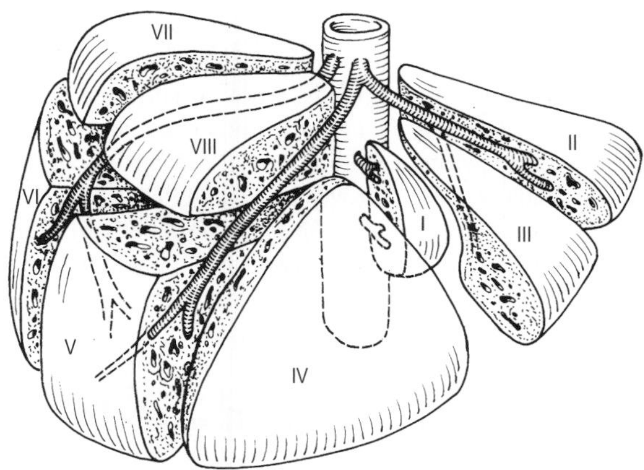

Fig. 25.1 Anatomy of the liver: diagrammatic representation of the segments of the liver. (Adapted from Launois B, Jamieson GG 1993 Modern operative techniques in liver surgery. Churchill Livingstone, Edinburgh, p 7.)

SURGICAL MANAGEMENT OF HAEMORRHAGE FROM OESOPHAGEAL VARICES

1 The most life-threatening complication of portal hypertension that requires surgical treatment is bleeding from oesophageal varices. Although most bleeding stops spontaneously, in-hospital mortality from the first bleed is approximately 50%. Resuscitate the patient with blood, platelets and clotting products and assess the severity of liver disease.

2 Endoscopically confirm the site of bleeding, if necessary injecting sclerosants into or around the varices or applying constricting rubber bands at their bases.

3 Alternatively or additionally, administer vasoactive drugs such as vasopressin (antidiuretic hormone; ADH), synthetic terlipressin, somatostatin or synthetic octreotide which reduce portal venous blood flow. If these fail, buy time for a maximum 24 hours by inserting a Sengstaken–Blakemore tube tamponade (French *tampon* = plug) with inflatable oesophageal and gastric balloons; gentle traction on the tube causes the gastric balloon to occlude veins at the oesophagogastric junction.

4 Radiologically-controlled transjugular intrahepatic portosystemic shunt (TIPSS) creates an artificial, stented passage between the portal vein through liver parenchyma to a hepatic vein, thus reducing portal venous pressure.

5 If this is not available or fails, oesophagogastric portacaval disconnection can be achieved by inserting a circular stapling instrument through a gastrotomy into the lower oesophagus, opening it, tying a ligature to draw in a ring of gastric cardia, closing and actuating it, thus excising a cuff of stomach to obliterate the varices, and then reunite the cut ends. In the Hassab procedure, the distal oesophagus and proximal stomach are devascularized, followed by splenectomy.

6 Decompress the portal venous system by connecting it to the systemic (whole body, somatic) veins such as portacaval, mesocaval (superior mesenteric vein) and splenorenal anastomoses (Fig. 25.2).

MANAGEMENT OF ASCITES

Management is mainly medical, consisting of a low-sodium diet, fluid restriction, diuretics and concomitant potassium

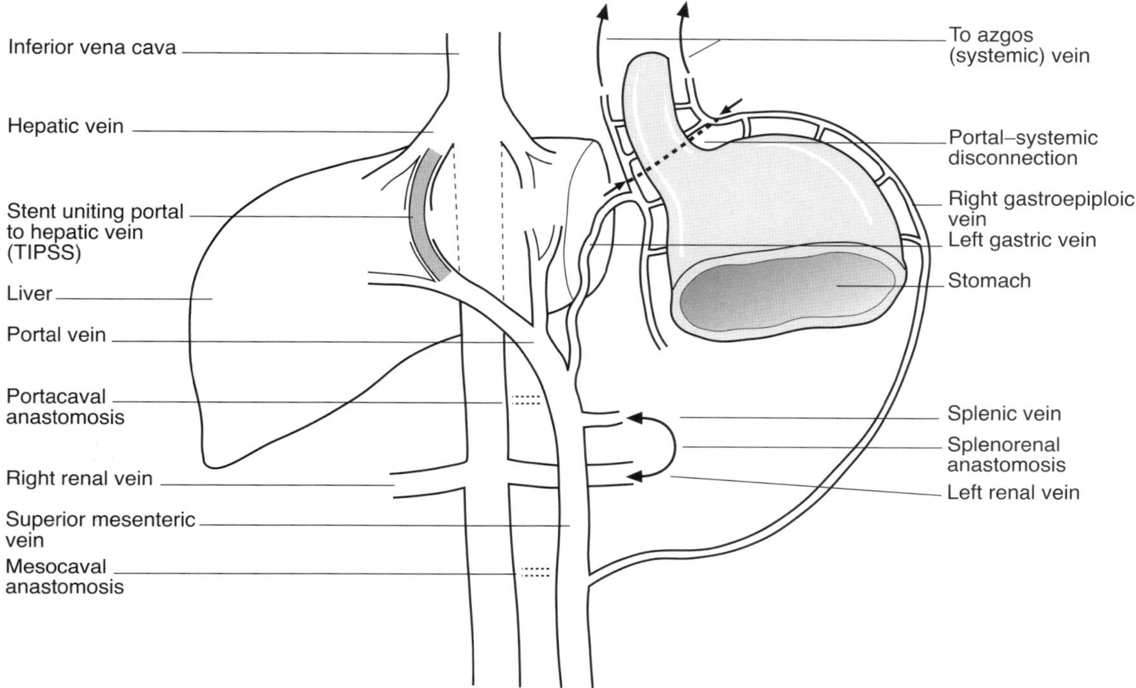

Fig. 25.2 Diagram demonstrating some methods of controlling or preventing bleeding from gastro-oesophageal varices. Gastro-oesophageal transaction and re-anastomosis interrupts the variceal-portosystemic connections. Under radiological control a transjugular intrahepatic portosystemic stent shunt (TIPSS) may be inserted. Portacaval, mesocaval and splenorenal venous shunts create portal-systemic anastomoses, bypassing the liver.

replacement if necessary. Paracentesis (Greek *para* = beside + *kenteein* = to pierce) with colloid replacement is the next step if medical management does not succeed. Monitor progress by weighing the patient daily, measuring urine volume and checking for electrolyte imbalances, azotaemia and encephalopathy. If repeated paracentesis proves difficult, consider ordering a TIPSS procedure.

In the LeVeen shunt a one-way valved ascitic drainage tube extends from the peritoneal cavity to the jugular vein.

FURTHER READING

Blumgart LH (ed) 2006 Surgery of the liver, biliary tract and pancreas, 4th edn. Saunders, Philadelphia

26

Spleen

R. C. N. Williamson, A. K. Kakkar

CONTENTS

ELECTIVE SPLENECTOMY

The spleen is an important organ. Do not lightly remove it. It has haematological functions in the maturation of red blood cells and the destruction of effete forms. Of greater importance in surgical practice, it has certain immunological functions, notably production of opsonins (tuftsin, properdin) for the phagocytosis of encapsulated bacteria. When possible, conserve at least part of the spleen, as opposed to total splenectomy. This may protect against serious post-splenectomy sepsis (see below). *Streptococcus pneumoniae* is the most common infecting organism, less commonly *Neisseria meningitidis* and *Haemophilus influenzae*. Laparoscopic splenectomy is an alternative with identical indications (Ch. 27).

Elective splenectomy may be indicated for certain lymphomas and leukaemias, haemolytic anaemias such as acquired autoimmune and hereditary spherocytosis, idiopathic thrombocytopenic purpura, for other types of splenomegaly with hypersplenism and occasionally for cyst, abscess, haemangioma or splenic artery aneurysm. It may be carried out as a part of total gastrectomy, radical proximal gastrectomy, distal pancreatectomy and 'conventional' splenorenal shunt.

Prepare

Patients with hypersplenism, anaemia, thrombocytopenia and coagulopathies require preoperative correction. Arrange for immunocompromised patients to receive prophylactic antibiotic cover. Risk of post-splenectomy sepsis necessitates prophylactic immunization against *Streptococcus pneumoniae, Haemophilus influenzae* type b and meningococcal strains A and C. Organize vaccination 3–4 weeks before operation, except in children under the age of 2 years or those who are immunocompromised, such as patients with Hodgkin's disease who have received extensive chemotherapy.

Make sure, in obtaining informed consent, that you have advised the patient of the risks of post-splenectomy sepsis.

Access and assess

1 As a rule make an upper midline, left upper paramedian or left subcostal incision. When removing a very large spleen, a left thoracoabdominal approach often facilitates the procedure. Use a long midline incision when carrying out a staging laparotomy.

2 Explore the whole abdomen, particularly noting the liver and any enlarged lymph nodes. Take appropriate biopsies. Search for accessory spleens (splenunculi), usually found near the splenic hilum, in the gastrosplenic ligament or greater omentum; remove all of them if you are performing splenectomy for a blood dyscrasia.

Action

1 If the spleen is enormous, first tie the splenic artery in continuity. Enter the lesser sac by dividing 8–10 cm of greater omentum between ligatures, keeping to the colic side of the gastroepiploic vessels. Divide the adhesions between the back of the stomach and the front of the pancreas. Palpate along the superior border of the body of pancreas for arterial pulsation. Incise the peritoneum

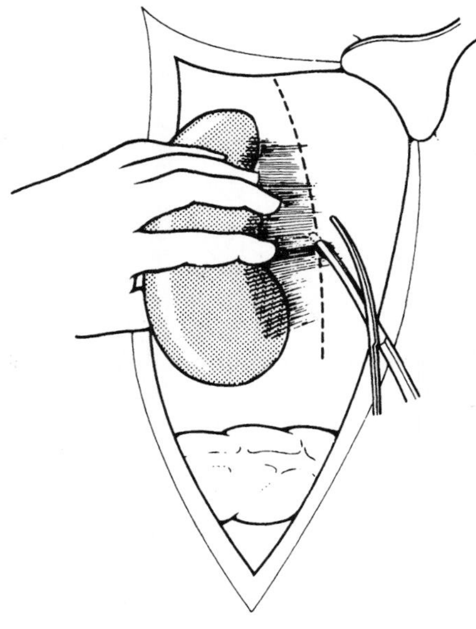

Fig. 26.1 Division of the left peritoneal leaf of the lienorenal ligament as a preliminary to mobilization of the spleen.

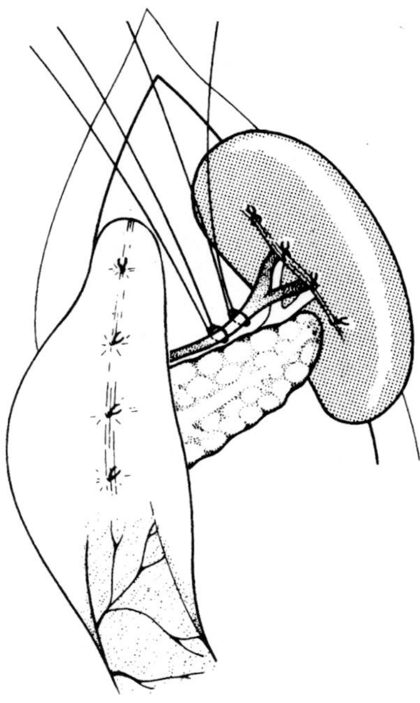

Fig. 26.2 Exposure of the splenic artery and vein after prior division of the gastrosplenic ligament. Two ligatures have been passed around the splenic artery.

at this point, mobilize the vessel with right-angled forceps and ligate it with 0 or 1 silk. Consider injecting 1 ml of 1:10000 adrenaline (epinephrine) into the splenic artery immediately before ligating it. This can shrink the size of a massive spleen and facilitate the subsequent dissection.

2 Pass your left hand over the top of the spleen to draw it medially, and have the left side of the abdominal wall retracted. Coagulate and divide any adhesions between the convex surface of the spleen and the parietal peritoneum. Swab any blood from the groove behind the spleen, and cut through the peritoneum just lateral to the spleen; this is the left leaf of the lienorenal ligament. Slit it upwards and downwards (Fig. 26.1).

3 Gently mobilize the spleen forwards and medially, and free the left colic flexure and tail of pancreas from the spleen. Free the spleen from the diaphragm (avascular) and greater curvature of the stomach, by identifying, ligating and dividing the short gastric vessels in the gastrosplenic ligament. To avoid damaging the stomach it may be easier to dissect out, clamp, doubly ligate and divide the splenic artery and vein separately (Fig. 26.2), avoiding injury to the tail of pancreas. Divide the right leaf of the lienorenal ligament and remove the spleen. Platelet transfusions may now be given in thrombocytopenic patients. Place a pack in the splenic bed, then remove the pack and obtain haemostasis.

4 Especially with a massive spleen (larger than 1.5 kg), enlarge the incision and ligate the splenic artery above the pancreas to avoid or control troublesome bleeding from vascular adhesions to the diaphragm or parenchymal tears. Alternatively, mobilize the spleen and bring it up to the surface as soon as possible.

5 Before closing, remove the pack, inspect the ligatures, splenic bed, adjacent viscera, and coagulate any oozing vessels. Place a suction drain in the splenic bed. If there is an enormous cavity or if the stomach or pancreas have been wounded, prefer a wide-bore tube drain until discharge is minimal and consider nasogastric intubation for 24–28 hours or until gastric aspirates diminish.

Aftercare

Check the blood haemoglobin, white cell and platelet counts postoperatively. Leucocytosis and thrombocythaemia nearly always ensue, with peaks at 7–14 days. Persistent leucocytosis and pyrexia suggest the possibility of a subphrenic abscess. Consider some form of prophylactic anticoagulation if the platelet count exceeds 1000×10^9 per litre. If not already started, begin immunization with antipneumococcal vaccine. Children should receive prophylactic penicillin for 2 years to prevent post-splenectomy sepsis. Advise adults to take an antibiotic such as amoxicillin at the first sign of any infective illness. Immunocompromised patients should receive either phenoxymethylpenicillin (250 mg b.d.) or amoxicillin (250 mg o.d.) as routine prophylaxis against post-splenectomy sepsis.

Complications

Chest infection may result from splinting of the left diaphragm causing atelectasis. You may avoid the need to give antibiotics if the patient receives vigorous physiotherapy. Occasionally a left pleural effusion requires aspiration. Suspect subphrenic abscess if there is fever and leucocytosis. Ultrasonography confirms the diagnosis and permits percutaneous drainage. Reactive haemorrhage may be caused by a slipped ligature, necessitating reoperation. Gastric or pancreatic fistula is rare. It may close with conservative management including parenteral nutrition, but otherwise reoperate to deal with it.

EMERGENCY SPLENECTOMY

Emergency splenectomy may be indicated for traumatic rupture. Enlarged spleens are at increased risk of rupture, which may even occur spontaneously. Most cases of ruptured spleen follow road traffic accidents. Classically, patients are shocked, with pain in the left hypochondrium and shoulder-tip and with evidence of left lower rib fractures. Diagnostic paracentesis may confirm a haemoperitoneum, and urgent laparotomy is normally required after initial resuscitation.

Some minor splenic injuries can be managed conservatively with vigilant monitoring and blood transfusion, in patients less than 60 years of age, haemodynamically stable, with a blood transfusion requirement not exceeding 3–4 units, and computed tomography (CT) scans demonstrating a spleen that is not fragmented. Perform laparotomy if there is renewed evidence of bleeding or spreading peritonism.

Accidental splenic injury sustained during operations such as vagotomy or left hemicolectomy was formerly an indication for splenectomy, but the bleeding can usually be controlled by lesser means (see below).

Access and assess

Use a midline upper abdominal incision. Do not hesitate to make a T-shaped extension towards the left costal margin if access is difficult and the patient is exsanguinating. A good view is essential. Have the left costal margin lifted by a retractor. Scoop and suck blood and clot from the left hypochondrium.

First check that a ruptured spleen is the source of bleeding. It is often easier to feel than to see whether the spleen is intact. Control the splenic hilar vessels with your hand if necessary to stop bleeding. Remove or repair a ruptured spleen without further ado, postponing exploration of the rest of the abdomen until later. Particularly in young children try to avoid total splenectomy if at all possible, because they are at particular risk of post-splenectomy sepsis. If the spleen is shattered or bleeding profusely, however, you have no alternative but to remove it promptly to save life.

Action

Quickly but carefully mobilize the spleen and bring it forwards into the abdominal wound. In ruptured spleen it is often possible to break down the left peritoneal leaf of the lienorenal ligament using your fingers. If splenic repair is at all likely, however, try to avoid further injury to the spleen during this manoeuvre and compress its vascular pedicle between finger and thumb to control the bleeding. Inspect the organ thoroughly and assess the extent of damage. If total splenectomy is inevitable, proceed as for an elective operation, securing the splenic artery and vein at an early stage. Consider placing thin slices of splenic tissue in omental pockets at the end of the operation to encourage splenic regeneration (splenosis). Conservative splenic operations are described later in this chapter. Determine to give triple vaccine immunization during the recovery period plus prophylactic penicillin as an additional precaution in children or the immunocompromised.

? DIFFICULTY

1. *The patient is bleeding to death from the spleen, but you cannot identify the precise source of haemorrhage.* There may not be time to summon senior help. Consider extending the incision as described. Place your hand over the top of the spleen, break down its posterior attachments and deliver it into the wound as quickly as possible. Now compress or clamp the pedicle, and you will bring the situation under control.
2. *You have inadvertently injured the stomach or pancreas during splenectomy,* usually because of inadequate mobilization of the spleen. Remove the spleen and place a pack in the splenic bed. Inspect the damage carefully. Repair a gastric defect in two layers. Repair or resect the tail of pancreas, using non-absorbable sutures. Ask the anaesthetist to insert a nasogastric tube. Drain the splenic bed.

CONSERVATIVE SPLENIC SURGERY

Following splenectomy there is a 1.0–2.5% risk of developing overwhelming septicaemia from encapsulated bacteria, especially the pneumococcus, usually within 2 years of operation. The mortality rate of post-splenectomy sepsis is high. The risk is higher in young children and after splenectomy for haematological disease, but fatal cases have occasionally been reported in adults after removal of a ruptured spleen. Non-operative management may be appropriate for lesser degrees of splenic injury, especially in children. Embolization therapy has been attempted in hypersplenism. With these exceptions, alternatives to total splenectomy can be assessed only at laparotomy, but they may be feasible in at least 40% of patients with blunt splenic trauma.

Assess

At operation for abdominal trauma, remove forthwith a spleen that is either fragmented or avulsed from its vascular pedicle. Under these circumstances consider autotransplantation of some splenic pulp into the peritoneal cavity. If the damage and bleeding are less severe, gently mobilize it to decide if topical haemostatic agents, partial splenectomy or some form of splenic repair (splenorrhaphy; Greek *rhaphe* = a seam) are feasible, with or without ligation of the splenic artery or its branches.

Capsular tears and other minor injuries to the spleen inadvertently sustained at operation seldom necessitate splenectomy. Retract or extend the incision adequately to inspect the spleen without mobilizing it. Application of a haemostatic agent usually suffices, with or without suturing. Removal of the entire organ can sometimes be avoided in certain elective operations on the spleen. Thus marsupialization (Greek *marsyppion* = a pouch) may be adequate for congenital splenic cysts and segmental splenectomy for tropical splenomegaly.

FURTHER READING

Clarke PJ, Morris PJ 1994 Surgery of the spleen. In: Morris PJ, Malt RA (eds) Oxford textbook of surgery. Oxford University Press, Oxford, pp 2121–2130

Cooper MJ, Williamson RCN 1983 Splenectomy: indications, hazards and alternatives. British Journal of Surgery 71:173–180

27

Laparoscopic splenectomy

S. J. Nixon, A. Rajasekar

DESCRIPTION OF OPERATION

A laparoscopic approach is now accepted as the standard procedure for elective splenectomy. Technical developments and surgical experience have overcome most of the practical difficulties. Long-term follow-up of patients with idiopathic thrombocytopenic purpura (ITP) and autoimmune haemolytic anaemia, the two most common indications, have shown identical results to open operation. The short-term benefits of laparoscopic over open surgery are those seen in other areas.

There are no absolute contraindications to laparoscopic splenectomy and few relative contraindications. Gross obesity, peritoneal adhesions and the presence of inflammation add to the technical challenges. Spleen size is a major factor. Massive splenomegaly presents you with difficulties of access to the vessels lying beneath it, difficulty in manoeuvring the spleen due to its physical size and weight, and problems with retrieval. The rate of conversion to open splenectomy varies from 0% to 19%; haemorrhage is the most common reason. Before elective splenectomy give Pneumovax (Pasteur Mérieux, UK) in an emergency, vaccinate after full recovery; give prophylactic antibiotics.

Action

We prefer an anterolateral approach. After mobilizing the spleen the hilar vessels are ligated using an EndoGIA with a 60-mm vascular cartridge introduced through a 15-mm Versaport (US Surgical Corporation; Fig. 27.1). The spleen is now free. Introduce a large retrieval bag (EndoCatch II, Auto Suture, UK) via the Versaport, open it and place the spleen within it. Withdraw the bag and remove the spleen piecemeal after morselating it with sponge-holding forceps, or an electromechanical morselator. If you require an intact spleen for histological examination or if it is too large to be placed in a retrieval bag, remove it through a small Pfannenstiel incision.

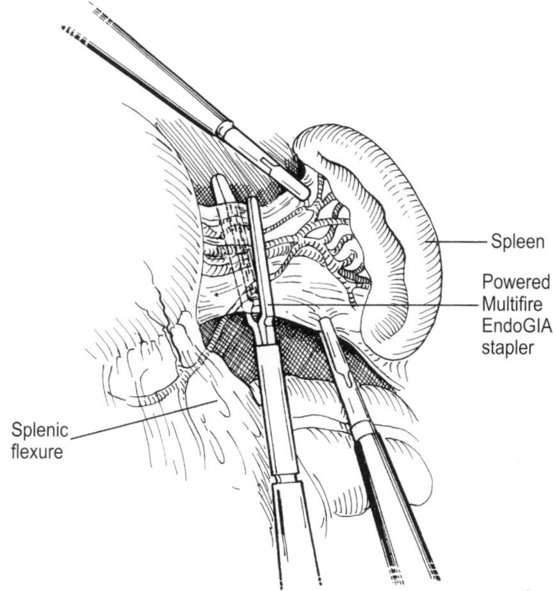

Fig. 27.1 Ligation of hilar vessels.

Complications

These include bleeding, injury to adjacent organs, subphrenic collections or abscess, thrombocytosis, portal vein thrombosis and overwhelming post-splenectomy infection (OPSI); give advice regarding immunization, foreign travel and lifelong prophylactic antibiotics. Advise patients to carry an information card at all times. If signs of infection develop, they should take a course of appropriate antibiotics immediately. If the infection does not settle, then admit and treat the patient with parenteral antibiotics.

FURTHER READING

Friedman RL, Phillips EH 1997 Laparoscopic splenectomy. In: Ponsky JL (ed.) Complications of endoscopic and laparoscopic surgery: prevention and management. Lippincott Raven, Philadelphia, pp 159–170

Rege RV, Merriam LT, Joehl RJ 1996 Laparoscopic splenectomy. Surgical Clinics of North America 76:459–468

Wu JM, Lai IR, Yuan RH 2004 Laparoscopic splenectomy for idiopathic thrombocytopenic purpura. American Journal of Surgery 187:720–723

Internet websites

http://www.edu.rcsed.ac.uk/video_album_menu.htm
An example of the lateral approach with a stapling gun.

http://www.edu.rcsed.ac.uk/gem%20videos.htm
An example of a more anterior approach using the harmonic scalpel.

28

Breast

R. Sainsbury

CONTENTS

MANAGEMENT OF BREAST SYMPTOMS

You need a scheme of management for patients presenting with a breast complaint (Fig. 28.1). Common symptoms include breast pain, lumps, lumpiness and nipple changes including inversion, bleeding and discharge. Be suspicious of carcinoma if an older woman presents with recent nipple inversion. Exclude carcinoma or other causes of breast pain and lumpiness before deciding on conservative management. Is a lump truly discrete? If there is diffuse nodularity, arrange ultrasound examination. If this is normal in a younger woman, re-examine her at a different point in the menstrual cycle and if this is also normal, reassure her.

Refer women over the age of 35 years for mammography and/or ultrasound to complement clinical examination of the 'difficult' breast. Select ultrasound for women below 35 years. For discrete lumps ultrasound differentiates cystic from solid lesions. Prepare a cytological smear from solid lesions. Completely aspirate a cyst then re-examine the breast to exclude a residual lump.

Breast cysts often appear suddenly and are of concern to the patient. They are most common before and around the menopause but occur at any age. Cyst drainage usually establishes the diagnosis and 'cures' the condition so the patient can be immediately reassured. Cytology of cyst fluid is worthwhile only if it is bloodstained or there is a residual mass after aspiration. If the fluid from the cyst is bloody, or if there is a residual lump, perform formal biopsy.

If the lump is solid, and declared benign on cytology, excise it if the woman is aged 35 years or older, if the lump increases in size or is associated with pain, if the cytology is equivocal or if the patient requests it. For a confirmed fibroadenoma in a younger patient, offer the alternatives of observation or ablation by means of laser thermocoagulation.

Perform triple assessment – examination, imaging and histology or cytology – on patients with discrete areas of breast abnormality. Histology of a core biopsy, usually taken using a spring-loaded device, may be helpful. If the diagnosis remains doubtful, determine to remove a biopsy as soon as possible. At open biopsy do not, as a rule, rely on frozen section histology; prefer to await paraffin section histology. Lesions that have defied diagnosis by standard triple assessment are also difficult to interpret by the pathologist and require an optimum specimen. Frozen section is occasionally valuable when imaging or cytology are equivocal in suspicious lesions.

Assess the risk for patients with a family history, and devise a stratagem for regular follow-up, or reassure and discharge them. Patients also present with cosmetic problems.

Operative steps and principles will be given to enable you, as a trainee, to follow the steps of complex procedures at which you will assist.

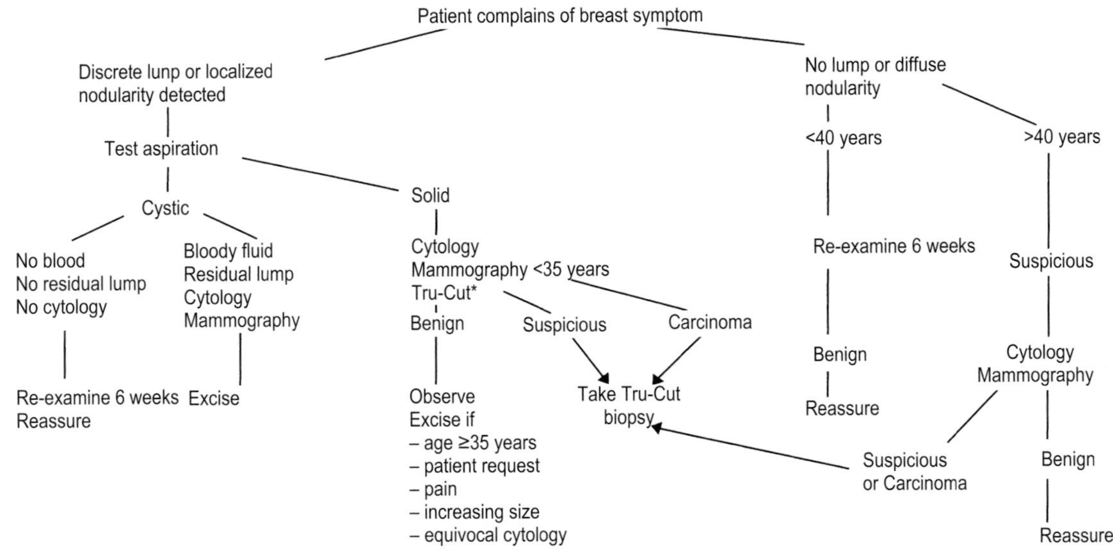

Fig. 28.1 Scheme of management for patients presenting with a breast symptom. *Tru-Cut is difficult unless lump is greater than 2 cm.

BIOPSY

Aspiration cytology

Aspiration cytology can be performed in the outpatient clinic, is applicable for all breast lumps and requires the minimum of special equipment. Interpretation requires expert cytology. The quality of the aspirate is operator-dependent, usually reported as containing no cells (C_0), blood and debris (C_1), benign epithelial cells (C_2), atypical cells (C_3), cells suspicious of carcinoma (C_4) or carcinoma (C_5). A preoperative diagnosis of carcinoma can usually be made by combining clinical assessment, cytodiagnosis and imaging, enabling appropriate patient counselling and planning of the operation list.

Attach a 21G (green) or 23G (blue) needle to a 10-ml syringe. You may wish to insert the syringe into an extractor 'gun'. Clean the overlying skin then fix the lump between thumb and index finger of the non-dominant hand. Insert the needle into the middle of the lump and apply suction to the syringe plunger. Move the needle in several different directions through the lump while maintaining negative pressure. Avoid penetrating the intercostal space. Do not allow the needle point to leave the skin or air enters the needle and the aspirated material is drawn into the syringe, becoming difficult to remove. Release the pressure and then withdraw the needle. Ask the patient or your assistant to apply pressure to the breast for 2 minutes to avoid haematoma formation.

Eject a drop of aspirate onto the end of a dry microscope slide. Gently spread this out with another slide to create a thin smear without repeated smearing, to avoid creating artefactual changes, which confuse interpretation. Immediately and accurately label the slide, ensuring that no material falls onto the table, which could then be picked up onto the back of the next set of slides. The slide may be sprayed with, or immersed in, a fixative. Send the slide for reporting. If you obtain no aspirate repeat the procedure.

Core-cut or Tru-Cut needle biopsy

Infiltrate the skin over the lump with 1% lidocaine. Introduce the needle into the breast, to inject local anaesthetic deep into the breast tissue to enter the tumour. Wait 2 minutes for the anaesthetic to work. Make a small nick in the skin with the tip of a sharp-pointed scalpel (no. 11 blade). Fix the tumour yourself or have an assistant fix the tumour within the breast between finger and thumb, to provide a static target. The best approach to the lump is often from the side to avoid firing the needle backwards. Push the needle, in its closed position, through the skin incision until you reach the edge of the tumour. A spring-driven biopsy needle can obtain a sample more rapidly than one obtained by hand and causes less discomfort for the patient. If microcalcification is a dominant feature, X-ray the specimen to ensure you have obtained the correct specimen.

Open biopsy

Open biopsy is rarely required to make a diagnosis. If a lesion is very large then a thin slice may be taken through the lesion, or part of the lesion may be taken if an operation is planned. The term 'lumpectomy' is best reserved for a definitive operation to remove a benign lump, and the term 'wide local excision' to remove a carcinoma with some surrounding normal tissue.

Needle-location biopsy

Needle-location biopsy is indicated when an impalpable, suspicious area is located on the mammogram. To mark it for accurate surgical removal, a percutaneous wire marker, such as a simple hook, Reidy or Nottingham needle, is inserted into it. An initial specimen radiograph ensures that you have removed the suspicious area, and subsequent radiographs of the sliced specimen ensure that the pathologist examines the radiologically abnormal sections. Plan a cosmetically satisfactory incision (Fig. 28.2). Have the mammograms and films available. You need paraffin section, not frozen section histology. Raise a skin flap between the chosen incision and the needle entry site until you reach the subcutaneous wire. Grasp the wire with an artery forceps and cut off the excess wire flush with the skin. Follow the wire down towards the site of the lesion by sharp dissection, gently moving the wire to facilitate the dissection. Once you reach the point of the wire, grasp it and adjacent tissue in order to excise the suspicious area. Mark the specimen with metal clips to facilitate orientation and send it to be X-rayed. Achieve perfect haemostasis, and search the cavity for any residual suspicious tissue. Examine the radiograph of the specimen to confirm that it contains the mammographic lesion. If the lesion is not present, excise a further specimen of breast tissue, searching particularly for areas that look or feel suspicious. Repeat the specimen radiography until you find the lesion. Close the wound as for excision biopsy. If the specimen was not calcified, make sure to inform the radiographer.

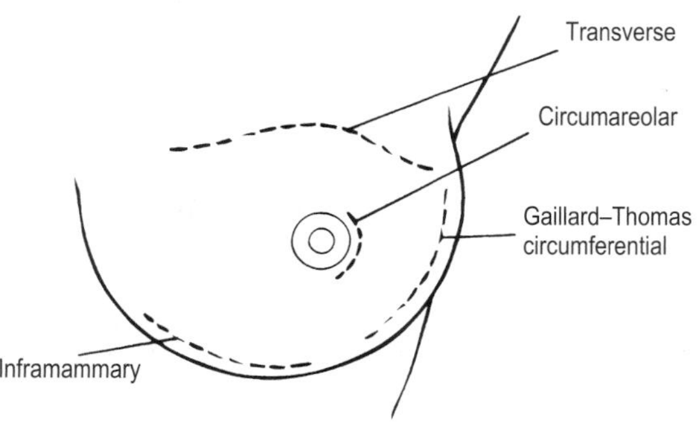

Fig. 28.2 Incisions for removal of a lump from the left breast.

Newer techniques are being developed for obtaining cores of tissue from impalpable lesions, or completely excising small impalpable lesions. The radiologist may insert a small metallic marker if he has removed all the microcalcifications to allow subsequent localization of an abnormal area.

BREAST ABSCESS

Breast abscess develops most commonly during lactation. Empty the affected breast by manual pressure, but encourage the mother to continue feeding. Treat early infection with antibiotics alone but do not delay until fluctuation develops when widespread destruction may have ensued. Aspirate with a wide-bore needle if a clinically or ultrasound detectable abscess is present, repeated as necessary. The abscess cavity can be washed out with a combination of antibiotic dissolved in local anaesthetic.

If the overlying skin is thinned, use open drainage under general anaesthesia. If the abscess is near the nipple use a peri-areolar incision. Explore the cavity with a little finger and send pus for culture and antibiotic sensitivities. Remove a specimen of the wall unless this is a lactational abscess to exclude carcinoma. Ensure that the incision is long enough to allow the wound to heal from the depths upwards, to avoid chronic abscess. As a rule, loosely pack the cavity. Advise the wearing of a supportive brassiere and allow bilateral breastfeeding to recommence as soon as it is comfortable.

DUCT ECTASIA AND MAMILLARY DUCT FISTULA

Duct ectasia (Greek *ex* = out + *tenein* = to stretch; dilatation) is the collection of thick, toothpaste-like material in the terminal ducts. It may become infected, causing areas of redness or abscesses. Occasionally, a fistula develops between a duct and the skin at the areolar margin. This discharges pus and often heals spontaneously before breaking down again. It is now acknowledged to be smoking-related, so dissuade the patient from smoking.

If a mamillary duct fistula does not heal, it may require laying open by inserting a probe, hooking it up though the nipple and cutting around the areola, extending to no more than a quarter of the nipple in order to excise the fistulous track to the back of the nipple.

Excision of the major ducts (Hadfield's operation), is performed through a longer incision.

NIPPLE DISCHARGE AND BLEEDING

Determine which duct the discharge or blood is coming from, send material for cytology and arrange an ultrasound scan and mammogram to exclude underlying malignancy. Surgically explore the breast for bleeding unless it occurs during pregnancy, frequently with bilateral bleeding, which stops spontaneously after parturition, or in someone who is taking anticoagulants. Infiltrate the area with bupivacaine 0.25% and adrenaline (epinephrine) 1:200000 to minimize bleeding and postoperative pain. Cannulate the affected duct with a fine lacrimal probe, expose the duct through a circumareola incision and excise it with a small amount of surrounding breast tissue.

CARCINOMA

Establish the diagnosis preoperatively in nearly all cases, by means of triple assessment – clinical examination, imaging by ultrasound scan or mammography, and histology or cytology. Counsel the patient about treatment options and arrange for a meeting with the Breast Nurse. Discuss the alternatives to primary surgery with wide local excision or mastectomy, for example primary medical treatment. Document your discussions.

When carcinoma has been detected as a result of screening, a preoperative diagnosis should have been made by percutaneous biopsy. Occasionally you need to perform a localization biopsy for diagnosis as opposed to therapy.

The local management of breast carcinoma demands excision of the tumour with clear margins. If the tumour is small in comparison with the total breast volume and sited peripherally, this can be achieved by wide local excision. Up to 10% of breast volume can be removed without significant cosmetic difference and long-term survival after wide local excision and radiotherapy equals that of a mastectomy. Some form of axillary dissection is still required to stage the patient and to treat the axilla. Adjuvant cytotoxic chemotherapy can reduce the relative risk of death by 20–25% in the node-positive population as can tamoxifen or newer aromatase inhibitors for hormone-responsive tumours. Sentinel node biopsy is replacing axillary dissection for staging the axilla.

Modified radical (or Patey) mastectomy provides good control if breast conservation is unsuitable and for central or large operable primary tumours and multifocal disease. Simple mastectomy is indicated only for isolated breast recurrence after breast-conserving surgery, multifocal duct carcinoma in situ and the elderly unfit, because axillary nodal staging is not carried out. Mastectomy with immediate reconstruction, using either an implant or a myocutaneous flap, is being increasingly used by trained breast surgeons (oncoplastic surgery) and with plastic surgery colleagues. Primary medical therapy with tamoxifen may be used in frail elderly patients, and primary cytotoxic chemotherapy may be appropriate for locally advanced cases such as 'inflammatory' carcinoma. Primary (or neoadjuvant) chemotherapy may be used to shrink a large operable tumour.

If you suspect Paget's disease, biopsy the nipple area under local anaesthetic to prove the diagnosis histologically. There is always an underlying intraduct carcinoma, which is invasive in 50% of cases, usually treated by mastectomy or wide local excision.

EXCISION BIOPSY AND WIDE LOCAL EXCISION FOR CARCINOMA

EXCISION BIOPSY

Normally reserve this for a solid breast lump that is clinically benign. Aim to extract the lesion with the narrowest margin and least cosmetic defect, consistent with establishing a histological diagnosis and removing the palpable abnormality. It is insufficient for removal of carcinoma but may be diagnostic if other methods have failed.

Check that the lesion is still present since they occasionally disappear, and that no new lesion has appeared in either breast. Mark the exact site of the lesion on the breast with the patient lying in the position she will occupy on the operating table. Obtain consent for the operation and carefully explain the potential risks.

Action (Fig. 28.2)

1 Did you check that this is the right patient in the anaesthetic room and that you are operating on the correct side?

2 Place the incision over the lump, sited to minimize scarring and to be within that for a subsequent mastectomy, if necessary. Periareolar incision scars are least visible, medial breast scars tend to keloid formation. Avoid radial incisions except medially.

3 If possible excise the lump completely without cutting into it and leave the specimen intact for the pathologist. No margin is necessary around benign lesions. When it is impossible to remove all the abnormal tissue, remove the most severely affected tissue and obtain a representative biopsy.

4 Finally obtain perfect haemostasis, so no drain is needed, using the diathermy spray setting, if there is one, with the electrode held 2–4 mm from the tissue so that the current jumps widely across the air gap. Close the skin using a subcuticular suture of 3/0 synthetic material. Support the closed wound with Steri-Strips for 10 days.

WIDE LOCAL EXCISION FOR CARCINOMA

This is a therapeutic operation for the excision of a carcinoma with clear surrounding margins. As an extra precaution the cavity walls can be re-resected, thus increasing the chance of achieving clear margins.

The breast-conserving operation against which other procedures are measured in the treatment of early cancer is the 'quadrantectomy'. It is upon this operation that most of the published data comparing breast-conserving therapy with mastectomy in randomized trials have been based. The local recurrence rate is higher in younger women.

QUADRANTECTOMY

Has the diagnosis of breast carcinoma been confirmed by cytology or biopsy, is the patient suitable for breast-conserving surgery, and are you sure that the mammogram does not reveal multifocal disease? Have you marked the side and site of the carcinoma? Did the Nurse Counsellor discuss the diagnosis and treatment with the patient? The principles of the excision are described.

Action

1 The patient lies supine on the operating table, with position of the lump marked on the skin equidistant between radial marks delimiting the quadrantectomy, and with access to the axilla as the arm on the operative side is extended on an arm board. Draw a circumferential incision, joining the radial lines approximately midway between the nipple and the breast periphery, ideally lying directly over the lump, allowing an ellipse or crescent of skin overlying the carcinoma to be removed in continuity. Remove skin only if the carcinoma directly involves it.

2 Through raised skin flaps centrally and peripherally, the segment can be lifted off the pectoral fascia from the periphery to the centre, excising the subareolar major duct system. Mark the specimen with sutures to denote its three planes: superior–inferior, medial–lateral and superficial–deep, and send it, uncut. After achieving complete haemostasis the cavity can be packed while axillary dissection is carried out.

3 Afterwards, confirm haemostasis and close the skin, usually without drainage. The air-filled cavity, subsequently fills with serous fluid which organizes into fibrous tissue. As a rule do not approximate the residual breast tissue at the edges of the cavity.

AXILLARY SURGERY

Axillary nodal status remains the most important prognostic factor for determining survival and is combined with size and grade to form the Nottingham Prognostic Index. If the patient presents with palpable nodes, then perform axillary clearance. Consider fine-needle cytology of palpable nodes and make a diagram. Ultrasound scanning and to some extent magnetic resonance imaging (MRI) demonstrate nodal status but, like clinical examination, do not rely upon them. In the absence of a palpable axillary node, apart from full clearance you may perform nodal sampling or a sentinel node biopsy. The main steps are described.

AXILLARY CLEARANCE

While a limited 'axillary sampling' operation to biopsy a few lymph nodes may give valuable staging information, more extensive clearance is also therapeutic, providing local disease control without the need for axillary irradiation. Because 70–80% of breast cancer patients have a negative axillary dissection, novel methods are being studied.

The technique most commonly practised is sentinel lymph node biopsy; the first node in the axilla draining the breast tissue around a tumour can be identified perioperatively using a combination of radioisotope and blue dye. This node can then be removed; if it is not involved it is unlikely that further axillary nodes are involved. Warn the patient about the possibility of postoperative numbness if the intercostobrachial nerve is damaged, and of lymphoedema. Encourage the patient to move the shoulder fully and arrange shoulder exercises postoperation. The axilla is shaved.

Axillary clearance performed through an oblique incision just behind, and parallel to, the lateral edge of the pectoralis major muscle provides good access but has the disadvantage of producing an ugly scar and limitation of shoulder abduction. Prefer a transverse incision with its anterior corner at the pectoral edge and the posterior angle just crossing the anterior border of latissimus dorsi, running 3 cm below and parallel to the axillary vein with the arm abducted at 90°. Cosmetically this produces an excellent result. The anterior limit of dissection is the lateral border of pectoralis major, the posterior limit is the lateral border of latissimus dorsi. Gently dissect the contents and lymph nodes up and down between these limits depending on the extent of the clearance. This may be to the insertion of pectoralis minor muscle into the coracoid process, or even involve dividing the muscle insertion. Preserve the thoracodorsal trunk down into latissimus dorsi muscle, and the medial pectoral, long thoracic and intercostobrachial nerves, although you may need to divide the last-named nerve. If there is heavy nodal involvement in the axilla, excise all the palpable lymph nodes together with any soft tissue disease. After achieving complete haemostasis, insert a vacuum drain into the axilla and suture the skin with subcuticular sutures. Before sending the specimen to the pathology laboratory, mark the apex of the specimen with a stitch to help the pathologist orientate around the specimen.

SENTINEL NODE BIOPSY

The sentinel (Italian *sentinella* = on guard) node is the first node to which the lymph drainage of the breast goes. With a patient who has a clinically uninvolved axilla, sentinel node biopsy is replacing conventional axillary dissection. The node is identified by injecting a radioisotope (usually technetium combined with colloidal albumin particles) some hours before operation, combined with a blue dye (Patent Bleu V) injected when the patient is on the operating table.

Discuss with the patient if you should proceed to a full axillary clearance if you discover positive nodes, so you have informed consent. Warn the patient about the need for a second operation if the sentinel node is found to be positive. Warn that the blue dye will cause green urine. Allow 5–10 minutes for the blue dye to reach the axilla, then make a short incision over the site of maximum radioactivity as detected by the gamma probe, usually revealing blue dyed lymphatics which lead you to the node which you gently remove. Check for other sentinel nodes, achieve haemostasis and close the wound using subarticular soluble stitches.

MODIFIED RADICAL (OR PATEY) MASTECTOMY

Has the diagnosis of breast carcinoma been confirmed by cytology, core-cut biopsy or previous excision biopsy? If the diagnosis rests on positive cytology, are you satisfied clinically and radiologically that this is invasive carcinoma prior to undertaking an axillary dissection? In case of doubt perform a preliminary biopsy for paraffin sections to be examined; the routine of 'Frozen section? Proceed' is no longer acceptable.

Confirm that the patient has seen the Nurse Counsellor and has had an opportunity to discuss her diagnosis and treatment fully. Breast reconstruction should be available for every patient undergoing mastectomy. Ensure that the patient is aware of this, offered either immediately or after an interval.

Mark the side and site of the carcinoma. It is unnecessary to cross-match blood but establish the patient's blood group.

Place the patient on the table supine arm extended on an arm board. Prepare the skin and place the towels to allow access to the breast and axilla. Wrap the arm separately to facilitate axillary dissection. With a skin-marking pen, mark the position of the lump and draw your chosen elliptical incision, lying transversely and encompassing approximately 5 cm of skin around the lesion and also the nipple (Fig. 28.3). If this is impracticable, make an oblique incision, but not taken up as far as the clavicle or across to the upper arm, which is ugly. Before cutting, will you be able to close your chosen incisions?

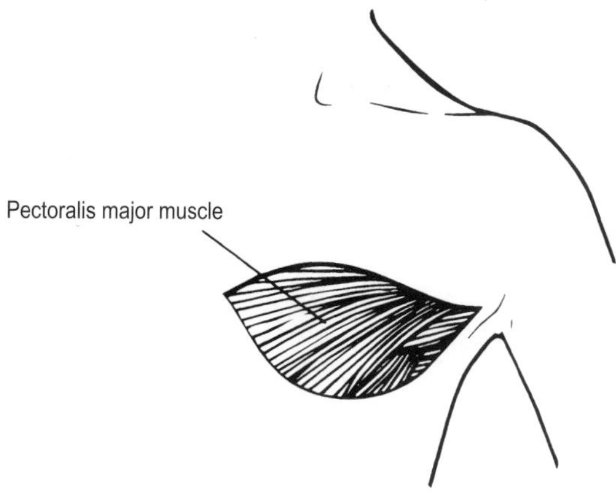

Fig. 28.3 Elliptical incision for Patey mastectomy.

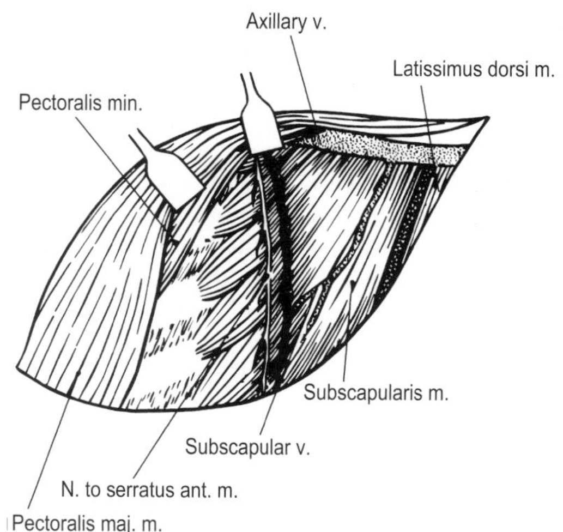

Fig. 28.4 Left Patey's operation with preservation of pectoralis minor.

Action

1 Elevate the skin flaps in the plane between subcutaneous fat and mammary fat. This can be facilitated by subcutaneous infiltration with 1:400000 adrenaline (epinephrine) in saline, or 0.25% bupivacaine (Marcaine) and adrenaline (epinephrine). Have your assistant hold up the skin flaps and check after every few cuts with the scalpel or scissors that you are not in danger of making the flap too thin, resulting in 'buttonholing'. However, ensure that you do not leave any breast tissue in the flaps. Do not traumatize skin by holding it with tissue forceps; use skin hooks inserted into the cut edges or Allis forceps applied on the rolled-back edges. Raise the upper flap to the upper limit of the breast – variable but usually 2–3 cm below the clavicle.

2 Catch any bleeding points with fine forceps and apply diathermy current to them. Take care not to burn the skin itself by contact with the diathermy needle. If skin is inadvertently burned, cut away the damaged area, bevelling it off so that it will not be demonstrable later. Burnt skin takes many weeks to heal and is painful. Raise the lower flap in a similar manner, to the lower limits of the breast. Place a large tissue forceps, such as Lane's, on the breast to be removed, to be held by an assistant.

3 Return to the uppermost part of the breast and dissect down until you see the fascia of pectoralis major. Introduce a finger covered by a swab and find a submammary plane of cleavage between the fascia and the breast, as discussed under quadrantectomy. Proceed downward in this plane, catching and ligating the perforating vessels as they appear, before cutting them; this reduces the amount of operative bleeding considerably. If the tumour appears to infiltrate into the pectoralis muscle, then excise a portion of this muscle with the specimen.

4 Continue downwards, elevating the breast alternatively laterally and medially but leaving the axillary tail of the breast in continuity with the axillary contents. The medial end of the dissection proceeds to the lower limit of the breast. Elevate the breast laterally to complete its removal from the chest wall. The breast is now only attached at the axilla. Take care to identify and ligate one or two major perforating vessels passing through the second and third intercostal spaces. Place dry packs under each skin flap.

5 Identify the lateral border of pectoralis major and clear the axillary tail of the breast and the axillary contents from along this border. Identify latissimus dorsi and clear the axillary contents from its anterior border. Proceed as for an axillary clearance; a satisfactory result can be achieved by preserving the pectoralis minor muscle and dissecting up to level II (Fig. 28.4). Insert

two vacuum drains, one for the flaps and a second for the axilla.

Closure

Suture the skin edges with subcuticular sutures. If there is a discrepancy between the lengths of the two flaps, close the wound using interrupted sutures placed halfway along the incision then halfway between these lengths and so on, thus avoiding a 'dog-ear' at one end. Now activate the vacuum drains and squeeze out all the fluid and air from beneath the skin flaps so that they adhere to the chest wall.

Rarely, you may need to apply a split skin graft to part of the wound if you cannot appose the skin edges without tension, possibly because the surgery was too radical or the case selection inappropriate. A myocutaneous flap gives a better cosmetic result in these circumstances.

Aftercare

Supplying and arranging the fitting of a breast prosthesis for the patient is really within the operation considerations.

Artificial breasts are now available that are of a weight and consistency comparable with the removed breast. They change shape with the patient's change of posture and they take on body temperature. It is almost impossible to tell which is the side of the mastectomy when feeling through a patient's clothes, and this is of very great importance to her as a woman. She can buy clothes as anyone else does, and also wear swimsuits and evening dresses without calling attention to her deficiency.

Make yourself aware of the range and variety of prostheses available. In the UK, under Health Service regulations, any woman is entitled to the type and size of prosthesis of her choice. In addition, these may be replaced as frequently as necessary. If you are unaware of the variety available, delegate the responsibility to the Appliance Officer.

Many centres now employ mastectomy counsellors who, as well as providing psychosocial rehabilitation of the patient, are responsible for the physical rehabilitation. This includes the prescription of a soft temporary prosthesis immediately postoperatively, which can be worn for about 6 weeks until the wound is no longer sore and then replaced by the permanent prosthesis worn within the brassiere.

No woman should leave hospital with a stiff shoulder following mastectomy. Commence active physiotherapy within 24 hours of operation and provide the patient with a list of exercises for abduction of the arm. Encourage her to brush her hair and fasten the back of her dress.

BREAST RECONSTRUCTION

In order to undertake breast reconstruction you need to assess the patient's suitability for the various procedures, in addition to the required technical skills. All patients undergoing mastectomy should be offered the option of a reconstruction, immediately or after a delay. The aim is to achieve symmetry, provide a lasting result and satisfy the patient's requirements. Techniques include insertion of a submuscular silicone implant, placement of a tissue expansion device with subsequent implant insertion, implantation of a 'permanent' expander, and autogenous tissue transfer using either the latissimus dorsi myocutaneous flap with a silicone implant or the transverse rectus abdominis muscle (TRAM) flap, which has the advantage of not requiring an implant. A new nipple complex may need to be constructed and the contralateral breast may need adjustment.

DEVELOPMENTAL ABNORMALITIES

Mastitis neonatorum occurs in the first few days of life, associated with maternal hormones; it subsides spontaneously. Extra or supernumerary breasts and/or nipples are encountered along the milk line from midclavicular region to groin; as a rule do not intervene. With the onset of puberty, one breast disc may enlarge in a young girl from the age of 8 years onwards. Avoid operation. Unevenness may cause embarrassment during this period of a girl's life.

OTHER BREAST PROCEDURES

Breast augmentation requires insertion of prostheses either in the submammary or subpectoral plane to enhance breast size (Fig. 28.5).

Breast reduction may be beneficial if the breasts are much oversized and various techniques are available.

Gynaecomastia is frequently unilateral and may occur in boys and young men, either following minor trauma or spontaneously. It usually settles without treatment. If it does not bilateral breast disc excision may be necessary. In old age it is associated with drugs given for hypertension or congestive cardiac failure, infrequently nowadays after

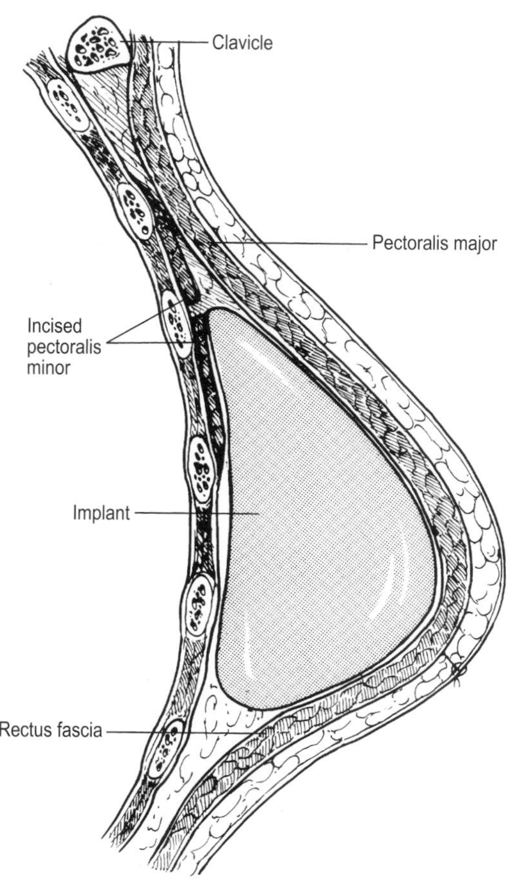

Fig. 28.5 Subpectoral silicone implant.

treatment with oestrogens for prostatic cancer and in men suffering from alcoholic cirrhosis.

FURTHER READING

Dixon M 1995 ABC of breast disease. BMJ Publishing Group, London

Hughes LE, Mansel RE, Webster DJT 1989 Benign disorders and diseases of the breast: concepts and clinical management. Baillière Tindall, London

Keshtgar MRS, Ell PJ 1999 Sentinel lymph node detection and imaging. European Journal of Nuclear Medicine 26:57–67

29

Thyroid

R. E. C. Collins

CONTENTS

INTRODUCTION

Thyroid disorders fall broadly into two categories: Swellings which can be solitary or multinodular, and Graves' disease, described by the Irish physician in 1835, which is usually, but not always, associated with diffuse enlargement of the gland. Thyroid surgery is increasingly performed by specialist surgeons as evidence-based, consensus management is introduced by the British Association of Endocrine Surgeons (BAES), which audits national results including complications such as damage to the recurrent laryngeal nerve and to parathyroid glands.

Operative complications are potentially so disabling that occasional thyroidectomy is increasingly deprecated. If you carry out thyroid surgery in the UK, you should submit your results to the national audit organized by BAES. If you do not, you expose yourself to adverse legal comment in the event of poor outcomes.

Investigate

- *Thyroid function tests* include levels of thyroid-stimulating hormone (TSH), thyroxine/tri-iodothyronine (T4/T3), calcium/albumin and thyroid antibodies.
- *Fine-needle aspiration cytology.* Ask the patient to lie supine. Gently extend the neck. Local anaesthesia is unnecessary. Perform the aspiration free hand, aiming at the dominant nodule. Smear the aspirate, from two or three passes to the nodule, onto a slide and allow it to dry in the air. Use either a 5-ml syringe and green no. 1 needle or a special 'aspiration gun'. Skin preparation is traditionally an alcohol swab but its value is uncertain. The cytologist may not be able to distinguish between benign and malignant disease.
- *Ultrasound-guided cytological biopsy* is valuable if the nodule is small and difficult to palpate, and is usually conducted by a radiologist in the X-ray department.
- *Ultrasound scanning*, performed by the radiologist, helps distinguish solitary from multiple nodules, solid from cystic lesions, and is a useful adjunct to cytology.
- *Computed tomography* (CT) scanning clearly defines the relationship of the gland to the trachea and its retrosternal progression, in cases where you suspect malignant disease with lymphatic involvement, or in the presence of large, multinodular goitres.
- *Routine radio-isotope imaging* of euthyroid multinodular goitres is unnecessary, but it is valuable in toxic disease to identify the site of the toxic focus, which is not always in the dominant nodule.
- *Laryngoscopy.* Many surgeons routinely employ this preoperatively but others confine themselves to doing it only when there is a history of voice change, previous thyroid surgery or when thyroid malignancy has been already established.
- *Pulmonary function tests* are valuable in the presence of multinodular goitre and indicate the degree of tracheal compression.

Prepare

Offer thorough counselling and consent prior to operation and record the precise discussion so it can be seen to have been done. Discuss the implications of recurrent laryngeal nerve damage and be prepared to give your own figures. BAES reports an incidence of approximately 5%; a higher rate is unacceptable. Damage from neurapraxia is transient. Subtle changes of timbre of the voice can occur in the absence of obvious damage to the recurrent laryngeal nerve, sometimes from external laryngeal nerve damage. Discuss the small but definite risk of postoperative haemorrhage. There is an inevitable visible scar, sometimes with temporary surrounding numbness. Following in particular total thyroidectomy, temporary or permanent hypoparathyroidism may develop, requiring vitamin D or calcium supplements. Lifelong T4 supplements are needed following total thyroidectomy and in about 20% of patients following hemithyroidectomy. If the operation is for malignant disease, warn that adjunctive treatment may be indicated. BAES supplies useful, simple, explanatory leaflets for your patients outlining the operation and its risks.

Low-dose heparin prophylaxis against deep vein thrombosis is of unproven value and it may increase perioperative bleeding. However, external pneumatic compression boots may be valuable.

THYROID NODULE DISEASE

Three conditions are included: multinodular goitre, a dominant nodule within a multinodular goitre and a solitary nodule. The predominant symptom is of swelling and, rarely, disorders of swallowing or breathing. Relatively moderate-sized multinodular goitres, particularly with a nodule behind the trachea, may produce a desire to cough or tracheal irritation and, particularly in possible malignancy, may cause voice changes from recurrent laryngeal nerve damage, and compression, rarely invasion, of the trachea. Dysphagia is rare – exclude globus hystericus and primary oesophageal disease. Sudden pain and swelling may be from haemorrhage into a cyst. Record the approximate size of the goitre, tracheal deviation or compression, or venous engorgement. Is there retrosternal progression?

Multinodular goitre is not an absolute indication for operation. These include: cytological features of a follicular adenoma or carcinoma, medullary cancer or papillary cancer, clinical suspicion of malignancy despite negative cytology, features of pressure on the trachea or venous return. Relative indications are toxicity if other treatments are rejected, progressive enlargement of a retrosternal goitre and continuing discomfort, as is patient preference.

GRAVES' DISEASE

Management of Graves' disease demands a multidisciplinary team, including an endocrinologist, a specialist in nuclear medicine, surgeon and anaesthetist. Operation is one of several options, including antithyroid drugs, beta-blocking drugs and radioactive iodine ablation. Eye signs, such as exophthalmos, may not regress postoperatively; it may temporarily worsen. Subtotal thyroidectomy designed to render the patient euthyroid leaves a total thyroid mass of about 4 grams, retaining 2–3-gram remnants of each lobe posteriorly. For fear of recurrent thyrotoxicosis there is a tendency for more radical surgery such as total thyroidectomy or hemithyroidectomy on one side, leaving a small remnant on the other side.

Render patients euthyroid preoperatively, with antithyroid drugs such as carbimazole or alternative regimens. Oral iodine, such as Lugol's iodine, 1 ml daily for 10 days preoperatively, reduces the vascularity of the gland at operation and in theory should reduce blood loss.

OPERATIONS ON THE THYROID

Access

1 Lay the patient supine on the table with a sandbag between the shoulders and a ring or some such securing device under the head so that the neck is extended. Take care in elderly patients not to over-extend the neck, since this is associated with postoperative neck stiffness. Raise the head to about 15° to minimize neck vein engorgement. Apply external pneumatic compression boots to the legs.

2 Infiltrate the fascia and platysma under the skin of the neck along the intended incision with 20–30 ml of 1:400000 adrenaline in physiological saline, checked by you, as 1 ml of 0.1% adrenaline (epinephrine) is mixed in 400 ml of saline; the resulting vasoconstriction reduces bleeding.

3 Inspect the neck and the goitre to estimate where the superior thyroid pedicle lies and place the incision (Fig. 29.1) such that this can be ligated comfortably and securely with Vicryl at an early stage in the procedure, thus controlling the vessels that may otherwise bleed throughout the operation. Deepen the incision through platysma and to the lateral border of the sternomastoid muscles. Achieve haemostasis using

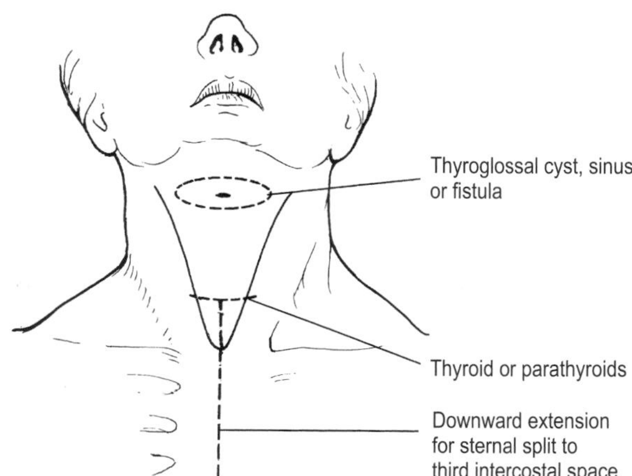

Fig. 29.1 Incisions for operations on the thyroid, parathyroids and thyroglossal lesions.

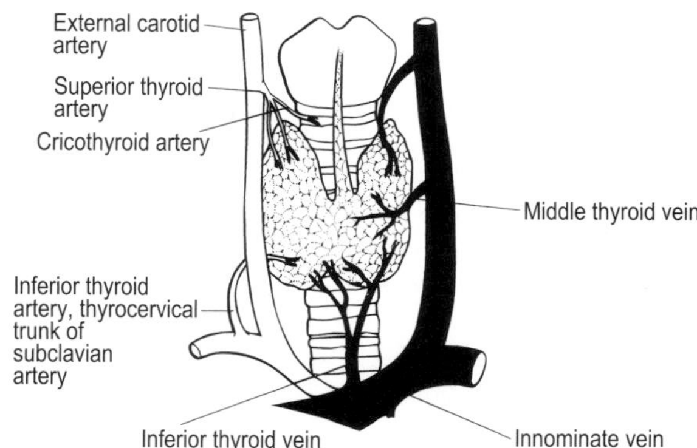

Fig. 29.2 Arterial supply and venous drainage of thyroid.

diathermy coagulation or by tying off the larger vessels with Vicryl.

4 Lift the platysma muscle of the superior flap upwards with Allis forceps, dissecting using coagulating diathermy in the subplatysmal plane. Identify and avoid damaging the anterior jugular veins and cutaneous nerves which lie superficial to the strap muscles. Raise the upper flap as far as the thyroid cartilage. Similarly, raise the lower flap as far down as the sternal notch. When this is completed insert a Joll's or similar self-retaining retractor to the platysma and subdermal tissues at the midpoint of each flap and open it fully to expose the strap muscles.

5 Identify and incise with diathermy the pale midline raphe between the strap muscles and separate the strap muscles, until you see the thyroid gland beneath. Apply Allis forceps on each side to the medial edge of the strap muscles on the side of the goitre or the dominant or bigger side, to be lifted vertically by an assistant while you draw the thyroid gland towards you.

6 Create a tissue plane between the strap muscles and the thyroid gland. There are several flimsy layers of fascia to divide, lifted off the gland. As the last flimsy layer is divided, the surface vessels on the thyroid bulge as the restraint is released. Now replace the Allis forceps with Langenbeck retractors.

7 Dissection should be completely bloodless. Achieve this by sealing small vessels with diathermy and ligating larger vessels using fine polyglycolic acid ligatures.

OPERATION FOR BENIGN NODULAR DISEASE

Subtotal lobectomy for nodular goitre results in a 15% recurrence rate, ultimately requiring reoperation. Recurrent nerve palsy rates are higher at reoperation. Subtotal lobectomy is not suitable for the majority of cases of benign nodular disease and its use is confined to Graves' disease. There is no place for enucleation of solitary thyroid nodules. Carry out total lobectomy with isthmusectomy. Frozen section is not recommended.

The steps of the operation will be described.

1 Identify and protect the inferior parathyroid gland and its blood supply; it is tongue-like, pink-brown, usually anterior inferior on the capsule but is variable. Identify the middle thyroid vein, also variable, sometimes multiple, along the anterolateral border of the thyroid gland. Now free the superior thyroid artery, doubly ligating and dividing it while preserving the cricothyroid muscle and external laryngeal nerve. Mobilize the superior pole of the thyroid gland, identifying and preserving the upper parathyroid gland, usually adherent to the upper posterolateral surface of the thyroid; ease it off, preserving the blood supply.

2 Secure the branches of the inferior thyroid artery for ligation in continuity (Fig. 29.2) on the capsule of the thyroid. First identify the white recurrent laryngeal nerve with its arteria commitantes, lying posteriorly

and medially in the tracheo-oesophageal groove but variable (Fig. 29.3).

3 Dissect across the front of the trachea, separating the gland, using diathermy when necessary; continue, to include the isthmus. There is frequently a pyramidal lobe going between the two main lobes superiorly, upwards high into the neck. Follow it as high as practical and as close to the hyoid bone as possible; then divide it between ligatures. The lobe to be removed, and the isthmus, are now free. Place an artery forceps across the contralateral side of the isthmus, divide the gland and remove the specimen. Oversew the remnant capsule with a running Vicryl suture.

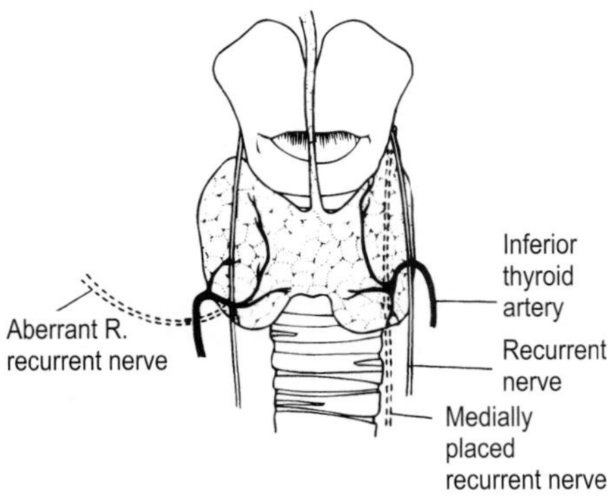

Fig. 29.3 Position of recurrent nerves in relation to inferior thyroid artery and some variations.

4 Check haemostasis, viability of the parathyroids, every step of the procedure, before approximating the strap muscles with Vicryl sutures, and the platysma muscle, and then the skin with staples or subcuticular absorbable sutures.

RETROSTERNAL MULTINODULAR GOITRE

Most extensions are into the anterior and superior mediastinum. Deliver them into the neck with gentle traction. Occasionally they extend behind the trachea, enter into the posterior mediastinum and become intimately related to major vascular structures within the chest. Rarely it is necessary to divide the sternum to mobilize an intrathoracic goitre.

SUBTOTAL THYROIDECTOMY FOR GRAVES' DISEASE

The principles will be described. Expose the whole thyroid gland as for total thyroidectomy, ligate both superior thyroid poles, tie the inferior thyroid artery in continuity, lateral to the recurrent laryngeal nerve avoiding damage to the nerve. Divide the isthmus and mobilize each lobe laterally.

You need to slice across each lobe from the lateral edge towards the trachea, leaving intact the posterior capsule with the attached remnant of thyroid gland. Leave the thickest part of the remnant laterally, so that it can be folded over medially, allowing the lateral capsular edge to be sutured to the medial capsule (Fig. 29.4).The remnant strip

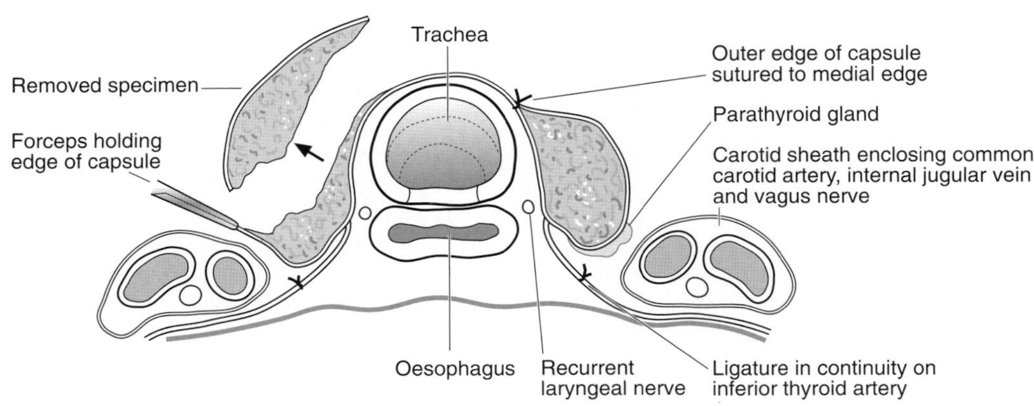

Fig. 29.4 Subtotal thyroidectomy. The diagram shows a transverse section. On the left is the posterior capsule and glandular remnant, thicker laterally. On the right, the posterior capsule and thyroid remnant have been folded medially and sutured to the medial capsular remnant and tracheal adventitia.

on each side is approximately 3 cm × 1 cm, thicker medially than laterally.

TOTAL THYROIDECTOMY

Repeat the process employed for a unilateral lesion on the other side. Follow exactly the same precautions as on the first side. Preserve at least one viable gland. In case of doubt, remove a doubtful gland, mince it and implant pieces into the sternomastoid or a forearm muscle.

MALIGNANT DISEASE

Well-differentiated tumours greater than 2 cm diameter and all medullary carcinomas demand total thyroidectomy. Treatment of papillary carcinoma, and follicular carcinoma, is controversial. Extensive lymph node dissection of the central inferior cervical compartment, skeletonizing the trachea and oesophagus, risks damaging aberrant low parathyroid glands with subsequent hypoparathyroidism. Central lymph node dissection is essential for medullary thyroid cancer. Screen preoperatively for a phaeochromocytoma as part of a MEN (multiple endocrine neoplasia) syndrome. Anaplastic carcinoma is rarely resectable.

MISCELLANEOUS

- *Minimal access techniques* can be successfully used in specialist units.
- *Local anaesthesia* is used in some centres.
- *Reoperative* surgery should be reserved for specialist centres.

POSTOPERATIVE

Close monitoring is essential to detect difficulty with breathing resulting from blockage of the airway during the 12 hours following thyroid surgery. This can be due to haematoma formation and subsequent laryngeal oedema. It is life-threatening and frightening for the patient and also the attendants alike. It requires immediate recognition and corrective action.

Keep clip-removing forceps by the bedside when clips have been used for closure. Remove clips immediately in order to evacuate the clot.

THYROGLOSSAL CYSTS

These are situated above the thyroid and below the hyoid bone, just off the midline, and usually present as painless lumps that move on swallowing or protruding the tongue. They are usually excised both for cosmetic reasons and because they occasionally become uncomfortable or infected. They may discharge in the neck, forming a thyroglossal sinus. They are usually excised as described by the American surgeon Walter Sistrunk in 1920. The cyst is excised through a crease incision, including a central portion of the hyoid bone since the cysts have a complex relationship with the bone. Follow the track up to the base of the tongue.

FURTHER READING

Col NF, Surks MI, Daniels GH 2004 Subclinical thyroid disease: clinical applications. JAMA 291:239–243

Surks MI, Ortiz E, Daniels GH et al 2004 Subclinical thyroid disease: scientific review and guidelines for diagnosis and management. JAMA 291:228–238

Internet websites

www.BAES.info

Guidelines for the surgical treatment of endocrine disease and training requirements for endocrine surgery. British Association of Endocrine Surgeons, 2004.

30

Parathyroid

R. E. C. Collins

CONTENTS

HYPERPARATHYROIDISM AND PARATHYROIDECTOMY

Hyperparathyroidism may be primary, usually from benign adenoma but occasionally from hyperplasia and very rarely from carcinoma. The effects of raised parathyroid hormone secretion are mobilization of calcium from the bone, enhanced calcium absorption from the small intestine and suppressed calcium loss from the kidneys, raising the blood calcium. Hyperparathyroidism may develop secondarily to renal failure with failure to excrete phosphate and inability to reabsorb calcium, raising the serum phosphate and lowering the blood calcium, both of which stimulate release of the hormone to maintain the blood level of calcium, resulting in decalcification of bone.

Classic symptoms of hypercalcaemia may be marked or very vague. They are classically described in a rhyming fashion.

Moans describes various neuropsychiatric disorders, *bones* describes skeletal pain from decalcification named 'osteitis fibrosis cystica', *stones* describes renal calculi or calcification, and abdominal *groans* are associated with abdominal pain, constipation, pancreatitis and a variety of vague, non-specific abdominal symptoms. Many patients are diagnosed coincidentally with hyperparathyroidism from serum chemistry performed for other medical conditions. A small percentage have hyperparathyroidism as a feature of one of the multiple endocrine neoplasia (MEN) syndromes.

The diagnosis is made by demonstrating persistently raised levels of serum calcium with an associated high serum parathormone (PTH) level or a level that is inappropriately normal in the presence of high serum calcium levels.

Serum calcium level in excess of 3.0 mmol/litre is considered to be an absolute indication for surgery. Because of the difficulty of predicting which patients are likely to deteriorate, operation is more freely offered than in the past, as it appears to reverse bone changes, depression and anxiety, and some cardiac changes.

Preoperative localization of enlargement or neoplasms is by technetium-99m-labelled sestamibi radionuclear scanning and high-resolution ultrasonography. Preoperative treatment with 1α-hydroxycholecalciferol for a few days may help 'hungry-bone syndrome' in the postoperative period by minimizing the risk of catastrophic falls in calcium.

The operation demands special training and experience.

STANDARD OPERATION

Incision and exposure are as for thyroidectomy (see Ch. 29).

To define the parathyroid glands (Fig. 30.1) dislocate the thyroid lobe medially and anteriorly whilst the strap muscles of the neck are retracted laterally in the opposite direction; if necessary divide the middle thyroid veins. Intraoperative localization of the glands by staining may be carried out using a methylthioninium chloride (methylene blue) total-body infusion technique. The lower gland usually lies at the anterior-inferior aspect of the thyroid capsule, the upper gland is usually high and posterior on the thyroid capsule near the cricothyroid muscle. Unstained, they appear tan colour, like little tongues, and cut like blancmange.

Remove a single enlarged gland. If all four are enlarged, first preserve half of one gland, remove the other half and

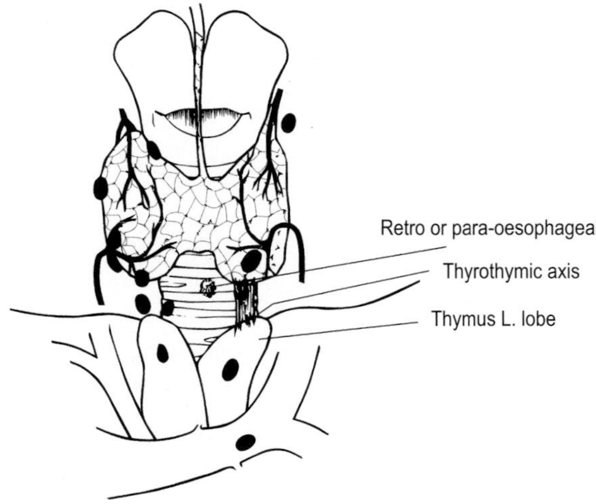

Fig. 30.1 Various positions for parathyroid glands.

the other three. Seal feeding vessels with diathermy current or with fine silver clips if they are near a laryngeal nerve.

A lateral approach or minimally invasive technique may be used.

PARATHYROID CARCINOMA

Parathyroid carcinomas are usually associated with extremely high calcium levels and sometimes with a palpable gland in the neck preoperatively. They invade especially the thyroid gland and may produce voice changes. As a rule perform a hemithyroidectomy on the same side and also remove any tissues nearby that are clearly macroscopically affected.

FURTHER READING

Irvin GL, Molinari AS, Figueroa C et al 1999 Improved success rate in reoperative parathyroidectomy with intraoperative PTH assay. Annals of Surgery 229: 874

Palazzo FF, Sadler GP 2004 Minimally invasive parathyroidectomy. British Medical Journal 328:849–850

Internet website

www.BAES.info

Guidelines for the surgical treatment of endocrine disease and training requirements for endocrine surgery. British Association of Endocrine Surgeons, 2004.

31

Adrenalectomy

R. E. C. Collins

CONTENTS

INTRODUCTION

Adrenalectomy is most commonly undertaken for a benign unilateral adrenal adenoma that is usually functional. Patients present with the consequence of excessive secretion of hormone rather than the mechanical effect of the adrenal tumour. Bilateral adrenal surgery is sometimes undertaken for simultaneously occurring bilateral adrenal tumours or for hypersecreting states associated with certain types of Cushing's syndrome associated with an excess of ACTH (adrenocorticotrophin) production. Carcinoma is rare. Laparoscopic approaches are increasingly used.

- *Phaeochromocytomas* (Greek *phaios* = dusky) arise in the adrenal medulla and secrete adrenaline, noradrenaline or dopamine. They present with episodic headaches, palpitations, hypertension and various syndromes involving apprehension and fear. There are raised levels of urinary catecholamines. Computed tomography (CT), magnetic resonance imaging (MRI) or meta-iodobenzylguanidine (MIBG) imaging are used to demonstrate a tumour. Ten per cent of phaeochromocytomas do not arise in the adrenal gland, 10% are bilateral, 10% are malignant and 10% occur in childhood.
- *Conn's syndrome* usually results from an adenoma arising from the zona glomerulosa – the outer layer of the adrenal cortex which secretes mineralocorticoids. Hyperaldosteronism produces hypertension with associated hypokalaemia (serum potassium less than 3.5 mmol/litre) and raised levels of plasma aldosterone with decreased plasma renin. Prepare the patient for 2–3 weeks before operation with spironolactone as an antagonist of aldosterone.
- *Cushing's syndrome.* Adenomas arise in the zona fasciculata and secrete excess glucocorticoids with raised plasma and 24-hour urinary cortisol. A dexamethasone suppression test helps confirm the diagnosis. In Cushing's disease, a pituitary adenoma produces ACTH with bilateral adrenal cortical hyperplasia. Plasma concentrations of ACTH are raised and can be suppressed by high-dosage dexamethasone. Preoperatively, metyrapone, a competitive inhibitor of 11β-hydroxylation in the adrenal cortex, inhibits production of cortisol, to control the symptoms.
- *Virilizing* (Latin *virilis* = man) *and feminizing syndromes* are rare and can be produced by excessive sex steroid secretion from an adenoma in the inner zona reticularis. There is a high incidence of malignancy.
- *'Incidentalomas'* are adrenal cortical tumours discovered by chance, often as a result of CT or MRI scans performed for the diagnosis of other conditions.
- *Adrenocortical carcinoma and other rare tumours.* Adrenocortical carcinoma is often highly malignant. Adrenalectomy is the one hope of cure but the 5-year survival rate is in the region of only 20–35%.

ADRENALECTOMY

As a rule treat solitary tumours by total removal of the affected adrenal gland. Where there is adrenal hyperplasia in Cushing's disease, remove all adrenal tissue. Subtotal excision of an adrenal tumour is inappropriate. Laparoscopic removal is increasingly employed for small tumours but open operation is preferred for large malignant tumours. Bring the patient to the best possible condition before operation. Order thromboprophylaxis during the perioperative period. Prescribe prophylactic antibiotics for patients with Cushing's disease or syndrome.

Laparoscopic approach

This may be performed transperitoneally after creating a pneumoperitoneum, or retroperitoneally after inserting ports posteriorly into the retroperitoneal fat just below the costal margin and creating an artificial space, either with an inflatable balloon or by using higher-pressure insufflation than that used in a transperitoneal (laparoscopic) approach, rising up to 19–20 mmHg. Identify the gland in the same manner as in the open approach, controlling the vessels with clips, diathermy or harmonic scalpel.

Open approach

For large or malignant tumours prefer the posterolateral approach through the bed of the 11th rib after dividing latissimus dorsi and serratus posterior muscles. Avoid damaging the intercostal neurovascular bundle and the underlying pleura. Cut through the rib costal cartilage with scissors and remove it. Sweep the pleura superiorly and posteriorly and similarly sweep the peritoneum anteriorly, using gauze swabs. Identify the kidney, lying inferiorly. Incise the deep fascia, allowing the retroperitoneal fat to bulge out. Have the kidney retracted inferiorly, while you proceed carefully by blunt dissection of the fat above and medial to the kidney, using light scissors (Fig. 31.1). The right adrenal tends to cap the upper pole of the kidney whereas on the left side it is more related to the upper medial border. Feel and see large tumours with small veins coursing away from the gland, particularly in phaeochromocytomas; they demonstrate that the dissection is adjacent to the adrenal gland. The adrenal gland has a characteristic golden colour quite distinctive from surrounding fat. Handle the gland carefully. On the right side concentrate on safely ligating the adrenal vein that empties directly into the inferior vena cava.

The posterior approach, with the patient prone and the table broken to flex the spine, is suitable for small benign tumours, also carried out through the bed of the 11th rib.

The anterior transperitoneal approach, through a rooftop (chevron) or long midline incision, is useful for bilateral phaeochromocytoma. Approach the right gland after performing Kocher's duodenal mobilization and elevating the liver. On the left incise the lienorenal ligament to release the splenic flexure and avoid injuring the spleen and tail of pancreas.

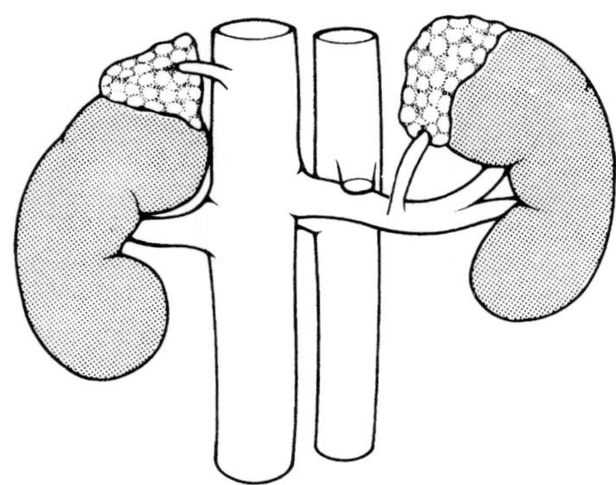

Fig. 31.1 Position and venous drainage of the adrenal glands.

Monitor the patient postoperatively in the intensive care unit, anticipating a liability to profound swings of blood pressure. Glucocorticoids are required following bilateral adrenalectomy for Cushing's disease. Following bilateral adrenalectomy, give fludrocortisone 0.1 mg orally.

FURTHER READING

Janetschek G 1999 Surgical options in adrenalectomy: laparoscopic versus open surgery. Current Opinion in Urology 9:213–218

Sidhu S, Gicquel C, Bambach CP et al 2003 Clinical and molecular aspects of adrenocortical tumorigenesis. Australia and New Zealand Journal of Surgery 73:727–738

Internet website

www.BAES.info

British Association of Endocrine Surgeons Guidelines for the Surgical Treatment of Endocrine Disease and Training Requirements for Endocrine Surgery, 2004.

32

Arteries

P. L. Harris

CONTENTS

INTRODUCTION

As a consequence of the high prevalence of arterial disease in Western countries, and the lack of effective medical treatment, arterial operations have come to represent a considerable proportion of the total surgical workload. Accordingly, this aspect of general surgery has evolved into a speciality with a degree of complexity that is recognized in the training programmes of those who wish to make the management of vascular disease a major part of their practice. However, given the ubiquitous nature of arteries, all competent surgeons should be familiar with the basic principles of arterial repair and reconstruction.

INDICATIONS FOR OPERATION

Injury

Injury resulting from sharp or blunt trauma; it may occur in association with fracture of long bones, especially the femur and humerus. Increasingly common are iatrogenic injuries resulting from the use of arterial access routes for various forms of investigation or treatment, and self-induced injury in main-line drug abusers.

Aneurysm

During the last few decades there has been a dramatic increase in the number of operations for atherosclerotic aneurysms of the abdominal and thoracic aorta. The incidence of aneurysms of the popliteal artery is also rising. Dissecting aneurysms of the aorta are a distinct pathological entity for which vascular surgical intervention is sometimes required. Mycotic aneurysms are seen occasionally.

Occlusion and stenosis

Most arterial occlusions result from thrombosis of a stenosed vessel, the underlying disease being atherosclerosis. This may be a slowly progressive condition, part of a natural ageing process, not always requiring surgical intervention. Critical limb ischaemia is a strong indication for operation, but intermittent claudication requires careful assessment to balance the potential benefits and risks of surgical intervention. Occasionally an artery becomes acutely occluded by an embolus. Sudden occlusion of an otherwise normal major artery is catastrophic, threatening both the viability of the limb and the life of the patient, requiring urgent removal or dissolution of the occluding embolus. The management of acute and chronic ischaemia is therefore quite different. Less commonly, acute limb-threatening ischaemia develops following sudden occlusion by thrombosis of a previously diseased artery or a bypass graft. The acute-on-chronic ischaemia that results makes management difficult, since it cannot usually be treated effectively by thrombectomy alone. Because of its inherently dangerous nature, the urgency which precludes detailed preoperative preparation, and the elderly frail condition of most of the patients, there is a high mortality risk associated with acute arterial occlusion. Furthermore, the urgency often makes it necessary to treat these patients in non-specialist units.

GENERAL PRINCIPLES

You do not need a large range of instruments but can produce good results provided you adhere closely to the basic principles described here. Prefer lightweight vascular clamps, control vessels with fine plastic loops, use atraumatic intraluminal catheters. To achieve perfection be willing to use 2.5× magnifying spectacles (loupes) when forming anastomoses.

Sutures, needle-holders and suture clamps

Arteries are always sewn with non-absorbable stitches. There are three types. Fine monofilament material such as polypropylene (Prolene) has the advantage of being very smooth and slipping easily through the tissues so that a loose suture can be drawn up tight. Compensate for its 'memory', tending to make it return to its original straight form. It is brittle; never handle it directly with metal instruments. Braided material coated with polyester to render it smooth, such as Ethiflex or Ethibond, does not slip so easily through the arterial wall but is pleasantly floppy to handle and knots easily. Tough atraumatic needles are swaged on to each end of the sutures. PTFE (polytetrafluoroethylene; Gore-Tex) sutures are used with PTFE grafts. PTFE is non-compliant so needle holes do not close around the suture to stop bleeding, so the diameter of the needles is made smaller than the suture – but also weakened, and so inappropriate for tough or calcified arteries. In general, use the finest suture that is strong enough for the job; as a rough guide, 3/0 for the aorta, 4/0 for the iliacs, 5/0 for the femoral, 6/0 for the popliteal and 7/0 for the tibial arteries are appropriate. For very fine work always use a monofilament stitch. When using double-ended sutures protect the 'idle' stitch by applying a small rubber-shod clamp. Have available a selection long and short, heavy and fine needle-holders.

Solutions

For local irrigation of opened vessels and instillation into vessels distal to a clamp, use heparinized saline – 5000 units of heparin in 500 ml of physiological saline.

Blood transfusion and autotransfusion

Arterial operations, particularly emergency procedures, may be associated with significant blood loss. An autotransfusion system or cell-saver reduces the requirement for banked blood and protects the patient from the risk of blood-borne infections.

Grafts

The best arterial substitute is the patient's own blood vessel, usually vein. However, quite often there is no suitable vein available, because it is either absent, too small for the job required or has itself been damaged by varicosities or thrombophlebitis. Under these circumstances a prosthesis has to be chosen and three types are currently available.

Dacron is an inert polymer spun into a thread, either woven or knitted into cloth graft and available in tubes from 5 mm to 40 mm in diameter, straight or bifurcated. Generally prefer the knitted variety with a velour lining as its porosity allows tissue ingrowth and better anchoring of the internal 'neointimal' surface compared to the original knitted grafts which needed to be preclotted with the patient's blood taken prior to heparin administration; in an emergency it was necessary to use a woven graft, which leaks less. Most vascular surgeons now use knitted grafts, presealed with bovine collagen, gelatin or albumen, with low porosity which do not require preclotting. Within 3 months the sealant is absorbed and replaced by natural fibrous tissue ingrowth, providing the advantages of both woven and knitted prostheses. Additional substances, for example antibiotics, anticoagulants or agents to prevent anastomotic myointimal hyperplasia, may in future be incorporated within the sealant. Dacron grafts perform extremely well when used to bypass large arteries with a high flow-rate such as the aorta and iliac arteries, making them the arterial substitute of choice in these situations.

Expanded polytetrafluoroethylene (PTFE) grafts are slightly more expensive than Dacron but their performance is superior for reconstruction of small arteries. In general, prefer Dacron grafts above the groin, PTFE below the groin, although some surgeons use Dacron rather than PTFE for above-the-knee femoropopliteal bypass. PTFE grafts are available with an external polypropylene support to prevent compression or kinking; always use this type if the graft crossed the knee or any other joint.

Biological substitutes in the past, such as arterial or venous allografts or xenografts, are rapidly degraded and were abandoned. Recently developed cryopreservation with dimethylsulfoxide (DMSO) and liquid nitrogen may reduce the host immunological response. They may be suitable for arterial bypass in the presence of infection when replacing infected prosthetic grafts in situ. Human umbilical veins can be treated to make them non-antigenic and then coated with an outer Dacron support to prevent aneurysmal dilatation; they have good patency rates even in distal sites, but are at risk of aneurysmal degeneration.

Preshaped vein cuffs, collars or patches interposed between PTFE grafts and small arteries below the level of the knee joint produce improved rates of patency. Possibly the configuration of a cuffed anastomosis promotes a pattern of blood flow inhibiting or redistributing the anastomotic myointimal hyperplasia that is the principal cause of graft failure. Preshaped grafts have been manufactured from PTFE to reproduce an anastomosis of 'ideal' configuration without the necessity of constructing a cuff from vein. An additional benefit is that the wall of the shaped end is thinner than that of the body of the graft and this facilitates suturing.

Grafts with a degree of compliance are available, and are thought to be more efficient conduits of pulsatile flow than stiff grafts. Their value in clinical practice is unproven.

Stents and stent/grafts

Metallic stents made from either stainless steel or nitinol may be used as an adjunct to balloon angioplasty in order to maintain patency of the vessel or as a framework to support an endovascular graft for exclusion of an aneurysm. They are of two types: balloon-expandable (e.g. Palmaz stent) and self-expanding (e.g. Wallstent). Stents for endovascular aneurysm repair are covered with Dacron, PTFE or other fabric. They are manufactured as straight tubes or bifurcated for repair of abdominal aortic aneurysms. Small stents 'covered' with PTFE are also available but are associated with a higher incidence of myointimal hyperplasia. Do not use them in preference to non-covered stents except for specific indications. Drug-eluting stents that release chemicals to inhibit myointimal hyperplasia such as paclitaxel and sirolimus have proved disappointing in clinical trials.

BASIC TECHNIQUES OF ARTERIAL REPAIR, ANASTOMOSIS AND TRANSLUMINAL ANGIOPLASTY

Arteriotomy

Longitudinal arteriotomy

Arteries are best opened longitudinally. They can be extended if necessary and are easily closed; any thrombus that accumulates on the suture line has minimal tendency to narrow the lumen. A transverse arteriotomy is difficult to close because the intima retracts away from the outer layers, increasing the risk of blood tracking in a subintimal plane, resulting in occlusion of the vessel.

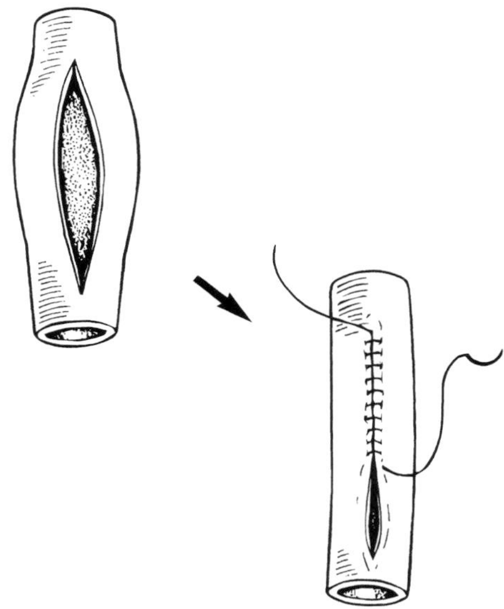

Fig. 32.1 Longitudinal arteriotomy closed by continuous everting arterial suture.

Simple suture

Longitudinal arteriotomies in large or medium-sized arteries can usually be closed by simple suture (Fig. 32.1).

Use the finest suture material compatible with the thickness and quality of the arterial wall. Aim to produce an everted suture line that is leak-proof. This is quite different from bowel suture, where the mucosa is deliberately inverted into the lumen and the tension on the sutures is kept low to avoid necrosis of the edges. Everting mattress sutures would narrow the lumen; a simple over-and-over stitch is adequate, provided you ensure that the intima turns outwards. You must pass the needle through all layers of the arterial wall with every stitch, including the inner layers to ensure good intimal apposition and to prevent flap dissection. Include the outer layers since the adventitia forms the main strength of the arterial wall. Keep a firm, even tension on the suture at all times. You will gain experience of the required spacing and size of each bite, which varies with the size and nature of the artery. Although evenly spaced stitching is usually best, on occasion, such as aortic aneurysm repair, you may need to insert large irregular stitches.

Closure with a patch

Close vessels of less than 4 mm in diameter with a patch in order to avoid narrowing of the lumen (Fig. 32.2) or widen

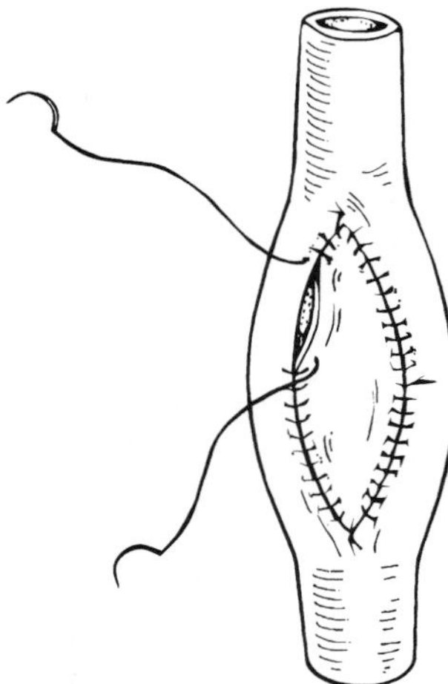

Fig. 32.2 Closure of longitudinal arteriotomy with a patch.

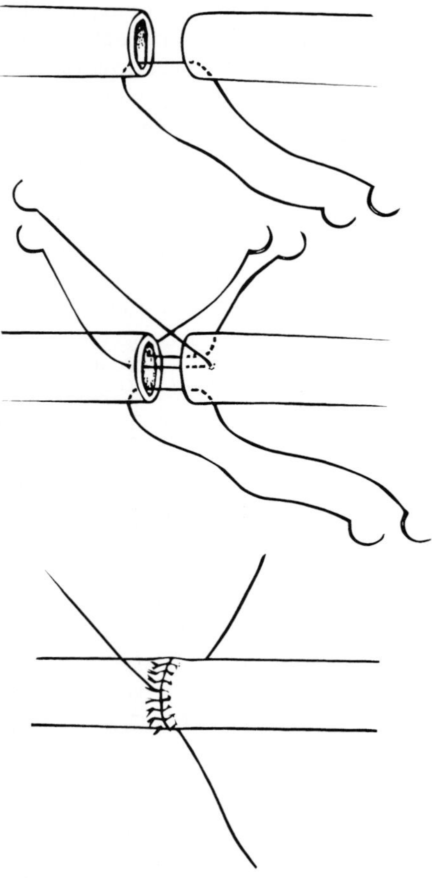

Fig. 32.3 End-to-end anastomosis by the triangulation technique.

the lumen of a vessel that has become stenosed by disease, such as the profunda femoris artery. For small vessels use a patch of autologous vein. Never sacrifice the proximal end of the long saphenous vein for this purpose. Use either a segment taken from the ankle, a tributary or a piece of vein from another site such as the arm. For larger vessels you may use prosthetic material, either Dacron or PTFE. When cutting the patch to shape, round the ends; do not leave sharp points which would cluster the sutures and cause narrowing. Use just one double-ended stitch commencing close to one end and working around each side. Do not finish the stitching at the apex but carry one of the sutures around to the other margin to complete the closure, so you can tie the knot a short distance to one side. Knots at the apex may be a cause of significant narrowing. This technique permits you to inspect the internal suture line and you can delay the final trimming of the patch until you have nearly completed the closure, to ensure a perfect match for size.

End-to-end anastomosis

For small delicate arteries this is accomplished most safely by applying the principles of the triangulation technique; join the vessels with a suture placed in the centre of the back or deepest aspect of the anastomosis (Fig. 32.3). Tie the knot on the outside. Place two more sutures to divide the circumference of the vessels equally into three. Compensate for any disparity in calibre at this stage. Always use interrupted sutures for small vessels, in which case keep the three original stay sutures long and apply gentle traction on them to rotate the vessel and facilitate exposure of each segment of the anastomosis in turn. Complete the back or deep segments first, leaving the easiest segment at the front to be finished last.

For larger vessels it is permissible to use continuous sutures. Cut the ends of the vessels to be joined obliquely, then make a short incision longitudinally to create a spatulate shape. Overlapping the two spatulate ends avoids any risk of narrowing at the anastomosis.

A different technique of end-to-end anastomosis can be employed with great effect in operation on aneurysms. This is the inlay technique (see Repair of abdominal aortic aneurysm, below).

End-to-side anastomosis

This is the standard form of anastomosis for bypass operations. It should be oblique with its length approximately twice the diameter of the lumen of the graft. Fashion the end into a spatulate shape, which will, on completion of the anastomosis, resemble a 'cobra-head'. The end of the anastomosis in the angle is referred to as the 'heel' and the other end as the 'toe'. The simplest way of completing it is to place a double-ended stitch at the heel and another at the toe and to run sutures along each margin, ending with a knot at the halfway point on each side. There is an advantage in keeping the inside of the suture line visible as much as possible. Achieve this by starting with a double-ended suture at the heel. Leave the toe free. Run the suture up each side to beyond the midpoint and then retain in a 'rubber-shod' clamp. Insert a further stitch through the toe and complete and trim the last two quadrants by tying to the previously retained threads. This is sometimes known as the 'four-quadrant technique' (Fig. 32.4).

The 'toe' and 'heel' are the most crucial points of an end-to-side anastomosis. To ensure that the toe is completed as smoothly as possible, offset the starting point of the 'toe', suturing a few millimetres to one side or the other of the apex. In order to further reduce the risk of causing a stricture at this point, you may prefer to place a few interrupted sutures around the toe.

Avoid a stricture of the heel by stenting the vessel with an intraluminal catheter of appropriate size until this portion of the anastomosis is complete. An alternative method is the 'parachute' technique (Fig. 32.5), for which you must use monofilament suture material. This is particularly useful where access is difficult and your view of the anastomosis is impaired, but it is applicable to most situations. With the graft and the recipient artery separated, place a series of running sutures between them at what will become the heel of the anastomosis. Then pull these sutures tight as you approximate the vessels.

Transluminal angioplasty

Approximately half of all patients with symptoms of peripheral arterial occlusion are now treated by this means and

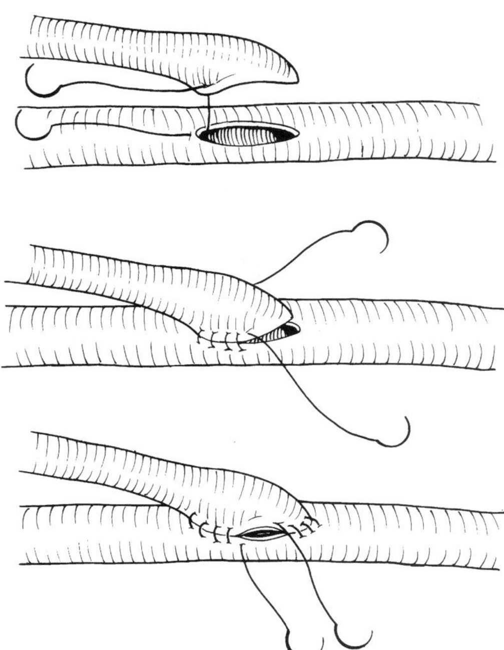

Fig. 32.4 End-to-end anastomosis by the four-quadrant technique.

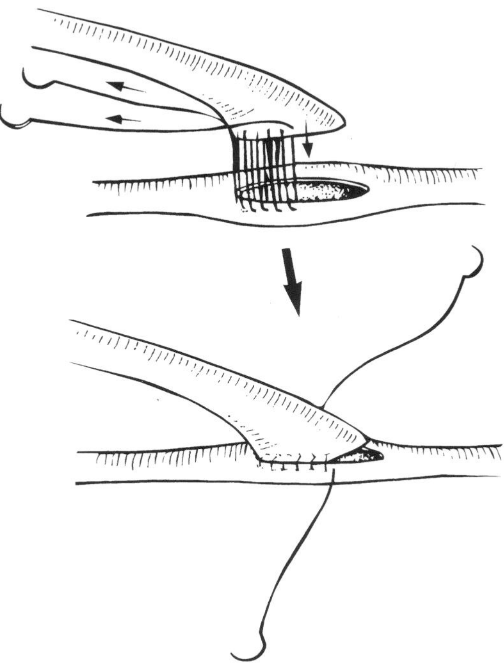

Fig. 32.5 End-to-side anastomosis by the parachute technique.

the proportion is increasing because it is minimally invasive, low risk, and often benefits patients with critical ischaemia but also serious co-morbidity. It may be performed percutaneously in a specialist radiology suite or open in the operating theatre. In principle, a guidewire is inserted, through a needle into the artery, and over this is passed a catheter carrying a special balloon which is manoeuvred under fluoroscopic control, to lie across the narrowing. The balloon is inflated to open up the stricture and then withdrawn.

EXPOSURE OF THE MAJOR PERIPHERAL ARTERIES

Common femoral artery

The common femoral artery needs to be exposed more frequently than any other vessel in the body and it is important to know how to do this swiftly and correctly. The surface marking of the artery is at the mid-inguinal point, halfway between the anterior superior iliac spine and the pubic symphysis – remember this, since the artery is not always palpable. The groin crease does not correspond in position to that of the inguinal ligament, but lies distal to it by 2–3 cm.

Provided that the saphenous vein will not be required during the operation, make a vertical incision directly over the artery. The midpoint of this incision should roughly correspond to the groin crease – do not make the incision too low. If you require only limited exposure of the common femoral artery, as for an endovascular intervention, use a transverse incision placed one finger's breadth above the groin crease. It is less painful and heals better. Deepen the incision through the subcutaneous fat, taking care not to cut across any lymph nodes. Expose the femoral sheath and incise it longitudinally to uncover the artery. Protect the femoral vein which lies medially; the laterally placed, and deeper femoral nerve is not usually at risk.

Pass a Lahey clamp behind the artery to draw through a plastic sling with which to gently lift the artery, helping to identify its branches and its bifurcation into the superficial and profunda femoral arteries. Isolate these similarly with slings. Avoid damaging the profunda vein, a tributary of which always passes anterior to the main stem of the profunda artery. To fully expose the profunda artery divide this vein between ties. If you need to expose the long saphenous vein at the same operation, make a 'lazy-S' incision, commencing vertically over the artery at the inguinal ligament and then deviating medially over the saphenous vein in the upper thigh.

You cannot avoid transecting the many lymphatics in the femoral triangle, sometimes causing a troublesome lymphocele or lymphatic fistula after the operation, so approach the artery from its lateral rather than its medial side and gently reflect any lymph nodes and visible lymph vessels off the femoral sheath with minimal damage.

Popliteal artery

Expose this above or below the knee by medial approaches. The most inaccessible part lies directly behind the joint line and if you need to expose it there a posterior approach is essential (see below).

To expose the suprageniculate artery, make a longitudinal incision over the medial aspect of the lower thigh. If you intend to perform a bypass with a saphenous vein graft, make this incision directly over the previously marked vein, otherwise make it along the anterior border of the sartorius muscle – but not too far anteriorly. Deepen it to expose, and retract posteriorly, the sartorius muscle, exposing the neurovascular bundle enveloped by the popliteal fat pad. The artery lies on the bone, the nerve lies some distance away, with the vein in between. The popliteal artery is always surrounded by a plexus of veins; separate and divide them carefully to avoid troublesome bleeding.

To expose the infrageniculate popliteal artery, make an incision on the medial aspect of the calf along the border of the gastrocnemius muscle. Dissect between its medial head and the tibia to reveal the neurovascular bundle. Expose the vein first, lift it carefully away to reach the artery. If you divide the soleus muscle along its attachment to the medial border of the tibia, you can expose the origin of the anterior tibial artery and the whole extent of the tibioperoneal trunk. Improve the exposure of the popliteal artery proximally by dividing the tendons of sartorius, semitendinosus and gracilis muscles and even completely divide the medial head of gastrocnemius – this leaves surprisingly little functional disability.

To expose the whole length of the popliteal artery use a posterior approach. With the patient lying prone, make a 'lazy-S' incision through the popliteal fossa and deepen it through the popliteal fascia and fat pad, defining the diamond between the hamstring muscles above and the two heads of gastrocnemius below; then follow the short saphenous vein into the neurovascular bundle.

Tibial arteries

The proximal end of the anterior tibial artery is relatively inaccessible but the remainder of this vessel and its terminal dorsalis pedis branch can be readily exposed through lateral or anterior incisions made directly over them. Retract the tibialis anterior and extensor digitorum longus muscles anteriorly to reveal the artery lying on the interosseous membrane.

Subclavian artery

Make a transverse incision 1 cm above the medial third of the clavicle; divide the platysma muscle in the same plane (Fig. 32.6), to expose and divide the clavicular head of sternomastoid muscle. Dissect and retract superiorly the fat pad containing the scalene lymph nodes from the surface of the scalenus anterior muscle. Identify the phrenic nerve, which passes obliquely across the front of this muscle to lie along the medial border of its tendon and usually separated from it by a few millimetres. Pass the blade of a MacDonald's dissector behind the tendon of scalenus anterior muscle, while protecting the phrenic nerve, and divide the tendon by cutting down on to the dissector with a pointed scalpel blade. Retract the muscle superiorly to expose the subclavian artery with its vertebral, internal mammary and thyrocervical branches. The first thoracic nerve root and the lower trunk of the brachial plexus cross the first rib above and posterior to the artery. The subclavian vein is deep to the clavicle and is not normally seen through this approach. On the left side, the thoracic duct enters the confluence of the internal jugular and subclavian veins; if you damage it, ligate it to prevent a troublesome chylous fistula developing. You can expose more of the subclavian artery by excising the inner two-thirds of the clavicle, although this is rarely necessary.

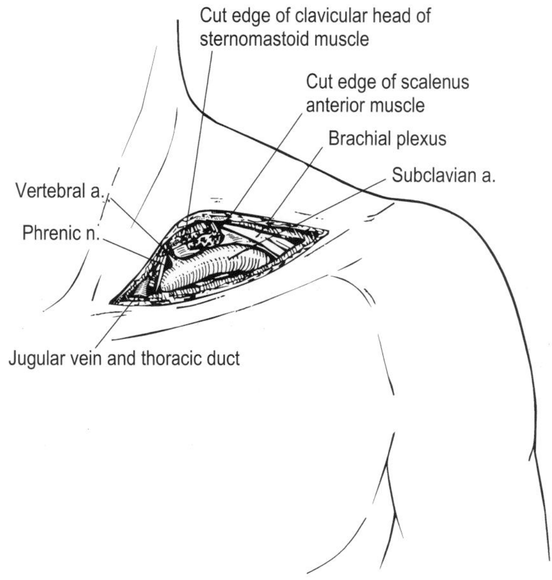

Fig. 32.6 Exposure of the subclavian artery.

The two most common operations on the subclavian artery are carotid–subclavian anastomosis or bypass for a proximal occlusion (subclavian steal syndrome) and repair of a subclavian aneurysm. Operations involving direct exposure of the origin of the subclavian artery are largely superseded by extrathoracic bypass procedures or, rarely, by splitting the manubrium and upper sternum.

The origin of the left subclavian artery, which arises far back on the aorta arch, can also be exposed through a posterolateral thoracotomy through the bed of the second or third ribs.

Axillary and brachial arteries

Access to the axillary artery is most often required for axillofemoral bypass and occasionally for subclavian aneurysm repair (see above). Make a horizontal incision 1 cm below the lateral third of the clavicle, split the fibres of pectoralis major muscle and divide the pectoralis minor tendon, lying beneath the fat pad, close to its origin. Divide obstructing branches of the acromiothoracic vessels to reveal the axillary artery surrounded by the cords of the brachial plexus, which must be carefully protected.

The proximal brachial artery lies in the groove between biceps and brachialis muscles on the inner aspect of the upper arm, still enclosed by cords of the brachial plexus joining to form the median nerve, which crosses it obliquely from the lateral to the medial side. Expose the bifurcation of the brachial artery through a 'lazy-S' incision in the antecubital fossa followed by division of the biceps aponeurosis (Fig. 32.7). Distal extension of this incision permits the radial, ulnar and anterior interosseous arteries to be followed into the forearm.

TYPES OF OPERATION

Techniques used to repair or bypass damaged or diseased arteries include direct repair, interposition grafting and

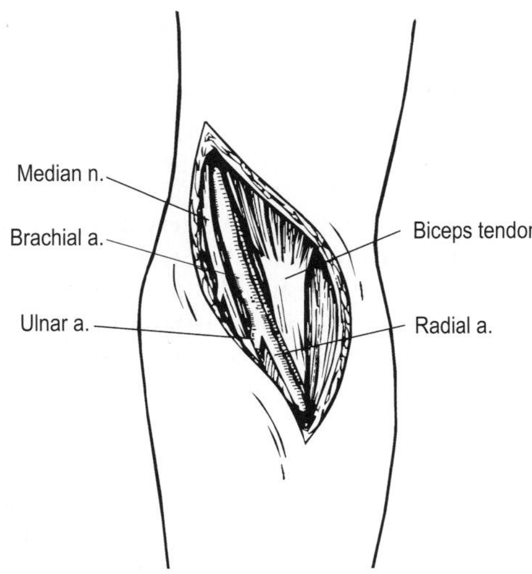

Fig. 32.7 Exposure of the distal brachial artery.

patch grafting for arterial trauma, surgical embolectomy or thrombectomy, thrombolytic therapy, percutaneous suction and mechanical embolectomy, bypass grafting and endarterectomy, which is now supplanted by bypass surgery, except for the carotids.

Percutaneous and intraoperative (adjunctive) dilatation angioplasty and endovascular stenting is available for occlusive arterial disease. Apart from balloon dilatation, recanalization of resistant occlusions can be achieved by including lasers, rotational guidewires, high-frequency electrocoagulation ablators and various types of atherectomy catheters. Inlay grafting for aneurysms is also available.

Endovascular stent/graft repair is valuable for aortic and peripheral aneurysms.

QUALITY CONTROL

Success in arterial surgery demands technical perfection. The presence of a palpable pulse is no guarantee of mean forward flow through the graft. Completion angiography or intraoperative Doppler flowmetry may be used. The return of palpable pulses to vessels downstream of the reconstruction, for example in the pedal arteries, is a valuable sign and I recommend that one of the simple and inexpensive devices available to supplement clinical assessment, including strain gauge and photoplethysmographs (digital pulse monitors), toe temperature probes, flat and hand-held Dopplers and pulse oximeters, is used routinely.

ARTERIAL OPERATIONS

There are three basic prerequisites for success in arterial surgery: an unimpeded inflow tract – the run-in; an adequate outflow tract – the run-off; and an efficient recanalization or bypass – the conduit. Appraise all three factors when planning any arterial reconstruction.

REPAIR OF ARTERIAL INJURY

Arterial trauma may occur as an isolated event but is usually associated with other injuries, for example fracture of long bones – and the symptoms of ischaemia may be masked until irreversible tissue damage has occurred. Always assess the distal circulation in cases of fractured long bones or disarticulation injuries, especially those that involve the elbow or knee.

Arterial injury is manifest by bleeding, either externally or with the formation of a haematoma, and by acute ischaemia with pallor, coldness, loss of sensation, muscle tenderness and weakness, absent pulses and absent or damped Doppler signals with reduced systolic arterial pressure in distal vessels. If you suspect arterial injury arrange urgent angiography. Angiographic discontinuity of a major limb vessel demands urgent surgical exploration. Occlusion of a single tibial or forearm vessel is usually tolerated without ischaemic damage and does not as a rule require reconstruction.

Beware the concept of 'arterial spasm'. Although smooth muscle of arteries contracts protectively in response to injury, revealed as narrowing angiographically and on inspection, luminal discontinuity indicates mechanical fault, demanding surgical repair, never reliance on vasodilator drugs.

Treat multiple injuries in close cooperation with colleagues of other specialities. Repair damaged major arteries in preference to orthopaedic fixation of fracture – but there is a danger that vascular anastomoses may become disrupted during the manipulation of fractures. It may be advisable to restore vascular continuity initially by inserting a temporary intraluminal plastic shunt, and completing the repair once the fractures have been stabilized, when the length of the arterial defect can be accurately measured.

Run-in is not usually relevant in arterial trauma. Run-off may be blocked by blood clot occluding vessels distal to the site of injury. Incorporate measures to deal with this problem; otherwise the run-off vessels are usually normal.

Conduit is either the original artery repaired directly or interposition of a short segment graft of autogenous vein. For closed injuries to major arteries, such as iliac or subclavian, with tearing or rupture of the vessel consider endovascular repair with a covered stent.

Once the presence of major arterial injury has been established, undertake surgical exploration without delay. Have cross-matched blood available and correct serious hypovolaemia.

Access

In the case of limb injury, prepare and drape the limb so as to permit direct inspection of skin perfusion and palpation of pulses distal to the site of injury. Anticipate the possibility that a segment of healthy undamaged vein of suitable size may need to be harvested for construction of a graft.

First, gain proximal control of the artery and then gain distal control through a skin incision that extends well beyond the confines of the injury, along the axis of the injured vessel and directly over it. Do not enter the haematoma until the vessel has been dissected and controlled by passing rubber slings around it proximally and distally.

Assess

On entering the haematoma there may be brisk fresh bleeding, in which case apply clamps at the proximal and distal control points already prepared. If there is complete disruption of the artery find the ends and apply soft clamps. It is unlikely that they will be actively bleeding at the time of exploration. It is always the case that the vessel is traumatized for some distance proximally and distally from the principal site of injury so trim both ends until you find undamaged intima. Can you achieve tension-free direct end-to-end anastomosis or should you insert an interposition graft of autologous vein, even only for one centimetre?

If the artery is in continuity there may be bruising of the adventitia at the site of injury and absence of downstream pulsation. These are sure signs of internal disruption. The intima and inner layers of the media split transversely and the edges roll back to form a flap, which obstructs flow, causing secondary thrombosis. Do not merely inspect the outer surface of such a vessel or apply topical vasodilator substances. Excise the damaged segment completely to healthy intima.

Active arterial bleeding usually signifies incomplete disruption or a lateral wall defect that inhibits protective retraction and constriction of the vessel.

Action

1 Before commencing repair of the artery, pass a Fogarty catheter distally and proximally to withdraw any propagated clot and then instil heparinized saline. If there are associated orthopaedic injuries consider inserting a temporary intraluminal shunt. The adventitia tends to prolapse over the end of a normal artery that has been cut across. Trim this back to prevent it intruding inside the anastomosis.

2 If direct end-to-end anastomosis is possible, accomplish it by the triangulation technique preferring interrupted sutures. If the defect is too great for direct repair, harvest a segment of vein of appropriate size. Complete the proximal anastomosis first, in end-to-end fashion, using the triangulation technique with interrupted sutures for small or inaccessible vessels or the oblique overlap technique for larger vessels. Reverse the vein to avoid obstruction to blood flow by competent valves. Apply a clamp to the distal end of the graft and allow arterial pressure to distend it in order to determine the optimum length to avoid both excessive tension and kinking. Finally, complete the distal anastomosis. You may repair a small puncture or lateral wall defect, as may result from iatrogenic injury following arterial access for investigation or treatment, by direct suture or by closing the arteriotomy with a patch.

3 Where possible, effect primary closure of the incision with suction drainage.

4 In the case of blast injuries and other causes of extensive skin and soft tissue damage, observe the general principles of wound management. Where primary closure is either not possible or inadvisable, always cover the arterial repair with healthy viable tissue, which in practice usually means a muscle flap.

? DIFFICULTY

1. Difficult access prejudices satisfactory end-to-end anastomoses; ligate the ends of the artery and bypass the traumatized area with end-to-side anastomoses at remote, more accessible, sites.

2. Magnification is advisable for small vessel anastomoses.
3. If there is any doubt about the effectiveness of the repair, obtain an on-table angiogram.
4. Recurrent thrombosis despite a technically satisfactory repair warrants immediate systemic heparinization.
5. Repair associated damaged veins? As a rule, repair major axial veins such as the femoral vein. In near-amputation of a limb, restore continuity to two veins for each artery repaired, constructing venous anastomoses obliquely and with interrupted sutures.

Aftercare

Except in cases where continued bleeding is a serious problem, maintain anticoagulation with heparin for several days. Arrange regular half-hourly observation of the distal circulation during the immediate postoperative period and be prepared to re-explore immediately in the event of recurrent occlusion.

Complications

Early thrombosis or bleeding at the site of the repair demands immediate re-exploration and reassessment. A false aneurysm may result from a contained anastomotic leak and this also requires early re-exploration and repair. The risk of associated deep venous thrombosis is high, so take appropriate preventative measures. Repair of arterial injuries in young, healthy people is usually very successful and long-term disability associated with ischaemia is rare.

SURGICAL EMBOLECTOMY

Embolic occlusion of a major artery results in acute ischaemia, which, if not relieved quickly, may progress to irreversible tissue damage and limb loss. The differential diagnosis is from acute thrombosis. Threatened viability signalled by muscle tenderness and paralysis, and loss of sensation demand immediate surgical exploration. But revascularization of an already non-viable limb is invariably fatal; urgent amputation may be life-saving.

Under other circumstances urgent angiography is indicated to establish the diagnosis and to permit proper appraisal of the various options for treatment.

Surgical embolectomy is indicated for embolic occlusion of the common femoral artery and vessels proximal to the groin such as saddle embolus, and for the brachial and axillary arteries. More distal emboli, such as in the popliteal artery, with no immediate threat to viability, can be appropriately treated by thrombolytic therapy.

Preoperative appraisal includes an assessment of the underlying cardiac disease. Surgical embolectomy can be performed under local anaesthesia but general anaesthesia is preferable in the absence of serious anaesthetic risk. Run-in, run-off and conduit usually are not relevant to surgical embolectomy in the absence of associated arterial disease. The urgency of the situation dictates that preoperative preparation must be limited. Treatment may be required for heart failure or dysrhythmia. Commence systemic anticoagulation with heparin.

Action

1 Expose and make a short longitudinal arteriotomy in the common femoral artery at the origin of the profunda artery for lower limb emboli, and the brachial artery in the antecubital fossa for upper limb emboli. Select an embolectomy catheter with a central irrigating lumen permitting injection of heparinized saline or X-ray contrast medium beyond the balloon; 3F for axillary and brachial arteries, 4F for the superficial and profunda femoral arteries and 5F for the aortic bifurcation.

2 Pass the uninflated catheter proximally through the vessel beyond the clot. Inflate the balloon and withdraw the catheter slowly while adjusting the pressure within the balloon to accommodate changes in the vessel diameter, avoiding friction between the balloon and the arterial wall which damages to the intima. Meanwhile instruct an assistant to control bleeding from the vessel by applying gentle traction to the rubber sling previously placed around it. Repeat the procedure until you can retrieve no more thrombus, and the vessel forcefully bleeds. Avoid unnecessary passages of the catheter.

3 Instil heparinized saline into the artery and gently clamp it. Repeat the same procedure distally. Fill the vessels with heparinized saline and close the arteriotomy. Directly suture the common femoral artery but always use a small vein patch for the brachial artery.

4 Arrange long-term anticoagulation to prevent recurrent embolization for younger patients; for the very elderly,

weigh the risks against the benefits. Determine to evaluate and treat the underlying cardiac disease.

5 If you cannot pass the catheter proximally or cannot obtain forceful forward bleeding, there is either pre-existing arterial disease or the catheter has passed into a subintimal plane. If the catheter will not pass distally obtain an on-table angiogram to find if an embolus has impacted at the popliteal bifurcation and beyond, or if there is atherosclerotic occlusion. Instil a small amount of a thrombolytic agent (streptokinase, urokinase or tissue plasminogen activator) through a small catheter advanced to the block. Pass a small Fogarty catheter 15 minutes later; more embolus may be retrieved. If you have available intraoperative fluoroscopy, pass the embolectomy catheter over a guidewire negotiated into each vessel in turn. Assess the result by angiography.

PERCUTANEOUS THROMBOLYTIC EMBOLECTOMY/THROMBECTOMY

Avoid thrombolytic therapy following a stroke, eliminate those with intracardiac thrombus by echocardiography and use streptokinase on a single occasion only. Administer systemic anticoagulation with heparin. Using the Seldinger technique, a guidewire is introduced through a percutaneously inserted needle, the needle is withdrawn and a small-bore catheter is passed over the guidewire, which is then also withdrawn so that a small amount of thrombolytic agent can be infused and repeated if clot lysis is radiologically seen to be incomplete after 30–60 minutes. Pulsed high-pressure thrombolytic spray technique is rapid and efficient, a mechanical technique breaks up the clot and adjuvant percutaneous angioplasty dilates stenosis from anastomotic intimal hyperplasia or progressive atheroma.

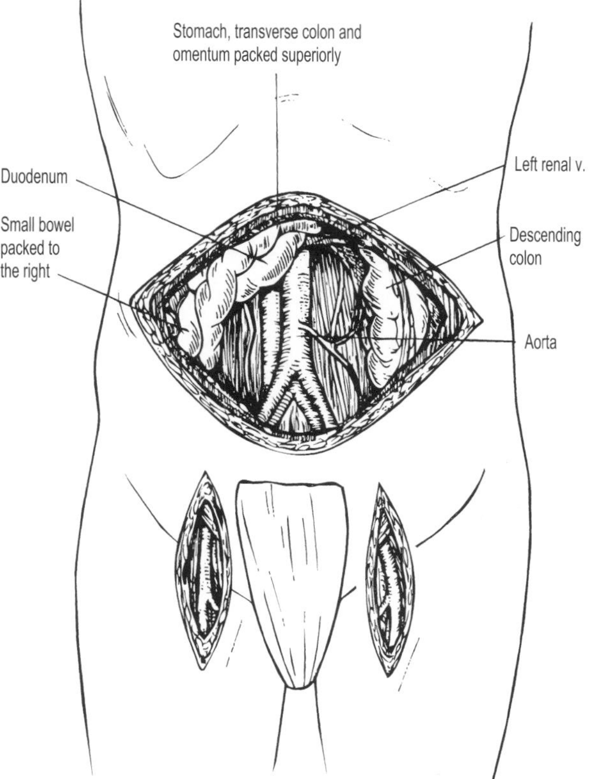

Fig. 32.8 Exposure of the abdominal aorta for aortofemoral bypass.

ILIAC ARTERY OBSTRUCTION

All aortic operations have features in common. Aortobifemoral bypass is increasingly replaced by percutaneous angioplasty except for total aortic occlusion, severe aortic bifurcation disease or diffuse widespread aortoiliac disease in patients with critical limb ischaemia or disabling claudication. Exclude cardiac disease, confirm an adequate outflow and use a preferably knitted bifurcated polyester Dacron graft. Access is shown in Figure 32.8. Select a correct sized bifurcated Dacron graft. As a rule occlude the aorta with a suprarenal clamp and transect the aorta 2 cm below the renal arteries closing the distal stump, and constructing an end-to-end anastomosis, with 3/0 polypropylene (Fig. 32.9) to the graft. Clamp the distal limbs and release the aortic clamp to test the anastomosis. Now pass the distal limbs retroperitoneally in order to create end-to-side anastomoses into the femoral arteries, if necessary extending them onto the profunda arteries, using 5/0 polypropylene. Minimally access techniques have been developed.

If one side only is affected, a unilateral aortofemoral, iliofemoral or cross-over iliofemoral bypass can be constructed. Femoro-femoral anastomosis can be performed under local anaesthesia, bringing the cross-over graft subcutaneously. Severe bilateral aortoiliac occlusive disease with critical lower limb ischaemia may be relieved by a Dacron graft extending from an axillary artery, tunnelled beneath pectoralis major then subcutaneous to the ipsilateral common femoral artery and across to the opposite

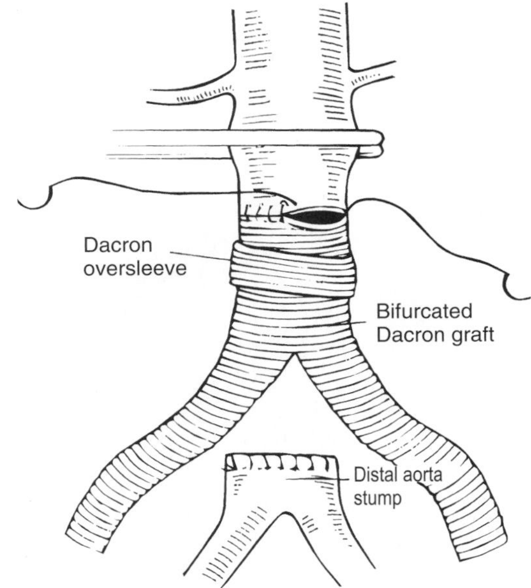

Fig. 32.9 Aortic anastomosis: end-to-end technique.

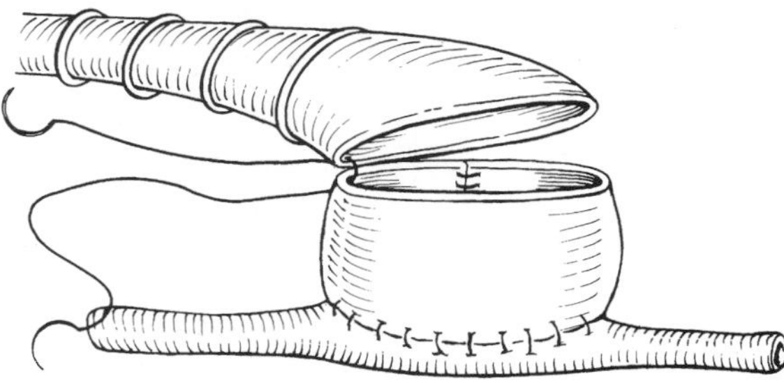

Fig. 32.10 The Miller cuff.

femoral artery. For short segments, iliac and femoral balloon angioplasty and stenting are often successful.

For longer femoral or distal stenoses, saphenous vein bypass is often indicated provided the run-off is adequate. This may be accomplished by totally removing the vein, tying off tributaries without narrowing it, reversing and inserting it to bridge the stenosis. Alternatively the vein may be left in situ but disconnected at top and bottom, to be connected to the artery above and below the stenosis after passing a valvulotome to destroy the valves. A prosthetic graft of PTFE tends to produce platelet adhesion with subsequent subintimal hyperplasia and blockage especially at the distal anastomosis. The tendency can be reduced by inserting a venous cuff (Miller), or patch between the end of the graft and the artery (Fig. 32.10).

REPAIR OF ABDOMINAL AORTIC ANEURYSM

The abdominal aorta is the commonest site for aneurysms. These are dangerous lesions, death being the likely outcome in the event of rupture. The rate of growth and the risk of rupture increase exponentially with the diameter of the aneurysm, with a watershed level for serious risk at about 5.5 cm. Therefore, unless the patient is gravely ill from other causes, any aneurysm wider than 5.5 cm should be operated upon electively. The mortality rate with elective aneurysm surgery is less than 5% in the best centres. The important surgical principles are minimal dissection, inlay technique of anastomosis and using straight rather than bifurcated grafts whenever possible.

Perform emergency operation for an aneurysm producing severe abdominal or back pain with or without circulatory collapse, unless the patient is already moribund. Mortality associated with emergency operation is 30–60% but the overall risk of death from a ruptured aneurysm is more than 90%, since 75% of patients die without reaching hospital.

Confirm the diagnosis by ultrasound scanning, or computed tomography (CT) if endovascular repair is contemplated. Assess cardiac, respiratory and renal risk. For emergency cases, insert vascular access lines and urinary catheter. Inject a broad-spectrum antibiotic with induction of anaesthesia as prophylaxis against graft infection. The principles only of technique will be described.

Action

1 Through a midline incision extending from the xiphisternum to the pubis skirting the umbilicus, exclude malignant disease which would alter your decision. Now displace the omentum and large bowel superiorly, small bowel and mesentery to the right including the mobilized duodenum, to display the neck of the aneurysm, crossed by the left renal vein. Incise the peritoneum longitudinally over the aneurysm passing down and to the right of the inferior mesenteric artery to expose the whole aneurysm and both common iliac arteries, having identified and protected the ureters. Carefully make a space on each side of the aneurysmal neck to accommodate the jaws of a straight clamp applied from the front, aiming to preserve the left renal vein. Similarly clamp each common iliac artery. Assess the aortic bifurcation and the iliac arteries. A minor degree of ectasia of the iliac arteries can be accepted and

it should be possible to use a straight graft in 60–70% of patients. A bifurcated graft is required if the common iliac ostia have been separated by the aneurysm or if one or both of the iliac arteries are grossly aneurysmal. Assess the inferior mesenteric artery. Usually it is totally occluded. However, if it is widely patent it is advisable to observe the effect of temporary clamping of this vessel on the bowel circulation before it is finally sacrificed.

2 Open the aneurysm longitudinally and scoop out the laminated thrombus and liquid blood, sending a specimen for culture. Control back-bleeding from patent lumbar and median sacral arteries with figure-of-eight sutures of 3/0 polypropylene applied from inside the sac. Infuse 60 ml of heparinized saline into each leg via a catheter inserted temporarily into the common iliac arteries to reduce the risk of intravascular thrombosis during clamping. If you need to insert a bifurcated graft, cut off all but 3–4 cm of the main trunk above the bifurcation.

3 Using 3/0 polypropylene sutures, construct an end-to-end anastomosis to the proximal aorta from within the sac by the inlay technique (Fig. 32.11). Start suturing, with the parachute technique, to one side of the midline at the back of the graft (see Basic techniques). Stitch from graft to aorta, taking large bites to include all layers of the aortic wall each time. Finish in the midline anteriorly. Apply a soft clamp to the graft and gently release the aortic clamp to test the anastomosis. Place additional sutures as required. If you use a straight tube construct a similar anastomosis at the aortic bifurcation. If you use a bifurcated graft it may be possible to construct an end-to-end anastomosis by the inlay technique to the iliac bifurcation on both sides. Before completion of the distal anastomosis flush the graft to eliminate any blood clots and also to ensure that the recipient vessels bleed back satisfactorily. If this is not the case pass embolectomy catheters to retrieve any distal blood clots.

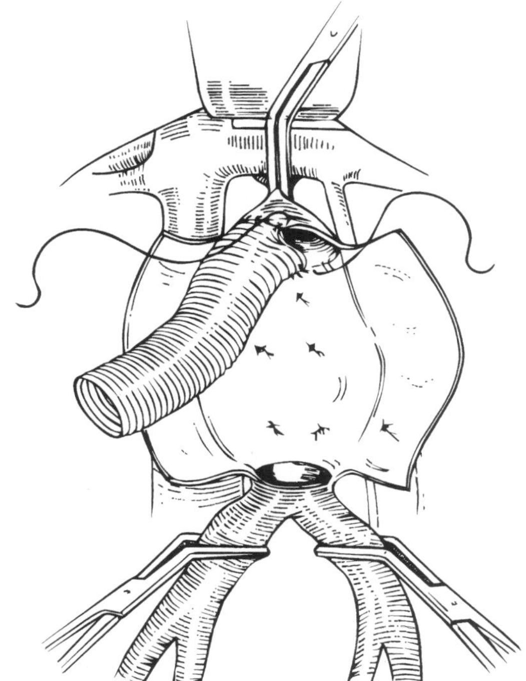

Fig. 32.11 The inlay technique of anastomosis.

4 Give the anaesthetist several minutes warning before releasing the clamps and re-perfuse one leg at a time in order to minimize the risk of declamping shock. In the case of a bifurcation graft the anastomosis on one side may be completed and this limb perfused before the second anastomosis is constructed. A slight fall in blood pressure on release of a clamp is reassuring evidence that the limb is in fact being adequately perfused.

5 Having made quite certain that all anastomoses are blood-tight and that there is no bleeding from any other source, fold the redundant aneurysm sac over the graft and fix it with a number of synthetic absorbable sutures. Make sure that the graft is covered completely.

Complications

Haemorrhage makes early re-exploration mandatory. Occlusion results from embolization or distal thrombosis. Renal tubular necrosis develops following prolonged hypotension. Adult respiratory distress syndrome (ARDS) usually follows emergency operations for ruptured aneurysms. Myocardial infarction and graft infection may also develop.

ENDOVASCULAR REPAIR OF ABDOMINAL AORTIC ANEURYSM

Endovascular aneurysm repair has the attributes of a minimally invasive operation. The procedure itself carries a very low risk and the recovery time is much shorter than that associated with conventional open operation. The main drawback of this approach at the present time is that the durability of non-sutured anastomoses and of the stent/grafts themselves is, as yet, unproven. For 'fixation' the endograft relies upon a stent with or without hooks or barbs attached, and for 'seal' to exclude the aneurysm sac from the circulation it relies upon firm contact between the fabric of the graft and the vessel wall at each end. These functions demand the existence of a 'neck' of at least 15 mm in length between the lowest renal artery and the start of the aneurysm and adequate distal 'landing zones'.

CAROTID ENDARTERECTOMY

The main indication for carotid endarterectomy is transient cerebral ischaemic attacks associated with a stenosis greater than 70%. Total occlusion of the internal carotid artery is a contraindication to surgery. Access is through an oblique skin incision along the anterior border of the sternomastoid muscle. The majority of patients will tolerate prolonged clamping of the internal carotid artery without suffering ischaemic damage to the brain. Operation can be performed under local or general anaesthesia, and with temporary plastic shunts. Through a longitudinal arteriotomy commencing on the common carotid and extending into the internal carotid, identify the plane between the arterial wall and the core composed of atheromatous material. Gently dissect out and remove the core. The termination of the plaque may require to be fixed before closing the artery, if necessary with a patch.

INTESTINAL ISCHAEMIA

Acute ischaemia results from acute thrombosis, sudden decompensation of an already narrowed mesenteric artery, 'non-occlusive infarction', where no arterial blockage is responsible or, rarely, from embolus. If the gut is infarcted, resect it. If it is viable it may be possible to carry out vascular reconstruction. After successful revascularization always perform a 'second look' operation next day.

Chronic intestinal ischaemia is difficult to define although genuine cases of 'intestinal angina' due to chronic obstruction of the visceral arteries do certainly exist.

33

Veins and lymphatics

K. G. Burnand, J. Tan

CONTENTS

VARICOSE VEIN SURGERY

Varicose veins are defined as tortuous dilated superficial veins. Small intradermal subcutaneous veins are excluded. Most patients seek treatment for their varicose veins because they dislike the appearance of the large, tortuous veins on their exposed legs. The greater number of varicose vein operations performed in women may reflect the greater importance they attach to attractive legs. Many patients complain that their veins ache – often worse at the end of the day or after prolonged standing. Patients also present with ankle swelling, itching, superficial thrombophlebitis and haemorrhage. Minor varicose veins and small intradermal subcutaneous veins can be made symptom-free by elastic support stockings.

Recurrent attacks of superficial thrombophlebitis or severe bleeding from a ruptured varix are clear-cut indications for surgical treatment. Surgical ligation and stripping remains the treatment of choice for major incompetence of the long and short saphenous (Latin *saphena* = visible) veins, since injection sclerotherapy provides only short-term benefit. Varicose branch veins may be avulsed through local incisions at the time of saphenous vein surgery, but, in the absence of saphenous incompetence, these are equally well treated by injection sclerotherapy. This may be by standard sclerosant such as sodium tetradecyl sulphate or by a foam sclerosant. Twenty to thirty per cent of varicose vein operations are for persistent or recurrent varicosities following saphenous surgery. These recurrent veins can be treated by injection sclerotherapy if there are no residual connections with the femoral or popliteal veins. Coincidental varicose veins are often erroneously diagnosed as the cause of painful or swollen legs, which may be the result of arthritis or other causes of leg oedema.

Most patients with uncomplicated and clear-cut varicose veins require little in the way of investigation beyond a careful history and an examination of the legs to determine the competence or incompetence of the major sites of communication between the superficial and deep venous systems. Inspection, palpation and the cough, percussion and tourniquet tests provide this information. Patients who have lipodermatosclerosis, past ulceration or history of limb fracture or deep vein thrombosis should undergo duplex scanning and bipedal ascending phlebography to enable an accurate assessment of the deep and calf communicating veins to be made. Do not carry out varicose vein surgery if the long saphenous vein forms an important collateral channel for obstructed deep veins. Arterial insufficiency is also a relative contraindication to varicose vein surgery.

Patients with complicated or recurrent varicose veins are more accurately assessed by varicography, in which low-osmolality contrast medium is injected directly into the surface veins to display their course and deep connections. Duplex examination of the reflux in the long and short saphenous trunks provides useful additional information. Carefully re-examine patients admitted for varicose vein surgery. Confirm or exclude incompetence in the long and short saphenous veins, and in the calf perforating veins. Mark with an indelible pen large branch varicosities and the sites of major communicating vein incompetence. Suspect incompetence of calf communicating veins in patients with lipodermatosclerosis. Preoperative marking with duplex scanning may be useful for locating the termination of the short saphenous vein and the sites of incompetent perforating veins.

A number of new minimally invasive alternatives to ligation and stripping are being assessed, including endoluminal radiofrequency ablation and laser ablation. These cannot be recommended at present until the results of properly conducted clinical trials are available.

HIGH SAPHENOUS VEIN LIGATION (TRENDELENBURG'S OPERATION) AND STRIPPING OF LONG SAPHENOUS VEIN

Perform the operation, which was described by Friedrich Trendelenburg (1844–1924) of Leipzig in 1890, on patients with varicose veins who have evidence of long saphenous reflux at the groin on clinical, Doppler or duplex examination. Avoid the operation if the long saphenous vein is a collateral channel for obstructed deep veins. Mark all sites of prominent varicosities with indelible pen as 'tram-lines' on either side of the vein to avoid the effect of tattooing. Have the skin of the groin and leg shaved before the operation.

Place the patient supine in the Trendelenburg position with approximately 30° of head-down tilt with both the legs abducted by 20° from midline and the ankles lying on a padded board. This allows easy access and reduces intraoperative haemorrhage. Prepare all exposed surfaces of the limb from the foot to the groin, up to the level of the umbilicus, with aqueous 0.5% chlorhexidine acetate solution, while an assistant elevates the leg by lifting the patient's foot.

Action

1 Approach the saphenofemoral junction through an oblique incision just below and parallel to the inguinal ligament in the groin crease, over the saphenofemoral junction, which is 2.5 cm lateral to and below the pubic tubercle. Deepen the incision through the subcutaneous fat, which is spread by digital retraction and held apart by the insertion of a self-retaining retractor such as Travers', West's or Cockett's. Modify the length of incision depending on the build of the patient. Bluntly dissect the long saphenous vein out of the surrounding fat and trace it upwards and towards the saphenofemoral junction. The perivenous plane is simple to open and is bloodless when entered.

2 You must dissect out all tributaries that join the long saphenous vein near its termination, ligating them with 2/0 polyglactin before dividing them. The superficial inferior epigastric vein, the superficial circumflex iliac vein, and the superficial and deep external pudendal veins all join the saphenous trunk near its termination. In addition, the posteromedial and anterolateral thigh veins terminate close to the saphenofemoral junction (Fig. 33.1). One or more of these veins may join together before emptying into the saphenous trunk. The long saphenous vein normally emerges as a dark-blue tube in the centre of dissection as you free the subcutaneous fat from its surface. Trace a smaller tributary back to the main trunk if it is hard to find. When you have divided these tributaries, approach the saphenofemoral junction. The long saphenous vein dips down through the cribriform fascia over the foramen ovale to join the femoral vein. Carefully separate the subcutaneous fat from the vein by blunt dissection to follow its path. Display the femoral vein for approximately 1 cm above and below the saphenofemoral junction, and clear any small tributaries entering from either side. Do not ligate or divide any large vessel until you have displayed the full anatomy of the long saphenous, its tributaries and its junction with the femoral vein. It is easy to mistake the femoral artery for the long saphenous vein, with disastrous consequences if it is inadvertently stripped. Be aware that a variable number of tributaries join the long saphenous vein as it approaches the femoral vein. Occasionally the anterolateral and posteromedial thigh veins terminate independently into the femoral vein, giving the appearance of a double saphenous vein. The long saphenous vein may occasionally be truly bifid with one channel joining the femoral vein below the saphenous opening.

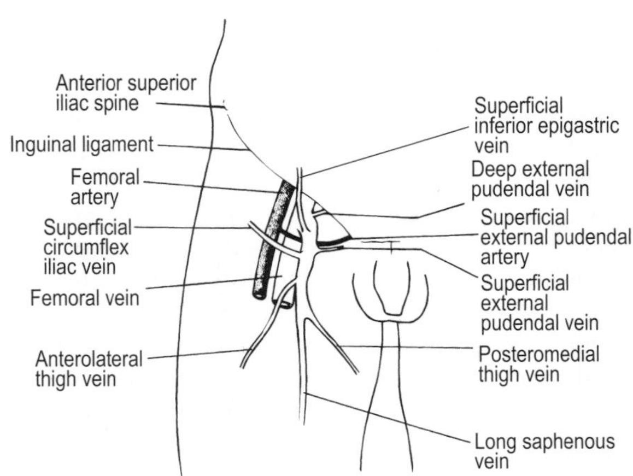

Fig. 33.1 The termination and tributaries of the long saphenous vein in the groin.

3 Ligate the long saphenous vein in continuity with 0 polyglactin, flush with the saphenofemoral junction, and divide it. For greater safety doubly ligate or transfix the saphenous stump. Alternatively, oversew the termination with a 3/0 polypropylene continuous suture. Place a strong ligature around the divided distal end of the long saphenous trunk and hold it up to occlude retrograde blood flow, then make a small transverse venotomy above the ligature through which to introduce the stripper. Use either a flexible intraluminal wire or a disposable plastic stripper with a blunt tip. Gently manipulate the tip of the stripper downwards until it is a hand's breadth below the knee, where it may remain in the saphenous vein or pass into a tributary (Fig. 33.2). If it will not pass, withdraw the stripper and reinsert it with a rotational action. Tie the ligature at the top end to prevent blood from leaking out of the divided long saphenous trunk. The alternative of a pin stripper does not appear to show any additional benefit. Take care not to damage the superficial external pudendal artery, which may pass either anterior or posterior to the saphenous vein; if you do, ligate and divide it.

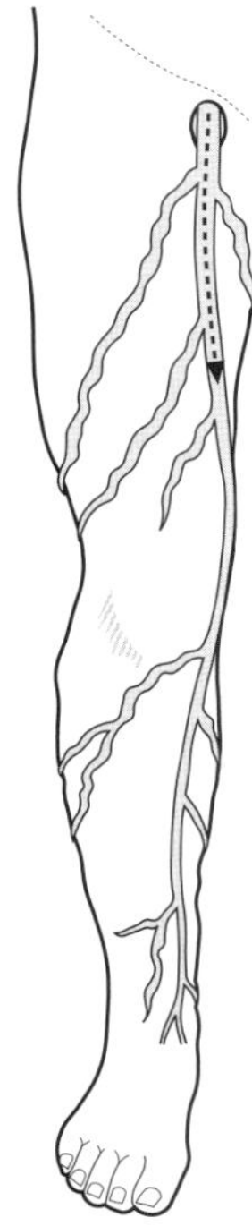

Fig. 33.2 Passage of a flexible intraluminal stripper in the long saphenous vein. Note the tributary below the knee into which the stripper may pass, leaving the main vein.

4 Make a short oblique incision in one of the skin crease tension lines, 1–2 cm in length, over the palpable tip of the stripper. Ensure that the incision is large enough to allow the head of the stripper to pass. Palpate the vein containing the stripper and dissect it off the saphenous nerve. Make a small side-hole in the vein through which the tip of the stripper can be delivered and attach the T-shaped handle to the stripper. Strip the long saphenous vein from the groin to the knee with steady downward traction. Ease the stripper and the bunched up vein through the lower incision. Clamp the attached long saphenous vein and any tributaries, divide and ligate it with 2/0 polyglactin.

5 Prevent excessive bleeding from the stripper track, either by tightly applying a sterile elasticated bandage while withdrawing the stripper, or by gently rolling a swab along the course of the vein before applying bandages. Some surgeons apply a sterile tourniquet to the leg to prevent excessive haemorrhage.

6 Appose the subcutaneous tissues and fascia with 2/0 polyglactin. Close the skin with 3/0 subcuticular sutures with Monocryl and Steri-Strip tapes. Apply compression bandages to the whole leg to avoid haematoma formation.

7 After operation keep the leg elevated 15° above the horizontal in bed. Encourage early mobilization after applying additional compression bandages over the bandages put on in the theatre. This reduces the haematoma formation and provides better support when the patient stands. Thromboembolism prophylactic stockings do not provide sufficient compression. Advise the patient to walk rather than stand still or sit with the feet down. Discharge fit patients on the first postoperative day, to re-attend for removal of any non-absorbable sutures a week later.

? DIFFICULTY

1. The passage of the stripper may be impeded by competent valves, varicosity or false passages into small tortuous tributaries. If you use force you will perforate the vein wall. Withdraw the stripper and repass it,

twisting the free end to rotate the tip and facilitate negotiating irregularities in the vein. If there is a hold-up around the knee, try flexing and extending the knee to aid the passage of the stripper, at the same time applying gentle external compression over the tip of the stripper to prevent it from passing into superficial tributaries. If these measures fail, leave the stripper in situ. Pass a second stripper into the long saphenous vein from below the knee, then gradually withdraw the first stripper ahead of the advancing stripper passed from below. If neither stripper will bypass the obstruction, cut down over the tips of both strippers. You may be able to redirect one stripper through the cut-down incision and pass it on down the vein, but if this fails, strip out the two halves of the vein leaving a short residual portion between the two incisions. Alternatively, forcibly avulse this segment of residual vein.

2. Control sudden massive haemorrhage in the groin by applying direct external pressure to the femoral vein above and below the saphenofemoral junction. Summon experienced vascular help. Never attempt to apply an artery forceps blindly.

SAPHENOPOPLITEAL LIGATION AND STRIPPING

This is indicated if there is gross dilatation and reflux in the short saphenous trunk or its tributaries. The location of the saphenopopliteal junction is very variable and, in a third of cases, the short saphenous vein enters the popliteal vein above or below the middle of the popliteal fossa. Preoperative varicography and duplex scanning or on-table saphenography all provide accurate information about the termination of the short saphenous vein and its proximal tributaries. When you identify the saphenopopliteal junction, mark it on the skin.

Carry out the short saphenous vein ligation first if you intend to strip the long saphenous vein under the same anaesthetic.

Action

1 Have the anaesthetized, intubated patient prone, with pillows under the chest, midriff and pelvis and the operating table in 30° of head-down tilt. Slightly abduct the legs to ease access and make a short transverse incision behind the lateral malleolus at the ankle. Find the short saphenous vein posterior to the lateral malleolus and dissect it from the fat and its accompanying sural nerve. Ligate the vein distally with 2/0 polyglactin. Pass another ligature proximally and use it to elevate the vein in order to create a venotomy to insert a stripper. The sural nerve is easily damaged unless you dissect it free from the vein.

2 Having inserted the stripper, pass it up the vein in an identical manner to that described for the long saphenous vein. Tie the ligature at the ankle to prevent blood loss. Now make a transverse incision 3–5 cm in length in the popliteal fossa over the saphenopopliteal junction, which was previously identified and marked. Divide the deep fascia in the popliteal fossa vertically and define the short saphenous vein containing the easily palpable stripper. Slightly withdraw the stripper and make sure it is not in the popliteal vein, having entered it through a connecting vein in the lower calf.

3 Gently expose the termination of the vein by blunt dissection, to separate it from the surrounding fat, until you identify the T-junction with the popliteal vein. Avoid damaging the popliteal artery, vein and nerve during popliteal dissection.

4 Apply deep retraction with a Langenbeck's retractor to help display the junction. There is often a tributary joining the short saphenous vein from above, known as the vein of Giacomini, in 2.5–10% of patients; carefully divide it between ligatures. Doubly ligate the stump of the short saphenous vein with 2/0 polyglactin, extract the head of the stripper from the lumen and tie the vein to the stripper. Strip out the vein, and firmly wrap the leg in an elasticated bandage.

5 Insert continuous 2/0 polyglactin into the subcutaneous tissue and fascia and close the skin with a 3/0 subcuticular suture and Steri-Strips.

INCOMPETENT PERFORATOR OR COMMUNICATING VEINS LIGATION

Communicating veins connect the branches of the saphenous system to the deep veins of the leg by crossing the deep fascia. Blood normally passes from the superficial to the deep veins, but reversal of flow may occur if the valves of the communicating veins become incompetent. Three almost constant communicating or perforating veins in the medial calf are particularly important in the development of venous ulceration (Cockett's veins).

Ligate these medial calf communicating veins in patients with clinical or duplex scanning evidence of incompetence and who have severe lipodermatosclerosis or healed ulceration. Your objective is to interrupt incompetent medial calf perforating veins, in order to obliterate deep to superficial venous reflux and reduce ambulatory venous hypertension in critical areas above the ankle where venous ulcers are most likely to develop.

Subfascial endoscopic perforating vein interruption is performed through an endoscope inserted through small ports placed well away from the active ulcer or area of diseased skin. This avoids making a long and often poorly healing wound.

AVULSION OF SUPERFICIAL VARICOSITIES

Occlude or excise large branch veins that are not in close proximity to the saphenous or perforator systems to prevent unsightly local recurrences and provide a satisfactory cosmetic result. Carefully mark out the superficial varicose veins on either side preoperatively, as varicosities are no longer visible when the patient is anaesthetized and the legs are elevated. Further reduce local blood loss by performing the avulsions after the limb has been exsanguinated with a tourniquet.

Action

Make minute stab incisions over the course of tributaries in the direction of skin tension lines. Draw out a loop of vein by gentle blunt dissection, using specially designed hooks or mosquito artery forceps. Divide the loop between mosquito forceps and tease out the vein in either direction by exerting steady traction and gentle blunt dissection under the skin with fine mosquito forceps. Employ a gentle circular motion on the forceps to help separate the tethering fibrous tissue from the vein. Release traction when the vein starts to stretch, and at this point ligate both ends. Alternatively, continue the traction until the vein breaks, controlling bleeding by local pressure until traumatic venospasm develops. Place incisions 5 cm apart along the course of each tributary. This technique can be used to remove a long segment of varicose vein through three to five small incisions.

NEW ALTERNATIVE TREATMENTS

Any alternative technique to high ligation and stripping of saphenous vein must produce as good as, or a better, outcome with, ideally, a reduced associated morbidity. Intimal damage by endoluminal radiofrequency ablation and endovascular laser treatment aim to result in fibrosis. Illuminated powered phlebectomy employs a suction needle containing a guarded blade which removes veins like a vacuum cleaner.

OPERATIONS FOR DEEP VEIN THROMBOSIS

First confirm the diagnosis with duplex scanning and obtain a venogram if you intend to carry out operative treatment. Unless they are contraindicated, anticoagulants are commonly given. Thrombectomy, for example through a femoral vein approach, may allow removal of fresh, loose, iliofemoral thrombus, using Fogarty balloon catheters.

Caval clipping – the application of a special plastic clip or placing of three or four sutures – converts the inferior vena cava into three or four smaller channels to prevent the passage of large thrombi.

Umbrella filters, resembling the ribs of an umbrella, can be inserted percutaneously under radiological control into the inferior vena cava to trap large loose thrombi.

LYMPHATIC SURGERY

If lymphoedema is a likely cause of chronic limb swelling, perform isotope or contrast lymphography to confirm the diagnosis. Most patients with primary and secondary lymphoedema respond readily to active conservative treatment with regular leg elevation, elastic support and massage. For severe lymphoedema from obstruction, bypass operations may be attempted. Reduction operations such as Homan's or Charles' aim to excise lymphoedematous skin and subcutaneous tissue, particularly between the knee and foot.

FURTHER READING

Adam DJ, Bello M, Hartshorne T et al 2003 Role of superficial venous surgery in patients with combined superficial and segmental deep venous reflex. European Journal of Vascular and Endovascular Surgery 25:469–472

Amarigi SV, Lees TA 2000 Elastic compression stockings for prevention of deep vein thrombosis. Cochrane Database of Systematic Reviews CD001484

Barwell JR, Davies CE, Deacon J et al 2004 Comparison of surgery and compression with compression alone in chronic venous ulceration (ESCHAR study): randomised controlled trial. Lancet 363:1854–1859

Browse N 1999 Diseases of the veins, 2nd edn. Arnold, London

Burnand K 1998 The new Aird's companion in surgical studies, 2nd edn. Churchill Livingstone, Edinburgh

34

Sympathectomy

J. A. Rennie

CONTENTS

SYMPATHETIC NERVOUS SYSTEM

The arteries to the skin and muscle of the limbs have a sympathetic innervation. The sympathetic nerves to the skin of the hands and feet are predominantly vasoconstrictor, but both vasoconstrictor and vasodilator fibres are present to the arteries in muscle. At rest there is a dominant vasoconstrictor tone to skin and muscle. Following sympathetic blockade, skin flow increases markedly and sweating is inhibited, and there is a modest rise in muscle flow. However, the increase in muscle flow during sympathetic blockade is only one-tenth the increase in flow seen during exercise of the muscle. This exercise-induced increase is mediated by the liberation of local metabolites from the contracting muscle fibres.

THORACIC SYMPATHECTOMY

Thoracic sympathectomy may be performed for hyperhidrosis, facial flushing, Raynaud's disease and digital artery thrombosis. The sympathetic fibres to the arm synapse in ganglia T2–3 (T2 for the hand and T2+3 for the axilla). The upper (T1) ganglion fuses with the inferior cervical ganglion to form the stellate ganglion. Damage to the stellate will produce a Horner's syndrome.

There are several approaches to the upper thoracic sympathetic chain: transaxillary or anterior (supraclavicular). However, the thoracoscopic method has become the standard method. In principle, under general anaesthetic, the appropriate lung is deflated and an artificial pneumothorax created with a Veress needle in the third intercostals space, replaced by a thoracoscope and also a pair of endoscopic shears. Dissect out and excise the sympathetic chain between the second and fourth ganglia inclusive. The stellate ganglion is not visible and so is safe from damage which would result in Horner's syndrome of eyelid ptosis, pupillary miosis (constriction) and facial anhidrosis. The anterior approach is through a 5-cm incision above the clavicle, transecting the insertion of the scalenus anterior muscle into the first rib, after securing and sparing the phrenic nerve, mobilizing and retracting the subclavian artery and incising the suprapleural (Sibson's) fascia.

LUMBAR SYMPATHECTOMY

Lumbar sympathectomy may be tried for peripheral occlusive vascular disease with absent 'run-off', pregangrene or dry gangrene of the toes. It does not increase blood flow to the muscle but dilates arteriovenous anastomosis, occasionally allowing trophic lesions to heal. Raynaud's syndrome may improve, diabetics often have autosympathectomy and rarely do, and improvement in Buerger's thromboangiitis obliterans is only temporary.

Chemical sympathectomy

Chemical sympathectomy (Fig. 34.1). A 21G spinal needle is inserted at the level of the upper border of L3, a hand's breadth from the midline, directed at the vertebral body. After radiological confirmation of the position, inject 7.5% phenol in 50% glycine and nurse the patient sitting for 6 hours.

Open operation

Open operation is now reserved for younger patients with hyperhidrosis, intractable vasospastic disease and

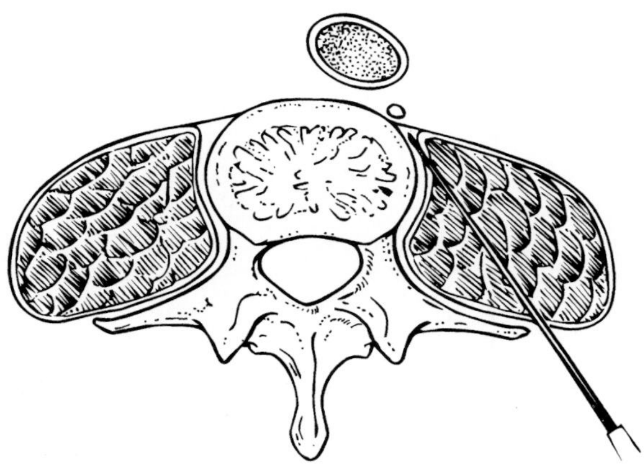

Fig. 34.1 In this posterior approach to chemical lumbar sympathectomy, the retroperitoneal space can be located by a sudden loss of resistance to air injection as the needle is advanced through the psoas fascia.

causalgia. There are usually four ganglia on each side and the second and third are removed. The approach is through an 8–10-cm transverse incision at the level of the umbilicus, starting just medial to the linea semilunaris, Carefully separate the transversalis fascia and muscle without entering the peritoneum and protect the ureters.

FURTHER READING

Cotton LJ, Cross FW 1985 Lumbar sympathectomy for arterial disease. British Journal of Surgery 72:678–683

35

Transplantation

K. Rolles

CONTENTS

INTRODUCTION

Solid whole-organ transplantation has been one of the main events in the evolution of 20th-century patient care. Within the field of general surgery a kidney transplant offers a quality of life unattainable by long-term dialysis, and the lack of long-term artificial support for end-stage disease of the liver, heart and lungs makes it likely that there will be a demand for organ transplantation into the foreseeable future. Immunosuppressive agents that reduce or abolish graft rejection are vital to the success of organ transplantation.

The donor pool comprises brainstem dead, heart-beating 'cadavers' – over 90% of solid-organ donors, usually providing multiple organs; non-heart-beating cadavers, providing suitable organs for kidney and increasingly for liver transplantation; living related donors, such as identical twins, siblings, parents, children, first-order cousins, providing excellent donor organs for kidney transplants and, with appropriate techniques, segments of livers, pancreas and lung which can be grafted; and living unrelated donors such as spouses, partners, friends, altruists and paid donors (illegal in the UK).

Brainstem death must be established by two independent medical practitioners, before organs are removed from a patient with irreversible cerebral destruction, determining that there are absent pupillary reflexes, corneal reflex, caloric response, gag reflexes and spontaneous breathing when disconnected from ventilator.

THE MULTIPLE ORGAN DONOR

It is possible to remove both kidneys, the liver, the pancreas, the small bowel, the heart and both lungs for transplantation from a single donor using techniques that will not interfere with the immediate function of the transplant organs in their respective recipients.

ORGAN PRESERVATION

Cool the organs in situ by infusing large volumes of isotonic cold crystallized solution such as Ringer's lactate, thus reducing the temperature of the perfused organs to 8–15°C (as above). Excise the organs and flush them through once more with approximately 1 litre of a preservation solution (University of Wisconsin solution for the liver and hypertonic citrate solution for the kidneys) and cool them to approximately 0°C in ice over the next few hours.

TISSUE TYPING

Despite 30 years of clinical organ transplantation, the role of human leucocyte antigen (HLA) matching remains controversial and enigmatic. At least four different gene loci on chromosome 6 code for the human major histocompatibility complex (MHC) and are known as HLA, B, C and D.

KIDNEY TRANSPLANTATION

Donor kidneys for transplantation may be obtained from living related donors, living unrelated donors, unrelated brainstem-dead heart-beating cadaver donors and unrelated non-heart-beating cadaver donors. Transplantation currently offers the best chance of long-term survival combined with near-normal quality of life for those suffering from end-stage chronic renal disease, which comprises the indications for transplantation. In living related kidney donation the donor has volunteered to undergo a major surgical operation.

Donor kidneys may be retrieved by the open approach, usually through a muscle-cutting loin incision or, increasingly more frequently, laparoscopically, extra- or transperitoneally. Carefully dissect the kidney free of its perirenal fat and the adrenal gland and gently draw it up into the wound to facilitate dissection of the renal pedicles. Ligate and divide the ureter distal to the pelvic bridge. After excising the kidney flush-cool it via the renal artery with preservation solution at 4°C and double-wrap it in sterile polythene bags placed in ice.

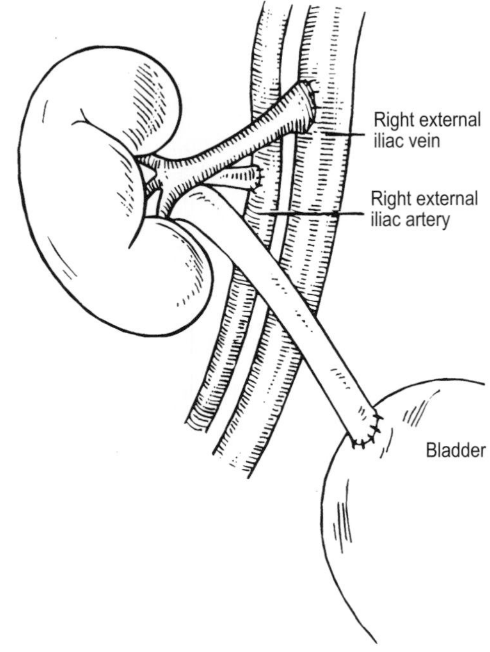

Fig. 35.1 Renal transplantation. The renal vessels have been united end-to-side to the external iliac vessels. The ureter is joined to the dome of the bladder.

KIDNEY TRANSPLANT OPERATION

The donor kidney is reimplanted into the right or left iliac fossa and vascularized from the iliac vessels. This is heterotopic (Greek *heteros* = other + *topos* = a place) transplantation, not into its normal anatomical – orthotopic (Greek *orthos* = straight, right) – position. Pass a urinary catheter and attach it to a 1-litre bag of saline via an infusion line.

Through a 'hockey-stick' incision starting 1 cm above the symphysis pubis and curving laterally to the pararectal line, expose the external iliac vessels extraperitoneally, ligating the inferior epigastric vessels, while controlling the spermatic cord with a nylon tape. Perform an end-to-side anastomosis between the renal vein and the external iliac vein using continuous 5/0 polypropylene or PDS and an end-to-side anastomosis between the donor renal artery and the external iliac artery.

Remove the clamps from the iliac vessels, to perfuse the graft, fill the bladder with physiological saline to distend it. Spatulate the end of the ureter, pass it below the spermatic cord and unite it through a submucosal tunnel to the dome of the bladder, using continuous 4/0 synthetic absorbable suture (Fig. 35.1). Take a renal biopsy before closing the wound in layers over a large silicone tube drain. Monitor the patient to detect and treat delayed function, vascular thrombosis, urinary leakage and acute cellular rejection.

For living related donor kidneys, graft survival is over 90% at 1 year and 80% at 5 years. Cadaver kidney graft survival is 80% at 1 year and 65–70% at 5 years.

LIVER TRANSPLANTATION

More than 125 000 liver transplants have been performed in over 200 liver transplant centres worldwide since Starzl reported the first liver graft in 1963. Ciclosporin has improved survival since 1979. I shall describe the original orthotopic liver transplant procedure.

In 70% of cases transplantation is for end-stage chronic liver disease due to cirrhosis arising from a variety of different causes such as primary biliary cirrhosis, primary sclerosing cholangitis, post-hepatic cirrhosis, autoimmune chronic active hepatitis and alcohol-related liver disease. In approximately 12% it is for primary hepatic malignancy and in another 10% for acute liver failure resulting from fulminant hepatitis, acute (drug) poisoning or idiosyncratic drug reactions. Metabolic diseases account for 6% of cases, including: Wilson's disease, α-antitrypsin deficiency and tyrosinosis, and where a hepatic enzyme defect damages other organs such as primary hyperoxaluria, familial hypercholesterolaemia and some forms of familial amyloidosis; liver transplantation is used as a highly effective form of gene therapy. An 85% 1-year patient survival and 65% 5-year patient survival are currently being achieved by most major liver transplant centres.

Action

1. Through a bilateral subcostal incision with upward extension to the xiphoid, excise the failed liver, retaining the common bile duct, hepatic artery, portal vein, and the cut ends of the inferior vena cava.
2. Begin the reimplantation with the suprahepatic vena caval anastomosis using a continuous 2/0 polypropylene, polydioxanone or polyester suture, then the infrahepatic vena caval anastomosis using 3/0 polypropylene. Anastomose the donor and recipient portal veins end-to-end using 5/0 polypropylene. Reconstruct the hepatic arterial supply as an end-to-end anastomosis between the donor and recipient common hepatic arteries using interrupted 6/0 polypropylene. Reconstruct the biliary tract as an end-to-end, duct-to-duct anastomosis using interrupted 5/0 PDS. Perform a donor cholecystectomy and a liver biopsy.
3. Check for haemostasis, inspecting all anastomoses then close the abdomen in layers over two large silicone tube drains; begin immunosuppressive therapy and antibiotics immediately and check liver function tests and coagulation profiles twice daily.
4. Monitor the patient for bleeding, right pleural effusion, vascular occlusion, acute rejection, and send urine, saliva, faeces, blood and appropriate skin swabs every 48 hours for bacteriological and virological surveillance.

PANCREAS TRANSPLANTATION

Microangiopathy, nephropathy and neuropathy may occur in individuals despite ostensibly good blood sugar control by exogenous insulin.

Transplantation of pancreatic tissue has been performed both clinically and experimentally by transplantation of the whole or part of the pancreas as a solid vascularized organ graft, which includes both endocrine and exocrine components of the gland and transplantation of the insulin-producing tissue only – the islets of Langerhans. Intraportal or intrasplenic injection appear to be the favoured sites of placement for islet grafts at present.

SMALL-BOWEL TRANSPLANTATION

Transplantation of the small bowel may be indicated for small numbers of adults and children who have suffered massive small-bowel loss and are unable to sustain body weight by either enteric feeding or total parental nutrition. In small children, transplantation of the liver together with the small bowel has produced better results than transplantation of the small bowel alone.

Major clinical problems include immunological rejection of the graft, septicaemia, fluid and electrolyte losses, graft-versus-host disease, and technical problems, including vascular thrombosis and torsion of the graft pedicle.

HEART TRANSPLANTATION

More than 50000 transplants have now been performed for ischaemic heart disease and its complications, cardiomyopathy and some cases of congenital heart disease.

Through a median sternotomy having established full cardiopulmonary bypass, excise the recipient's heart across a transatrial plane just dorsal to the atrial appendages, leaving the posterior atrial wall with the orifices of the systemic and pulmonary veins intact. Divide the aorta and pulmonary trunk just distal to their respective valves.

Implant the new heart, which consists of more of the donor atria in order to preserve the sinoatrial node. On completion of the anastomoses, release the aortic clamp and allow the heart to fill via the coronary circulation, displacing air through the left ventricular vent. Place temporary pacing wires in the donor right atrial wall and stop bypass. Remove cannulas, repair the pericardium and close the chest with pericardial drainage.

HEART–LUNG TRANSPLANTATION

Heart–lung transplantation is now a well-established therapy for primary pulmonary hypertension, pulmonary hypertension secondary to Eisenmenger's syndrome, cystic fibrosis and emphysema.

Through a median sternotomy, with cardiopulmonary bypass, excise both lungs and heart of the recipient, avoiding damage to the phrenic nerves or the vagal trunks. Leave the posterior wall of the right atrium intact and in continuity with the superior and inferior venae cavae. Insert the donor heart–lung block. Anastomose right atrium, trachea and aorta in that order, using polypropylene sutures and venting the right and left ventricles as described for the heart graft. On filling the heart by releasing the aortic clamp, the cardiac cycle usually starts spontaneously.

FURTHER READING

Couinaud C 1981 Controlled hepatectomies and exposure of the intrahepatic bile ducts. Couinaud, Paris

Lancet 1976 Diagnosis of brain death (editorial). Lancet ii:1069–1070

Strong RW, Lynch SV, Ong TH et al 1990 Successful liver transplantation from a living donor to her son. New England Journal of Medicine 322:1505–1507

Warnock GL, Kneteman NM, Ryan EA et al 1992 Long term follow-up after transplantation of insulin producing pancreatic islets into patients with type I (insulin dependent) diabetes mellitus. Diabetologia 35:89–95

36

Thorax

T. Treasure, R. R. Kanagasabay

CONTENTS

INTRODUCTION

Acquire an intimate three-dimensional knowledge of the thorax and its contents; you will be dissecting within and around vital structures. If you need to deal with trauma, you should, therefore, be competent to open the chest safely, through an appropriate incision, and perform well-judged surgery. Thoracic and cardiac surgery, however, are highly specialized, depending heavily not only on your competence but also on the supporting team and facilities. If a patient is stable for a while, or can be stabilized, prefer to arrange transfer to an expert centre as the best way to save life and preserve function. In this chapter we aim to guide both your judgement that something surgical needs to be done, and, once embarked upon, how to do it.

The safety margin during intrathoracic dissection is small. The bronchi and vessels are short, their branches close together and they are therefore vulnerable. The patient's respiratory reserve is often compromised. Main pulmonary veins have strong walls but pulmonary arteries are fragile walls, at risk of rupture with sudden heavy loss of blood; gain proximal control if dissection is difficult. For closure of main vessels rely on suture-ligatures or staples not simple ligatures. Avoid breakdown following bronchial closure by accurately closing it, perhaps with staples. Carefully site chest tubes to achieve full re-expansion of the lung and drain fluid and air in the postoperative period.

KEY POINTS Cardiac function

- Learn how to avoid the formation of air embolism by preventing air being sucked into empty veins.
- Familiarize yourself with the speedy, effective management of cardiac arrest.

BRONCHOSCOPY AND MEDIASTINOSCOPY

Fibreoptic bronchoscopy provides tissue for histology, microbiology and to assess operability. It can be passed through the nostril or the mouth, using local anaesthesia augmented with intravenous benzodiazepine sedation and has few contraindications but monitor oxygen saturation. Be wary of taking biopsies from vascular lesions and in patients taking anticoagulants. Aspirate retained secretions not responding to physiotherapy and transnasal or per-oral suction and perform lavage with saline or sodium bicarbonate solution in order to prevent or treat pulmonary atelectasis (Greek *ateles* = incomplete + *ektasis* = stretching out; collapse).

Rigid bronchoscopy requires general anaesthesia; angled telescopes or a flexible bronchoscope can be passed to extend the range of observation. Large biopsies can be removed and effective suckers passed. Pass the bronchoscope with the bevel facing posteriorly over the middle of the tongue until you see the tip of the epiglottis, protecting the teeth from pressure. If you cannot remove an inhaled foreign body carry out thoractomy and bronchotomy.

Mediastinoscopy allows assessment of nodes and masses through a small incision in the suprasternal notch following blunt finger dissection to create a space anterior to the pretracheal fascia then opening and entering within it. The mediastinoscope can be introduced into the space to view, biopsy and remove tissue. Alternatively the mediastinum can be entered through the second intercostal space.

PERIOPERATIVE MANAGEMENT

Preoperatively, following the history and examination, investigate the extent of the disease and exclude or assess co-morbidity, especially to exclude or correct anaemia, diabetes and cardiorespiratory function.

Stop the patient from smoking, order preoperative physiotherapy to increase diaphragmatic movement and clear sputum, if necessary giving antibiotics and bronchodilators such as salbutamol. Prescribe subcutaneous heparin, to be continued until the patient is fully mobile.

Postoperatively, aim to restore full lung expansion by relieving pain and by physiotherapy, antibiotics and early ambulation, with progress assessed by chest X-rays usually on the first, third and fifth postoperative days. Pain relief may be by extrapleural catheter-infused local anaesthesia, patient-controlled and oral analgesics. Apical and basal underwater-sealed chest drains may or may not require gentle suction at 10–15 mmHg to keep the lung expanded and they can be removed when drainage and air leaks stop. Monitor and treat cardiac irregularities – atrial fibrillation may signal hypoxia or mediastinal shift. Expect minimal air emphysema but sudden and severe accumulation suggests a blocked drainage tube or fresh air leak.

If bleeding exceeds 200–300 ml in the first 2–3 hours check blood coagulation, replace the loss, and re-explore if it continues. Empyema is infection of retained pleural fluid; drain it, employ lavage, instil antibiotics and be prepared to create open drainage if necessary. Bronchopleural fistula is rare; drain the space and re-suture the bronchial stump. Treat respiratory failure in a dependency unit; continuous positive pressure airways pressure (CPAP) may help.

CHEST DRAINS

Avoid morbidity from inappropriate, imperfect insertion of chest drains, which are usually inserted to drain air or liquids such as blood, effusion, pus or chyle. Air can be drained by placing the tube in the apex and fluid is drained basally. Provided the pleural space is not loculated the actual position is probably not important. To avoid injury to underlying structures, insert drains into the 'triangle of safety', bounded by the anterior axillary line, the mid-axillary line and the level of the nipple. Remember how high the diaphragm rises.

Lie the patient back on a pillow with the arm abducted, providing access to the target triangle. Clean the skin, infiltrate local anaesthetic generously but within the limits imposed by the patient's weight. Wait for at least 10 minutes. Make a short skin incision sufficient to admit a finger. Using a blunt dissector or artery forceps, dissect down to the pleura immediately above a rib and enter the chest by blunt dissection. Feel the pleura 'give' as a distinct 'pop'. Insert a finger to confirm that you are safely in the chest. Place a simple suture across the midpoint of the incision to close the wound when the drain is removed and tie a knot in the end. Place another suture at the corner of the incision to secure the drain. Now insert the drain, with the aid of a Roberts clamp if necessary.

UNDERWATER SEAL DRAINAGE

Connect the outer end of the drainage tube to a long tube passing well below the level of a measured amount of water in the bottle so that the fluid provides a seal preventing entry of air into the chest. Check that drainage is free by noting the fluid swing in the long tube on inspiration, provided no suction is connected. Resistance to drainage increases as the bottle fills with fluid. Change the bottle once it is more than half full to ensure good continued drainage.

Suction may be helpful where there is a pneumothorax and the lung does not inflate with simple drainage, after performing a pleurodesis (Greek *desis* = a binding together) or when draining a haemothorax or empyema, to help avoid the drains blocking. Connect the short tube, which allows escape of air, to a source of suction; this can be increased up to a negative pressure of 20 cmH_2O or 20 mmHg (3–5 kPa). Suction is never important in immediate management and has its own dangers. Never turn off suction while leaving the apparatus connected to the bottle, since the drain is effectively blocked. Ensure that the suction device is low-pressure, high-volume to prevent obstruction. Wall suction with a regulated adapter is ideal. Never apply suction to drains inserted following pneumonectomy since it produces mediastinal shift.

Clamping a chest drain is almost never indicated and is potentially dangerous. Never clamp drains while patients are being transferred. Never raise the drainage bottle above the patient or fluid may enter the chest.

POSTEROLATERAL THORACOTOMY

This is the usual route of access for pulmonary operations, some oesophageal operations, posterior, middle mediastinal and mainly unilateral anterior mediastinal lesions and for repair of coarctation, division of patent ductus arteriosus, and thoracic aneurysms.

Access

1 Place the patient in the lateral position with the chest arched over a soft pad, such as a Holmes Sellors support. Position the arms and legs as in Figure 36.1. Approach all standard lobectomies through the fifth interspace. Modify the approach if you predict specific problems such as pleural involvement or adhesions at the apex. Cut the skin in a smooth curve, running from midway between the midline and medial border of the scapula posteriorly, skirting the angle of the scapula by 2.5 cm, and passing forward to the anterior axillary line. Divide the muscles using the diathermy point, coagulating cut vessels. They are arranged in two layers: the superficial layer of trapezius and latissimus dorsi, the deeper layer of the rhomboid and serratus anterior. Preserve the serratus anterior muscle almost intact by dividing this layer through the aponeurosis below the muscle fibres, right to the anterior extent of the wound. We usually leave it completely intact.

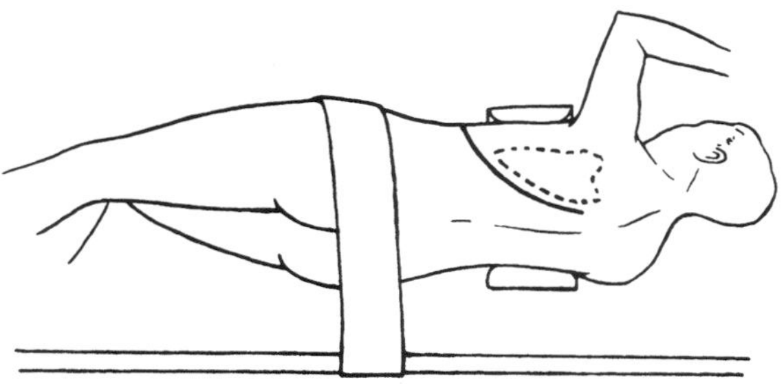

Fig. 36.1 Position for posterolateral thoracotomy.

2 Count the ribs from the apex by passing a hand up under the scapula. It is difficult to identify the first rib and the uppermost rib you can feel is usually the second. The third rib has a characteristically flatter, broader shape. Divide the periosteum of the upper border of the sixth rib with the diathermy point. Strip the periosteum from its upper border, using a curved rougine, working posteroanteriorly. Alternatively divide the intercostal muscle above the rib using diathermy without stripping the periosteum.

3 Rib resection or division is rarely necessary provided you free the costotransverse ligament posteriorly using a notched chisel and then open the retractor gradually and gently. Open the pleura along the length of the wound after warning the anaesthetist to allow the lung to fall away. The periosteal separation may be extended anteriorly deep to the wound. Insert a rib spreader. Divide light or filmy adhesions with scissors or diathermy. Use a mounted gauze swab and blunt dissection to strip the lung in the extrapleural plane when widespread marked adhesions are present. Having found the plane of dissection, stay in it. A hot pack controls diffuse oozing; coagulate bleeding points with diathermy. The extrapleural strip needs be over an area of dense localized adherence only if the rest of the lung is free.

Closure

1 Insert an anterior apical drain for air and basal drains anterolaterally two or three spaces below the wound. with the skin and pleural holes offset to direct the drain and create a tunnel for a better seal. Pass the apical tube up the apex of the chest, usually sited anteriorly to the basal drain (Fig. 36.2). Position the drain exit sites sufficiently far anterior so that the patient will not lie in discomfort on them.

2 Use a Holmes Sellors approximator to draw the ribs together and close the intercostal layer with a continuous suture of absorbable synthetic suture, approximating the edge of the stripped intercostal layer above to the intercostal muscle below the rib that has been stripped. This intercostal closure is usually sufficient, avoiding the need for pericostal sutures which often cause chronic post-thoracotomy pain from nerve

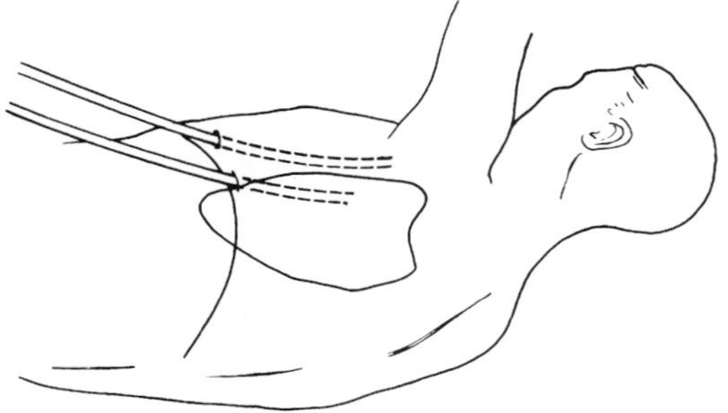

Fig. 36.2 Siting of drainage tubes.

entrapment. Unite each muscle layer with a continuous absorbable suture.

ANTEROLATERAL THORACOTOMY

This provides access to the heart, pericardium and lung and may be used for open cardiac massage in cardiac arrest and for pericardial drainage. Use a shorter version for open-lung biopsy in diffuse pulmonary disease. Lay the patient rotated obliquely with the ipsilateral (Latin *ipse* = self, same) hip and shoulder supported on pillows or sandbags. Elevate the ipsilateral arm, carefully avoiding nerve traction. Usually employ the fifth intercostal space and follow the line of the appropriate rib, which can readily be counted anteriorly. In the female, curve the incision below the breast. Start the incision close to the midline and extend it to the axilla, passing 2.5 cm below the angle of the scapula if you need additional length. Divide pectoralis major muscle in the line of the incision; split the serratus anterior muscle along the line of the rib selected. Divide the periosteum using the diathermy point and strip it from the upper border of the rib posteroanteriorly. Open the pleura in the depth of this layer. Take care to avoid the internal mammary vessels close to the sternum. Open the pericardium anteriorly to the phrenic nerve, as this gives better access.

MEDIAN STERNOTOMY

This usually provides best access for cardiac operations using cardiopulmonary bypass, producing less postoperative pain and respiratory upset. A shorter version allows exposure of the trachea for resection of a stricture or tumour. Use it to remove anterior mediastinal tumours such as thymomata, germ cell tumours and rarely for retrosternal goitre. Bilateral bullous lung disease and pulmonary metastases may be approached but access to the left lower lobe is limited by the heart. The incision can be performed rapidly using appropriate equipment. In an emergency if a sternal saw is unavailable, prefer an anterior thoracotomy.

Place the patient supine with the arms by the side. For cardiac surgery attach ECG electrodes to shoulders and chest wall, percutaneously insert a radial artery catheter for arterial pressure monitoring and a central venous pressure line via the internal jugular vein. Insert a urinary catheter, rectal and nasopharyngeal temperature probes. Prepare the skin to allow access to groins and also to the leg in coronary artery bypass operations. In a patient with a stocky neck place a sandbag under the shoulder blades and extend the neck to improve exposure.

Action

1. Incise from the lower margin of the suprasternal notch to the xiphoid process. Divide the subcutaneous tissue with the diathermy point down to the sternal periosteum to maintain haemostasis. Keep between the pectoralis major muscles and precisely mark the midline of the sternum with the diathermy. The sternum is least wide at the second space. Carefully avoid veins that lie in the immediate suprasternal region by keeping close to the upper border of the bone. There is also a large vein frequently crossing the xiphisternal junction; control it with diathermy. Free tissues from the deep surface of the xiphisternum by passing a finger up from below, avoiding the danger of catching a fold of pericardium in the saw with risk of injury to the heart.
2. Divide the sternum longitudinally using a reciprocating saw, hugging the posterior surface to avoid damaging the heart, ascending aorta or left innominate vein. You may use a Gigli saw, drawing it down from above after passing up extra-long Roberts forceps behind the sternum hugging its posterior surface. You may also use an oscillating saw. Seal periosteal vessels on both aspects of the sternum with diathermy. If possible, avoid pressing in bone wax to control bleeding from exposed marrow. Insert a self-retaining retractor, dissect between the lobes of the thymus and carefully incise the pericardium in the midline. If the heart is not visible, moving freely behind the pericardium, suspect

pericardial adhesions. Extend the incision up to the reflection on the aorta, avoiding the left innominate vein, and down to the diaphragm. Sew the pericardial edges to the skin to form a well and improve the exposure of the heart.

Closure

If you opened the pericardium, introduce pericardial and anterior mediastinal drains (24–28F catheter) through separate skin incisions below the xiphoid process and through separate openings in the rectus sheath. Using a heavy trocar-pointed needle, or awl if the specialized sutures are not available, pass non-ferrous wire sutures through each side of the sternum. Firmly close the sternum by twisting the wire. Alternatively, pass the needle close to the edge of the sternum, from the second space caudally, avoiding the internal mammary vessels. Approximate the muscle and the subcutaneous layers with polyglactin 910 (Vicryl) sutures, 1 and 00, respectively. Suture the linea alba accurately to avoid an incisional hernia.

PNEUMONECTOMY

This is commonly performed for carcinoma involving upper and lower lobes, either because it crosses the fissure or because it impinges on both lobar bronchi. It is rarely necessary nowadays for destruction of a lung by tuberculosis, other infections or bronchiectasis. Employ a posterolateral thoracotomy through the fifth space. If the chest wall is fixed, be prepared to excise the pleura to free the lung. Rarely you need to resect a portion of the chest wall before assessing the site, extent and involvement of disease.

Dissect inside the adventitia and divide the pulmonary artery between ligatures or preferably oversew with 4/0 vascular suture. We recommend using a vascular clamp such as a Satinsky. If necessary, divide the left artery close to the main trunk after dividing the ligamentum arteriosum while preserving the recurrent laryngeal nerve. Beware! The left pulmonary artery is very short. Divide the pulmonary veins, extrapericardially or after opening the pericardium for easier access, between ligatures. Isolate and divide the bronchus close to the carina using a stapler, a bronchus clamp or open division with direct suture. Divide the inferior pulmonary ligament. Do not routinely insert a drain; if you do, never apply suction to it following pneumonectomy; remove it on the first morning postoperation.

Carefully close the intercostal layer to avoid leakage of fluid into the muscle layers. Routinely examine the patient to assess the position of the mediastinum and order a postoperative chest X-ray to confirm your findings. If there is gross shift towards the operated side, instil air under strict aseptic precautions, using a syringe, filter and three-way tap.

LOBECTOMY

This is the preferred operation for bronchial carcinoma, ideally when the lesion is sited peripherally in the lobe, for resection of localized bronchiectasis not controlled by conservative measures and for resection of tuberculous disease which has not responded fully to antituberculous chemotherapy. Each lobectomy has individual variations dependent upon the relevant anatomical features. As an example, perform a right posterolateral thoracotomy through the fifth intercostal space. Check for enlarged nodes and assess the disease before dissecting the hilum anteriorly to expose the superior pulmonary vein. Find the middle lobe vein inferiorly and isolate the main portion of the upper lobe vein superiorly for ligation. Ligate the segmental branches distally and divide the vein. Take care posteriorly in the dissection as the main right pulmonary artery trunk lies deep to the vein. Display the upper branch of the right pulmonary artery superiorly to the vein and separate it from the superior vena cava anteriorly. Dissect the artery in the subadventitial plane and divide it between ligatures; this branch supplies the apical and anterior segments. Display the main trunk. Look for the recurrent branch to the posterior segment and, if you see it, divide it between ligatures. Expose the right upper lobe bronchus by dissecting the pleura over its posterior aspect. Ligate the bronchial artery branch to the upper lobe bronchus and ligate it or seal it with diathermy. Pass an O'Shaughnessey forceps around the upper lobe bronchus as close to the main bronchus as possible to divide it, using staples or sutured closure, before separating the lobe from the lower lobe posteriorly and the middle lobe anteriorly. Lightly suture the middle lobe, if it is freely mobile, to the lower lobe to prevent it from becoming rotated and necrotic.

Other lobectomies are left upper, left lower and middle. Sleeve resection may avoid pneumonectomy if carcinoma extends too close to the main bronchus. Segmental resection allows the removal of wedges for small peripheral carcinomas, metastases, tuberculosis, abscess and bronchiectasis.

COMPLICATIONS OF CHEST TRAUMA

Patients with chest injuries frequently have multiple injuries that all require treatment. Immediately decide the correct priority for treating multiple injuries. A valuable system is the advanced trauma life support (ATLS) protocol.

Rib fractures usually require only adequate analgesia, if necessary with intercostal nerve block or patient-controlled intravenous analgesia, and physiotherapy.

Multiple fractures may result in a *flail or paradoxical segment*. A portion of chest wall becomes completely mobile, embarrassing respiration, often associated with underlying pulmonary contusion. Treatment of the flail segment and the underlying contusion are supportive. Ventilation is often required.

A breach of integrity of the chest wall producing a *sucking chest wound* leads to a pneumothorax. Tension pneumothorax is signalled by absence of air entry, shift of the mediastinum to the contralateral side, raised jugular venous pressure and incipient circulatory collapse. Cover any sucking chest wound with an airtight dressing once you have established adequate intercostal chest drainage.

Lung lacerations may be caused by fractured ribs protruding into the chest cavity. The resulting pneumothorax often responds to simple drainage, but large air leaks may require open repair, particularly if the lung remains collapsed. Repair the laceration.

Diaphragmatic injury is often overlooked and should be suspected in any patient presenting with major chest trauma who has a poorly defined hemidiaphragm, or basal chest shadowing. Repair it using direct suture, augmented if necessary with polypropylene mesh.

Major vascular trauma is usually associated with multiple injuries. The most serious is aortic transection. Approach it through left thoracotomy. If you do not have the expertise or equipment, you can only clamp above and below the tear.

Penetrating stab wounds or perforating wounds demand exploration only if there is clinical evidence of serious internal damage or bleeding and the chest X-ray is satisfactory. Note the direction of the wound to estimate which structures are at risk.

Wounds of the heart and pericardium produce haemopericardium and evidence of cardiac tamponade. Pericardial aspiration is a temporary measure before exposing the heart through a left anterior, median sternotomy or clamshell approach to suture the defect or apply a Dacron, Teflon or pericardial patch.

ASPIRATION OF THE PERICARDIUM

Perform this for cardiac tamponade resulting from the accumulation of blood following trauma, or fluid developing as a result of pericardial inflammation. Sit the patient up at 45° (Fig. 36.3). Confirm the clinical diagnosis with echocardiography. Infiltrate the skin below the xiphisternum and to the left of the midline with local anaesthetic. Advance the needle towards the right shoulder; the inferior aspect of the pericardium has a definite resistance. Push the needle through the pericardium and aspirate the fluid. It is possible to introduce a plastic catheter such as Intracath through a larger-bore needle or a small cannula if aspiration needs to be maintained. Leave a pericardial drain in situ for at least 24 hours to limit further re-accumulation, and to encourage obliteration of the space.

MISCELLANEOUS

Empyema thoracis

Empyema thoracis is pus in the pleural cavity following pneumonia, oesophageal perforation or thoracic operations. Antibiotic therapy has modified the presentation of this condition. Confirm the diagnosis radiologically, by ultrasound and by aspiration. An intercostal catheter may effectively drain thin pus, as is often the case in postoperative patients.

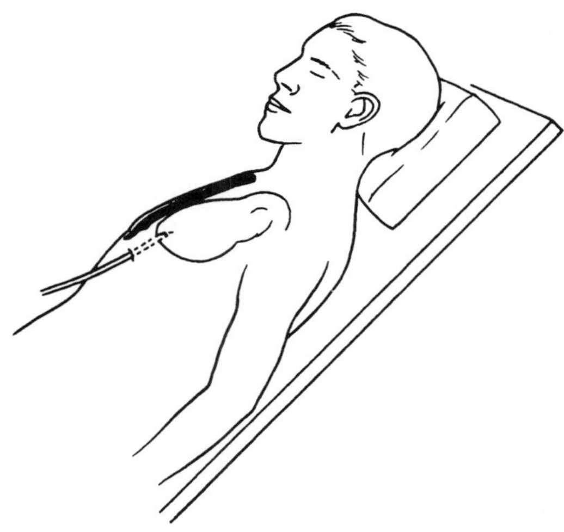

Fig. 36.3 Technique of aspiration of the pericardium.

Insertion of intercostal catheter

Use the chest X-ray, ultrasound or CT scan to establish the most dependent point of the cavity to be drained. The patient is semirecumbent, rolled away from the affected side. Under local anaesthesia, insert the tube anterior to the mid-axillary line and tunnelled into the bottom of the cavity, which is usually more posterior. Connect the catheter to the drainage bottle and underwater seal. Apply suction if necessary.

Open drainage by rib resection

Open drainage by rib resection is largely being replaced by modern tube drains and antibiotics. Ensure that the lung is adherent to the chest wall around the cavity. Make a 5-cm incision in the line of a rib, insert a self-retaining retractor and divide the muscles with diathermy to expose the ribs. Resect 2–3 cm of the lowest appropriate rib after checking by aspiration. Open the cavity, remove the coagulum and thickened pleura for histological examination, and pus for bacteriological culture. Suck out and remove fibrin masses, insert a multiply fenestrated drain tube securely, and subsequently apply suction.

Excision of the empyema and decortication

Through a posterolateral thoracotomy free the lung and empyema in the extrapleural plane.

Spontaneous pneumothorax

Spontaneous pneumothorax is commonly seen in tall, thin, young adults usually from ruptured apical bullae in the upper lobe. Closure of the leak is by stapling or sutures, or pleural adhesions are induced, for example by chemical pleurodesis.

Lung biopsy

Lung biopsy is often useful in diagnosis of suspected interstitial lung disease. An open procedure may be carried out by the posterior approach through the auscultatory triangle. For a very sick patient use a submammary approach.

Pulmonary embolectomy

Pulmonary embolectomy is rarely required, although pulmonary embolism is relatively common, from multiple risk factors for deep venous thrombosis such as immobility, malignancy, pelvic or orthopaedic surgery. Surgery may benefit patients with incipient or established circulatory collapse although interventional radiology and catheter disobliteration of emboli is an alternative. Through a median sternotomy place two stay stitches side by side on the main pulmonary artery and vertically incise between them. Extract the clot and close, before aggressively replacing circulating volume, and achieving adequate oxygenation and anticoagulation.

Thoracoscopy

Procedures that can be performed in this manner include diagnostic pleural biopsy, drainage of pleural effusion and pleurodesis, lung biopsy, evacuation of a haemothorax and drainage of an empyema. Sympathectomy is described in Chapter 34. Make a short skin incision, and with blunt artery forceps, dissect down to the pleura immediately above a rib and enter the chest by blunt dissection. Insert a finger to confirm that you are safely in the chest. Insert the port and thoracoscope. Drain pleural effusions and break down thin loculi or adhesions with the sucker tip. Take pleural biopsies. If the diagnosis of malignancy is obvious from the macroscopic appearance then a pleurodesis can be performed by insufflating talc at the same operation.

37

Head and neck

M. P. Stearns, R. W. R. Farrell, M. Hobsley

CONTENTS

GENERAL PRINCIPLES

Detailed knowledge of anatomy is crucial since many important structures are crowded into a small volume such as the facial nerve, recurrent laryngeal nerve and internal carotid artery. Always refresh your memory before performing a new or unfamiliar operation and be willing to seek advice and help from a plastic, thoracic, dental colleague, neurosurgeon or otolaryngologist.

Anticipate risks of airway blockage by insisting on endotracheal intubation for all but the simplest procedures; respiratory problems are infrequent and infective, gastrointestinal and thromboembolic complications are rare.

Because of the generous blood supply, even massive tissue resections are well tolerated, healing is usually by first intention and skin grafts survive well but primary haemorrhage is an increased risk. Hypotensive anaesthesia may reduce blood loss but delay closure until the patient's blood pressure has returned to normal. Control large vessels by doubly ligating them before dividing them. Venous pressure is kept low by maintaining a clear airway, keeping arterial carbon dioxide low, by raising the patient's head, thus minimizing venous bleeding. Use diathermy carefully, preferring cutting diathermy which restricts the zone heated by it. Anticipate likely blood loss and be prepared to replace it. After operation use suction drainage to obliterate the dead space.

PAROTIDECTOMY

Assess a parotid lump before operation to identify pain and facial nerve palsy suggestive of malignancy, to be confirmed with fine-needle aspiration cytology; needle biopsy is debatable. Most parotid neoplasms are benign. The facial nerve and its five main branches run through the substance of the parotid salivary gland (Fig. 37.1) and are at risk in any parotidectomy. Plan to expose the nerve and its branches at an early stage, although you may need to sacrifice a nerve to excise a lump with a wide margin of normal tissue, in which case repair the gap with a graft from the great auricular nerve. Warn the patient of the possibility beforehand and monitor the nerve with electromyography. Access the gland with an S-shaped cervicomastoid–facial incision. Deepen it along the anterior surface of the cartilaginous external auditory meatus to identify the facial nerve.

Action

As a rule dissection is carried out after exposing, preserving and mobilizing the branches of the facial nerve over the

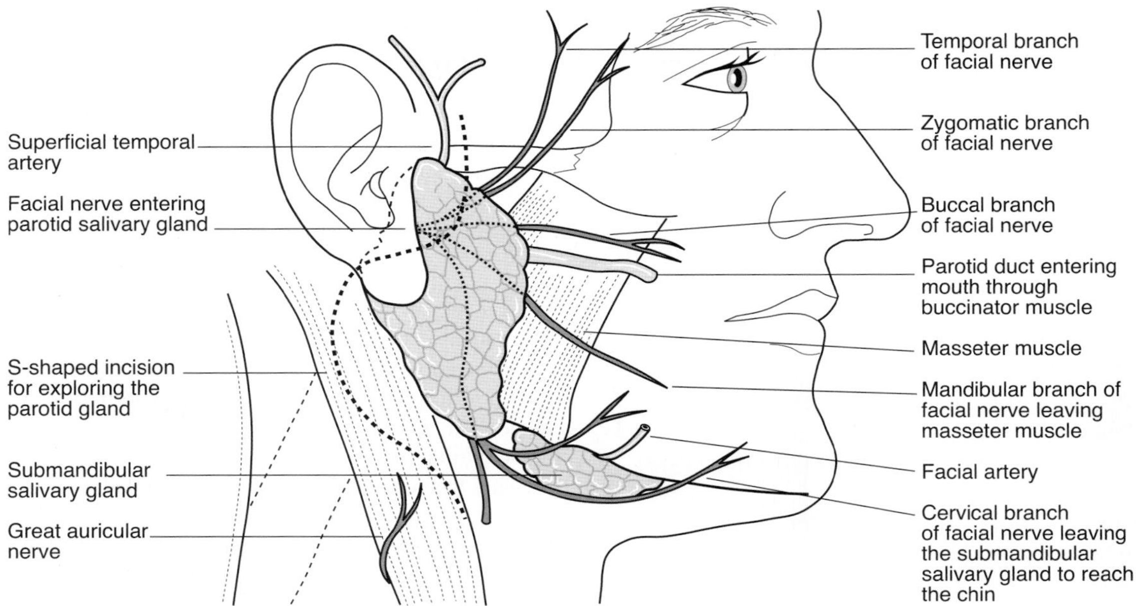

Fig. 37.1 Parotid and submandibular salivary glands. The facial nerve enters from the depths posteriorly into the parotid salivary gland, dividing into temporal, zygomatic, buccal, mandibular and cervical branches within the gland. The heavy broken line indicates the incision for parotid exploration.

area to be resected. This may be over the whole surface for a superficial parotidectomy for recurrent parotitis from a stone in the salivary duct; it may be localized to the area when excising a lump such as an adenoma with the widest possible margin of healthy tissue to avoid spilling and implanting adenoma cells, risking recurrence.

You may explore the lower pole of the parotid to determine if a lump is, or is not, in the parotid gland.

Radical parotidectomy entails the sacrifice of the facial nerve if this, or its main divisions, are surrounded by tumour. You also need to doubly ligate and divide the external carotid artery and the accompanying vein below the gland and the superficial temporal and maxillary vessels.

OPERATIONS ON SALIVARY DUCTS WITHIN THE MOUTH

Parotid duct

Parotid duct stone impacted at the orifice can be removed from within the mouth after cutting down on it (Fig. 37.2). Do not let it slip back. You have cut through at the oral and ductal mucosa; sew them together (stomatoplasty)

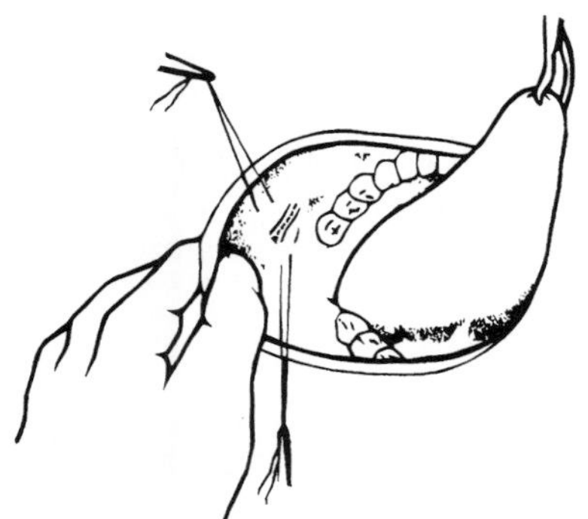

Fig. 37.2 The approach to the right parotid duct orifice. The dental prop in the left side of the mouth is not shown. The tongue is retracted to the opposite side with the towel clip. The operator pulls the angle of the mouth towards himself and at the same time pushes the cheek inwards to make the papillary region prominent inside the mouth; the assistant helps in achieving the latter effect by pulling on the two stay sutures. The dotted line indicates the incision to be made through the mucosa of the cheek and the mucosa of the wall of the duct.

to enlarge the parotid duct orifice, either to enable a calculus in the parotid duct to be passed more easily or to prevent a stricture forming. Do not pass sutures or ligatures round the duct for fear of injuring branches of the facial nerve.

Submandibular duct

Submandibular duct stone can be prevented from falling back from the intraoral orifice by under-running the duct behind it with a suture which is gently lifted to kink the duct. Cut down onto the stone, lift it out, remove the ligatures and leave the duct open.

SUBMANDIBULAR SIALOADENECTOMY

Submandibular sialoadenectomy (Greek *sialon* = saliva) may be necessary if a deeply placed, inaccessible stone causes chronic infection. Access is through crease incision through skin and platysma about 5 cm below the lower border of the mandible. The mandibular branch of the facial nerve is at risk. You need to include the facial artery and vein with the gland, and the gland extends on the deep aspect of the mylohyoid muscle, beyond which you must transect the duct. Sialoadenectomy for tumour includes resection of a segment of the mandible.

EXCISION BIOPSY OF A BASAL CELL CARCINOMA OF THE FACE

A rodent ulcer may be treated by resection with a wide margin of normal tissue both in depth and around it, preferably 1 cm but near the eye, 0.5 cm, or by radiotherapy. Refer tumours near the eye and nostril to specialists. Primary closure is possible after excising a small ulcer, otherwise apply a cosmetically preferable full-thickness skin graft. Plan and mark out an oval aligned with the skin tension lines.

Cut vertically through the skin along the oval line to expose fat. Working from alternate ends excise the tumour with adequate depth. Stop bleeding. Cut a petroleum gauze pattern of the defect to use in planning a full-thickness graft from just below the clavicle or in the groove between the back of the pinna and the scalp. Excise all fat from the graft and sew it into the defect, intending to have sufficient tension to prevent haematoma formation.

LOCAL EXCISION OR BIOPSY OF AN INTRAORAL LESION

Totally excise small lesions in the surface of the oral mucosa of cheek, tongue, palate, floor of mouth or inner surface of the lips, with an appropriate margin of normal tissue. Obtain absolute haemostasis before closing, in this very vascular tissue. For larger lesions perform biopsy in continuity with normal tissue. You may insert sutures of 3/0 absorbable material beforehand, to tie after excising the biopsy.

PARTIAL GLOSSECTOMY

Excise small lesions of the anterior two-thirds of the tongue using laser-cutting. Excise larger lesions with a wide 0.8 mm margin, since tumour planes in the tongue are indiscrete. Preserve length in preference to width and also mobility. Control bleeding during wedge excision of the tip of the tongue by compression between fingers and thumb and approximate the muscles with absorbable 3/0 stitches before closing the mucosa.

WEDGE EXCISION OF THE LIP

Early tumours can be removed with a wide margin. Close the defect with 3/0 absorbable sutures for the muscles and mucosa, and fine non-absorbable stitches for the skin and vermillion border.

EXCISION OF CYST, SINUS AND FISTULA IN THE NECK

Submental cyst

Submental cyst in the midline above the hyoid may be a dermoid cyst but if it rises on swallowing it is a thyroglossal cyst. Remove the cyst through a transverse crease incision centred over it, raising upper and lower skin flaps and underlying fascia to expose the superficial surface. Now elevate the cyst; watch for fibrous extensions down to the hyoid or upwards between the mylohyoid muscle from a thyroglossal cyst. Close with a suction drain.

Thyroglossal sinus and fistula

The thyroid isthmus and part of the lateral lobes migrate down from the foramen caecum (Latin = blind) of the tongue, intimately related to the hyoid bone. Excise a sinus opening within a horizontal ellipse of skin and follow the track up, excising a 1-cm portion of the anterior part of the hyoid bone, coring out a cylinder of muscle of the tongue for a further 2 cm while your assistant pushes down the back of the tongue with a finger in the patient's mouth.

Branchial cyst, sinus or fistula

Branchial cyst, sinus or fistula (Greek *branchion* = a gill) develops if a gill cleft remains patent. A cyst lies deep to the junction of the middle and upper thirds of the sternomastoid muscle, usually the second cleft. The complete lesion is a fistula with one opening in the pharynx near the posterior pillar of the fauces and the other in the skin at the junction of middle and lower thirds of the anterior border of the sternomastoid muscle. In branchial sinus there is a lower opening but no communication with the pharynx.

Excise a branchial cyst through a horizontal, skin crease incision over the swelling, through platysma muscle and deep cervical fascia to reach the thin surface of the cyst. Gently sweep away the surrounding areolar tissue to excise it, guarding the division of the common carotid artery, vagus and hypoglossal nerves deep to it, and avoid rupturing the cyst.

Include the external opening of a branchial sinus or fistula in an ellipse of skin, and follow a fistulous track usually between the internal and external carotid arteries to the middle constrictor muscle.

EXCISION BIOPSY OF CERVICAL LYMPH NODE

First revise the anatomy (Fig. 37.3); the accessory nerve in the posterior triangle is often at risk. Prefer general anaesthesia. Make a skin crease incision over the lump, through the fascia to the surface of the gland, gently inserting small curved artery forceps tips under the overlying fascia, separating and lifting it to cut safely. Do not manipulate the gland with instruments or damage it. Seal the vessels feeding it, using diathermy. Cut the removed node into two equal parts, one into formol saline for histology, the other sent sterile for culture, including for tuberculosis.

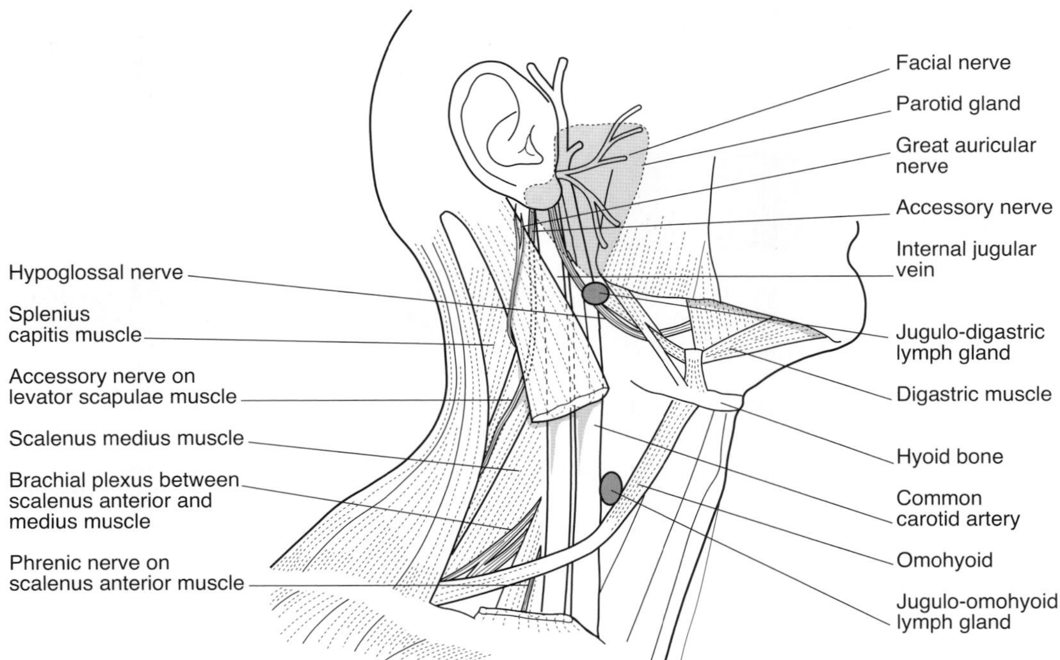

Fig. 37.3 Structures within the neck. The sternomastoid muscle has been resected.

SCALENE NODE BIOPSY

Nodes lie in a pad of fat, superficial to the lower end of the anterior scalenus (Greek *skalenos* = uneven; triangle with unequal sides) muscle, often involved by diseases of the lungs or mediastinum. Unless the disease is on the left, biopsy the right nodes through a 5-cm horizontal skin-crease incision 2.5 cm above the clavicle, between the sternal head of sternomastoid and medial border of trapezius muscles, through the clavicular head of sternomastoid muscle and through platysma muscle. Doubly ligate and divide the external jugular vein – the internal jugular vein is at risk just beneath.

Identify scalenus anterior muscle with overlying transverse cervical vessels, fat pad covering lymph nodes, then fascia covering phrenic nerve. Elevate and free the fat pad containing the lymph nodes from the fascia overlying the phrenic nerve, retracting omohyoid muscle; medially lies the internal jugular vein, laterally lies the brachial plexus. If lymph accumulates, find and tie off the divided duct.

OPERATIONS ON TUBERCULOUS CERVICAL LYMPH NODES

Tuberculous cervical lymph nodes occur as undiagnosed lumps and as cold abscesses. Never start chemotherapy without bacteriological diagnosis. Aspirate a fluctuant mass through healthy skin and a long track. Operate on a mass increasing in size, not responding to chemotherapy, or involving skin. Excise mass, drain and scrape out abscess cavity. Take care; nodes in the anterior triangle may be adherent to the jugular vein, the common carotid artery and its two branches, and the vagus nerve. The jugulodigastric group may be adherent to the hypoglossal, accessory and glossopharyngeal nerves. Involved lymph nodes in the posterior triangle may lie around the lower part of the accessory nerve.

BLOCK DISSECTION OF CERVICAL LYMPH NODES

Many carcinomas of the head and neck metastasize to the cervical lymph nodes. Whatever is the best mode of treatment for the primary, control of affected cervical lymph nodes is best obtained by excising them, but only if the primary is cured or curable, and there are no distant metastases. Your intention is to remove en bloc the connective tissue containing the nodes from the anterior and posterior triangles, extending from the clavicle below to the base of skull above. You may perform it as an extension of parotidectomy, glossectomy, mandibulectomy, laryngectomy appropriately, to create flaps that lay open the neck on the side of the growth.

As a separate procedure following apparent cure of the primary tumour, create a Y-shaped incision with equal limbs from the submental, mastoid and midclavicle. Divide the clavicular and sternal heads of sternomastoid muscle, inferior belly of omhyoid muscle. Doubly ligate and divide internal jugular vein, preserving the thoracic duct on the left. If indicated, divide the thyroid isthmus, and associated vessels to include in the block. Strip up the sternomastoid muscle, internal jugular vein, with contents of the submental and submandibular triangles, dividing Wharton's duct but usually preserving the brachial plexus, vagus and phrenic nerves, and carotid arteries. Dissect the block up to the base of the skull to excise it.

FURTHER READING

Jones AS, Cook JA, Phillips DE 1993 Squamous cell carcinoma presenting as an enlarged cervical lymph node: the occult primary. Cancer 72:1756–1761

Radkowski D, Arnold J, Healy GB 1991 Thyroglossal duct remnants: pre-operative evaluation and management. Archives of Otolaryngology Head and Neck Surgery 117:1378–1381

38

Orthopaedics and trauma: amputations

N. Goddard, G. Harper

CONTENTS

INTRODUCTION

Approximately 5500 amputations are performed each year in England. The number steadily increases as the population ages; 75% of the patients are over 60 years of age, and 65% are men. The intention is to excise all disease and restore maximal limb function. The main indications for amputation are arterial or venous vascular disease, diabetes (diabetes and vascular disease together account for about 85% of amputations), trauma (10%), tumours (3%), infection (now only 1.5%), neurological causes such as nerve injury and its secondary effects, and congenital problems. Major upper limb amputations are rarely required (only 3% of the total).

In case of doubt about the necessity for amputation obtain advice from a senior colleague. Before elective operations ask advice from the regional limb-fitting centre on the best level and type of procedure and involve the skills of nurses, physiotherapists, occupational therapists, prosthetists and social workers. Operate using general anaesthesia whenever possible.

The level of amputation and type of prosthesis are influenced by the viability of soft tissues, underlying disease, functional requirements including comfort and appearance. Energy conservation is important when planning lower-limb amputation and bilateral below-knee amputation is less tiring than unilateral above-knee amputation. Try to preserve the knee joint and the epiphysis in children, appraise the blood supply from skin colour changes, shiny atrophic appearance, lack of hair growth and skin temperature. Be willing to order transcutaneous Doppler recordings and measurement of the ankle–brachial index, thermography, radioactive xenon clearance and transcutaneous PO_2 measurement.

Assess the bone from radiographs taken in two planes at right angles to each other, tomograms or a radioisotope bone scan. Confirm malignancy with a biopsy and stage it with computed tomography (CT) and magnetic resonance imaging (MRI) since accurate staging may make possible limb-sparing surgery. Obtain informed consent after explaining possible complications including the possible need to perform a higher amputation than intended.

Mark the proposed skin flaps, approximately as long as the base is wide at the level of bone section, leaving them too long rather than too short; following trauma, preserve all viable skin to create an adequate stump. In the presence of vascular disease do not undermine the edges of the flaps and always handle the flaps gently.

Order prophylactic antibiotics: penicillin (or erythromycin) plus one other broad-spectrum antibiotic. Swab and culture any wounds preoperatively. Mark and clean the limb and seal off the infected or necrotic areas and arrange for the disposal of the amputated limb.

Use a tourniquet except in peripheral vascular disease. Exsanguinate the limb by elevation for 2–4 minutes rather than an Esmarch bandage. Prepare the skin and apply the drapes.

Action

1 Wherever possible include underlying muscles in the flap (myoplastic flap), to maximize skin blood supply

and covers and protects the stump. Muscles provide power, stabilization and proprioception to the stump but remove all dead muscle to avoid gas gangrene, leaving viable, red, bleeding and contracting muscle. In elective cases cut the muscle with a raked incision angled towards the level of bone section.

2 Double-ligate major vessels with strong silk or linen thread. Ligate other vessels with absorbable material such as polyglycolic acid. Gently pull down nerves, divide them cleanly and allow them to retract into soft tissue envelopes. Ligate major nerves with a fine suture just above the site of division to prevent bleeding, and reduce neuroma formation.

3 Prepare to cut the bone at the appropriate level. Remember that the stump must be long enough to gain secure attachment to the prosthesis and to act as a useful lever but short enough to accommodate the prosthesis and its hinge or joint mechanism. Divide the periosteum and cut the bone with a Gigli or power saw. During bone section, cover the soft tissues with a moist pack and irrigate them afterwards to remove bone dust and particles. Round-off sharp bone edges with a rasp.

4 Check that the flaps will approximate easily. Release the tourniquet and secure haemostasis. Insert a suction drain then suture the flaps together without tension, starting with the muscle. Handle the skin carefully and close it with staples if available, or interrupted nylon sutures. In the presence of infection or if you have any doubt about the viability of the flaps, approximate the muscles loosely over gauze soaked in saline or proflavine to prevent them from contracting. Do not close the skin. Plan delayed primary closure at 5–7 days.

5 Apply a well-padded compressible but not crushing dressing, using either cotton wool or latex foam and aim to leave it undisturbed for 10 days. Hold this in place with crepe bandage taking care to avoid fixed flexion or other deformity of neighbouring joints. Except in cases with infection or doubtful flap viability, apply a light shell, a maximum four layers of plaster of Paris over the dressing to make the patient comfortable and able to be mobile in bed. In specialist centres a rigid dressing can be applied, to which a temporary pylon can be attached, allowing early ambulation.

6 Inspect the wound if there is increasing pain, seepage of blood or pus through the dressing, or a rising temperature and pulse.

7 Order regular physiotherapy to prevent joint contractures and encourage the patient to become mobile and use the stump early. When the wound has healed and sutures have been removed, apply regular stump bandaging to maintain its shape and refer the patient to the local limb-fitting centre.

Special situations

Children's amputations present special problems, since growing bones will overgrow by apposition, not related to growth at the proximal growth plate, often needing revision of the bone to prevent skin problems. If possible, always preserve epiphyseal growth plates. Perform a disarticulation more distally rather than an amputation through a long bone at a more proximal level if at all possible. The disarticulation prevents terminal overgrowth of the bone. Children suffer less than adults from the complications of amputation such as phantom pain, neuroma, etc. They adapt amazingly well to prostheses if fitted correctly at an early age.

Decision-making for amputations in major trauma may be assisted by the Mangled Extremity Severity Score (MESS), using four significant criteria of skeletal/soft-tissue injury, limb ischaemia, shock and patient age to help discriminate between salvageable limbs and those better managed by primary amputation.

Facilitating the use of a prosthesis demands earliest possible application. In specialist centres, rigid casts are applied to the stump to which a prosthesis can be attached. Patients are mobilized within 48 hours of operation. Early application is facilitated if there is minimal postoperative oedema and pain; it offers psychological benefits, reduces immobility, joint contracture, osteoporosis and hospital stay, with earlier maturation of the stump and earlier return to full social activities.

Complications

Haematoma in the stump predisposes to infection, delaying prosthetic fitting. Avoid it by meticulous haemostasis, releasing the tourniquet before closing the stump and doubly ligating major vessels. Prevent infection, which causes secondary haemorrhage. Aspirate or drain collections of blood, usually under local anaesthesia. Elevate the limb and apply pressure to control severe haemorrhage while arranging surgical exploration under general anaesthetic.

Infection is an important risk because the tissues are often poorly vascularized, there is often infection in the distal extremity, and patients are often frail, elderly, with poor resistance to infection. Give prophylactic antibiotics that are active against gas gangrene organisms, *Escherichia coli* and staphylococci to all lower-limb amputees. Handle soft tissues gently and avoid leaving dead muscle and long sections of denuded cortical bone in the stump. Treat infections promptly with antibiotics, drain pus. Explore under general anaesthesia a chronic sinus failing to dry up after a 6-week course of antibiotics, seeking a focus of infection such as a small bony sequestrum or infected suture material.

Flap necrosis can be avoided by preoperative assessment of skin viability, gentle handling and preferring a myoplastic flap which carries a better blood supply when possible. Treat small defects conservatively, allowing granulation tissue to form beneath, and detach the skin slough. Treat major flap necrosis by wedge resection down to and including bone or by higher re-amputation.

Joint contractures are common in elderly, immobile patients, those in chronic pain, and especially following head injuries or coma. The hip and knee are particularly affected. Prevent or treat mild contractures with early active and passive exercises, positioning them in a corrective posture, and fitting a prosthesis that retains the position and encourages movement. Apply serial plasters or surgically release severe contractures.

Neuromas form at the ends of all cut nerves but they are painful only if trapped in scar tissue or exposed to repeated trauma. Ensure that transected nerves lie within normal tissues proximal to the stump end. Resect painful neuromas with a length of affected nerve, well away from scar tissue.

Phantom limb sensation is likely; warn the patient but do not mention phantom pain. Reassure a patient who still feels the missing limb that this will gradually fade and warn against attempts to use a missing limb.

Phantom pain is most common with proximal rather than distal amputations, following severe preoperative pain and in those who have been in contact with others experiencing phantom pain for no known reason, and is untreatable even by nerve section or chordotomy. Be optimistic and supportive and involve the whole team in this. Patient distress occasionally leads to suicide.

Failure to use a prosthesis is common in those with a physical or mental disability and those determined not to do so. The most adaptable are those who were able to stand and walk, with or without aids, shortly before operation. In both the upper and lower limbs, the higher the amputation the less likely it is that a prosthesis will be used. If the energy expenditure in a wheelchair is less than on a prosthesis, it requires a determined patient to get out of the wheelchair.

HINDQUARTER AMPUTATION

This radical operation, usually performed for malignant disease of bone or soft tissue of the pelvis or upper thigh, involves removal of the lower limb and hemipelvis. It requires the division of the external iliac, deep epigastric and internal iliac branch vessels and femoral, obturator and sciatic nerves.

ABOVE-KNEE AMPUTATION

Leave the femoral stump long to improve control of the prosthesis but leave at least 15 cm above the knee for the prosthetic knee mechanism, otherwise the artificial knee joint is lower than on the normal leg, most marked when the patient sits. Always perform a myodesis (Greek *desis* = a binding together), anchoring a muscle group to the femur, to prevent the femur from migrating through the stump. Make equal anterior and posterior flaps.

BELOW-KNEE AMPUTATION

Carefully assess the viability of the soft tissues of the lower leg when considering amputation at this level, looking for evidence of peripheral vascular disease, diabetic gangrene or trauma. Do not perform the operation in a non-ambulant patient but otherwise try to preserve the knee joint.

Use a long posterior flap, or a skew flap, in peripheral vascular disease, diabetes and trauma. Equal flaps are suitable for amputating tumours or for severe acute infection.

In case of fixed flexion knee deformity of 5° the tibia can be more than 20 cm, if 15° it should be 10–15 cm and if 35° only 6–10 cm.

The optimal length of tibia is one third of its full length. There is insufficient muscle in the flaps to maintain the viability if it is any longer. The minimum length is 6 cm.

Access

1. Seal off any infected, gangrenous areas by enclosing them in a polyethylene bag.
2. Employ general or epidural anaesthesia.
3. Apply a tourniquet to the thigh unless the amputation is for peripheral vascular disease.

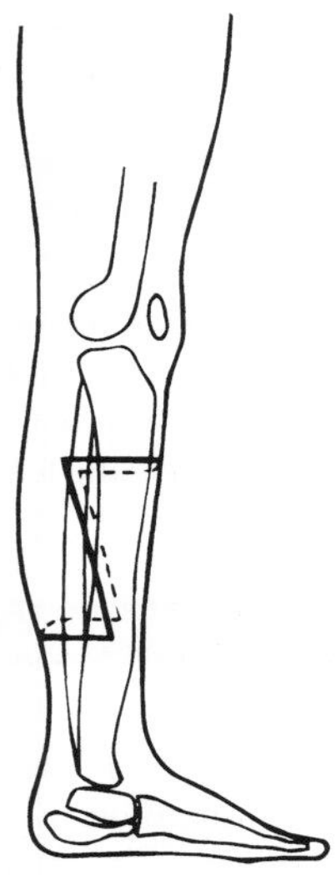

Fig. 38.1 Incision for below-knee amputation.

4 Place the patient supine on the operating table with a padded, inverted bowl underneath the proximal tibia.

5 Mark the skin flaps (Fig. 38.1).

Action

1 Start the anterior incision at the base of the proposed bone section, cutting transversely round each side of the leg to a point two-thirds of the way down each side. Then take the incisions distally on each side, passing slightly anteriorly to a point well below the length that is likely to be required. Join the two incisions posteriorly.

2 Deepen the longitudinal incisions down to deep fascia. Anteriorly incise straight down to bone and then on to the interosseous membrane. Ligate the anterior tibial vessels at this point.

3 Elevate the periosteum of the tibia for 1 cm proximal to the level of section. Divide the tibia using a Gigli or amputation saw. Bevel the anterior half of the tibial stump with the saw and a rasp. Divide the fibula 1 cm proximally and bevel the bone laterally.

4 Use a bone hook to distract the distal part of the tibia. Divide the deep posterior muscles of the calf at the same level as the tibia. At this stage identify and ligate the posterior tibial and peroneal vessels. Cleanly divide the posterior tibial nerve, allowing it to retract.

5 Use a raking cut through the soleus and gastrocnemius muscles down to the end of the posterior flap. Remove the limb.

Close

1 Complete the smoothing and bevelling of the tibia and fibula using bone nibblers and a rasp.

2 Bevel gastrocnemius and soleus medially and laterally, and trim the excess skin to fashion a rounded, slightly bulbous stump.

3 Release the tourniquet and secure haemostasis. Insert a suction drain brought out medially through the wound.

4 Bring the posterior flap forwards over the bone and suture it anteriorly to the deep fascia of the anterolateral group of muscles, using a strong absorbable suture.

5 Close the skin, preferably with closely placed staples, or with interrupted nylon sutures and adhesive strip such as Steri-Strip tapes. Do not leave any 'dog ears' laterally.

6 Apply a dressing of gauze and sterile plaster wool, then apply gentle compression of the stump with a crepe bandage. Apply a further layer of plaster wool and then a light plaster cast to mid-thigh level. Mould the plaster over the femoral condyles to prevent it from slipping down. Do not use plaster if there is any infection.

Aftercare

1 Elevate the leg, remove the drain at 48 hours by gently pulling it out of the top of the plaster cast and mobilize the patient early but retain the plaster cast undisturbed for at least 10 days.

2 Remove the sutures at 14 days, then apply a daily stump bandage and arrange for daily hip and knee physiotherapy.

3 As soon as the wound has fully healed, arrange for the fitting of a temporary pylon, either patellar-tendon-bearing or ischial-bearing, depending on the quality of the stump. Now arrange for definitive limb-fitting.

SYME'S AMPUTATION

Amputation of the foot just above the ankle joint, covering the stump with a heel flap, is an alternative to below-knee amputation. The stump is end-bearing with good proprioception and the modern cosmetic prostheses are very light and comfortable. Transmetatarsal and tarsometatarsal amputation is occasionally required for severe trauma.

AMPUTATION OF THE TOES

Use a tourniquet and amputate single toes through a racquet incision but neighbouring toes often develop secondary deformity. Remove all the toes (the 'Pobble' operation) if there are multiple painful, fixed deformities or if several toes are gangrenous. If you need to amputate the great toe, try to preserve the attachments of the short flexor and extensor tendons on the proximal phalanx. Disarticulate the toes or preserve the base of the proximal phalanx with the joint capsule if possible.

THE UPPER LIMB

Many of the indications for amputation in the hand have changed in recent times as a result of improvements in surgical method, prosthetics and plastic surgery. These techniques require special expertise. Here we shall consider only some of the common and simpler procedures.

AMPUTATION OF FINGERS

Use an exsanguinating tourniquet. Mark the incision, placing the scar dorsally, covering the stump with volar skin. Do not suture together the ends of the extensor and flexor tendons over the end of the bone. Isolate and cleanly divide the digital nerves 1 cm proximal to the stump. Round off the end of cut bone; following disarticulation, remove articular cartilage and prominent condyles.

Amputation through the distal phalanx

Ablate the nail bed if less than a quarter of the nail remains to prevent a hooked nail remnant forming.

Disarticulation through the distal interphalangeal joint

Incise the skin in the midlateral line on either side of the neck of the middle phalanx and join them across the dorsum at the level of the joint and across the volar pulp 1 cm distal to the flexor crease (Fig. 38.2). Dissect back the fibrofatty tissue, divide the extensor and flexor tendons at the level of the neck of the middle phalanx and allow them to retract, ligate the digital vessels and divide the nerves proximally and finally divide the capsule and collateral ligaments. Shape the head of the middle phalanx using bone nibblers and close the wound.

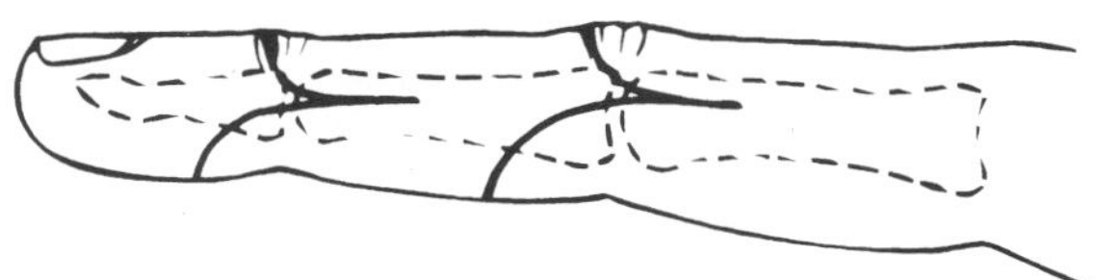

Fig. 38.2 Incision for disarticulation through interphalangeal joints.

Disarticulation through the metacarpophalangeal joint

Disarticulation through the metacarpophalangeal joint is best restricted to the middle and ring fingers.

Amputation through the shaft of the metacarpal

Amputation through the shaft of the metacarpal for the index or little finger is through the radial or ulnar border respectively, also dividing the nerves on the radial and ulnar side respectively. Divide the bone obliquely through the junction of the distal and middle thirds and smooth the edges of bone.

MAJOR UPPER-LIMB AMPUTATIONS

These are fortunately rarely required, usually for trauma, occasionally for malignancy, severe infection and congenital abnormalities or deformities. Except in an emergency, obtain a second opinion. Whenever possible operate using general anaesthesia and an exsanguinating tourniquet.

Below-elbow amputation is carried out through equal dorsal and volar flaps at the junction of the middle and lower thirds of the radius and ulna, with the arm supinated.

Above-elbow amputation is carried out through equal anterior and posterior flaps at 20 cm from the tip of the acromion.

Forequarter amputation, carried out for extensive tumours, necessitates dividing the clavicle, subclavian artery and axillary vein and trunks of the brachial plexus, followed by all the attaching muscles. The forequarter, including the scapula, is then removed.

FURTHER READING

Angel JC, Weaver PC 1979 Amputations. In: Bentley G, Greer RB III (eds) Rob and Smith's operative surgery, 4th edn. Orthopaedics Part 1. Butterworths, London

Anonymous 1991 Symposium on Amputations. Annals of the Royal College of Surgeons of England 73:133–176

Tooms RE 1987 Amputations. In: Crenshaw AH (ed.) Campbell's operative orthopedics. Mosby, St Louis, pp 597–646

39

Orthopaedics and trauma: general principles

N. Goddard

CONTENTS

PREOPERATIVE PREPARATION

Assess fitness for operation beforehand. Following trauma first resuscitate the patient, correct blood loss and dehydration. Postpone elective operations until you have corrected any concomitant illness such as a chest or urinary infection or hypertension, especially if you intend implanting a prosthetic device such as total joint replacement.

Usually administer an antibiotic intravenously at induction of anaesthesia, followed up by two further doses at 8-hourly intervals. The choice of antibiotic depends upon the nature of the operation, the likely infecting organism and the patient's potential sensitivity but a broad-spectrum antibiotic (cefradine 500 mg t.d.s.) or an agent with potent anti-staphylococcal activity is often given.

KEY POINT Avoid bone infection at all costs

- Infection of bone and non-living implants is a potentially catastrophic complication. Give prophylactic antibiotics for all but the most minor operations on bone, when an implant is used, and if there is an open wound.

Routine prophylactic anticoagulants are controversial for major orthopaedic operations, particularly on the hip joint. Heparin and warfarin may reduce the incidence of deep venous thrombosis but fatal pulmonary embolus is not reduced.

General anaesthetic is appropriate for most orthopaedic procedures, especially for prolonged operations when a tourniquet is used but regional block (spinal, epidural, axillary), or local anaesthetic wound infiltration are sometimes appropriate.

TOURNIQUETS

Most orthopaedic operations on the limbs, especially the hand, are facilitated if performed in a bloodless field using a pneumatic tourniquet but take care in the presence of peripheral vascular disease or impaired blood supply following trauma. Do not exsanguinate the limb in the presence of distal infection, suspected calf vein thrombosis or foreign bodies, so as to avoid propagating the infection, dislodging any blood clot or shifting the foreign body. Take care when exsanguinating a fractured or injured limb.

Apply a pneumatic tourniquet of appropriate size over a few turns of orthopaedic wool around the proximal part of the upper arm or thigh. Exsanguinate the limb by elevation (Bier's method) or with a soft rubber exsanguinator (Rhys-Davies); if this is not available, use an Esmarch bandage applied over stockinette to protect friable skin. Secure the cuff and inflate to just above systolic blood pressure for tourniquets on the upper limb, such as 200 mmHg but not over 250 mmHg, and to twice the systolic blood pressure for the lower limb such as 350 mmHg but not over 450 mmHg. If the tourniquet is accidentally deflated during the operation, deflate the cuff completely, reposition, refasten it, and elevate the limb before reinflating the cuff.

Record the time of inflation of the tourniquet and the duration of its application, which must be kept to a minimum by careful planning of the operation. Save 5 minutes of ischaemic time by exsanguinating the limb after preparing the skin. It is regarded as safe to leave the tourniquet for 60–90 minutes on the arm and up to but not desirable, 3 hours for the leg. If necessary, temporarily release and then reinflate the tourniquet, but be prepared for a poorer operative field.

I prefer to release the tourniquet and achieve satisfactory haemostasis before closing the wound, rather than first closing and dressing the wound. On completion ensure that the circulation has returned to the limb. Locate and mark the position of the peripheral pulses to facilitate subsequent postoperative observations. Reduce the likelihood of swelling by applying bulky cotton wool and crepe bandage dressing for at least 24 hours after the operation. Encourage and supervise active exercises.

SKIN PREPARATION

Elective surgery

If there is a break or superficial infection in the skin be prepared to postpone the operation. The patient should bathe using antiseptic soap within 12 hours. Shaving is optional but should be as late as possible. Apply iodine or chlorhexidine in spirit or aqueous solution.

Emergency surgery

Prepare the skin in the anaesthetic room after induction of anaesthesia and cover open wounds. Clean the surrounding skin with a soft nail brush and warm cetrimide (Savlon) solution, removing ingrained dirt and debris, then clean the wound similarly, controlling bleeding by digital pressure. Irrigate the wound copiously with physiological saline.

OPEN WOUNDS

Resuscitate the patient, if necessary, according to ATLS (advanced trauma life support) principles and guidelines before dealing with an open wound. Stop the bleeding by applying local pressure. Elevate the limb if necessary. Do not attempt blind clamping of any bleeding vessels, to avoid damaging adjacent structures.

Take a culture swab from the wound; this may be useful in the management of later infection.

Clean open wounds in the accident and emergency department and cover them with an iodine-soaked dressing, left undisturbed until the patient is in theatre, to reduce wound infection.

If possible take a Polaroid or digital photograph of the wound prior to the dressing being applied to provide a record of the extent and configuration of the wound and so avoid disturbing the dressings.

For clean, recent wounds in a fully immunized patient, you need not give a further tetanus booster. You may be in doubt about full immunization in which case give a deep subcutaneous or intramuscular dose of absorbed diphtheria [low dose], tetanus vaccine. The wound may be more than 6 hours old, punctured, devitalized, with foreign bodies, likely to be contaminated with manure, and in an immuno-compromised patient or one in whom you are uncertain about the immunization status. Primarily concentrate on cleaning the wound and removing devitalized or foreign material to leave it clean and healthy. Give an antibiotic such as benzylpenicillin or metronidazole. Give a tetanus booster now, to start or continue full immunization, and through a different site, give an intramuscular injection of tetanus immunoglobulin.

Assess damage to arteries, nerves, tendons and bones, initially estimate skin loss or damage and look for exit wounds following penetrating injuries. X-rays show the extent of bone damage and the presence of radio-opaque foreign bodies – but remember, not all foreign bodies are radio-opaque. Depending on the extent of the wound, carry out further assessment and treatment without anaesthesia or with regional or general anaesthetic. Avoid local infiltration anaesthesia.

Always request X-rays of the skull, lateral cervical spine, chest and anteroposterior views of the pelvis in multiply injured patients, but do not let this delay treatment.

Assess

Apply a proximal tourniquet when appropriate, before gently exploring the wound, examining the skin, subcutaneous tissues and deeper structures. Follow the track of a penetrating wound with a finger or probe to determine its direction and to judge the possibility of damage to vessels, nerves, tendons, bone and muscle. If you suspect muscle damage, slit open the investing fascia and take swabs for an anaerobic bacterial culture. Decide into which category the wound falls, since this determines the subsequent management.

Simple clean wounds have no tissue loss, although all wounds are contaminated with microorganisms, which may already be dividing. In clean wounds seen within 8 hours of injury, the bacteria have not yet invaded the tissues.

Simple contaminated wounds have no tissue loss. However, they may be heavily contaminated and if you see them more than 8 hours after the injury, they can be assumed to be infected. Late wounds show signs of bacterial invasion, with pus and slough covering the raw surfaces, and redness and swelling of the surrounding skin. Although there is no loss of tissue from the injury, the infection will result in later soft-tissue destruction.

Complicated contaminated wounds result when tissue destruction (e.g. loss of skin, muscle or damage to blood vessels, nerves or bone) has occurred, or foreign bodies are present in the wound. Recently acquired low-velocity missile wounds fall into this category since there is insufficient kinetic energy to carry particles of clothing and dirt into the wound.

Complicated dirty wounds are seen after heavy contamination in the presence of tissue destruction or implantation of foreign material, especially if the wound is not seen until more than 12 hours have elapsed.

High-velocity missile wounds deserve to be placed in a category of their own. For instance, when a bullet from a high-powered rifle strikes the body it is likely to lose its high kinetic energy to the soft tissues as it passes through, resulting in extensive cavitation. Although the entry and exit wounds may be small, structures within the wound are often severely damaged. Muscle is particularly susceptible to the passage of high-velocity missiles and becomes devitalized. It takes on a 'mushy' appearance and consistency and fails to contract when pinched or to bleed when cut. If the bullet breaks into fragments or hits bone, breaking it into fragments, the spreading particles of bullet and bone also behave as high-energy particles. The whole effect is of an internal explosion. In addition, the high-velocity missile carries foreign material (bacteria and clothing) deeply into the tissues, causing heavy contamination.

The risk of tetanus and gas gangrene is increased when the wound is sustained over heavily cultivated ground in which the organisms abound. Devitalized ischaemic muscle makes an excellent culture medium. As haematoma and oedema formation develop within the investing fascia, tissue tension rises, further embarrassing the circulation and causing progressive tissue death. Although handgun bullets, shotgun pellets, shrapnel from shells and fragments from mine, grenade and bomb explosions have a relatively low velocity, they behave as high-velocity missiles when projected into the tissues from nearby. When a shotgun is fired from close to the body, the wad and the pellets are carried in as a single missile.

Open fractures can be classified in a variety of ways.

Action

1. Stop all bleeding. Pick up small vessels with fine artery forceps and cauterize or ligate them with fine absorbable sutures. Control damage of major arteries and veins with pressure, tapes or non-crushing clamps, so as to permit later repair.
2. Irrigate clean simple wounds with copious volumes of sterile saline solution without drainage. Do not attempt to repair cleanly divided muscle with stitches but simply suture the investing fascia. Close the skin accurately.

KEY POINTS Infected wounds

- Never close an apparently simple infected wound immediately. Take a swab for culture. Remove any retained foreign material, radically excise and debride any dead or devitalized tissue and drain any potential pockets of infection. Systemic antibiotic or local instillations may be started but will not make up for poor technique.
- Pack the wound with gauze soaked in sterile isotonic saline solution and cover with an occlusive dressing. Plan to renew the packing daily until the wound is clean and produces no further discharge. Provided there is no redness or oedema of the surrounding skin, close the wound by delayed primary suture, usually after 3–7 days.

3. Complicated contaminated wounds can be partially repaired after excising the devitalized tissue. Once bone stability has been achieved, damaged segments of major arteries and veins should be repaired by an experienced surgeon using grafts where appropriate. Loosely

appose the ends of divided nerves with one or two stitches in the perineurium, so that they can be readily identified and repaired later when the wound is healed and all signs of inflammation have disappeared. Similarly, identify and appose the ends of divided tendons in preparation for definitive repair at a later date. Do not remove small fragments of bone that retain a periosteal attachment, or large fragments whether they are attached or unattached. Excise devitalized muscle, especially the major muscle masses of the thigh and buttock. Remove foreign material when possible. Some penetrating low-velocity missiles are better left if they lie deeply, provided damage to important structures has been excluded. Remove superficial shotgun pellets. Low-velocity missile tracks do not normally require to be laid open or excised, but do not close the wound. Excise damaged skin when the deep flap can be easily closed, if necessary by making a relaxing incision or applying a skin graft. Do not lightly excise specialized skin from the hands; instead leave doubtful skin and excise it later, if necessary, on expert advice.

4 Stabilize any associated fracture. It may be possible merely to immobilize the limb in a plaster cast, cutting a window into it so that the wound can be dressed. An open fracture, however, is not an absolute contraindication to surgical stabilization using the appropriate device (plates and screws, intramedullary nails), but should be undertaken only by an experienced trauma or orthopaedic surgeon. In an emergency situation it is preferable to use temporary skeletal traction and an external fixator.

5 Complicated dirty wounds require similar treatment of damaged tissues such as nerves and tendons, but do not attempt to repair damaged structures other than major blood vessels. Pack the wound and change the dressing daily until there is no sign of infection, then close the skin by suture or by skin grafting.

6 Lay open high-velocity missile wounds extensively. Foreign matter, including missile fragments, dirt and clothing, is carried deeply into the wound, so contamination is inevitable. Explore and excise the track, since the tissue along the track is devitalized, lay open the investing fascia over disrupted muscle to evacuate the muscle haematoma and excise the pulped muscle, leaving healthy contractile muscle that bleeds when cut. This leaves a cavity in the track of the missile.

7 Mark divided nerves and tendons for definitive treatment later. Excise the skin edges and pack the wound with saline-soaked gauze. Treat any associated fracture as described above. Change the packs daily until infection is controlled and all dead tissue has been excised. Only then can skin closure be completed and the repair of damaged structures be planned.

EXTERNAL FIXATION

There are many types of external fixator, ranging from the simple unilateral frame (Denham, Orthofix), multilateral frames (Hoffman) through to the more complicated circular frames (Ilizarov) and hybrid devices. The essential feature of the external fixator is that it provides a stable reduction of any fracture by using percutaneously introduced wires or pins into the bone, which are then attached to an external frame. In an emergency you should be familiar with the principles involved, and the techniques of applying a simple unilateral frame. Such a frame is constructed from one or more rigid bars, which are aligned parallel to the limb, to which the threaded pins that are drilled into the fragments of bone are attached. In the simplest form, here described, the pins are held to the bar with acrylic cement (Denham type; Fig. 39.1).

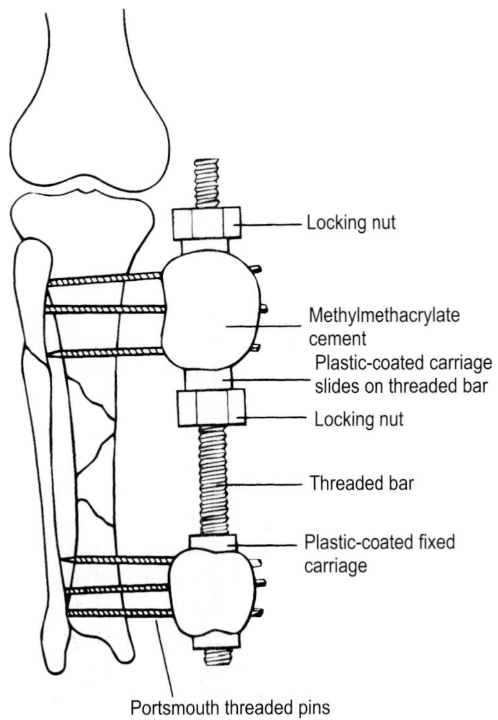

Fig. 39.1 The Denham external fixator.

Action

1 After treating the wound, and reducing the fracture – either open under direct vision, or closed using an image intensifier, maintain the reduction using bone clamps, traction or temporary wires. Make a stab wound through healthy skin proximal to the fracture site, bearing in mind the possible need for subsequent skin flaps. Drill a hole through both cortices of the bone approximately at right angles to the bone with a sharp 3.6-mm drill. Take care in drilling the bone that the drill bit does not overheat, which may in turn cause local bone necrosis leading to the formation of ring sequestra with subsequent loosening and infection of the pins. Measure the depth of the distal cortex from the skin surface.

2 Insert a threaded Schantz pin into the drill hole so that both cortices are penetrated. If possible insert two more pins approximately 3–4 cm apart into the proximal fragment and three pins into the distal fragment in similar fashion. Biomechanically the stability of the fixator is enhanced if there are three pins in each of the major fragments with the nearest pin being close to the fracture line.

3 Loosen the locking nuts that hold the carriages onto the rigid bar and hold the bar parallel to the limb and 4–5 cm away from the skin. Place one carriage opposite the protruding ends of each set of three pins and adjust the locking nuts to hold the carriages in position. Fix the pins to the carriages with two mixes of acrylic cement for each carriage, moulding the cement around the pins and the carriage, maintaining the position until it is set. Remove any temporary reduction device and carry out the final adjustment on the locking nuts to compress the bone ends together and dress the wound.

Aftercare

Keep the pin tracks clean and free of scabs and incrustations by daily cleaning with sterile saline or a mild antiseptic solution. A rigorous regimen will minimize the risk of pin-tract infection and premature pin loosening. An external fixator is essentially only a temporary measure before definitive treatment can be carried out. It is seldom used as the sole method of fracture management and should therefore be removed at a time when the wound is healthy, at which time it may be possible to definitively stabilize the fracture. Fixator removal is simple. Cut the pins with a hacksaw or bolt cutters and then unscrew them. The acrylic cement can be removed from the carriages, which may be used again.

OPEN (COMPOUND) FRACTURES

Assess the patient according to ATLS principles and resuscitate as necessary. After managing the wound as outlined above, X-ray the bone to determine the pattern of the fracture and to decide on the appropriate method of reduction and fixation.

Anaesthetize the patient, prepare the skin and clean the wound.

Action

1 Explore and reassess the wound and expose and assess the fracture. Remove only small and completely unattached fragments of bone. Retain any bone that has a remaining periosteal attachment, as this bone is potentially still viable. Free the bone ends from any adjacent fascia and muscle through which they may have buttonholed. Wash away any blood clot and other debris.

2 Strip the periosteum for 1–2 mm only from the bone ends to allow accurate reduction without the interposition of soft tissues. Using a combination of traction, bone clamps, levers and hooks, reduce the major fragments into an anatomical position. If necessary, extend the original wound to improve access.

3 If the fracture is stable, immobilize in a plaster cast after definitive treatment of the wound. Leave a window in the cast to permit wound inspection and changes of dressings. Apply an external fixator when the wound is contaminated or there is extensive skin loss. If the fracture is unstable and there is a simple, clean wound, then it may be appropriate to internally fix the fracture. If there are multiple injuries or if the wound is contaminated an external fixator may be more appropriate. Do not forget the possibility of immediate amputation if the limb is severely mutilated with associated neurovascular injuries.

SKELETAL TRACTION

Temporary skeletal traction can be applied using skin traction, and indeed this is the method of choice when using a Thomas splint for immobilization of a femoral fracture as a first aid measure. For prolonged treatment insert a traction pin through the tibia or calcaneus. Other sites such as the olecranon or metacarpals are occasionally used. Skeletal traction is a simple and safe method of immobilizing a limb after injury or operation. It may be a temporary measure, definitive treatment, or a supplement to treatment. With the more widespread use of increasingly sophisticated internal fixation devices, skeletal traction is less frequently employed as a definitive method of treating long-bone fractures. Skeletal traction requires careful supervision and adjustments to remain effective.

There are two types of pin in common usage. Each has a triangular or square butt, which inserts into a chuck, and a trocar point. The Steinmann pin is uniform throughout but the Denham pin has a short length of screw thread wider than the main shaft near its centre, which screws into one cortex of the bone and minimizes sideways slip during traction.

Action

1 Clean the skin and drape the limb, leaving about 10 cm exposed on either side of the site of entry. Anaesthetize the skin, subcutaneous tissue and periosteum on both sides of the bone at site of entry and exit of the pin with 1% lidocaine.

2 Make sure that the pin selected fits the sockets in the stirrup. To insert the pin through the upper tibia, make a 5-mm stab incision in the skin on the lateral side of the bone 2.5 cm posterior to the summit of the tibial tuberosity; this avoids damage to the common peroneal nerve when a medial approach is used. If the tibial plateau is fractured, make the nick and insert the pin 2.5–5.0 cm distally.

3 To insert the pin through the calcaneus, make a 5-mm stab incision in the skin on the lateral side of the heel 2.5 cm distal to the tip of the lateral malleolus.

4 Introduce the point of the pin through the nick at right-angles to the long axis of the limb and parallel to the floor with the limb in the anatomical position. Avoid obliquity in either plane.

> **KEY POINT Care inserting pins**
>
> - Drill the pin through both cortices of the bone with a hand drill until the point just bulges under the skin on the opposite side of the limb. Take care that the pin does not suddenly penetrate the skin to impale your hand or the opposite limb. This is particularly likely if the bone is thin and porotic.

5 Incise the skin over the exit point and gently push the pin through until equal lengths are protruding on either side. When using the Denham pin, screw the threaded section into the cortex a further 6–8 mm so that the thread engages the bone. Make sure that the skin is not distorted where the pin passes through by making tiny relieving incisions if necessary.

6 Dress the punctures with small squares of gauze soaked in tincture of benzoin.

7 Attach traction cords or a traction stirrup to the pin. Three types of stirrup are available: Bohler stirrup, for general use, Nissen stirrup, for more accurate control of rotation and Tulloch–Brown 'U'-loop for Hamilton Russell traction. Place guards on the ends of the pin. Attach a length of cord to the centre of the stirrup through which the traction will be applied.

8 Keep the pin tracks clean and free of scabbing and incrustation as described above. Continually monitor the position of the fracture and adjust the traction as necessary so as to maintain an accurate reduction. Monitor the patient to ensure the enforced recumbence does not predispose to chest infection and pressure sores.

SIMPLE SKELETAL TRACTION

Simple skeletal traction over a pulley fixed to the end of the bed usually suffices for relatively stable fractures (e.g. of the tibial plateau). Unstable fractures need the support of a splint. Support the calf on two or three pillows with the point of the heel clear of the bed. Have the traction string horizontal and apply sufficient traction weights so as to reduce the fracture and restore alignment and length of the bone. Usually 4–5 kg is sufficient depending upon the weight of the patient.

HAMILTON RUSSELL TRACTION

This is a convenient method for fractures and other conditions around the hip (e.g. dislocation or acetabular fractures). It controls the natural tendency of the leg to roll into external rotation and avoids the use of a Thomas splint, the ring of which causes discomfort if the hip is tender. Set up the apparatus as in Figure 39.2, passing the cord through the pulleys as indicated. The sections of string 'x' and 'y' must be parallel to the horizontal and the section 'z' must lead in a cephalic direction. Support the calf either on two ordinary pillows or on slings of Domette bandage attached to the 'U'-loop with safety pins.

Attach between 2 and 5 kg of weight to the end of the cord and make sure that it is clear of the floor. Remember that the effective traction is doubled as a result of the pulley arrangement. Keep the point of the heel clear of the bed to avoid pressure sores. Place a foot rest between the bars of the loop to maintain the foot at a right angle to the leg. A separate cord running from the Nissen stirrup through the more proximal pulley can be attached to a handle so facilitating knee flexion exercises.

SLIDING SKELETAL TRACTION

Sliding skeletal traction with the leg supported on a Thomas or similar splint is a standard method of conservative treatment for femoral shaft or supracondylar fractures. It allows the knee to be flexed (20° for shaft fractures and 40° or more for supracondylar fractures), with suspensory weighted pulleys to facilitate nursing.

CALCANEAL TRACTION

Use calcaneal traction with the leg supported on a Bohler–Braun frame in the conservative treatment of unstable fractures of the tibia. It may be combined with a padded plaster cast to provide more lateral stability. Apply 2–4 kg of weight. Support the calf and thigh from the side-bars of the frame with slings of Domette bandage. Pad under the limb with cotton wool.

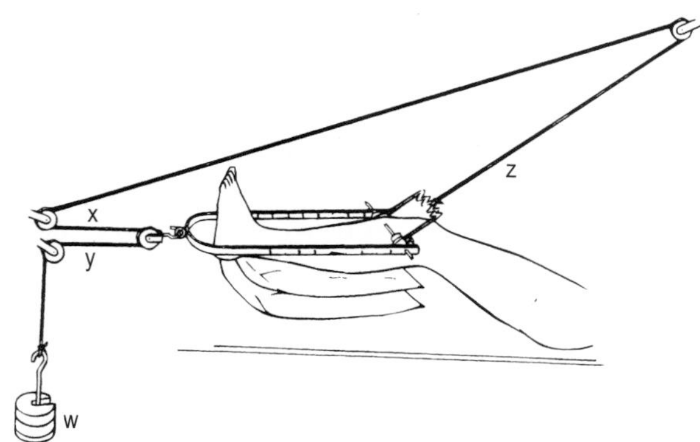

Fig. 39.2 Hamilton Russell skeletal traction.

SKULL TRACTION

Skull traction is often employed to immobilize the cervical spine after injury (fracture, subluxation or dislocation) and sometimes after operations on the neck. It is applied through skull tongs inserted under local anaesthetic prior to the administration of any general anaesthetic. The caliper is inserted at the point of maximal diameter of the skull in a line running across the vertex of the skull from one mastoid process to the other. In practice this is usually 2–3 cm above the top of the ear. After making a stab incision under local anaesthesia down to the pericranium, introduce the pins on each side to abut the outer table of the skull and tighten down through the outer table.

PERIPHERAL NERVE REPAIR

Complete disruption of a peripheral nerve may be associated with both open and closed injuries and recovery will not take place unless continuity is re-established surgically. Peripheral nerve repair (Fig. 39.3) is a specialist technique but, faced with it in the field, you should be aware of the principles. If you feel unable to attempt a primary repair then mark the nerve ends with a non-absorbable suture to assist their location at the time of the definitive operation. Always assume that a peripheral nerve injury in the presence of an open wound results from complete division of the nerve fibres (neurotmesis), so examine it when you treat the wound to check its integrity. If it is divided, either mark or appose the ends in their correct orientation for secondary repair later. Magnification is essential; if an operating microscope is not available, simple magnifying loupes usually suffice.

It is entirely acceptable to treat a peripheral nerve injury conservatively in the absence of an open wound. Neurapraxia (block to conduction of nerve impulses without disruption of the axon or its supporting cells) usually recovers spontaneously in days or weeks, and an axonotmesis (the axon undergoes Wallerian degeneration) in the time it takes for the axons to regenerate. This is calculated by measuring the distance from the site of injury (e.g. a fracture) to the point at which the motor nerve enters the first muscle innervated distal to the lesion. Axons regenerate at a rate of

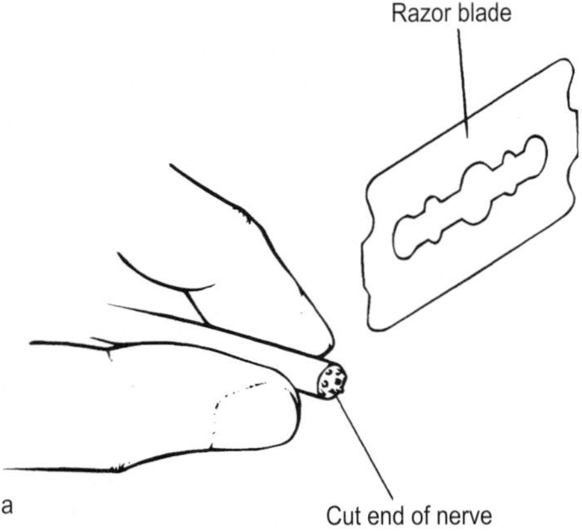

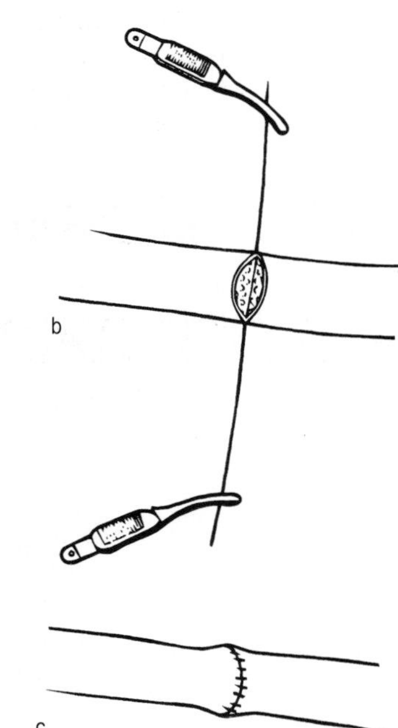

Fig. 39.3 Nerve suture: (a) cutting back to pouting fibres with a razor blade; (b) first and second sutures in place; (c) sutures completed.

1 mm/day and so it will take approximately 90 days, for example, for re-innervation of the brachioradialis to occur following an injury to the radial nerve at the distal end of the spiral groove of the humerus. Electrophysiological studies (EMG, nerve conduction) may give pointers as to the likely nerve lesion and help in documenting recovery. If recovery fails to occur in the predicted time and if the nerve conduction studies show no improvement then explore the course of nerve and treat any lesion appropriately.

Do not attempt immediate primary nerve repair unless you have adequate magnification (loupes or operating microscope) and are sufficiently experienced in the techniques involved. If in doubt, mark or appose the nerve ends for later exploration and repair.

KEY POINTS When to repair?

- Primary repair undoubtedly gives the best results and may sometimes be undertaken in specialist centres. If the patient is stable and fit for transfer, then do so.
- Secondary repair is safer and sometimes easier when the wound is soundly healed and the danger of infection has passed.

Action

1. Clean and explore the wound. If there is a previous wound that has healed, excise the previous scar if necessary, and extend the wound proximally and distally along the course of the nerve. If there was no wound, make an incision 15 cm long along the course of the nerve centred at the site of injury. Use a 'lazy-S' incision if the incision crosses the flexor crease of a joint.
2. Always begin by exposing the nerve in normal tissue on either side of the site of injury and then work towards the site of the injury, carefully dissecting along the course of the nerve. In the case of an open wound there may be extensive scar tissue and adhesions.
3. Decide whether repair is possible or not. If repair is possible but beyond your competence, what action should you take?

KEY POINT Repair not possible, or beyond your competence?

- Free the ends of the nerve from the surrounding soft tissues and place a marker suture of 4/0 nylon or other non-absorbable material, through the perineurium 2–3 cm proximally and distally from the site of injury to facilitate later alignment of the ends. If possible, appose the ends now, with two or three stitches for ease of later identification. If the ends cannot be apposed without tension, tack them to the underlying soft tissues to prevent retraction until definitive repair can be undertaken.

4 If this is a delayed repair there may be fibrous scar tissue at the cut ends, or joining the ends. If necessary, cut transversely across fibrous scar tissue that may be joining the ends together. Hold one end of the nerve firmly using a special nerve-holding clamp (a finger and thumb will suffice in extremis) and carefully cut thin slices of tissue from the exposed end with a sharp razor blade at right angles to the long axis of the nerve until all the scar tissue has been excised and the nerve bundles can be seen pouting from the cut surface (Fig. 39.3a). Repeat the procedure on the other end of the nerve. It may be necessary to resect a centimetre or more from each end of the nerve because of the intraneural fibrosis (neuroma) caused by the initial injury.

5 If this is a primary closure place the nerve ends in their correct rotational orientation. If this is delayed closure similarly identify the correct rotational alignment. Mobilize the nerve from the surrounding soft tissues proximally and distally as far as is necessary to bring the ends together without tension, carefully preserving and dissecting out the main branches. Flex a neighbouring joint if necessary. If it proves impossible to appose the nerve ends then an interposition graft may be necessary.

6 Release the tourniquet and achieve perfect haemostasis. Ensure again that the ends of the nerve are correctly orientated. Place an 8/0 nylon stitch through the perineurium on one side of the nerve. Cut the suture 3 cm from the knot and hold the ends in a small bulldog clip (Fig. 39.3b). Place a second suture directly opposite the first and place another bulldog clip on the ends. These act as stay sutures and facilitate rotation of the nerve while placing further sutures. Place further sutures through the perineurium, 1.5 mm or so apart, around the circumference of the nerve. After completing the repair of the superficial surface, turn the nerve over by passing one bulldog clip suture under and then other over the nerve. Complete the repair. Cut the first pair of sutures and turn the nerve back to the correct position (Fig. 39.3c).

7 Close the soft tissues and skin without altering the position of the limb if there is any danger of putting tension on the suture line. Apply a padded plaster without increasing the tension on the repair. Remove plaster and skin sutures after 3 weeks and gently mobilize the limb. If joints were flexed to avoid tension they must only be extended gradually over the next 3 weeks, if necessary by applying serial plasters at weekly intervals, or by incorporating a hinge with a locking device to allow flexion but no more than the set amount of joint extension.

TENDON SUTURE

Tendons are relatively avascular structures and heal by the ingrowth of connective tissue from the epitenon. When the tendon is divided within a fibrous sheath on the flexor surface of the hand, for example, the sheath is also damaged and the connective tissue from the healing sheath grows into the healing tendon, causing adhesions. For this reason injuries to the digital flexor tendons within the sheath should preferably be treated by experienced hand surgeons. Tendons may also require suturing as part of another procedure such as tendon transfer.

KEY POINT Delayed repair?

- It is entirely safe to perform a delayed primary repair of a divided flexor tendon up to 14 days post-injury without adversely affecting the final outcome.

Examine the wound. As with nerve injuries, if it is in the vicinity of a tendon and there is no distal action, assume that the tendon is divided until it is shown to be intact on clinical examination. If no action is demonstrated or if there is doubt, explore the wound.

Action

1 Prepare the skin, apply the tourniquet and explore the wound, extending it if necessary in order to identify any divided tendons. If the wound is suitable for primary closure then proceed to repair the tendons. If not, delay the repair until the wound is healed and is no longer indurated, maintaining full mobility of the joints in the meantime by physiotherapy. When several tendons are divided (e.g. at the wrist), make sure that the cut ends are correctly paired. It is not unheard of to suture the proximal end of one tendon to the distal end of another or even to the cut end of a nerve! Draw the cut ends together after picking up the paratenon round each end of the tendon with fine mosquito forceps, flexing neighbouring joints if necessary.

2 Secure the cut ends of the tendon by passing one needle into an exposed tendon end and bring it out of the side of the tendon about 1.5 cm from the cut end. Now pass this needle transversely through the tendon 3–4 mm nearer to the cut end. Reinsert this needle on the other side of the tendon to create a mirror image and bring it out through the cut end (Fig. 39.4a). Freshen the ends of the tendon by cutting them with a no. 15 blade. Use a 3/0 braided non-absorbable (Ethibond) suture with a 15-mm straight needle at both ends using a modified Kessler core stitch (Fig. 39.4a). Repeat this process using the second needle on the other tendon end. Make a half-hitch and approximate the tendon ends till they just meet. Complete the knot with at least six throws. Cut the knot flush; this should now have been buried within the tendon (Fig. 39.4b).

3 Complete the repair with a simple running suture of 6/0 monofilament nylon with a small curved needle. It is helpful to begin the running stitch on the posterior face, leaving the cut end of the suture long with which to turn the tendon through 180° for ease of access. The final repair must be smooth, with no bunching at the repair site.

4 Release the tourniquet and secure haemostasis. Close the wound with suction drainage if necessary. Apply a padded plaster so that the suture line is not under tension and remove after 3 weeks in the upper limb and 6 weeks in the lower limb.

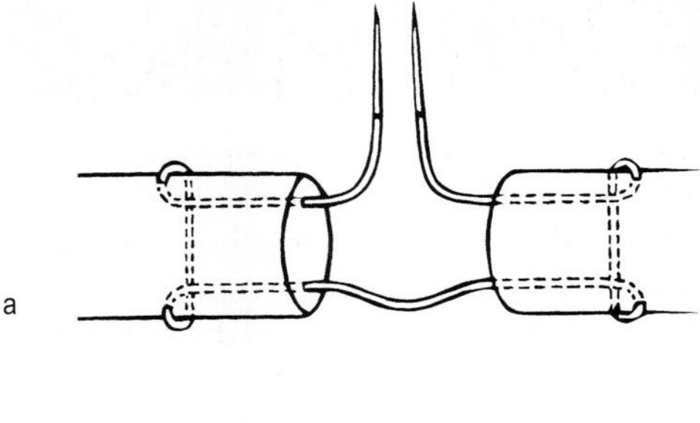

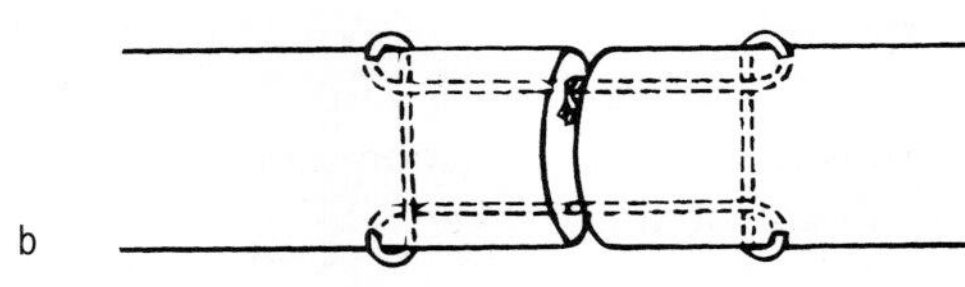

Fig. 39.4 End-to-end suture of a tendon.

BIOPSY

Biopsy of bone or soft tissue may be taken at an open operation or by aspirating material through a needle (closed biopsy). Closed biopsy is now usually performed by interventional radiologists, who are able to take specimens with extreme accuracy aided by the modern imaging techniques at their disposal. In both cases material is taken from the margin of the lesion, for the tissue in the centre is often necrotic and difficult to identify. Take at least two specimens – one for culture and the other for histological examination.

Bone biopsy is indicated in order to investigate a potential bone tumour (benign or malignant) or where infection is suspected. In the case of a potential malignant tumour ask a surgeon experienced in bone tumour management for advice on the technique and also the siting of the biopsy and scars so that it will not interfere with any later surgery.

A wedge-shaped piece of tissue is taken from the margin of the lesion approximately 1 cm long by 0.5 cm thick and 0.5 cm deep and place in formol saline unless specific staining techniques are required. Further similar specimens are taken for immediate culture and a culture swab is taken if pus is present.

DRAINAGE OF ACUTE OSTEOMYELITIS

Assume that any unwell infant or child with an area of local bone tenderness has osteomyelitis until proved otherwise and treat as such. For drainage of joints in the case of septic arthritis see the appropriate chapter. If an abscess is present on initial clinical examination, or if pain, temperature, local swelling and tenderness fail to improve within 12 hours of starting antibiotic therapy, undertake operative treatment immediately. However, an isotope bone scan may be helpful in determining the site of infection. Magnetic resonance imaging (MRI) can show the extent of the problem.

Take blood for culture, haemoglobin, ESR (erythrocyte sedimentation rate), CRP (C-reactive protein), WBC (white blood cell count) and differential white cell count. Give flucloxallin 100–200 mg/kg of body weight daily in divided doses intravenously until there is clinical improvement, usually apparent within 24 hours. If the patient is intolerant of penicillins give cefradine 100 mg/kg of body weight daily. Change antibiotic as necessary when sensitivities are known, as a result of blood culture or operation. Otherwise continue with oral flucloxacillin 50–100 mg/kg, when there is clinical improvement. If operation proves to be necessary (see above), perform it under a general anaesthetic. Apply a tourniquet if possible but do not exsanguinate the limb for fear of propagating the infection. Mark the most tender point on the limb before premedication.

At operation the incision is carried to the periosteum; pus may already be escaping, otherwise drill a single hole to detect pus and repeat this if necessary. Take pus for culture, irrigate the wound with saline and insert a suction drain before closing the skin.

CHRONIC OSTEOMYELITIS

Chronic pyogenic infection of bone may give rise to a recurrently discharging or permanent sinus and be associated with an underlying sequestrum. Identify a sequestrum radiologically by tomography, CT scanning or MRI. In the case of a chronically discharging wound a sinogram may determine the extent of the sinus. It is the sequestrum (a piece of dead bone) that is generally the source of the chronic infection. Therefore operative treatment is not indicated in the absence of a sequestrum or sinus.

Under general anaesthetic apply a tourniquet to the elevated limb but do not exsanguinate it. Centre the skin incision on the mouth of the sinus and excise it and the sinus track. Extend the incision in the direction of any sequestrum to remove it, excising any previous scars and unroof the cavity to curette out granulation tissue. Irrigate the cavity thoroughly, with a mixture of half-strength hydrogen peroxide and alcoholic Betadine and then physiological saline. Insert one or more chains of gentamicin-impregnated methyl methacrylate beads to fill the cavity without kinking, leaving the last bead of each chain protruding above skin level to facilitate later removal. Close after inserting a drain.

ACUTE SEPTIC (PYOGENIC) ARTHRITIS

In all cases of acute arthralgia, especially in children who are systemically unwell, suspect septic arthritis. If possible, attempt to aspirate the joint (it may be difficult to aspirate a hip) when the signs and symptoms of infection are present in association with a leucocytosis or a raised ESR. A negative aspiration, however, does not exclude infection.

Take blood for culture, haemoglobin, CRP, WBC count and ESR. X-ray the joint, but it may appear normal. Give flucloxallin intravenously.

Under general anaesthesia insert a wide-bore needle attached to a syringe into the joint through the site of easiest access, maximum tenderness or fluctuation and aspirate any fluid present for culture, cell counts, Gram stain and an immediate microscopy. If the aspirate is free from pus and no organisms are seen on the smear, treat by antibiotics and immobilization alone, until the results of cultures and all cell counts are available. Open the joint in all doubtful cases involving the hip, if the aspirate is obvious pus, if organisms are visible on the smear or are subsequently grown and if the cell counts exceed 100000/mm^3.

FURTHER READING

Dixon RA 1978 Nerve repair. British Journal of Hospital Medicine 20:295–305

Gelberman RH, Berg JSV, Lundborg GN et al 1983 Flexor tendon healing and restoration of the gliding surface. Journal of Bone and Joint Surgery 65A:70–79

Klenerman L, Miswas M, Hughland GH et al 1980 Systemic and local effects of the application of a tourniquet. Journal of Bone and Joint Surgery 62B:385–388

Müller ME, Allgöwer M, Schneider R et al 1979 Manual of internal fixation. Techniques recommended by the AO group, 2nd edn. Springer-Verlag, Berlin

Seddon H 1975 Surgical disorders of the peripheral nerves, 2nd edn. Churchill Livingstone, Edinburgh

40

Orthopaedics and trauma: upper limb

N. Goddard

CONTENTS

THE ANTERIOR (DELTOPECTORAL) APPROACH TO THE SHOULDER

The glenohumeral joint may be exposed through anterior, posterior or transacromial approaches, but most procedures can be carried out satisfactorily through the anterior approach (Fig. 40.1), particularly suited for exposure of the upper humerus for internal fixation or draining a potentially infected joint. The deltopectoral groove runs obliquely across with the cephalic vein which may need to be ligated. Open the groove to reveal the coracoid process; if you divide this and retract coracobrachialis and the short head of biceps you reach subscapularis. Divide this and reach the joint capsule. Extend the wound distally, lateral to biceps, to expose the entire humeral shaft.

APPROACHES TO THE UPPER ARM

Orthopaedic operations on the upper arm are infrequent but access to the humerus is occasionally required for internal fixation of fractures or exposure of the radial nerve.

ANTEROLATERAL APPROACH

This approach to the humeral shaft avoids the major neuromuscular structures except for the radial nerve, which winds in the spiral groove. Expose the humerus through an incision along the lateral border of biceps from the deltoid above down to the elbow (Fig. 40.2). Expose and split brachialis muscle. The outer strip of brachialis protects the radial nerve. The incision can be extended upwards in the deltopectoral groove, detaching deltoid from the clavicle, folding it back and detaching pectoralis major muscle from the humerus.

APPROACHES TO THE ELBOW

The elbow joint may be exposed from the anterior, posterior, medial or lateral aspects. The posterolateral approach allows drainage of the elbow or exposure of the head of the radius (Fig. 40.3). If necessary it can be extended distally to expose the upper proximal third of the radius and adjoining ulna. Minimize risk to the posterior interosseous nerve by pronating the forearm to move the nerve away from the operative field.

SUPRACONDYLAR FRACTURES

No matter how experienced you are, be circumspect when treating a displaced supracondylar fracture, especially in a child because of potential damage to the neurovascular

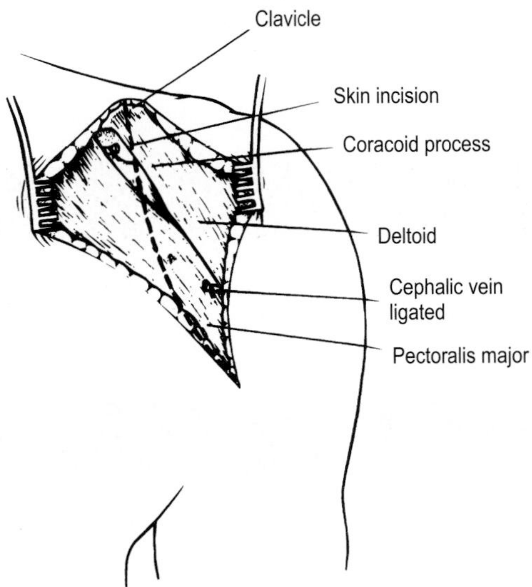

Fig. 40.1 Anterior exposure to the shoulder joint: the skin incision – location of the deltopectoral groove and coracoid process.

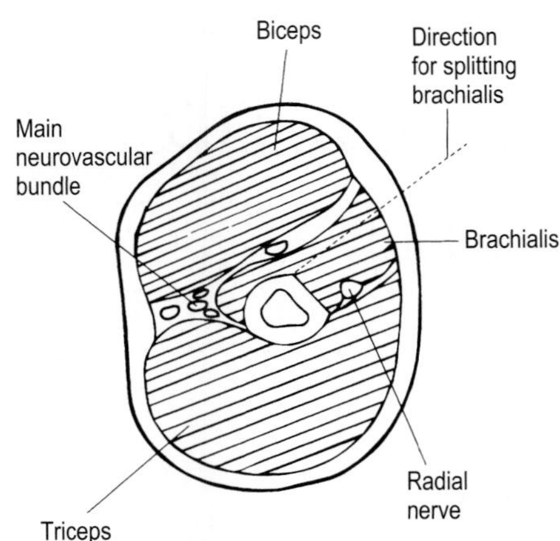

Fig. 40.2 Cross-section through the middle third of the arm showing the lateral part of the brachialis that is not covered by the biceps. This is split in the direction of the dotted line to expose the front of the distal half of the humerus. The cut slopes in to reach the midline of the shaft.

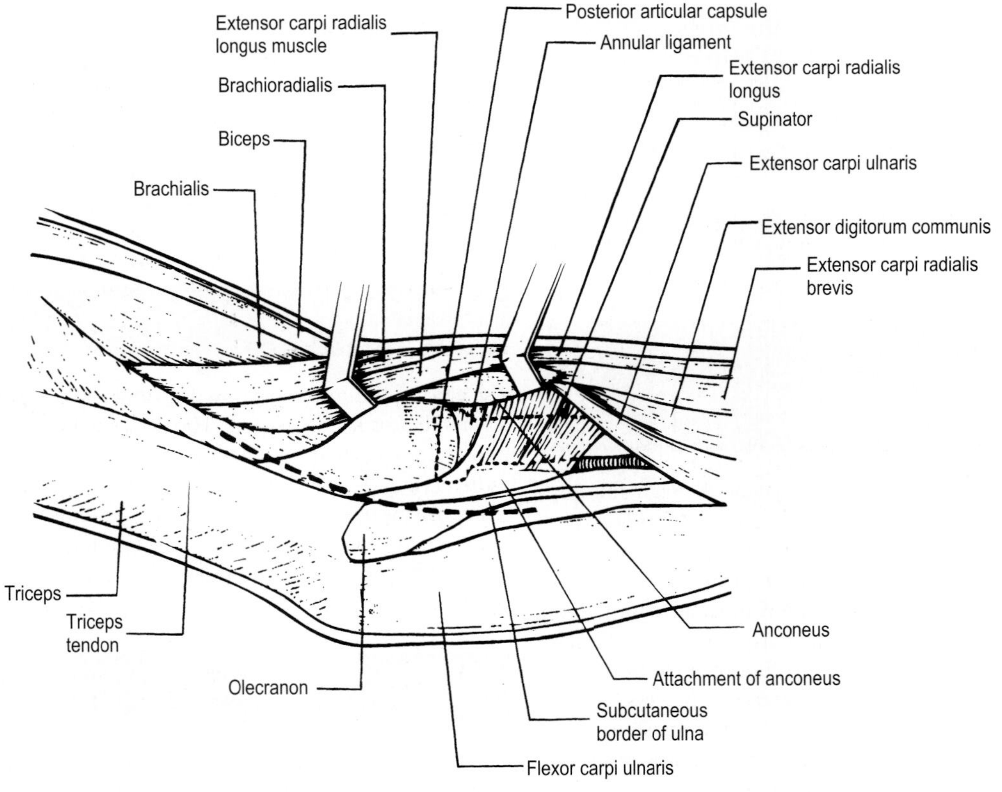

Fig. 40.3 Exposure of the head of the radius.

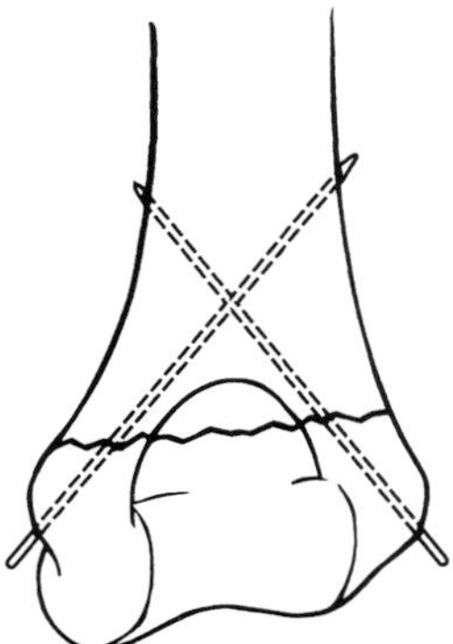

Fig. 40.4 Supracondylar fracture of the humerus held by crossed Kirschner wires.

structures from ischaemia, nerve damage and consequent long-term complications.

This fracture can be treated conservatively by manipulation or olecranon traction in children. Take anteroposterior radiographs of both elbows in a comparable position, usually acutely flexed, to check after closed reduction.

The open approach is midline posterior, turning down a flap of triceps muscle to reduce the fracture, allowing K-wire fixation (Fig. 40.4).

KEY POINT Circulation intact?

- Check the circulation and leave instructions that the radial pulse is monitored every hour for the next 12 hours.

DECOMPRESSION OF THE ULNAR NERVE

Decompression of the ulnar nerve may be carried out for relieving ulnar neuritis or nerve entrapment. Occasionally it needs to be transposed anteriorly so as to gain length to repair the nerve following injury, or as part of another procedure. If operating for a compression neuropathy, it is advisable to obtain preoperative nerve-conduction studies.

Use a medial approach. Identify the nerve, expose it through the investing fascia and mobilize it. If necessary transpose it anteriorly by dividing the common flexor origin, placing the nerve deep to the muscle mass and reattaching the common flexor origin.

APPROACHES TO THE FOREARM

Preferably approach the shafts of the radius and ulna through separate incisions – the ulna from behind and the radius from the front.

Posterior approach to the ulna

Posterior approach to the ulna is generally simple since it is immediately subcutaneous. Separate muscles from the bone with a periosteal elevator.

Anterior (Henry) approach to the radius

Incise the skin from the radial styloid in the interval between the brachioradialis and the flexor carpi radialis muscles, proximally in a straight line as far as the lateral side of the biceps tendon, to expose the whole radial shaft. To expose the proximal radial shaft, supinate the forearm, ligate and divide the large superficial vein crossing the incision, divide the deep fascia lateral to the biceps tendon. Retract the belly of brachioradialis muscle and separate the short radial extensors and flexors medially to expose and ligate the vessels passing laterally from the radial artery. Sweep the supinator laterally off the bone with a periosteal elevator, protecting the posterior interosseous nerve which lies within it, by supinating the forearm.

APPROACHES TO THE WRIST

The *anterior volar approach* is through an 'S' shaped incision (Fig. 40.5) exposing the transverse carpal ligament distally, and continuous proximally with the deep fascia of the forearm. Carefully incise the palmar fascia and incise the transverse carpal ligament to expose the median nerve and its recurrent, motor branch to the thenar eminence. Retract the median nerve and palmaris longus towards the ulnar side, exposing flexor pollicis longus tendon with pronator quadratus in the floor beneath, which is the lower end of the radius and the radiocarpal joint.

The *posterior (dorsal) approach* is longitudinal, centred on Lister's tubercle.

The *lateral approach* gives access to the distal radius.

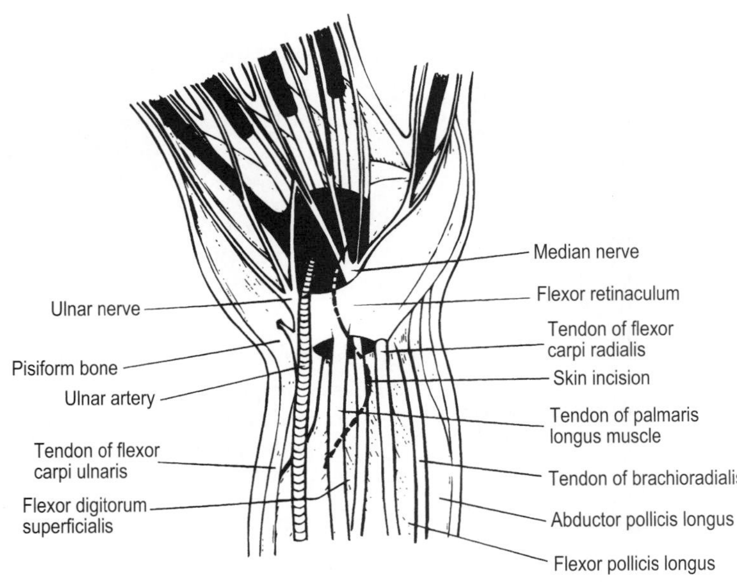

Fig. 40.5 Anterior approach to the wrist. The skin incision is indicated by the broken line.

GANGLION OF THE DORSUM OF THE WRIST

This results from cystic degeneration of fibrous tissue, commonly arising from a synovial joint or tendon sheath on the dorsum of the wrist.

Make a skin crease transverse incision over the apex of the swelling onto the surface. Dissect round it to identify and divide the attachment, with a small fragment of capsule or tendon sheath.

MEDIAN NERVE DECOMPRESSION IN THE CARPAL TUNNEL

Decompress the median nerve if conservative treatment with night splints, steroid injections and diuretics fails to relieve the symptoms of carpal tunnel syndrome, or if abnormal neurological signs develop, such as wasting and weakness of the thenar muscles and dryness of the skin over the radial two-thirds of the hand. Carry out preoperative nerve conduction studies. Use the anterior approach, carefully preserving the palmar cutaneous branch of the median nerve. Deepen the incision down through the longitudinal fibres of the palmar aponeurosis to expose the transverse fibres of the flexor retinaculum. Incise this longitudinally to expose the median nerve. Protect the nerve with a McDonald's dissector while fully dividing the remaining transverse fibres to release the nerve.

APPROACHES TO THE HAND AND FINGERS

The unique sensibility and mobility of the hand and fingers call for special care whenever surgical treatment is contemplated.

Palmar approach to the hand can be made anywhere (Fig. 40.6) but cross skin creases obliquely, not at right angles, and take the creases into account when dealing with pre-existing lacerations and injuries. Employ general anaesthesia or regional block and apply a tourniquet. Incise the skin and subcutaneous tissue, obliquely crossing the skin creases at their apices. Extend the incision proximally and distally over the structure to be exposed. Carefully dissect the skin and subcutaneous tissue from the underlying fascia and retract the edges with skin hooks. Expose the deeper structures with incisions made according to anatomical

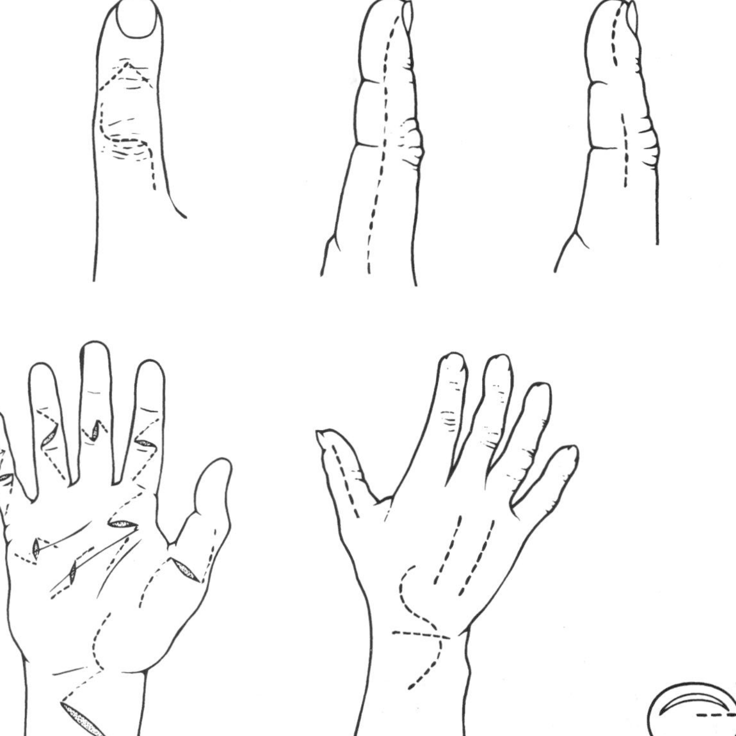

Fig. 40.6 Skin incisions in the hand and fingers.

considerations and not necessarily following the skin incisions. If there is a pre-existing contracted scar, or if you need additional length, consider inserting a Z-plasty of the skin (Ch. 42).

Dorsal approach incisions are not as critical as those on the palm.

Mid-lateral incisions on the digits can be made on either side.

Release of trigger finger or thumb

Remember that the condition often occurs in diabetics. Avoid damaging the radial digital nerve when operating for trigger thumb, and damaging the digital nerves in the fingers. The thickening of the tendon and flexor sheath usually lies deep to the distal palmar crease or over the metacarpal joint. Make a transverse or short oblique incision in the skin over the thickened tendon sheath 1.5 cm long and deepen it to reach and incise the thickened portion, then lift up the tendons and confirm that they are free.

PYOGENIC INFECTIONS OF THE HAND

These are common, present with cellulitis alone, and most resolve with antibiotics, elevation and rest.

Incise and drain as soon as an abscess develops or if you detect pus or because of increasing pain and tenderness. Open subcuticular, intracutaneous and subcutaneous infections where they are most superficial and take a swab for bacteriological analysis.

With superficial infections accurately localize the most tender point with the tip of an orange stick before inducing anaesthesia. Make a cruciate incision over the most tender point and cut away the corners of the skin to saucerize the lesion. Take a swab for bacteriological analysis. If pus extends under the nail, remove only that portion of the nail that has been raised from the nail bed.

Web and palmar space infections are rare. Very little swelling is obvious in the palm, but the back of the hand is oedematous and pain is severe. Tendon sheath infections cause swelling and tenderness along the line of the sheath, and the finger cannot be extended passively because of excruciating pain. Incise in the line of the skin crease over the most tender part when a web or palmar space is infected. Do not incise the web itself. Carefully explore between the deeper structures (Fig. 40.7) by blunt dissection and follow the track to the abscess cavity. Insert a small latex drain. Cut back the skin edges to ensure adequate drainage but do not insert a drain.

Drain tendon sheath infections through transverse incisions at either end of the sheath. Irrigate the sheath with antibiotic solution through a fine ureteric catheter until the effluent is clear. Leave the catheter in place for subsequent irrigation if necessary. Local anaesthetic can also be instilled for postoperative pain relief.

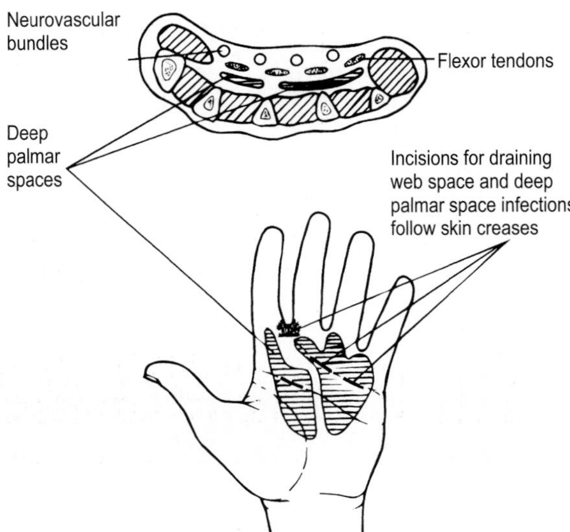

Fig. 40.7 Incisions for the drainage of web and deep palmar space infections.

Palmar space infections can be drained through a dorsal incision between the first and second metatarsals. When the infection is superficial, make a cruciate incision over the most tender point and cut away the corners of the skin to saucerize the lesion. Take a swab for bacteriological analysis.

OPERATIONS ON THE NAILS

Partial avulsion of a nail

It may be necessary to remove a portion of the nail in the presence of infection or trauma but preserve as much of the nail as possible to splint any associated soft tissue or bony injury, removing only that part of the nail that is separated from the nail bed, using fine scissors.

Evacuation of a subungual haematoma

This is often associated with a distal phalanx fracture, making it an open fracture, in which case give antibiotics. It is a simple matter to trephine the nail using a red-hot needle or paper clip. The blood spurts out under pressure. Cover the hole with a sterile dressing.

FURTHER READING

Bailey DA 1963 The infected hand. HK Lewis, London.
Barton NJ 1984 Review article. Fractures of the hand. Journal of Bone and Joint Surgery 66B:159–167
Fisk GR 1984 Review article. The wrist. Journal of Bone and Joint Surgery 66B:396–407
Henry AK 1957 Extensile exposure applied to limb surgery, 2nd edn. E&S Livingstone, Edinburgh
Keon-Cohen BT 1966 Fractures at the elbow. Journal of Bone and Joint Surgery 48A:1623–1639

41

Orthopaedics and trauma: lower limb

N. Goddard

CONTENTS

APPROACHES TO THE HIP AND PROXIMAL FEMUR

The hip joint is deeply placed and relatively inaccessible but can be exposed by several routes that are variations of the anterior, posterior and lateral approaches. The anterolateral approach is an extensile approach, providing access for draining a potentially septic hip as well as more complex procedures such as total hip arthroplasty. The lateral approach is usually used for open reduction and internal fixation of femoral fractures. Understand the anatomical approaches to benefit and be able to assist intelligently.

Anterolateral approach

Anterolateral approach (Fig. 41.1). Make a straight incision extending from the anterior superior iliac spine towards the tip of the greater trochanter, following the junction between gluteus medius and tensor fascia lata muscles. Incise the fascia overlying the interval between the two muscles and develop the plane proximally towards the anterior superior iliac spine. You should now be able to see the tendon of gluteus minimus and the capsule of the hip joint. Retract the gluteus minimus posteriorly and incise the capsule of the hip joint, draining any accumulated intra-articular fluid. Send a sample for bacteriological analysis.

Lateral approach to the proximal femur

Lateral approach to the proximal femur can be carried proximally to expose the hip joint. Use the distal approach to access the proximal femur and femoral neck for treatment of fractures. Make a 15-cm, straight longitudinal incision from the posterior superior corner of the greater trochanter, split the fascia lata longitudinally, posterior to the insertion of the tensor fascia lata muscle, to expose the vastus lateralis and identify its posterior attachment.

APPROACHES TO THE UPPER LEG

The femoral shaft may be approached from the anterior, medial or lateral aspects but the posterolateral approach is the most convenient and most commonly used. It can be extended proximally and distally if necessary and is most commonly employed to reduce and internally fix fractures of the femoral shaft.

Posterolateral approach

Palpate the tendon of the biceps femoris at the level of the lateral femoral condyle and also the posterior margin of the greater trochanter and make an incision joining these two points, deepened through fascia lata to locate the lateral intermuscular septum immediately anterior to the biceps femoris. Insert a finger between the septum and the bulk of the vastus lateralis lying anteriorly and continue the dissection down to the bone in this plane with a knife. Ligate the perforating branches of the profunda femoris vessels as you encounter them.

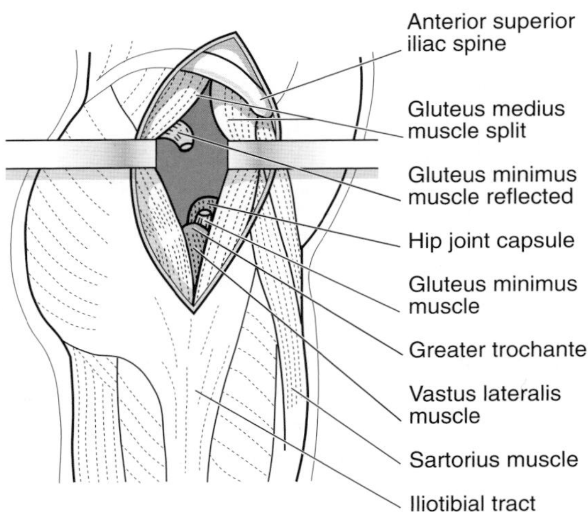

Fig. 41.1 Diagrammatic view of anterolateral approach to the right hip, viewed from the patient's right side. After identifying the opening up of the interval between the tensor fascia lata and gluteus medius muscles, retract them. You may not see the gluteus minimus muscle beneath the gluteus medius but if you do, you may retract it posteriorly. Below is the joint capsule and greater trochanter.

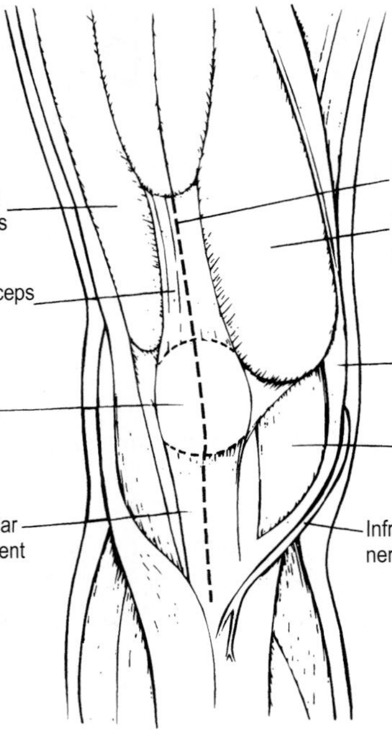

Fig. 41.2 Anterior approach to the knee joint.

APPROACHES TO THE KNEE

Most operations on the knee joint are carried out from the front, but many do not require a full and formal exposure of the whole joint, and a more limited exposure is adequate. Use the anterolateral and anteromedial approaches when you require limited access, for example to carry out meniscectomy or removal of loose bodies.

Anterior approach

Anterior approach (Fig. 41.2). Use this for operations on the extensor mechanism of the knee joint and to gain wide access to the inside of the joint itself. Make a straight incision 15 cm long in the midline, extending proximally from the upper margin of the tibial tubercle, and deepen it to expose the patellar ligament, the anterior surface of the patella and the quadriceps tendon, and the distal fibres of the rectus femoris. Reflect the skin and subcutaneous fat as a single layer medially to expose the junction of the quadriceps tendon and the vastus medialis, the medial border of the patella and the patellar ligament.

Make an incision along the medial edge of the quadriceps tendon and through the capsule along the medial margin of the patella and medial edge of the patellar ligament into the joint. If required, evert the patella, retract it laterally, and flex the knee at the same time. Extend the incision proximally into the rectus femoris if this proves to be difficult.

Posterior approach

Posterior approach is used to gain access to the popliteal fossa and occasionally to the posterior part of the knee joint to expose the popliteal vessels. The skin incision is 'S'- shaped.

Simple knee arthrotomy

Simple knee arthrotomy is suitable for open knee drainage, open meniscectomy and removal of a loose body. Incise the skin on the medial or lateral margin of the patella, down and slightly backwards to 1 cm below the articular margin of the tibia. Pick up and open the synovium.

APPROACH TO THE LOWER LEG

The shafts of the tibia and fibula are subcutaneous and may therefore be exposed by incisions through the overlying skin.

Anterior approach

Anterior approach gives access to the shaft of the tibia and the anterior compartment of the lower leg. Expose the fibula through a separate lateral incision if required. Incise the skin longitudinally 1 cm lateral to the crest of the tibia, from the tibial tubercle to the ankle. Reflect skin flaps medially and laterally to expose the subcutaneous surface of the tibia and the tibialis anterior muscle.

TIBIAL COMPARTMENT FASCIOTOMY

Decompression of the fascial compartments of the leg may be indicated after extensive closed soft-tissue injuries of the lower leg, proximal vascular reconstruction following arterial injury, and chronic exertional compartment syndrome. Measure the individual compartment pressures prior to operation and suspect impending ischaemia when the pressure reaches 10–30 mmHg below the diastolic pressure; higher pressures indicate an urgent need for fasciotomy. Impending or established compartment syndrome is a surgical emergency.

To measure the compartment pressure, you require a slit catheter (14G intravenous cannula), a length of plastic manometer tubing connected to a pressure transducer (a sphygmomanometer suffices if necessary). Prepare and sterilize the skin. Instil 2 ml of 1% lidocaine into the skin and insert the catheter into the anterior compartment. When it is satisfactorily positioned withdraw the trocar. Inject a small quantity of saline into the catheter to fill the dead space. Prefill the manometer tubing with saline and connect this via a three-way tap to the slit catheter and the pressure monitor, ensuring that there are no air bubbles in the system. Now connect the three-way tap to the pressure recorder and measure the compartment pressure.

Action

The anterior and lateral compartments can be decompressed through a full-length longitudinal anterolateral skin incision lateral to the crest of the mid-tibia extending from the level of the tibial tuberosity to just proximal to the ankle. Incise the fascia covering the tibialis anterior muscle and extend the incision in the fascia subcutaneously both proximally and distally so completely decompressing the anterior muscle group. By slightly undermining the skin it is also possible to decompress the lateral compartment, avoiding damage to the superficial peroneal nerve. In cases of exertional compartment syndrome only, it may be possible to perform a limited decompression through a short skin incision and then extend the fascial incision with a Smillie meniscectomy knife. The superficial and deep posterior compartments can be decompressed in a similar fashion using a single longitudinal posteromedial incision made just medial to the posteromedial border of the tibia. Incise the deep fascia and extend the incision proximally to the level of the tibial tuberosity and distally to a point 5 cm proximal to the medial malleolus, using the same technique.

Close only the skin following release of chronic exertional compartment syndrome. In acute compartment syndrome leave the wounds open and plan to suture the skin 3–5 days later when the swelling has subsided. If necessary apply a split skin graft. Be willing to inspect the wound in the interim period. Apply a compression dressing and elevate the leg.

KEY POINT Emergency decompression

- In an emergency excise the middle half of the fibula; this provides decompression of all compartments.

APPROACHES TO THE ANKLE

Anterior approach

Anterior approach (Fig. 41.3) is usually employed for operations on the ankle joint. Make an incision in the skin 10 cm long in the midline, centred over the middle of the ankle joint, avoiding the superficial peroneal nerve crossing diagonally, deepened through the deep fascia and extensor retinaculum, identifying the anterior tibial artery and deep peroneal nerve between the tendons of tibialis anterior and extensor hallucis longus. Retract the neurovascular bundle, extensor hallucis longus and extensor digitorum laterally and the tibialis anterior medially and incise the

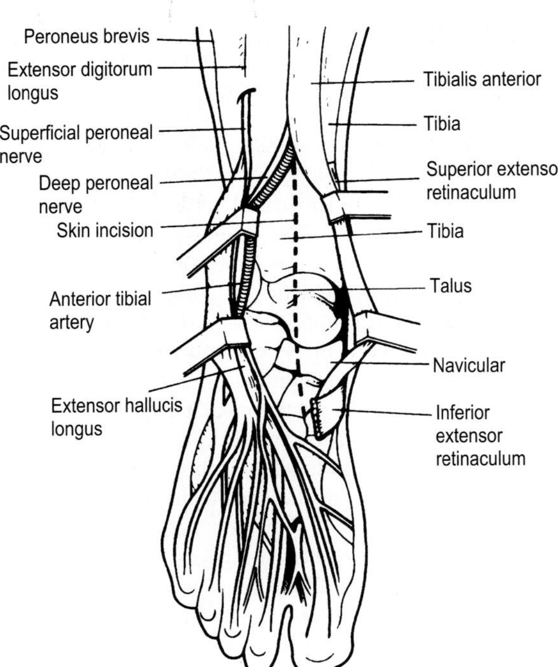

Fig. 41.3 The anterior approach to the ankle joint.

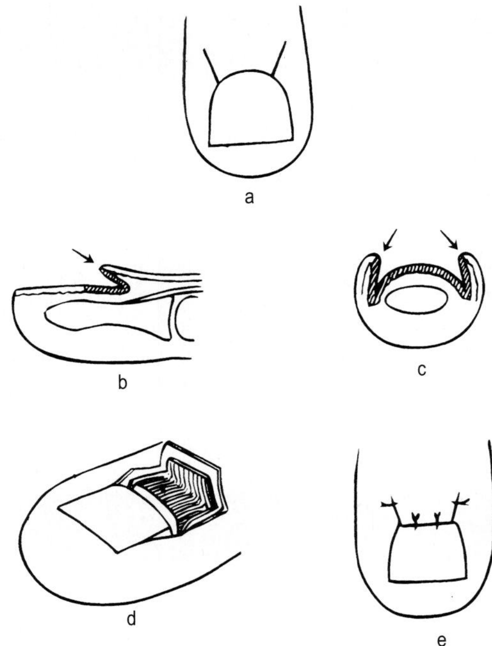

Fig. 41.4 Radical resection of the nail bed.

joint capsule longitudinally to open the ankle joint. Do not confuse the ankle joint with the talonavicular joint, which is unexpectedly close to it.

Posterior approach

Posterior approach gains access to the Achilles tendon, posterior aspect of the ankle joint and distal end of the tibia. Make an incision 15–20 cm long in the midline of the calf ending at the calcaneum, exposing the lateral side of the Achilles tendon, and retract the sural nerve and short saphenous vein laterally with the skin flap.

REPAIR OF RUPTURED ACHILLES TENDON

Rupture of the Achilles tendon is frequently missed and the choice between surgical repair and plaster immobilization in debatable. Access is through the posterior approach. Open the paratenon and expose the ends of the ruptured tendon, which are usually very ragged, like a shaving brush. Plantar-flex the foot and insert an absorbable size 0 core suture in a modified Kessler pattern, as described in Chapter 39 (p. 314, Fig. 39.4). Pull the suture tight to close the gap in the tendon. Insert a 4/0 running suture around the ragged ends of the repaired tendon and then suture the paratenon. With the ankle in full plantar flexion apply a plaster-of-Paris slab to the front of the ankle from the upper tibia of the toes and bandage it in place. Elevate the leg. Do not allow full sporting activities for at least 3 months after the repair.

RADICAL RESECTION OF THE NAIL BED (ZADEK'S OPERATION) (Fig. 41.4)

This operation is suitable for chronic ingrowing toenails and can be performed under local ring-block anaesthesia with a rubber band as a digital tourniquet. If it is infected remove the nail and wait for 2 months until the sepsis has subsided. Do not perform the operation in the presence of peripheral vascular disease. Remove the nail by separating it from the underlying nail bed with a MacDonald's elevator. Make two incisions, 1 cm long, extending proximally from each corner of the nail to the transverse skin crease just distal to the interphalangeal joint. Lift the skin and subcutaneous tissue as a flap and dissect this proximally. Carry the dissection under the edges of the skin incisions on either side of the terminal phalanx to the midlateral line to complete the clearance of the germinal matrix of the nail. Cut across the nail bed transversely at the site of the lunula (Latin diminutive of *luna* = moon; the opaque whitish half-moon at the root of the nail) and join this transverse incision to the dissections under the nail folds. Remove the block of nail bed from the surface of the proximal phalanx as far back as the insertion of the extensor tendon. Do not leave behind any fragments of germinal matrix. Draw the skin flap distally and carefully insert and tie one or two stitches to attach it to the nail bed. The tissues are fragile and the sutures easily cut out. Close the incisions on either side.

FURTHER READING

Antrum RN 1984 Radical excision of the nail fold for ingrowing toenails. Journal of Bone and Joint Surgery 6B:63–65

Henry AK 1957 Extensile exposure applied to limb surgery, 2nd edn. E&S Livingstone, Edinburgh

Rorabeck CH, Bourne RB, Fowler PJ 1983 The surgical treatment of exertional compartment syndrome in athletes. Journal of Bone and Joint Surgery 65A: 1245–1251

Zadik FR 1950 Obliteration of the nail bed of the great toe without shortening the terminal phalanx. Journal of Bone and Joint Surgery 32B:66–67

42

Plastic surgery

M. D. Brough (Deceased), P. Butler

CONTENTS

GENERAL PRINCIPLES

Plastic surgery (Greek *plassein* = to mould) is concerned with the restoration of form and function of the human body. It is used in the repair and reconstruction of defects following damage or loss of tissue from injury or disease or from their treatment. It is used in the correction of congenital deformities. It also includes aesthetic or cosmetic surgery, which involves the treatment of developmental or naturally acquired changes in the body.

There have been many advances in plastic surgery in recent years, giving rise to a multitude of new methods of reconstruction. These include improved techniques in microsurgery, tissue expansion, liposuction and craniofacial surgery. The most important development has been the recognition and application of axial pattern flaps. Several hundred cutaneous, myocutaneous and other flaps have now been identified but only those used more commonly will be described.

Prepare

KEY POINTS Planning repair

- Plan for repair and reconstruction of tissue defects well in advance of operation.
- Carry out the simplest procedure to achieve wound healing.
- If you need to reconstruct a defect in stages ensure that one stage does not jeopardize a subsequent one.

Identify the lines of tension within the skin described by the Professor of Anatomy in Vienna, Carl Ritter von Langer (1819–1887), which encircle, not cross, joints. Try to make all incisions parallel to these lines and if this is not possible, consider using a Z-plasty or local flap in closing the wound to help prevent the formation of scar contracture postoperatively. When planning a large flap, mark out a plan on the patient with a skin marker the day before operation. For smaller flaps and simple incisions, mark out the area of incision on the patient after preparing the area, before incising the skin. Use a fine pen and ink for marking out the lines of incisions on the face and a broad proprietary marking pen in other areas. Try to follow these lines, as they provide a useful guide once the skin has been incised and tension in the surrounding skin has changed. Be prepared, however, to make adjustments on occasions according to the circumstances.

General anaesthesia is now very safe but do not forget that many operations can be carried out under regional or local anaesthesia (see Ch. 2). Many operations on the hand, for example, can be performed under regional anaesthesia, including cases of replantation. Large areas of split skin graft can be taken from the lateral aspect of the thigh by infiltrating the lateral cutaneous nerve of the thigh in the region of the inguinal ligament with local anaesthetic. Many other procedures can be carried out under regional anaesthesia, if necessary with the assistance of a sedative. Many simple skin lesions can be excised under local anaesthesia with 1% lidocaine. To excise small lesions in the head and neck region, where the skin is highly vascular, use 2% lidocaine with 1:80000 adrenaline (epinephrine). Wait 5 minutes after injecting the mixture, to provide a relatively avascular field as well as anaesthesia. When carrying out extensive excisions of the face or scalp under general anaesthesia, inject a dilute solution of 0.5% lidocaine with 1:200000 adrenaline (epinephrine).

Technique

Sutures

On the face, approximate the deep dermis of the skin edges with interrupted 5/0 polyglactin 910 sutures. Accurately appose the skin edges with 6/0 interrupted nylon sutures. Remove them on the third or fourth postoperative day. If they remain longer, suture marks form which may prove impossible to remove without producing an ugly scar. Elsewhere on the body, approximate the deep dermis of the wound edges with 3/0 polyglactin 910 sutures and use subcuticular polypropylene sutures whenever possible, tying a knot at either end to prevent slipping. Leave these sutures in for 10 days or longer if there is a tendency for the scar to stretch because of its site.

Instruments

Respect tissues and their viability by handling them with care and using the appropriate instruments. Control and steady the skin with skin hooks or fine-toothed forceps; do not crush it by grasping it with non-toothed forceps.

For accurate suturing, use a fine needle-holder with a clasp that feels comfortable. Practise using needle-holders with their own cutting edges for cutting sutures so you can use them effectively. They are particularly useful when you are inserting many interrupted sutures, the accuracy of which is not crucial to the overall result.

Microvascular surgery requires specialized instruments.

Drains

For general principles see Chapter 1.

When moving large flaps introduce large suction drains at the donor site, which has a large potential cavity.

Diathermy

Beware of unipolar diathermy when coagulating vessels near the skin. The burnt tissue may be visible and painful.

Always use a bipolar coagulator for fine work and flaps. The current from a unipolar machine could destroy the vessels in the base of a flap as it is being raised.

SKIN COVER

Close skin wounds primarily to provide ideal cover following incisions of the skin, excisions of skin lesions and simple lacerations.

Use split skin grafts to repair wounds with significant skin loss, to avoid skin closure with tension, or following trauma with an appreciable degree of crush injury to the local tissues. Skin graft survival depends on adequate vascularity of the base of the wound.

Use skin flaps, which carry their own blood supply and are temporarily self-sufficient, in primary or secondary repair or reconstruction. Use them as primary cover for vital structures such as exposed neurovascular bundles or for structures that have an inadequate blood supply to support a graft, such as bare bone, bare cartilage, bare tendons and exposed joints.

SKIN CLOSURE

Employ primary skin closure following simple skin incisions, surgical excision of small skin lesions and to repair simple lacerations.

Do not carry out primary closure if the tension in closing the wound causes blanching of the skin.

Action

1. Whenever possible, make incisions following the direction of the tension lines, particularly on the face.
2. For excisions, mark the skin in ink, planning to excise the minimal necessary amount of tissue. Draw an ellipse with pointed ends around this mark, parallel to the tension lines.
3. On the face, inject the surrounding tissue with 2% lidocaine and 1:80000 adrenaline (epinephrine), and wait 5 minutes for both components to take effect.
4. Make a vertical cut through the skin along the lines of the ellipse. Ensure that you adequately clear the lesion in depth.

5 Undermine the skin edges beneath the layer of subcutaneous fat to facilitate approximating the edges without tension.

KEY POINTS Skin viable?

- If the skin edges have been crushed, do not further insult them by inserting sutures, but carefully trim away dead skin and apply a simple dressing. Close the skin after a delay of 24–48 hours.
- Beware of skin that has been degloved or torn from its fascial base. Resect it primarily.
- If damaged skin is possibly viable, replace it, re-examine it at 48 hours, and then resect it if it does not bleed when it is cut.

6 Place a skin hook in each end of the wound and ask your assistant to draw them apart. This manoeuvre approximates the edges.

7 Close the wound in layers and apply a small dressing, or use no dressing at all if practical.

SKIN GRAFTS

A skin graft (Greek *graphion* = a style; something inserted) is a piece of skin completely detached from its donor site and transferred to a recipient site. It may contain part of the thickness of the skin (a split skin graft described by the German surgeon Karl Thiersch in 1874) or the full-thickness graft of skin, described in 1874 by the Austrian ophthalmologist John Wolfe, who settled in Glasgow. A skin graft depends for its survival on receiving adequate nutrition from the recipient bed. Thus, thin split skin grafts survive more readily than thick split skin grafts or full-thickness grafts. If there is a poor vascular bed, or infection, no graft will survive. In these cases prepare the graft bed appropriately with dressings (see below), or consider using a flap. Choose an appropriate donor site for each individual patient.

SMALL SPLIT SKIN GRAFT

A split skin graft is a sheet of tissue containing epidermis and some dermis taken from a donor site. It is obtained by shaving the skin with an appropriate knife or blade. A layer of deep dermis is preserved at the donor site and, when dressed appropriately, this is re-epithelialized from residual skin adnexae.

Use a small split skin graft to repair traumatic loss of small areas of skin from the hand or fingers, and occasionally in other parts of the body. Avoid using them on the tips of the thumb and index fingers since they tend to become hyperaesthetic.

Choose the donor site carefully. On the upper limb prefer skin from the medial aspect of the arm where the donor site is inconspicuous; on the forearm an ugly resultant scar may be visible.

Action

1 Mark out on the medial aspect of the arm an area of skin which is more than sufficient to cover the recipient site.

2 Inject 2% lidocaine and 1:80000 adrenaline (epinephrine) intradermally into and beyond the marked area and wait for 5 minutes.

3 Lubricate the marked area with liquid paraffin.

4 Grip the arm on the lateral aspect with your left hand so that the skin which is marked out becomes tense, with a convex surface.

5 Cut the graft from the marked area using a Da Silva knife.

6 Dress the donor site with a calcium alginate dressing, one layer of paraffin gauze, several layers of dressing gauze and a crepe bandage.

7 Apply the split skin graft directly onto the recipient site, spread it and anchor it using a minimal number of sutures.

8 Apply paraffin gauze, dressing gauze and a crepe bandage.

9 Re-dress the graft at 5 days.

10 Re-dress the graft donor site at 10 days.

LARGE SPLIT SKIN GRAFT

Use these grafts following extensive skin loss from burns, trauma or radical excisional surgery.

Adequately prepare the recipient site to ensure a good 'take' of the graft. Grafts take best on exposed muscle or well-prepared granulation tissue. They do not reliably survive on exposed fat where there is a poor vascular supply.

The take of a graft can be improved in certain circumstances by meshing it, quilting it, or by delaying its application and then exposing it. These are described below.

Use an electric dermatome, if available, to harvest the graft using the same principles outlined below.

Prepare

1 Following 'elective' surgical excisions apply pressure to obtain haemostasis. Avoid diathermy if possible since skin grafts do not take over diathermy burns.

2 Where subcutaneous fat is exposed, suture the overlying skin down to the muscle or deep fascia to cover it.

3 For infected wounds, take swabs for bacterial culture and prepare the recipient site with dressings of Eusol (Edinburgh University solution of lime) and paraffin. Change them 3–4 times a day. The recipient site is ready to receive a graft when it appears healthy and compact and has red granulation tissue with minimal exudate.

> **KEY POINT Haemolytic streptococci**
>
> - Do not apply grafts in the presence of beta-haemolytic streptococci, group A. First eradicate the infection with regular dressing changes and appropriate systemic antibiotics.

4 Choose the donor site most readily available to provide a large area of skin graft; this is usually the thigh. In young people, use the inner aspect of the thigh, where the donor site will be hidden. In elderly people, use the outer aspect of the thigh, where the skin is slightly thicker, so that if healing is delayed the wound is accessible and is easily managed.

Action

1 Prepare both recipient and donor sites by applying skin antiseptic.

2 Have your assistant spread a large swab on the side of the thigh opposite to the proposed donor site. With a hand on the swab it is possible to support the thigh and tense the skin at the donor site by gripping the skin firmly with the swab.

3 Set the blade on the Watson knife to take the appropriate thickness of skin graft. Use a medium setting at first and then adjust it accordingly. Apply liquid paraffin on a swab to the donor site and along the knife blade.

4 Ask your assistant to hold the edge of a graft board at the starting point with the other hand (Fig. 42.1).

5 Cut a skin graft with the Watson knife, holding a board in your non-cutting hand and advancing this a few centimetres in front of the knife. Start with the knife at 45° to the skin and once the blade has entered the dermis rotate it axially so that it runs just parallel with the skin surface. Use a 'sawing' action with the knife, advancing the blade only a few millimetres at a time. When you have harvested an adequate length of skin, turn the blade upwards and cut the graft off with one firm movement. If the graft is not detached with this movement, cut along its base with a pair of scissors.

6 Place the skin graft, outer surface downwards, on a damp saline swab and make sure that you have obtained sufficient skin; in case of doubt, take another strip of split skin.

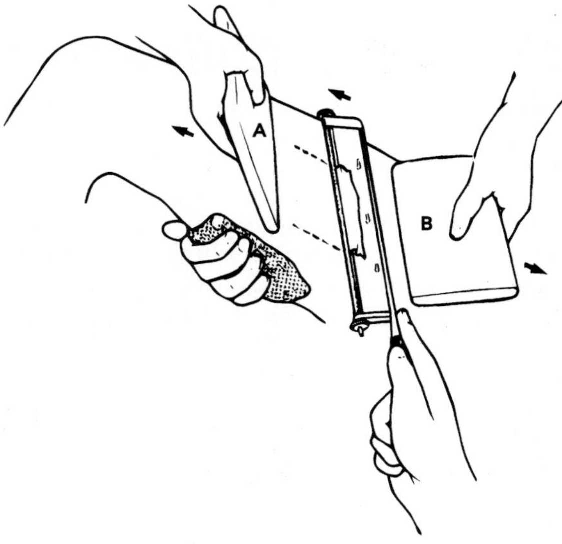

Fig. 42.1 Taking a large split skin graft from the thigh, the surgeon advances board A in front of the knife as it progresses along the thigh. The assistant tenses the skin of the thigh in his right hand, using a large swab to prevent his hand from slipping, and tenses the skin behind the knife using board B.

7 Dress the donor site with calcium alginate dressing, one layer of paraffin gauze, dressing gauze, cotton wool and a crepe bandage.

8 Apply the skin graft to the recipient defect, ensuring that it is placed with its cut surface applied to the wound. The outer surface is opaque, the inner surface is shiny. Spread it, using two pairs of closed non-toothed forceps.

9 Cut off the surplus skin at the wound edge, leaving a margin of 3 mm around the periphery.

10 If the skin has been applied on a site to which you can apply a satisfactory compression dressing, do not use sutures.

11 Dress with several layers of paraffin gauze, dressing gauze, wool and crepe bandage, immobilizing the joints above and below the graft with a bulky dressing.

12 In areas where it is difficult to apply a compression dressing, immobilize the graft with interrupted sutures at the edge or insert a circumferential continuous suture around the graft.

13 Dress with paraffin gauze, dressing gauze, wool and strips of adhesive dressing.

14 Keep the graft site elevated postoperatively.

15 For grafts on the lower limb below the knee, do not allow the grafted area to be dependent for 7 days; fluid will collect between the graft and the base unless the graft is meshed. Then arrange progressive mobilization with compression support to the leg and foot including the graft.

DELAYED EXPOSED GRAFTS

Use a delayed graft when haemostasis is difficult to establish peroperatively. Prepare the recipient site by excising all dead or doubtful tissue and any foreign material. Achieve haemostasis and dress it. Harvest adequate split skin grafts and dress the donor site (see below). Spread the graft on paraffin gauze with the external opaque surface on the gauze, fold and wrap it in a saline-soaked swab, place it in a sterile jar to be stored in a refrigerator at 4°C.

On the following day expose the recipient site and apply the skin graft, spreading it to cover all areas and trim excess marginal skin. Remove the paraffin gauze, leave the graft exposed and observe it regularly. If serum collects beneath it, extrude it to the edge or through a small incision made in the graft. Ensure that the exposed area is well protected.

MESHED GRAFTS

These are useful for covering large areas if donor skin is limited, as following extensive burns. Any underlying seroma that collects escapes through the interstices of the graft. They can be moulded to cover irregular surfaces but the resulting appearance is not ideal.

Prepare the donor site in the usual way. Harvest long, thin strips of split skin graft, as described above and dress the donor site.

Pass the skin graft through the skin mesher. It may need to be placed on a carrier for this, depending on the type of instrument. Apply the mesh graft directly onto the recipient site using two pairs of non-toothed forceps, spreading the skin to cover all suitable recipient areas and suturing the graft with continuous sutures at the periphery if the area is difficult to dress. Dress the area with a calcium alginate dressing, one layer of paraffin gauze, dressing gauze, cotton wool and crepe bandage. Re-dress it at 4 or 5 days and continue at approximately 3-day intervals until the interstices have epithelialized.

QUILTED GRAFTS

These are most usefully applied to large areas of the tongue or any other highly vascular area. Any method of graft fixation is liable to cause bleeding beneath the graft, lifting it off. If multiple sutures are inserted over the whole area of the graft, giving it the appearance of a bed quilt, at each suture site a small area of graft take is ensured. Epithelialization subsequently spreads out from each of these.

FULL-THICKNESS GRAFTS

These give better cosmetic results than split thickness grafts as they contract less. The quality of the skin is better but they need a very good vascular bed in order to survive. They are most commonly applied on the face following excision of small lesions, and the best results are achieved in the eyelid region and around the medial canthus. They can occasionally be used on the hand, but are not generally used elsewhere, as large grafts leave a large primary defect. The best donor sites are those with surplus skin so that the skin can be closed primarily with an insignificant scar. The most common donor areas are post-auricular, pre-auricular, upper eyelid, nasolabial and supraclavicular skin.

Action

1 Mark the area of skin to be removed and measure it.

2 Mark out a similar area in the donor site, allowing an extra 2.5 mm or more at each margin for the contour difference that will be present at the recipient site. Plan an ellipse at the donor site around the proposed graft to allow primary closure.

3 Inject local anaesthetic at the excision and donor sites.

4 Create the defect at the recipient site.

5 With a size 15 blade, cut around the margins of the planned donor skin. Raise the full ellipse of skin and subcutaneous tissue. Undermine the skin edges at the donor defect and close this primarily.

6 Place the skin graft onto a wet saline swab, skin surface down. Using small, curved scissors, cut the subcutaneous fat off the skin graft and excise the redundant skin.

7 Place the skin graft into the defect and suture the edges at the periphery. Leave the suture ends long.

8 Use tie-over sutures to fix the dressing of paraffin gauze and proflavine wool. Apply a pressure dressing for 24 hours, if possible.

9 Dress the donor site and plan to re-dress the recipient site at 1 week.

COMPOSITE GRAFTS

These consist of skin and other tissue, usually subcutaneous fat and some underlying cartilage. They are most commonly used where there is significant loss of a nostril rim or the periphery of the pinna of the ear.

RANDOM PATTERN SKIN FLAPS

Skin flaps are used to repair or reconstruct defects at sites with inadequate local blood supply to support a skin graft. Flaps differ from grafts by remaining attached, surviving by bringing their own blood supply, which may be beneficial to the recipient site. It may introduce a new blood supply to an avascular area following irradiation, or to a delayed union fracture site.

The skin quality in a flap is almost normal and its texture and cosmetic appearance are much better than a graft. It may, however, lose its nerve supply and the transfer may compromise the vascular supply and lymphatic drainage.

Until relatively recently, all skin flaps were based randomly because the underlying blood supply was not studied. It was, however, recognized that in certain areas, flaps with a length greater than their base would survive. This is now known to result from the fact that these flaps were unwittingly based on an axial pattern. If a flap has an adequate artery and vein passing down its central axis, it may be safely transferred with a very large length-to-breadth ratio. Indeed, the breadth need be the artery and vein alone, providing they remain patent. Such flaps are termed axial pattern flaps and have been identified in many areas.

Many of the superficial muscles of the body have one principal vascular hilum, and these muscles can be rotated about the hilum on a single pedicle. It has further been realized that the skin overlying these superficial muscles receives its vascular supply from them. Consequently the muscle with its overlying skin can be transposed as a single unit, forming a myocutaneous flap. A large number of these flaps have been described. We shall describe only the more commonly used ones.

Special terms are traditionally used in relation to flaps. Delay indicates partial division of a flap at its base and re-suturing. This procedure encourages an improved blood supply to the flap from the opposite attachment. Complete division at the base carried out a few days later is then usually safe. After a flap has been transferred safely, the bridging portion may be divided. The two ends are trimmed and one is sutured into the new recipient area while the other is replaced in the donor site. This is referred to as in-setting.

When planning a flap, it is useful to employ a sheet of sterile paper or other similar material to act as a template. This can be cut to shape and used as a trial flap.

Z-PLASTY

These are used for releasing linear contractions that usually develop along linear scars that traverse Langer's lines. They are often most evident when crossing the concavity of the flexor aspect of a joint, but they can occur on extensor surfaces and in other areas unrelated to joints. In effect, skin is drawn in from the sides to increase the length.

1 Draw a line along the full extent of the contracture (Fig. 42.2). From one end, draw a line at 60° to the first line and of the same length. From the opposite end, draw a line at 60° on the opposite side of the line for the same length.

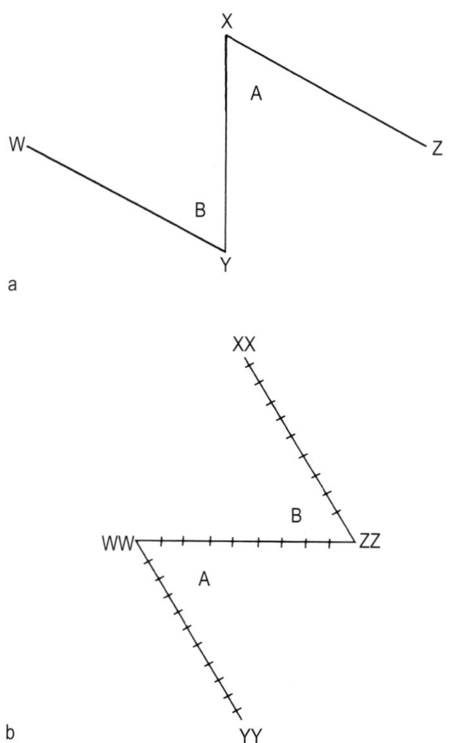

Fig. 42.2 Z-plasty. Contracture along X–Y is released to XX–YY by raising and interchanging flaps A and B. The distance W–Z is shortened to WW–ZZ.

2 Cut along the central line and excise any scar tissue. Cut along the two lateral lines through the full thickness of skin and subcutaneous tissue. Raise the flaps so formed, lifting the skin and subcutaneous tissue as one, holding the tip of each flap with a skin hook.

3 Interchange the two skin flaps. If they do not meet comfortably, undermine the skin and subcutaneous tissue around the periphery of the wound to allow them to lie correctly.

4 Suture the tips of the two flaps into place first then suture the remaining edges of the flaps.

5 Dress the wound.

The angle of the Z-plasty can be varied according to circumstances.

If the scar contracture is particularly long, use two or more Z-plasties, either in series or at intervals along the length of the contracture. For scar contractures across a web space, use a W-plasty. This consists of two Z-plasties, placed in reverse direction to each other, meeting at the base of the web space.

TRANSPOSITION FLAP

Small transposition flaps on the face have long been used. It is well recognized, that in this region, because of the vascularity of the skin, flaps with a large length-to-breadth ratio can be used safely. They allow skin from an area of abundance to be moved to a defect where primary closure is inappropriate. On the face there is an abundance of skin appropriate for transposition flaps in the nasolabial area, the glabella (Latin *glaber*=smooth, bald); between the eyebrows and the upper eyelid. In other parts of the body, many axial pattern flaps are used as transposition flaps.

RHOMBOID FLAP

Rhomboid usually signifies lozenge shape; such a flap is most useful when the appropriate ellipse for excision of a defect is at right angles to Langer's lines. It has a similar effect to a transposition flap carried through 90°.

ROTATION FLAP

These are large flaps used to close relatively small defects, using excess skin at a distance from the defect and borrowing small amounts of skin from a large area. They are principally used to borrow skin from the neck to take up to the face. They can be used on the scalp and for treating sacral pressure sores.

ADVANCEMENT FLAP

Advancement flaps are most commonly used on the face to preserve feature lines or structures of the face. They can be used on the forehead or for defects of the eyebrow. Frequently, in these situations, bilateral advancement flaps are used simultaneously to reconstruct one defect.

1 Mark out the defect. Mark out the smallest possible square or rectangle enclosing this defect, with lines parallel and at right-angles to Langer's lines. Extend the marks of the sides running parallel to Langer's lines in each direction from the defect, thus delineating two flaps.

2 Create the defect. Elevate the flaps and advance them towards each other. Suture them together and suture their sides.

EXPANSION FLAP

These flaps are used specifically for repairing and reconstructing defects of the scalp, which are notorious for their inability to stretch because the galea (Latin = a helmet) is inelastic. Raise a wide-based flap including the galea and make multiple vertical and transverse incisions in the galea with a no. 15 blade.

CROSS-LEG FLAP

This used to be the most commonly used flap to cover fractures of the tibia and fibula with extensive overlying skin loss. It is usually replaced with fasciocutaneous and free flaps. In principle the flap, including deep fascia, is raised from the other leg.

CROSS-FINGER FLAP

Cross-finger flaps are a convenient means of obtaining good-quality skin cover for defects on the flexor aspects of the fingers, where split skin grafts would contract.

ABDOMINAL TUBE PEDICLE FLAP

These flaps were formerly used for transferring a large amount of skin and subcutaneous tissue from the abdomen to a distant site such as the foot, the face, or elsewhere. They have been superseded almost totally by the introduction of axial pattern flaps.

AXIAL PATTERN SKIN FLAPS

A flap designed around a recognized artery and vein, with these vessels passing down its central axis, can be safely transferred, and may have a large length to breadth ratio. The breadth of the base need be the artery and vein alone, provided they remain fully patent.

Many of the superficial muscles have a single vascular hilum so that the muscle can be rotated about this pedicle. Moreover, superficial muscles offer vascular supply to overlying skin, so that the combined muscle and overlying skin can be moved together as a myocutaneous flap.

LATISSIMUS DORSI FLAP

The flap is based on the thoracodorsal vessels, and these enter the muscle just below its insertion into the humerus (Fig. 42.3). Its most useful application is as a myocutaneous flap in breast reconstruction and reconstruction of chest wall defects. It can be used in pharyngeal reconstruction and for defects of the back up to and just above the nape of the neck. It can be used as a muscle flap alone to cover a large defect, or the muscle can be used to transfer a small island of skin, as in breast reconstruction, or a large island of skin. If a large island is transferred, primary closure of the donor site is not possible.

The flap has wide application in free tissue transfer.

TRAM FLAP

The transverse rectus abdominis muscle (TRAM) provides an alternative flap for breast reconstruction to the latissimus dorsi muscle. It has the advantage that it can normally transfer sufficient autologous tissue to avoid the necessity of using an implant.

The flap can also be used for reconstructing chest wall defects and defects of the perineum. In either of these circumstances the skin paddle may be taken in the vertical plane (a vertical rectus abdominis muscle or VRAM flap), with the skin paddle lying completely over the muscle.

The flap may be used as a pedicled flap based either on the superior deep epigastric vessels for breast reconstruction or chest wall defects, or on the inferior deep epigastric vessels for perineal defects.

It can be used as a free flap, most commonly for breast reconstruction by using the inferior deep epigastric vessels, which are larger and more reliable.

OTHER AXIAL PATTERN FLAPS

Forehead and scalp flaps

The forehead flap survives on the anterior branch of one superficial temporal artery while the scalp flap depends on the posterior branch of the superficial temporal artery.

Tongue flap

Tongue flap, used for closing large palatal fistulas, and lip, pharynx and oral defects, relies on the rich vascular supply rather than on a single vessel.

Deltopectoral flap

Deltopectoral flap, sometimes known as a Bakamjian flap after its innovator, is used for providing skin flap cover to the chin, the cheek, the region of the pinna and the neck. It is now rarely used to provide lining to the oral cavity and pharynx.

Pectoralis flap

Pectoralis flap, based on the pectoral vessels, is a versatile myocutaneous flap that can reach the head and neck.

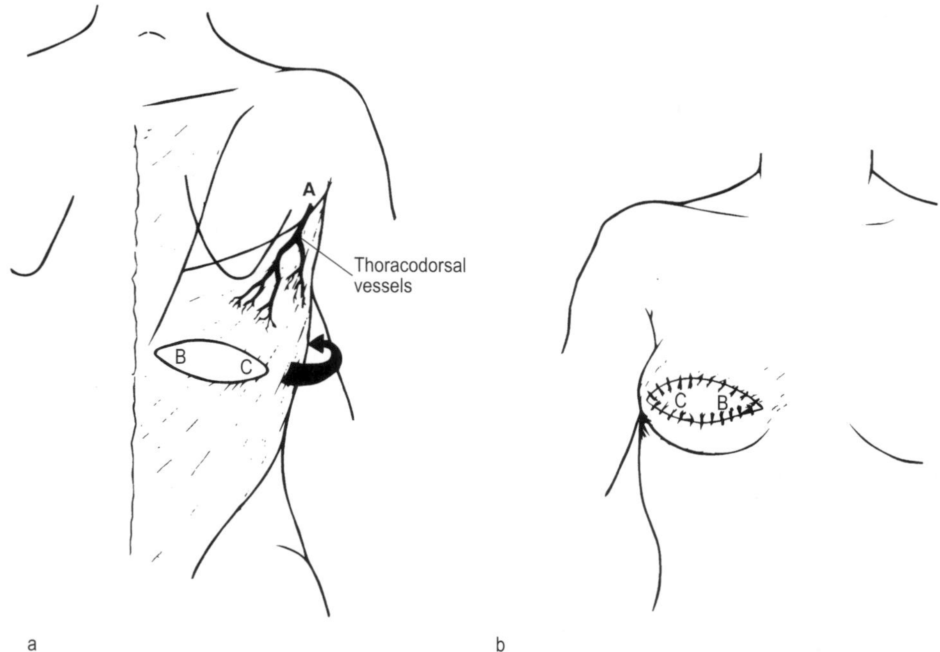

Fig. 42.3 Latissimus dorsi flap. The skin overlying the right latissimus dorsi flap is elevated from the muscle, leaving a central elliptiform island of skin attached to the muscle. The muscle is freed from its peripheral and underlying attachments and passed subcutaneously to the defect on the anterior chest wall, pivoted on its insertion (A) where the thoracodorsal vessels enter the muscle (a). In breast reconstruction, the muscle is sutured into the region of the reconstructed breast and the island of skin inserted into the mastectomy scar. A prosthesis is inserted beneath the flap (b).

Groin flap

Groin flap can be used for defects of the lower abdominal wall, but its greatest application is providing skin cover for severe injuries to the hand or wrist. It is therefore most useful when the skin over the iliac crest is relatively thin.

Tensor fascia lata flap

Tensor fascia lata flap is useful in treating trochanteric and ischial pressure sores and defects of the upper thigh, lower abdominal wall and the groin, particularly when the femoral vessels are exposed. It is a myofasciocutaneous flap, based on the vessels to the tensor fascia lata muscle. Inclusion of the lateral cutaneous nerve of the thigh within the flap allows it to be used as a sensory flap.

Biceps femoris flap

Biceps femoris flap receives branches of the profunda femoris artery and is a myocutaneous flap or can be a simple muscle flap. It is particularly useful for ischial pressure sores.

Gastrocnemius flap

Both heads can be used separately for covering defects on the anterior aspect of the leg, as simple muscle flaps or as myocutaneous flaps.

Fasciocutaneous flaps

Fasciocutaneous flaps have their greatest use in providing skin cover to exposed bone in the middle third of the leg.

TISSUE EXPANSION

The principle is exemplified by the stretched abdominal wall resulting from pregnancy. An expander (Fig. 42.4) is inserted beneath the deep fascia or superficial muscle and expanded serially by injections of saline into an attached reservoir to stretch the overlying skin. Following expansion, the expander is removed and the surplus skin used to cover the adjacent defect.

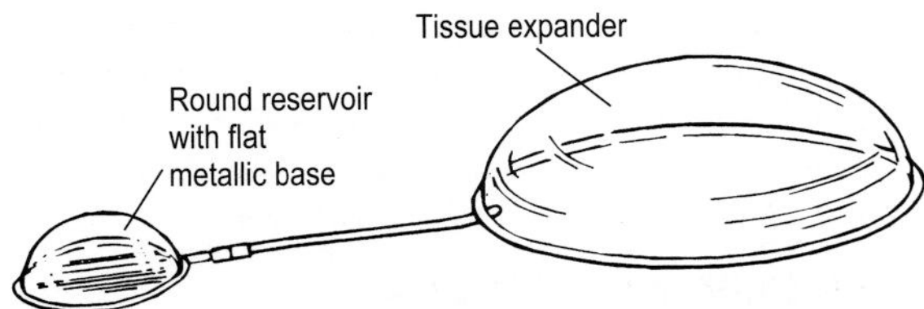

Fig. 42.4 Tissue expander and reservoir.

Expanders are most effective when placed on a bone base. They are particularly effective when placed on the calvaria (Latin = skull) to expand scalp, and on the chest wall to expand skin for breast reconstruction. They have limited value in limbs. Do not use tissue expanders under badly scarred or irradiated skin.

GRAFTS OF OTHER TISSUES

Cartilage grafts

Cartilage grafts are used in reconstructing cartilaginous defects of the nose, large defects of the lower eyelids and major defects of the ear.

Nose

Composite defects of skin and cartilage at the nostril margin can be reconstructed using composite grafts from the ear. Most other small cartilaginous defects of the nose can be reconstructed using cartilage from other parts of the nose during a corrective rhinoplasty.

Eyelids

Large defects of the lower eyelid often require the introduction of cartilage for support and the best donor site for this is the septum of the nose. This provides a composite graft of cartilage and mucous membrane. The latter is used to reconstruct the conjunctival surface.

Ear

Costal cartilage is used for total ear reconstruction. Reconstruction of a major portion of the ear may be difficult. It is sometimes justifiable to discard those cartilaginous segments already present and perform a total ear reconstruction; you may need to employ preoperative tissue expansion or use a temporoparietal flap.

Vascular grafts

Vascular grafts (see Ch. 32). Employ small-vessel grafts for replanting and free-flap transfer. Vein grafts can be used to replace damaged arteries and veins; choose one that matches the vessel to be repaired. Use magnification and microscopy for small vessels.

Nerve, tendon and bone grafts

Nerve, tendon and bone grafts are described in Chapter 39. Homograft (Greek *homos* = same; from the same species) bone, xenograft (Greek *xenos* = strange, foreign; from a different species) cartilage and xenograft collagen are all used, after appropriate preparation, in reconstruction. Theoretically, they act as a scaffold into which the patient's own tissue grows.

Homograft and xenograft skin

Homograft and xenograft skin may be used as temporary biological dressings but they are eventually rejected.

MICROVASCULAR SURGERY

Microvascular surgery involves the anastomosis and repair of small vessels.

It has clinical application in cases of replantation and free tissue transfer.

The surgery is highly specialized. Operations may take many hours and require special instruments in addition to an appropriate microscope.

This type of operation should be carried out only in specialized units.

REPLANTATION

Consider replantation following accidental amputation or devascularization of limbs proximal to the ankle or wrist joints (macroreplantation) and distal to the ankle or wrist joint (microreplantation). Control bleeding from the amputation stump by simple pressure and elevation. Avoid clamping vessels to stop haemorrhage unless essential, as this may cause unnecessary damage. Cool but do not freeze the part to be implanted; place it in a polythene bag and lay it on ice.

Replantation may also succeed for the ear, scalp, penis and for composite facial tissues.

Contact the nearest microvascular surgery unit and take advice.

Prepare the patient and amputated part for urgent transfer.

FREE TISSUE TRANSFER

Free tissue transfer is used in many forms of reconstruction. Isolate the tissue on a recognized vascular pedicle. After transfer to its distant site, anastomose the vessels of the vascular pedicle to appropriate nearby vessels, either directly or with vein grafts, usually with an end-to-side anastomosis so that the distal flow of the donor artery is not prejudiced. Venous drainage is usually via end-to-end anastomoses to superficial veins or to venae comitantes of a nearby artery.

Most free flaps currently used in reconstruction consist of cutaneous or myocutaneous flaps. Apart from the flaps described above there are many other cutaneous and myocutaneous flaps which are occasionally used.

Other free tissue transfers include vascularized bone grafts from rib, iliac crest, fibula, radius and metatarsal, osseocutaneous flaps from the iliac crest, fibula, radius or metatarsal with overlying skin, sensory cutaneous flaps, muscle flaps with motor innervation and fascial flaps. Other transfers include small bowel for oesophageal reconstruction, and omentum for soft tissue defects. A high undescended testis can be re-sited in the scrotum. Digits or parts of digits can be transferred from toe to hand.

One of the most common free flaps used in reconstruction is the radial forearm flap, based on the radial artery and either the venae comitantes or superficial veins.

BURNS

The treatment of patients with extensive burns is complex and ideally these patients should also be treated initially in an intensive care unit.

KEY POINTS Special circumstances

- Treat patients with burns involving 15% of the body surface area (10% in children), or severe burns of the face or hands in a specialized burns unit.
- Treat patients with any significant inhalation burn in a specialized unit.

SUPERFICIAL BURNS

1. Clean the burn wound, remove the roof of all blisters. Expose superficial burns of the face but apply sterile liquid paraffin to reduce crusting.
2. Clean and expose burns of the perineum but apply silver sulfadiazine (Flamazine) cream. Nurse the patient without dressings on a sterile sheet on a low-air-loss or water bed but keep him warm.
3. Cover superficial burns of other areas with two layers of paraffin gauze and a bulky absorptive dressing and leave it unchanged for 1 week unless it becomes soaked. Then change the dressing at 1 week and subsequently twice per week until the wound is healed.

DEEP DERMAL BURNS

1. Tangentially shave with a graft knife between the second and fifth day. Continue to shave until you observe punctate bleeding from the surface. Achieve haemostasis with pressure, apply a split skin graft and re-dress at 4 days.
2. When fully healed, measure and apply a pressure garment. This is an elasticated garment individually measured for the individual to cover the area of the burn wound, to be worn for at least 6 months, to minimize hypertrophy and contracture of the resulting scars.
3. Treat areas that are not healed at 3 weeks as full-thickness burns.

EXTENSIVE FULL-THICKNESS BURNS

ESCHAROTOMY

Identify areas of full-thickness burns that are circumferential around digit, limb or trunk. If the viability of the distal part is jeopardized, or if respiration is hindered as with partial circumferential burns of the chest wall, carry out an escharotomy (Greek *eschara* = a hearth; the mark of a burn). Give an appropriate intravenous dose of diazepam. Take a scalpel and incise the full length of the full-thickness burn, allowing subcutaneous fat to bulge out of the escharotomy wound.

Repeat the longitudinal escharotomy at different sites of the circumference until you have restored satisfactory perfusion of the distal part then dress the wounds with paraffin gauze or silver sulfadiazine (Flamazine).

Action

1. Identify a suitable area, not exceeding 20% of the body area, to treat primarily.
2. Identify a suitable donor site for the skin graft.
3. Excise the chosen area of full-thickness burn with a scalpel and be sure that the resultant bed consists of

viable tissue. It is often safer to excise all subcutaneous fat to leave a graft bed of deep fascia. Achieve haemostasis.

4 Harvest a split skin graft and mesh this (see above).

5 Apply the mesh graft to the burn wound site and dress with several layers of paraffin gauze and an absorbent dressing.

6 Re-dress after 4 days. Do not excise burn tissue between the fifth and the twelfth day post-burn, as the patient may be in an unsuitable catabolic state. Do not excise further burn until the donor site has healed and is ready for reharvesting, or another donor site is available.

Small areas

1 Operate between the second and fifth day to excise all burn tissue and apply a split skin graft.

2 If the viability of subcutaneous fat is in doubt, excise this down to the deep fascia.

3 If the viability of the tissue is still in doubt, dress the wound and bring the patient back to the theatre 48 hours later. Reassess viability at this second operation and extend the excision if necessary and graft. Re-dress after 4 days.

OTHER WOUNDS

Infected wounds arise in a multitude of different situations. Do not close them primarily.

Two common causes presenting to plastic surgeons include pressure sores and necrotizing fasciitis. Their management is described below.

WOUNDS FROM PRESSURE INJURIES

Pressure injuries are common and difficult to detect in the early stages of development. The tissues between the skeleton and an external surface are compressed, causing a variable degree of ischaemia, which may be sufficient to cause necrosis involving superficial skin, full thickness of skin or all the tissues overlying the skeleton.

The most frequent sites are well-recognized 'pressure areas' over the backs of the heels and around the pelvis, over the ischial tuberosity, the sacrum and the greater trochanter, resulting from the patient lying on or against a hard surface for a prolonged period. Particular risks include coma, general anaesthesia, loss of sensation as in diabetic neuropathy or paraplegia, and patients who are thin, poorly nourished, cachectic and relatively immobile. Some surgical patients are therefore at particular risk.

The first sign is erythema in the damaged area. Blistering usually indicates a superficial injury only. If the damage is deep the skin colour changes to blue and then to black as a thick eschar develops over a period of many days. This remains dry for several weeks before the necrotic tissue starts to separate and spontaneous separation may take many weeks or months. After separation the wound will heal by secondary intention. A residual sinus persists if necrotic tissue remains buried or if the underlying bone becomes infected.

As many patients with these injuries are debilitated, the above process may take many months and treatment is aimed at accelerating the healing process without insulting the patient further with unnecessary surgery.

Action

1 Avoid these injuries by identifying those patients particularly at risk and attend to their general health, specifically their nutrition and other medical disorders.

2 Take appropriate precautions when they are on the operating table and when in bed on the ward. Use one of the many specialized mattresses or beds to distribute the weight of the patient where possible. If these are not available the nursing staff may need to assist a change of position of the patient at least every 2 hours.

3 Cover superficial wounds with non-adherent dressings such as paraffin gauze and change on alternate days until healed.

4 Cover hard eschar with simple protective dressings only, or leave exposed if appropriate.

5 When the eschar starts to separate use a debriding agent such as Eusol and paraffin dressings changed daily.

6 Assist separation of the eschar by using a forceps and scissors during a dressing change. Repeat this with every change of dressing and avoid formal debridement in theatre and an unnecessary general anaesthetic.

7 Take wound swabs at regular intervals to monitor the organisms present but use antibiotics sparingly, for example if there is evidence of surrounding cellulitis.

8 Advise the patient to have a regular bath or shower, if appropriate, to help clean the wound and improve the patient's morale.

9 When a cavity is established use a vacuum dressing. After irrigating and cleaning the wound with saline, insert the foam dressing, introduce the drain and cover with an occlusive dressing. Apply negative pressure to the drain via the pump and leave for 2–3 days before repeating.

10 If a vacuum pump is not available, change the dressings to calcium alginate when the necrotic tissue has separated and a surface layer of red granulation tissue is evident. Change this daily.

11 If a large cavity persists consider introducing a large cutaneous or myocutaneous flap (see above, Rotation flap, Biceps femoris flap, Tensor fascia lata flap).

12 Also consider continuing with dressings until healed, avoiding surgery and allowing uninterrupted mobilization.

NECROTIZING FASCIITIS

KEY POINT Recognize and act

- If the patient is to survive you must make an early diagnosis and act immediately.

This is a rare condition but you must recognize it immediately as serious and life-threatening.

There is a focal point where the infection commences, and this often arises from a surgical intervention.

The condition results usually from the symbiotic effect of the coincidental occurrence of an aerobic staphylococcus and an anaerobic streptococcus.

The bacteria appear to spread initially and preferentially along fascial planes. The overlying subcutaneous fat and skin are subsequently rendered ischaemic and necrotic.

Action

1 Look out for unexpected local cellulitis, rapidly expanding cellulitis – mark the area of erythema on the skin, deteriorating general condition.

2 Take wound swabs and blood specimens for culture of organism and sensitivities and commence appropriate antibiotics.

3 If the area of erythema is seen to progress beyond the marked line within a few hours, take the patient to theatre immediately.

4 Use a cutting diathermy to remove all skin showing erythema as well as underlying subcutaneous fat and deep fascia.

5 Remove any tissue suspicious of being involved in the infective process.

6 Dress the wound with gauze soaked in saline and further absorbent dressings, leaving the skin adjacent to the wound available for inspection.

7 Take the patient back to theatre after 24 hours or earlier if there are signs of progression of the disease.

8 Carry out further debridement of infected tissue.

9 Repeat this after a further 24 hours, remaining vigilant until all signs of infection have been eradicated.

10 When the patient is stable, consider covering the residual defect with split skin grafts or skin flaps or a combination of these.

SCARS

HYPERTROPHIC SCARS

These present as red, raised, broad, hard, itchy scars that are unsightly and uncomfortable. They develop a few months after the wound has healed.

Beware of excising or revising them unless there was failure of primary healing or unless a marked contraction has developed. Simple excision of the scar alone will probably cause a larger one to develop.

Inject the scar tissue only with triamcinolone. Repeat the injections at monthly intervals for 3–6 months or longer if necessary until the scar is soft.

Avoid excessive injections and avoid injecting the triamcinolone into the surrounding skin. This may cause skin atrophy.

If the scars are extensive, fit and apply a pressure garment as early as possible. Advise the patient to wear this garment for 6–12 months. A pressure garment is a synthetic elastic garment that is specifically measured to fit part of an individual. In applying pressure to a scar, it modifies the maturation and limits hypertrophic scar formation, provided it is applied early.

Pressure garments are most useful in reducing hypertrophic scar formation and preventing the development of contractures, particularly from burn wounds. They are also used in controlling progressive lymphoedema.

KELOIDS

Keloids (Greek *kelis* = scar + *eidos* = like) have a different histological appearance from hypertrophic scars. They are most commonly found in patients of African origin but can be found in all races.

Excision of keloids, like excision of hypertrophic scars, only temporarily cures the problem. A larger lesion will develop in its place and this treatment is to be condemned.

Treatment with triamcinolone, as used for hypertrophic scars (see above), reduces the size of most keloids but does not eliminate them. This may, however, be the best treatment.

Excision of the whole keloid followed by radiotherapy to the resultant scar can be very effective. This requires expertise in radiotherapy but may not be suitable for young patients.

AESTHETIC SURGERY

You should undertake these operations only if you are an expert. Aesthetic (Greek *aisthanesthai* = to feel, perceive) operations demand specialist management, since they are intended to be pleasing to the patient. They can nearly always be deferred until specialist treatment is available.

Within the generality of surgery, you are most likely to encounter these operations following surgical excision of breast lumps. Augmentation can be achieved by inserting prostheses in the submammary plane or in the subpectoral plane.

Breast reduction may be carried out for symptoms of large breasts or to reduce the size of a breast after, for example, excisional surgery on the other breast.

Liposuction can be carried out by inserting a cannula through a small incision and applying suction to draw out fat from, for example, the superficial tissues of the abdominal wall.

LASER SURGERY

Lasers are being used to treat an increasing number of skin lesions. These fall into four principal groups:

1. *Vascular lesions.* Many cutaneous vascular lesions can be eradicated without leaving any significant scarring. These include all types of telangiectasia, capillary haemangiomata, including port wine stains, pyogenic granulomata and other small vascular lesions. Many of the small lesions can be treated successfully with a single treatment with one of the pulsed dye lasers. While the larger lesions can be eradicated, treatment may leave a residual area of variable pigmentation.
2. *Pigmented lesions.* Several lasers with short wavelengths, such as the Q-switched lasers, remove pigmented lesions limited to the epidermis and basal layer, such as lentigo simplex, solar lentigines and ephilides. They also remove pigment from the superficial dermis. Pigment in the deeper dermis requires a laser with a longer wavelength, but treatment of these lesions is less satisfactory and surgical excision may be the better treatment option.
3. *Tattoos.* Removal of professional as well as accidental tattoos with lasers is now much more effective than surgical excision because of the absence of scars. The Q-switched ruby, Nd-YAG and Alexandrite lasers are all effective in removing blue-black pigment, but complete excision can be difficult to achieve even with multiple treatments and pigmentation changes may occur.
4. *Skin resurfacing.* The carbon dioxide laser in effect causes a predetermined superficial burn to the skin and has a similar effect to dermabrasion, which causes a physical burn, and a chemopeel, which causes a chemical burn. Treatment of wrinkles and irregular scarring of the skin surface with the carbon dioxide laser is more accurate and predictable than these treatments and is therefore replacing them. The occasional complication of a change in pigmentation remains unresolved.

PROSTHETIC IMPLANT MATERIALS

All implants must be inserted under strict aseptic techniques.

Implants require good-quality soft tissue cover to prevent ulceration of the overlying skin.

If subsequently exposed, most implants will become infected and require removal. It may be possible to replace the implant when the infection has been eradicated.

All implants develop a surrounding fibrous capsule. This may be useful but is a disadvantage with a breast prosthesis as the fibrous capsule may contract and distort the prosthesis.

Several inert metals are used in reconstruction. Titanium plates are used in cranioplasty, gold weights are inserted into the upper eyelid in facial palsy to improve function by assisting closure, and stainless steel, vitallium and tantalum are occasionally used.

Hard plastics used in reconstruction include: methyl methacrylate, used in cranioplasty; polyethylene, used as a mesh in abdominal wall repair; and polypropylene. Proplast, a combination of two polymers (polytetrafluoroethylene and pyrolytic graphite), is used to augment the cheek and the chin.

Silicone is a general term for a class of polymers with long chains of dimethylsiloxane units [$—CH_3—Si—O—CH_3$]. These are manufactured in many forms, including liquids, gels, resins, foams, sponges and rubbers.

Silicone implants are used in facial bone augmentation, small-joint replacement in the hand and as a stent to reconstruct tendon sheaths prior to tendon grafting.

Silicone implants are commonly used in breast augmentation or reconstruction. Some breast implants consist of a silicone gel contained within a silicone elastomer shell. Others are made using a cohesive gel that maintains their shape. A textured surface modifies the fibrous reaction of the body and capsule contracture is reduced. There is no scientific evidence to show that any silicone breast implant has a significant carcinogenic risk and although these implants may leak there is no evidence that the silicone that does leak causes any serious complication.

FURTHER READING

McGregor AD, McGregor IA 2000 Fundamental techniques of plastic surgery and their surgical applications, 10th edn. Churchill Livingstone, Edinburgh
An excellent manual of basic techniques in plastic surgery, ideal for young trainees in the specialty and general surgeons.

43

Paediatric surgery

L. Spitz, I. D. Sugarman

CONTENTS

GENERAL CONSIDERATIONS IN NEONATAL SURGERY

INTRODUCTION

Neonatal surgery is best practised by fully trained paediatric surgeons working in large specialist centres. They see many patients, gaining wide experience, and have the support of experts in nursing, anaesthesia, radiology and pathology.

The neonatal period was defined as the first 28 days of extrauterine life, but this is obsolete now babies are surviving birth at gestational ages as low as 22 weeks – but survivors of very premature birth have an increased risk of multiple sensory and neurodevelopmental handicaps. Some require surgery within the first 28 days of life. Infants less than 44 weeks beyond conception (the current definition of the neonatal period) have a marked tendency to apnoea and day-case surgery in such infants is contraindicated.

The neonate differs widely from the adult in both structure and function. Full adaptation to independent life takes several weeks and during this time any severe stress may cause the ductus arteriosus to reopen and the circulation to regress to a 'persistent fetal circulation', resulting in shunting of deoxygenated blood into the systemic circulation with resulting hypoxia. The neonatal circulation is unstable and any noxious stimulus may result in renal or intestinal ischaemia or intracranial haemorrhage. The ratio of surface area to weight in the neonate is twice that of the adult and this exposes the infant to genuine risks of dehydration from excessive insensible fluid loss accompanied by hypothermia, the latter enhanced by radiated losses, especially from the head. The neonatal kidney is immature and can only function within a limited homeostatic range. The diuretic response is weak and circulatory overload can easily occur following excessive intravenous fluid administration, which may also cause reopening of the ductus arteriosus resulting in hypoxia and severe heart failure. Liver functions, particularly detoxifying enzyme systems, are restricted and hyperbilirubinaemia easily develops. Low immunoglobulin levels and reduced leucocyte activity result in poor resistance to infection, bacteraemia rapidly progressing to meningitis. Infection compounds any cardiac, renal or hepatic failure. Progressive multi-organ failure rapidly develops, the correction of which is difficult. Although techniques of assisted respiration have improved dramatically in recent years, haemodialysis and cardiac support still present difficulties.

Recognize congenital abnormalities

External abnormalities are easily recognized at birth but there are a number of clinical features indicative of concealed anomalies that require further amplification. Bilious vomiting suggests mechanical intestinal obstruction. X-ray the chest if there is respiratory distress to exclude pneumothorax, diaphragmatic hernia, lobar emphysema or oesophageal atresia. Failure to pass meconium within 24 hours of birth suggests the possibility of Hirschsprung's disease. Investigate failure to pass urine. Exclude abdominal masses, and look for passage of blood in the stools. Remember congenital abnormalities are frequently multiple; if you find one, look for others.

Neonatal transport

Newborn infants can be transported safely over long distances for specialist treatment provided adequate precautions are taken to maintain body temperature and deal with any cardiorespiratory emergency. In oesophageal atresia keep the blind upper pouch empty, manage diaphragmatic hernia in an oxygen-rich environment, and restrict fluid losses from exomphalos or gastroschisis by wrapping the intestine in plastic film.

Intravenous fluids

Use peripherally sited cannulas whenever possible. Have available tables of requirements for different ages and weights.

Laparoscopy

Laparoscopy can be utilized in infants and children now suitable instruments are available for operations including fundoplication, pyloromyotomy cholecystectomy, Meckel's diverticulectomy, splenectomy, and also for management of intrathoracic conditions.

LAPAROTOMY IN INFANTS AND CHILDREN

Preoperative preparation

Cross-match 1 unit of fresh packed cells. Administer vitamin K, phytomenadione 1 mg intramuscularly, if this was omitted immediately postnatal. Check and if necessary correct the blood glucose using Dextrostix. Correct any fluid and acid–base imbalance. In all emergencies, keep the stomach empty through a large (8FG) nasogastric tube. Use ECG, pulse, blood pressure and oxygen saturation monitors. Keep the infant normothermic, reducing radiant heat losses with aluminium foil and a thermostatically controlled warm air blanket.

THE ABDOMINAL OPERATION

Access

Greater access is afforded by transverse rather than longitudinal incisions. A general purpose incision is transverse, muscle-cutting, supra-umbilical, extending across right and left rectus abdominis muscles. Divide the subcutaneous fat and fascia with cutting diathermy to limit blood loss, the anterior sheath of left and right rectus abdominis muscles and then the muscle bellies, coagulating the superior epigastric vessels on the deeper surface of each rectus abdominis muscle.

Divide the posterior sheath and fascia down to the peritoneum, open the peritoneum on either side of the midline. Identify, clamp and divide the relatively large umbilical vein. Ligate both ends of the vein with 0000 polyglycolic acid suture.

If necessary extend the incision using cutting diathermy into the oblique muscles of the abdominal wall at either, or both, ends of the incision.

Closure

It is unnecessary to close the peritoneum separately. Close the muscles and fascia en masse with either continuous or interrupted sutures of 000 or 0000 polyglactin, polyglycolic acid or polydioxanone. Close the skin with a continuous subcuticular suture of 00000 polyglycolic acid, polydioxanone or polyglactin.

If you expect wound infection, omit the subcuticular suture and close with adhesive tapes, such as Steri-Strips. Do not use tension sutures or through-and-through skin sutures because the cosmetic results are unacceptable.

ABDOMINAL WALL DEFECTS

When present at birth, these are associated with longstanding evisceration of the abdominal contents into a hernial sac, thin external membrane, or the thoracic cavity. As a result, the abdominal cavity is relatively small, and repair of the defect causes a rise in intra-abdominal pressure, poor circulation in the lower parts of the body, splinting of the diaphragm and hypoxia. Prevent the cycle of deterioration by assisted endotracheal ventilation with high concentrations of oxygen.

CONGENITAL DIAPHRAGMATIC HERNIA

The infant has respiratory distress with tachypnoea more than 60/minute, tachycardia more than 160/minute and cyanosis. Chest X-ray shows intestinal gas shadows in the involved hemithorax with displacement of the mediastinal structures to the contralateral side. Resuscitate including ventilation using endotracheal positive-pressure, and if necessary a chest drain.

At laparotomy the intestines, stomach and spleen are withdrawn from the chest, the sac is excised and the defect closed, if necessary using a plastic mesh patch.

EXOMPHALOS AND GASTROSCHISIS

Exomphalos is herniation of abdominal viscera into a persistent fetal umbilical hernia, often associated with other abnormalities. If it is minor, operation may not be necessary, but if the sac is ruptured, management may require repair with prosthetic material. Gastroschisis is evisceration of the intestine through a slit-like defect in the anterior abdominal wall immediately to the right of an apparently normal umbilical cord. Primary repair can often be carried out.

INGUINAL HERNIA

In the paediatric age range, inguinal hernia is generally due to failure of closure of the processus vaginalis. The hernia may be complete (to the scrotum) or incomplete (confined to the inguinal region). Operation is indicated in all cases. Inguinal hernias may become irreducible; pressure upon the spermatic cord causes testicular ischaemia, and infarction may occur. They can often be reduced following sedation and 'taxis' – gentle to-and-fro pressure applied to the neck of the hernial sac at the level of the external inguinal ring. Strangulation is rare. Premature babies are particularly prone to develop complications.

In infants under the age of 6 months, the tissues are thin and friable so operative difficulties are common. Preoperatively ensure that the ipsilateral testis is in the scrotum; if not, perform orchidopexy with the herniotomy but do not attempt it in an infant under age 6 months. Except in children with neuromuscular disorders, herniotomy rather than herniorrhaphy is the treatment of choice but it is a difficult procedure for a trainee.

Herniotomy at the external ring

1 Through a skin crease incision 2 cm long over the external inguinal ring, dissect through the subcutaneous fat, Camper's and Scarpa's fascia to reveal the spermatic cord as it passes from the external inguinal ring. Split the external spermatic fascia and cremasteric fascia or muscle in the long axis of the cord and deliver the cord, surrounded by the internal spermatic fascia, from the wound.

2 Rotate the cord to bring its posterior surface into view, split the internal spermatic fascia longitudinally, allowing the vessels and vas to be separated from the sac. Exert traction upon the sac, withdrawing as much as possible from within the inguinal canal. Transfix and ligate the sac with a suture of either 0000 polyglycolic acid or polyglactin. Divide the neck of the sac distal to the suture. Bring together the superficial fascia with one or two sutures of 0000 polyglycolic acid or polyglactin and close the skin with a subcuticular suture of polyglycolic acid or polyglactin or apply skin-closure tapes.

Herniotomy through the inguinal canal

This can be carried out as a day case except in infants less than 44 weeks post-gestational.

1 Make an incision 2 cm long in a skin crease midway between the deep ring and pubic tubercle. Divide the subcutaneous fat, Camper's fascia then Scarpa's fascia using scissors, and retract it.

2 Clear a small patch of external oblique aponeurosis over an area of 2 cm^2, at least 1 cm above the inguinal ligament, and incise the external oblique aponeurosis and retract the edges. Do not open the external inguinal ring. Dissect into the inguinal canal, keeping close to the posterior surface of the external oblique aponeurosis to reveal the ilio-inguinal nerve, providing a useful landmark. Using a mosquito artery forceps, split the fibres of the cremaster muscle overlying the spermatic cord just inferior to the ilio-inguinal nerve. Gently grasp the internal spermatic fascia and deliver the spermatic cord from its bed whilst pushing away the adherent fibres of the cremaster muscle with delicate non-toothed dissecting forceps.

3 Pass the index finger of your non-dominant hand behind the cord and use it and the thumb to rotate the

cord so that its posterior aspect comes into view. Using non-toothed dissecting forceps, split the internal spermatic fascia overlying the vas and vessels in a longitudinal direction. Gently sweep the vas and vessels away from the sac. Do not hold the vas or vessels with the forceps or you risk crushing them.

4 Place an artery forceps across the sac, and divide the sac distal to the forceps. Allow the distal part of the sac to fall back into the wound. Dissect the vas and vessels from the proximal part of the sac, until you see the inferior epigastric vessels. Rotate the artery forceps to twist the neck of the sac, so ensuring that there is no bowel or omentum within it.

5 Ligate the sac flush with the deep ring using a 0000 polyglycolic acid suture, and then transfix the sac just distal to this tie. Ligation prior to transfixation and ligation prevents the needle from causing a split in the sac that may spread across the deep ring and onto the peritoneum of the anterior abdominal wall, and prevents the escape of intestines or omentum at a difficult site to repair.

6 Allow the vas and vessels to drop back into the inguinal canal, close the inguinal canal with two or three sutures, approximate the Scarpa's fascia with one or two sutures and close the skin with a subcuticular stitch. If you use 0000 polyglycolic acid you can accomplish the whole operation using but one suture. Alternatively, close the skin with adhesive skin tapes.

7 Gently pull the testis to the bottom of the scrotum to ensure that it does not become caught in the superficial inguinal pouch, necessitating an orchidopexy.

8 A slight fever on the first postoperative night is a normal response to surgery.

? DIFFICULTY

As a trainee do not continue if you are uncertain. Stop immediately and call for advice and help from a senior colleague.

ORCHIDOPEXY

Incidence of undescended testis is approximately 3% at birth, falling to 1% at 1 year. If the condition is either bilateral or unilateral associated with a hypospadias, investigate the chromosomes to rule out intersex. If a testis is impalpable, laparoscopy is the investigation of choice to assess its presence and site, or absence. If there are bilateral impalpable testes confirmed at laparoscopy to be intra-abdominal, bring one down at a time. This can either be by a Fowler–Stephen's procedure (ligating the testicular vessels and relying on the spermatic fascia for vascularity of the testis), or microvascular transfer. The operation for the undescended testis should be performed between the ages of 1 and 2 years.

If the testis is palpable, explore it through a crease incision midway between the pubic tubercle and deep ring, mobilize it together with the vas and testicular vessels and divide the gubernaculums. Create a pouch within the scrotum between the skin and the dartos muscle in which to place the testis, taking care not to twist the vessels (see also Ch. 46).

If there is an inadequate length of vas and vessels, try dividing the lateral fibres which may be tethering the vas, or gently sweep the peritoneum off the vas and vessels deep to the internal ring, or pass the vas, vessels and testis under the inferior epigastric vessels in the hope of gaining the extra length.

OESOPHAGEAL ATRESIA

Surgery for the repair of oesophageal atresia is seldom an emergency so there is adequate time for referral to a specialist centre. As a result, in the absence of other severe congenital anomalies (especially cardiac malformations) nearly all infants weighing over 1500 g survive. Establish the diagnosis with a plain X-ray to reveal arrest of a radio-opaque nasogastric tube in the upper oesophagus. Include the abdomen on the radiograph. Air in the stomach indicates a distal tracheo-oesophageal fistula, for which primary repair is usually possible. Absence of an abdominal gas shadow usually indicates isolated oesophageal atresia in which the distance between the proximal and distal segments is too long to permit primary oesophageal anastomosis, so a feeding gastrostomy and an end cervical oesophagostomy may be required.

Repair is carried out through a right thoracotomy. Find the lower segment which opens into the trachea (Fig. 43.1), detach it and close the hole in the trachea. Now identify the blind upper end of the oesophagus, open it at the lower extremity and unite it to the lower end.

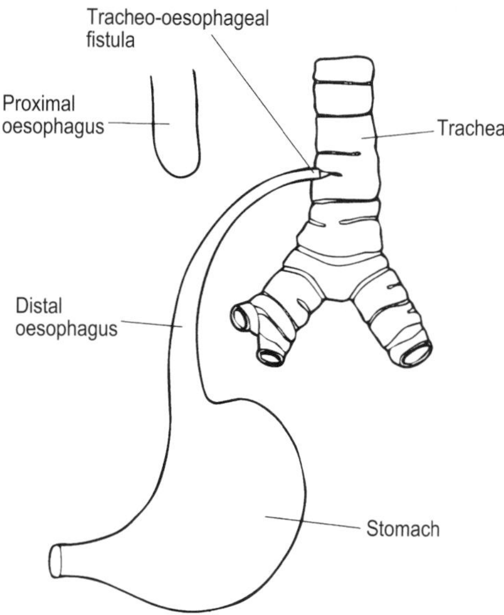

Fig. 43.1 Oesophageal atresia: the most frequent (90%) condition with distal tracheo-oesophageal fistula. The distal oesophagus is detached from the trachea and united to the blind upper segment.

GASTROSTOMY

Through a transverse incision 3–4 cm long in the left hypochondrium, midway between the umbilicus and the costal margin, identify the stomach and create a stab wound on the anterior wall into which insert a Malecot catheter, held with two or three inverting purse string sutures. Bring the catheter out through the stab wound and close the incision after anchoring the stomach to the inner wall of the abdomen.

Percutaneous endoscopic gastrostomy (PEG) has become the preferred method of gastrostomy insertion as it avoids an 'open' procedure. This cannot be used in a child with an unrepaired oesophageal atresia.

The indications are mainly for long-term nutrition in the handicapped child or hyperalimentation in children with either cystic fibrosis or chronic renal failure. See also Chapter 16.

PYLORIC STENOSIS

This occurs predominantly in male infants (male-to-female ratio = 4 : 1) around the second to fourth week of life, producing projectile non-bilious vomiting, failure to thrive and constipation. Establish the diagnosis by palpating the pyloric 'tumour' in the right hypochondrium. Measure serum urea, electrolytes and acid–base status and correct hypochloraemia and hypokalaemia with intravenous infusion of half-normal saline adding potassium (10–15 mmol KCl per 500 ml of 0.45% saline).

The operation can be performed laparoscopically with equally good results.

It is never an emergency. Do not operate until the serum bicarbonate is 26 mmol/litre or less and serum potassium above 3.5 mmol/litre. Prohibit all milk feeds and leave a nasogastric tube on free drainage, replacing losses millilitre for millilitre with normal saline and potassium (10 mmol KCl per 500 ml of 0.9% saline).

General anaesthesia is now preferred to local anaesthetic. Access may be through a transverse incision, 3–4 cm long, in the right hypochondrium midway between the costal margin and the palpable inferior margin of the liver; the medial end of the incision ending 1–2 cm from the midline, or a supra-umbilical incision of adequate length to allow delivery of the 'tumour'. Divide the deep tissues with diathermy and open the peritoneum.

Action (Fig. 43.2)

1 Retract the inferior margin of the liver, identify the greater curvature of the stomach, if necessary after gently applying traction on the transverse mesocolon. Do not attempt to withdraw the pyloric tumour by applying direct traction on the mass; this results in serosal tears and haemorrhage. Deliver the greater curvature of the body of the stomach into the wound. Draw the firm, white, glistening pyloric tumour into view by applying gentle traction on the gastric greater curvature and ease it out of the peritoneal cavity and into the wound. Identify the pyloric vein of Mayo, marking the distal end of the pyloric canal.

2 Make an incision 1–2 mm deep with a scalpel on the anterior surface of the pyloric tumour in the relatively avascular plane midway between the superior and inferior borders. Extend the incision from the pyloric vein of Mayo, through the pyloric canal and onto the hypertrophied body of the stomach. Using firm but gentle pressure on the incised pylorus with a MacDonald dissector, the blunt handle of a scalpel or a blunt artery forceps, split the hypertrophied muscle down to the submucosa. Ensure that you split all the fibres of the

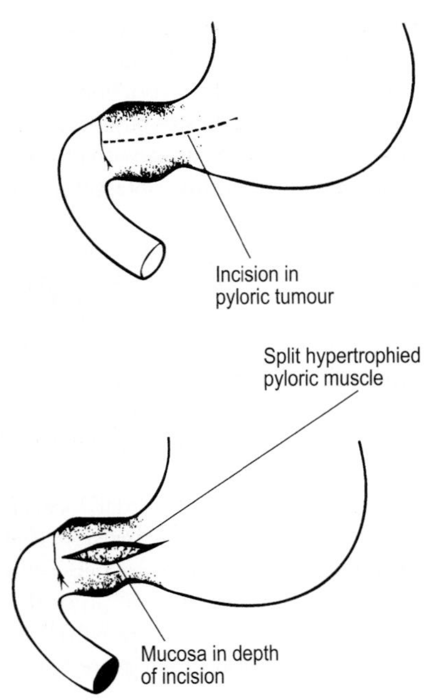

Fig. 43.2 Ramstedt's pyloromyotomy.

pyloric tumour from end to end using a pyloric spreader (Denis Browne) or blunt artery forceps.

3 Bubbles of air or bile at the duodenal end of the incision signify a perforation of the mucosa, most common in the duodenal fornix; close it with a few interrupted 00000 absorbable sutures and cover it with omentum. Haemorrhage from the incised pylorus is mainly due to venous congestion. Bleeding usually ceases once the pylorus is returned to the abdominal cavity. If bleeding persists, use diathermy coagulation.

4 Close the wound en masse using interrupted 0000 polyglycolic acid sutures; approximate the skin with a continuous subcuticular 00000 absorbable suture.

5 Intend to commence feeds within 4–6 hours of operation but continue intravenous fluids for 12–24 hours. Starting with 15–20 ml of milk, reintroduce feeds cautiously 12 hours after operation. Gradually increase the volume until normal milk feeds are being offered at 24–48 hours. As a rule discharge the infant on the second or third day.

INTESTINAL OBSTRUCTIONS

The infant with intestinal obstruction is best managed in a specialist centre for paediatric surgery, not just for the operative treatment but especially for the postoperative care which often entails prolonged parenteral nutrition, particularly when massive resection results in 'short-bowel syndrome'.

The main causes of intestinal obstruction are intraluminal such as meconium ileus; intramural such as atresias, stenoses, necrotizing enterocolitis and Hirschsprung's disease; extramural such as malrotation with or without volvulus, duplication cysts, peritoneal bands, adhesions from necrotizing enterocolitis and tumours; and functional such as paralytic ileus secondary to septicaemia, urinary infection, hypoglycaemia, hypocalcaemia, endocrine disorders, and prematurity.

Meconium ileus

Perform enterotomy and attempt to disimpact the obstructing inspissated mucus with warm saline, Gastrografin or Tween 80. If this fails create a double barrelled ileostomy.

Intestinal atresia

Intestinal atresia (Greek *a* = not + *tresis* = perforation; no lumen). Resect the affected segment and unite the ends using a single layer of interrupted 00000 or 000000 extramucosal sutures of polyglactin 910, polydioxanone or polypropylene. Perform an end-to-end or end-to-back anastomosis. Avoid side-to-side anastomosis.

Hirschsprung' s disease

Hirschsprung' s disease confirmed prior to laparotomy by suction rectal biopsy requires initial loop colostomy in the dilated segment. The definitive treatment is highly specialized and should be performed only by experienced paediatric surgeons.

Duplication cysts

Duplication cysts on the mesenteric border of the intestine obstruct by stretching and compressing the lumen of the adherent normal bowel. Resect the cyst en bloc with the adjacent intestine.

MALROTATION WITH OR WITHOUT MIDGUT VOLVULUS

The midgut develops within the physiological umbilical hernia in early intrauterine life. Between the tenth and twelfth weeks of development, the midgut loop returns to the peritoneal cavity, rotating in an orderly manner beginning with the jejunum and ending with the ileocaecal region. Malrotation results when this process of rotation and fixation is incomplete, forming abnormal bands that cross, and may compress, the second part of the duodenum, and twisting (volvulus) around the narrow base of the midgut, causing intestinal obstruction with bilious vomiting.

The surgical procedure described by the American surgeon W.E. Ladd is division of the peritoneal bands, placing the caecum in the left upper quadrant of the abdomen, duodenal flexure to the right of the midline, mobilization of the duodenal loop, division of the fibrous bands at the base of the mesentery to broaden its base, resection of any gangrenous bowel and returning the intestine to the abdomen after untwisting it.

NECROTIZING ENTEROCOLITIS

This is now the most common abdominal emergency in the neonatal intensive care unit, presenting with bilious vomiting, rectal bleeding and radiological pneumatosis intestinalis caused by transmural inflammation of the intestine, and is of unknown aetiology. It may affect any part of the gastrointestinal tract from stomach to rectum, most commonly the terminal ileum and splenic flexure. Management in the acute phase is intensive medical care but operation is required if there is any deterioration. At operation, resect gangrenous ischaemic intestine and oversew perforations, reuniting healthy ends or exteriorizing doubtful bowel.

INTUSSUSCEPTION

Between the ages of 6 months and 2 years, most intussusceptions are 'idiopathic', possibly caused by viral infections. The vast majority originate in the ileocaecal region. If pneumostatic reduction or hydrostatic reduction by means of a barium enema fails, operation is required. Withdraw the colon distal to the mass and gently attempt to push out the intussusceptum by squeezing the intussuscipiens in an antiperistaltic direction towards the caecum. Never try to pull out the intussusceptum.

ANORECTAL ANOMALIES

It is essential to differentiate the high (supralevator) anomaly from the low (translevator) lesion. If you are uncertain perform a colostomy.

Anoplasty involves widening a pinhole anus by advancing a 'V' shaped skin flap into the canal.

Colostomy is a loop colostomy preformed in the right transverse or left iliac colon. In Nixon's technique, to avoid the need for a glass rod, a 'V'-shaped skin flap is brought through a small gap made in the juxtacolic mesocolon to form a bridge and sutured to the skin of the opposite side.

MYELOMENINGOCELE

Failure of the spine (spina bifida) and the spinal canal to close, may, in severe cases, result in exposure of the covering membranes. Because of the naturally declining incidence and increased availability of termination of pregnancy, this has become an uncommon condition in Britain during the last 5 years, but remains common in other parts of Western Europe.

FURTHER READING

Ashcraft KW, Holcolm GW III, Murphy JP (eds) 2005 Paediatric surgery, 4th edn. Elsevier Saunders, Philadelphia

Beasley JW, Hutson JM, Myers NA (eds) 1993 Paediatric diagnoses. Chapman & Hall, London

Puri P (ed.) 2003 Newborn surgery, 2nd edn. Arnold, London

Rowe MI, O'Neill JA, Fonkalsrud EW et al (eds) 1995 Essentials of pediatric surgery. Mosby Year Book, St Louis

Spitz L, Coran AG (eds) 1995 Operative surgery: paediatric surgery, 5th edn. Chapman & Hall, London

44

Neurosurgery

R. S. Maurice-Williams

CONTENTS

GENERAL PRINCIPLES

Central nervous tissue is easily damaged and, once damaged, cannot regenerate. Patients may make remarkable recoveries from injuries to the central nervous system, mediated by the compensatory action of intact neural tissue, rather than by local repair of the damaged areas. Unnecessary damage must be avoided even in the simplest neurosurgical procedure. Wound haemorrhage or infection may have appalling consequences so perfect haemostasis is imperative. In most developed countries it is possible to obtain telephoned expert neurosurgical advice within minutes and most neurosurgical emergencies do not deteriorate during transfer to a neurosurgical centre. Over-treatment is counterproductive; a patient with very severe head injuries commonly has extradural and subdural haematomas which are incidental to the main injury to the brain and removal of an intracranial haematoma would be of no benefit. Rapidly developing arterial extradural haemorrhage, however, is an exception and needs to be dealt with urgently.

Prepare

Have adequate quantities of blood cross-matched; the patient may have lost blood and bleeding may occur during operation. Prefer general anaesthesia; have the patient paralysed and ventilated to lower the intracranial pressure. Do not allow systolic blood pressure to fall below 70–80 mmHg. When the patient is prepared, administer intravenously 250 ml of 20% mannitol for a teenager or an adult, or 100 ml for a child aged 3–10 years, given over 5–10 minutes. This lowers intracranial pressure for up to 3–4 hours, causing a brisk diuresis, so insert a urinary catheter. It 'buys time' if rising intracranial pressure causes rapid deterioration. Do not be tempted into delay if there is dramatic improvement; when the effects wear off, the rebound rise in intracranial tension may cause sudden deterioration. Cerebral venous pressure can be reduced, so minimizing cerebral swelling, by tilting the patient feet-down by 20°. Shave the whole head; unexpected negative findings may demand further exploratory burr holes elsewhere. Mark out intended incisions with a light scratch on the scalp, and then infiltrate beneath them with adrenaline (epinephrine) 1:200000 in physiological saline to reduce blood loss.

Access to the brain

Burr holes can be carried out rapidly if preoperative computed tomography (CT) is not available, to establish whether there is any haematoma on the brain surface in that part of the head or whether the brain is under tension. They expose only a tiny surface of the intracranial contents; nearby or deep pathology may not be detectable and they seldom provide sufficient access for definitive treatment of important lesions. For this reason they should be placed so that they can be converted into an osteoplastic flap or craniectomy.

Craniotomy

An osteoplastic flap is turned and then replaced at the end of the operation. It is the best way of exposing a wide area of the intracranial contents above the tentorium (Fig. 44.1).

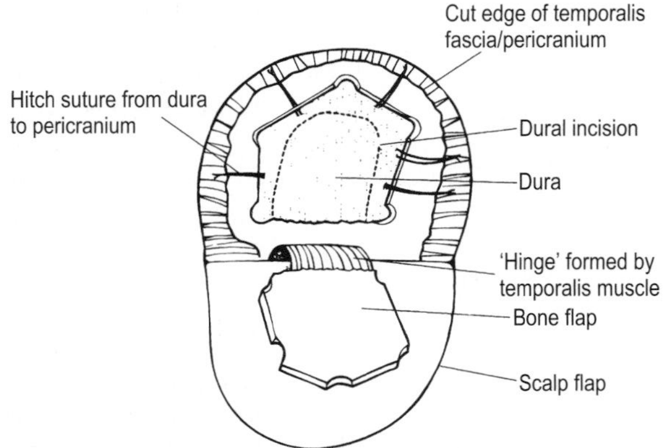

Fig. 44.1 Craniotomy with an osteoplastic flap. A scalp flap has been reflected and the underlying muscle cut through to leave it attached to the bone flap. Burr holes are then made and joined up by Gigli saw so the bone flap can be turned back, hinged on the muscle, and replaced at the end of the procedure.

Craniectomy

A burr hole is extended by removing bone around it, leaving a defect which remains at the end of the operation. A craniectomy is the usual mode of exposing the posterior fossa contents and the defect is covered over by the thick suboccipital muscles. The outer wall of the middle fossa may be removed by a 'subtemporal craniectomy', to provide access to an arterial extradural haematoma or a swollen temporal lobe. At the end of the operation the defect is concealed by suturing the temporalis muscle over it.

MULTIPLE EXPLORATORY BURR HOLES

Multiple burr holes may be required after a head injury, when a deteriorating level of consciousness and/or the appearance of focal neurological signs suggests an expanding intracranial haematoma and a diagnostic CT scan is not available. Mark out for frontal, parietal and temporal burr holes on each side of the head. Cut down to the bone, retract the edges and create the hole. Start with the perforator in a brace until it begins to wobble as it exposes the dura mater. Now use the burr to expose a wider area of dura. An extradural haematoma is apparent immediately inside the bone. To open the dura and release a subdural haematoma, first lift the exposed centre with a sharp hook. A brain cannula can be introduced into the ventricle to relieve pressure from acute hydrocephalus and to aspirate a cerebral abscess.

SUBTEMPORAL CRANIECTOMY FOR EXTRADURAL HAEMATOMA

If an exploratory temporal burr hole reveals an appreciable extradural clot, you will need to extend the burr hole into a craniectomy to remove it. After scraping the temporalis muscle from the bone, nibble around the burr hole to improve the access. Suck out the haematoma and seal the bleeding middle meningeal artery with diathermy current. Cover the defect with temporalis muscle before closing.

SCALP LACERATIONS

Arrest severe bleeding with temporary single-layer through-and-through sutures. X-ray the skull following a heavy blow. Minimally excise contused edges. Repair the galea if it is breached before closing the scalp.

DEPRESSED SKULL FRACTURE

The purpose of elevating a depressed skull fracture is to reduce the risk of infection, so elevate only compound depressed skull fractures. Leave alone depressed fractures with intact overlying scalp. Excise a badly contused scalp laceration extended to give full access and clear off the pericranium. Make a single burr hole just outside the edge of the visible depression to expose dura. Insert a periosteal elevator and gently ease out the depressed fragments, removing any dirt and small bone fragments. Leave intact dura but explore beneath tears to remove pulped necrotic brain; diathermize bleeding points. Take care not to damage venous sinuses.

MISSILE WOUNDS OF THE BRAIN

If active treatment is likely to lead to a worthwhile outcome, resuscitate the patient; obtain good quality X-rays. Anaesthetize, intubate and hyperventilate the patient to reduce any cerebral oedema. Start a broad-spectrum antibiotic.

Expose the entry hole and extend it, opening the dura to remove debris, missile fragments and pulped brain, and stop bleeding. Close while controlling swelling with hyperventilation and intravenous mannitol.

REPAIR OF DEFECTS IN THE SKULL VAULT

Leave bone defects in the skull vault unless they are very large and cause intracranial contents to be unprotected. Large disfiguring defects or those exposing cranial contents may require titanium or tantalum plates, best inserted after an interval.

The defect is exposed by a scalp flap placed so that its edges are well clear of the defect. The defect may be covered by a premoulded titanium or tantalum plate, or by titanium strips. Holes in the metal permit it to be sutured to the surrounding pericranium. Alternatively, after the scalp flap has been reflected, a methyl methacrylate plate may be moulded to fit the defect and held in place by thick braided silk sutures. The sutures are passed through drill holes in the plate and the surrounding bone, after the bone edge round the defect has been cleared of tissue.

AFTERCARE FOLLOWING INTRACRANIAL SURGERY

Do not give opiate analgesics, which depress consciousness and respiration. Start antibiotic parenterally and continue for 5 days. Give prophylactic anticonvulsants following cerebral cortical damage. The commonest complication is cerebral compression from bleeding or oedema at the operation site producing deterioration in consciousness, progressive focal neurological deficit such as ipsilateral fixed dilated pupil, and rising blood pressure and falling pulse rate. Be willing to re-explore the wound.

FURTHER READING

Collins REC, Cashin PA 1999 General surgeons and the management of head injuries. Annals of the Royal College of Surgeons of England 81:151–153

Connolly ES, McKhann GM, Huang J et al 2002 Fundamentals of operative techniques in neurosurgery. Thieme, New York

Greenberg MS 2001 Handbook of neurosurgery, 5th edn. Thieme, New York

Jennett WB, Lindsay KW 1994 An introduction to neurosurgery, 5th edn. Butterworth-Heinemann, London

This is a good basic guide to neurosurgery, suitable for the medical neurologist, general surgeon, or for the house officer on a neurosurgical unit.

45

Upper urinary tract

C. G. Fowler, I. Junaid

CONTENTS

INTRODUCTION

Urology has developed as a separate discipline in part due the sophistication of endoscopic procedures which demand specialist skills. Major open operations for urological cancer, stone disease and reconstruction are increasingly performed by specialists. Routine inguinoscrotal and genital procedures are performed by both urologists and general surgeons. You should know the principles of treating acute retention, impacted ureteric stone, torsion of the testes, priapism, urinary tract trauma and urinary extravasation.

ACUTE PYONEPHROSIS (OBSTRUCTED INFECTED KIDNEY)

Septicaemia resulting from obstruction by a stone, a congenital hold-up at the pelviureteric junction or rarely a tumour, is a particular risk in diabetics and immunologically compromised patients. Confirm the diagnosis with plain abdominal X-ray, which may display air from gas-forming organisms in the system, and ultrasound examination. The urine contains organisms that can also be cultured from the blood. Ultrasound-guided percutaneous nephrostomy is the preferred method of draining an obstructed infected kidney. Aspiration of the tube confirms its position and provides a specimen of pus for culture.

Open operation is indicated only if a satisfactory percutaneous drain cannot be inserted or if the pus is too thick to be aspirated. If you undertake open operation when the cause of obstruction is a calculus in the ureter or renal pelvis, remove it.

OPEN NEPHROSTOMY FOR ACUTELY OBSTRUCTED KIDNEY

Mark the side of operation, rehydrate the patient, administer a broad-spectrum antibiotic intravenously and be prepared to monitor a severely ill patient in an intensive care unit. With the patient lying on the side and the table broken, make an incision below the 12th rib of sufficient length to expose the convex border of the kidney. Perirenal tissues appear oedematous and the kidney is swollen and friable. Incise pus-filled calyces pointing on the surface, releasing pus. Otherwise insert and aspirate a large-bore needle on a syringe to locate pus to incise and drain it – pyelotomy (Greek *pyelos* = trough, pelvis + *tome* = a cutting). Through this introduce an eyed malleable silver probe and manoeuvre it to puncture the cortex from within a lower pole calyx. Attach and draw through a size 18F tube drain or a Foley catheter (Fig. 45.1) and close the pyelotomy with absorbable sutures. Bring out the nephrostomy tube through the abdominal wall with as straight a course as possible, to facilitate changing the tube if necessary.

OBSTRUCTED KIDNEY CAUSED BY AN IMPACTED STONE

Obstruction for a few days is not usually harmful but demands urgent release if the kidney is infected for fear of

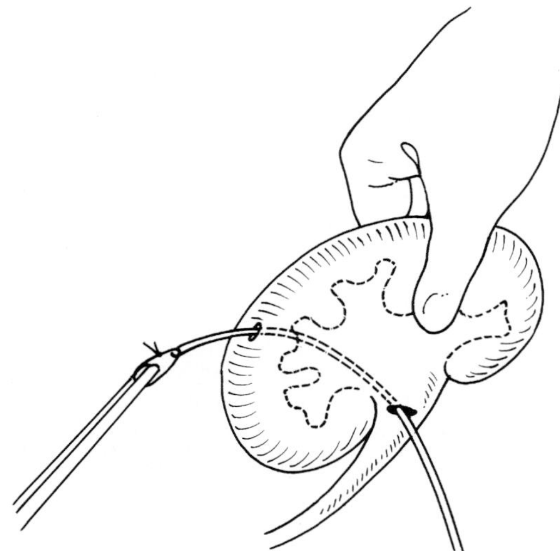

Fig. 45.1 Technique of open nephrostomy tube insertion.

septicaemia, or if the other kidney is diseased or obstructed. The obstruction may be due to an impacted stone at the pelviureteric junction or in the lower ureter. Make the diagnosis with a plain abdominal X-ray, ultrasound scan or intravenous urogram. Renal failure and uraemia develop rapidly from solitary obstructed kidney or bilateral obstruction; relieve it using a percutaneous nephrostomy or failing this, open nephrostomy. For bilateral upper tract obstruction, urgently insert bilateral nephrostomy tubes to retrieve the patient from renal failure. If the patient is seriously ill with associated Gram-negative septicaemia, urgently transfer the patient to an intensive care unit or renal unit to save life.

The current management of upper urinary tract stones is by extracorporeal shock-wave lithotripsy (ESWL), percutaneous nephrolithotomy (PCNL) with or without ESWL, and laser fragmentation of ureteric stones. Open ureterolithotomy is rarely required.

URETEROLITHOTOMY FOR A LOWER URETERIC CALCULUS

Make an oblique muscle-splitting or muscle cutting incision on the lateral side of the anterior abdominal wall down to peritoneum. Sweep the peritoneum medially to expose the retroperitoneal structures. Identify the ureter and impacted stone within it. The ureter crosses the common iliac vessels at the pelvic brim. Avoid dislodging the stone. Place a wetted nylon tape around the ureter proximally and be prepared to place one distally. Make a vertical incision in the ureter directly over the stone, a few millimetres longer than the calculus and ease out the stone using a Watson–Cheyne dissector.

RUPTURE OF THE KIDNEY

The majority result from blunt trauma following falls, road traffic accidents and sports injuries. Penetrating injuries are associated with gunshot and stab wounds. These injuries are often associated with trauma to bowel, pancreas and spleen. Resuscitate the patient and thoroughly assess the damage. Trauma associated with haematuria is an indication for spiral computed tomography (spiral CT) or intravenous urography (IVU), combined with angiography if the renal pedicle may be involved. If the IVU is normal or there is some contrast extravasation, employ monitored conservative management. Penetrating injuries and damage to other organs demand exploration.

Perform abdominal exploration and palpate the retroperitoneal structures. If you encounter a large pulsatile expanding haematoma, gain control of the renal pedicle before opening the perirenal fascia of Gerota. Eviscerate the small intestine and incise the peritoneum over the aorta, exposing the vena cava and aorta. Identify the renal artery(ies) and vein(s). Place vessel loops around the vessels of the injured kidney to gain control. You may be able to repair the kidney if the parenchymal damage is not great. Close the defects with continuous sutures of 4/0 Monocril, excise devitalized tissue, preserving as much capsule as possible. If it is badly traumatized perform nephrectomy. If the contralateral kidney has been confirmed as intact, perform a nephrectomy rather than exposing the patient to unnecessary risk by attempting a difficult repair.

NEPHRECTOMY FOR TRAUMA

Double ligate the artery(ies) and the vein(s) with 2/0 Vicryl suture in continuity and then divide the vessels. Carefully ligate and divide any adrenal vein and artery(ies) arising from the main renal vessels. On the left, also ligate and divide gonadal vein draining into the renal vein. Complete any required remaining dissection to free the kidney from the surrounding tissues. Remove the kidney by dividing the ureter between clamps. Ligate the distal ureteric stump with 2/0 Vicryl suture.

REPAIR OF A DAMAGED URETER

If you operate in the vicinity of the ureter, always check for damage. If you recognize inadvertent surgical ureteric injury at the operation, repair it immediately. Mobilize both ends of the divided ureter to make sure that they are accessible for anastomosis. Place a double pigtail stent with one end in the renal pelvis and the other in the urinary bladder. Open out the ends like a broad, flat-bladed spatula, hold the ends between stay sutures (Fig. 45.2) and anastomose them using fine interrupted sutures of 4/0 or 5/0 Monocril or any other available absorbable suture. Leave a size 18F tube drain in the vicinity of the ureteric anastomosis. Remove the stent or tube splint after about 10 days.

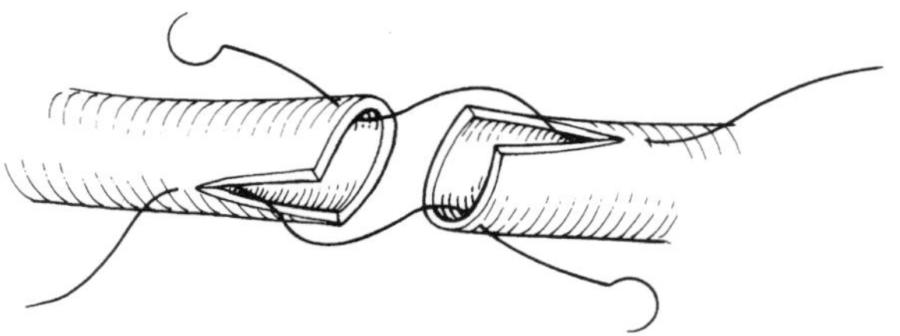

Fig. 45.2 Spatulated uretero-ureterostomy.

DRAINAGE OF A PERINEPHRIC ABSCESS

Is the patient diabetic? Immunocompromised? Debilitated? Suffering from renal cortical abscess or pyonephrosis?

The safest procedure is preliminary drainage followed by nephrectomy. Radiologically directed percutaneous drainage is the best option, otherwise undertake open drainage.

Through a small incision below the 12th rib or where the abscess is pointing on the surface, deepen it into the perinephric space. Pus usually starts to pour out. Sweep your forefinger around in the perinephric space to break down all the septa. Leave in a wide-bore soft plastic tube drain in the cavity and secure it to the skin.

FURTHER READING

Ghali AM, El-Malik EM, Ibrahim AI et al 1999 Ureteric injuries: diagnosis, management, and outcome. Journal of Trauma 46:150–158

Krane RJ, Siroky MB, Fitzpatrick JM (eds) 2000 Operative urology: surgical skills. Churchill Livingstone, London

Santucci RA, Wessells H, Bartsch G et al 2004 Evaluation and management of renal injuries: consensus statement of the Renal Trauma Subcommittee. BJU International. 93:937–954

46

Lower urinary tract

C. G. Fowler, I. Junaid

CONTENTS

URETHRAL DILATATION

KEY POINTS Avoid damage

- Stricture dilatation is one of the most delicate procedures you will perform. Do not attempt it without first watching and receiving monitored instruction from an expert.
- Small-gauge dilators have sharp-pointed tips with which it is easy to make a false passage. Initially choose a medium-sized metal dilator.

You may encounter an unforeseen urethral stricture when attempting urethral catheterization to relieve acute urinary retention or as a prelude to major pelvic surgery. Preferred treatment is internal visual urethrotomy with the Sachse urethrotome but urethral dilatation is an alternative for short strictures just behind the urethral meatus or in the bulbar urethra. An ascending urethrogram characterizes the stricture. Use general anaesthesia, or empty a tube of 1–2% lidocaine gel into the urethra, massaging it into the posterior urethra, leaving it for at least 10 minutes held in with a penile clamp. The most commonly used dilators are bullet-tipped curved metal rods ('sounds'), plastic or gum-elastic bougies or dilators in graduated sizes.

We shall describe only the preparation for, and principles of, urethral dilation. Under strict sterile conditions, with the patient supine, clean and drape the penis. For topical anaesthesia gently empty a 15–20 ml tube of 2% lidocaine gel into the urethra, massaging the gel back into the posterior urethra. Apply a penile clamp for at least 10 minutes. Firmly elevate the penis and insert the dilator with the concavity facing the patient's head to reach the stricture and gently negotiate it. If you fail, try a smaller size. If you succeed, continue into the bladder by depressing the handle of the sound between the patient's legs. You may try gradually larger dilators but do not over-dilate. In case of difficulty prefer suprapubic catheterization.

SUPRAPUBIC CYSTOSTOMY DRAINAGE

A suprapubic tube can be used to drain the bladder if it is impossible or inappropriate to pass a urethral catheter and is particularly indicated when the urethral route is closed by trauma causing urethral disruption, or stricture. Use local anaesthesia unless the patient is already under general anaesthetic or deeply unconscious.

KEY POINT Full bladder needed

- A 'stab' suprapubic cystostomy can be performed safely only if the bladder is full. If it is empty, wait for it to fill.

Action

Prepare and drape the patient, who lies supine. Infiltrate local anaesthetic through the skin 2–3 cm above the pubic symphysis, subcutaneous tissues and linea alba. There is a 'give' as the needle enters the bladder and clean urine can be drawn back into the syringe. A variety of disposable suprapubic catheters come packaged with instructions for use. Insert the catheter noting again the 'give' as it enters the bladder. Confirm this by noting when urine flows back between the catheter and its introducer. Now advance the tube well into the bladder before removing the needle. Secure the catheter – some have a balloon or a pre-formed 'pigtail'.

KEY POINTS Careful control

- Be wary of the sudden loss of resistance that indicates that the end of the introducer is in the bladder.
- If you use too much force, you risk impaling the posterior wall of the bladder and may even penetrate the rectum!

CYSTOSCOPY

Passing a rigid cystoscope is very similar to passing a metal urethral dilator. Use general anaesthesia when possible. With the cleaned and draped patient in the lithotomy position, insert the cystoscope under direct vision, using a 0° or 30° rod-lens telescope, with the irrigation running. The whole of the urethra can be visualized as you insert the instrument and so you are less likely to cause damage.

PROSTATECTOMY

Operation may be required for patients with chronic retention and overflow, or chronic retention with back pressure on their upper urinary tracts. Men with urgency, frequency and urge-incontinence with primary bladder instability are often not improved by operation. Urologists select transurethral resection (TUR) almost exclusively. Open approaches to the prostate are via the retropubic or transvesical routes.

Retropubic prostatectomy is performed through a Pfannenstiel incision, between the separated rectus muscles and behind the symphysis pubis. Through a transverse incision in the prostatic capsule the prostate is separated, with transection of the urethra below. The bladder neck is widened by resecting a 'V' posteriorly and after attaining haemostasis and passing a three-way catheter, the prostatic capsule is closed.

MANAGEMENT OF SUPERFICIAL URINARY EXTRAVASATION

Superficial urinary extravasation may follow injury during urethral dilatation or develop behind an anterior urethral stricture. It produces extensive necrosis of subcutaneous tissues and eventually of the skin. The leaked urine remains within Colles fascia, which is the lower and posterior extension of Scarpa's deep abdominal wall fascia into the perineum. This attaches to the ischiopubic rami and posterior edge of the perineal membrane, and the attachment of Scarpa's fascia to the fascia lata just below the inguinal ligament in the thighs limits migration of fluid posteriorly and into the thighs. Urine therefore fills the subcutaneous tissue of the scrotum and the penile shaft and ascends up the anterior abdominal wall. The clinical context and the distribution of swelling distinguish it from the far more common dependent perineal oedema that is sometimes seen in cardiac failure.

If the urine is not already infected, the necrotic tissues will certainly become so.

Action

Divert the urinary stream by draining the bladder by the suprapubic route. Make as many incisions as are necessary in the perineum, scrotum, penile shaft and anterior abdominal wall to let out the infected urine and necrotic tissue. Never be afraid to open up the spaces widely. Use a specific antibiotic if you know the microorganism, otherwise administer a broad-spectrum one.

KEY POINTS Fournier's gangrene

- Watch for the spreading, fulminating streptococcal gangrene described by Jean Fournier (1832–1914), the Parisian Professor of Dermatology.
- If present, you must radically excise all necrotic tissue and start an intensive course of antibiotic therapy in order to save the patient's life.
- Even in expert hands, the outlook is very poor.

EMERGENCY TREATMENT OF RUPTURED URETHRA

Such injuries are often seen in victims of multiple trauma. There are essentially two varieties:

- *Direct perineal injury* which damages the bulbous or penile urethra. The injury may be partial or complete.
- *Associated with pelvic ring fracture.* This is either a partial or complete tear of the posterior urethra associated with fracture of the pelvic ring; a distracting force pulls the prostatic urethra away from the membranous urethra.

The first imperative is to save life; dealing with the urethral injury is subordinate to coping with other more immediately threatening conditions. The extent of the urethral injury can often be deduced from the pattern of bony injury to the pelvis. Wide distraction of the anterior part of the pelvic ring is very often associated with complete urethral disruption. If circumstances allow, gently perform an ascending urethrogram, using an aqueous contrast solution, to give useful information about the state of the urethra. If the contrast medium enters the bladder, then rupture is either insignificant or incomplete, and in this instance institute simple suprapubic drainage if the patient is unable to void.

Ruptured bulbous urethra

With 'falling astride' injuries, the patient's general condition is usually good and the ends of the damaged urethra are close together. Seek the help of a specialist if at all possible. Intervention is necessary only if the patient cannot pass urine. Very gentle attempts to pass a small-calibre urethral catheter risks converting a partial into a complete rupture. It is probably safer to avoid instrumentation of the urethra unless you have extensive experience and this is unlikely, since such injuries are relatively uncommon. In case of need, insert a suprapubic tube into the bladder and refer the patient to a specialist.

Rupture of the posterior urethra

Rupture of the posterior urethra that results from pelvic trauma requires expert attention if the patient is to avoid lifelong disability. If the patient cannot pass urine following lower abdominal or pelvic trauma, the differential diagnosis lies between bladder rupture and posterior urethral injury. Urethral injury is more likely if there is significant bony deformity of the pelvis. Stabilize the urinary tract condition by inserting a suprapubic catheter while life-threatening injuries receive attention.

Traumatic rupture of the bladder

Extraperitoneal rupture can follow blunt trauma to the lower abdomen when the bladder is full. It is easily diagnosed by a cystogram, using aqueous contrast medium, which also indicates the existence of associated urethral injury. Treat it conservatively by inserting a urethral catheter, giving broad-spectrum antibiotics and monitoring the patient. Operative repair of the bladder is indicated if there is a failure to drain urine through the catheter, increasing lower abdominal distension or evidence of intraperitoneal rupture. Rupture of the bladder into the peritoneal cavity is an unusual injury in isolation, though it may occur as a complication of transurethral surgery to a bladder lesion. If it results from external trauma, there are commonly associated injuries that need attention.

Action

Expose the bladder intra- and extraperitoneally. This enables you to perform an exploratory laparotomy at the same time. Clean the peritoneal cavity using saline lavage. Open the bladder anteriorly to detect other bladder injuries that may have escaped notice. Close the bladder incision and injuries in two layers using an absorbable suture. Drain the bladder urethrally if there is no urethral injury, and suprapubically if there is any doubt.

DRAINAGE OF PERIURETHRAL ABSCESS

This usually results from a urethral stricture. It may be necessary, before draining the abscess, to establish adequate urinary drainage with a suprapubic catheter. It is hazardous to use force to dilate the stricture under these conditions.

Make an incision over the most prominent part of the abscess and lay it completely open, break down any loculi and pack the cavity with a Eusol or similar dressing.

Once healing is proceeding well, it is safe to pass a dilator and establish urethral drainage if necessary. When healing is complete, perform a urethrogram to establish the extent of the stricture; use this information to decide on future management.

FURTHER READING

Blandy J 1986 Cystoscopy. In: Blandy J Operative urology, 2nd edn. Blackwell Scientific, Oxford, pp 6–9

Blandy J 1986 Dilatation of a stricture. In: Blandy J Operative urology, 2nd edn. Blackwell Scientific, Oxford, pp 216–219

Blandy J 1986 Suprapubic cystostomy. In Blandy J Operative urology, 2nd edn. Blackwell Scientific, Oxford, pp 117–120

Blandy J, Fowler C 1996 Bladder: trauma. In: Blandy J, Fowler C Urology, 2nd edn. Blackwell Scientific, Oxford, pp 265–271

Blandy J, Fowler C 1996 Urethra and penis: trauma. In: Blandy J, Fowler C Urology, 2nd edn. Blackwell Scientific, Oxford, pp 460–471

47

Male genitalia

C. G. Fowler, I. Junaid

CONTENTS

CIRCUMCISION

Circumcision is most commonly performed for cultural reasons. Medical indications include phimosis (Greek= muzzling), paraphimosis, recurrent balanoposthitis (Greek *balanos*=acorn, glans+*posthe*=prepuce+*itis*=inflammation) and carcinoma of the penis. Phimosis may be infantile, to be distinguished from normal failure of the foreskin to retract because of physiological adhesions between the prepuce and glans penis. In later life it is almost invariably due to balanitis.

Circumcision in infants is traditionally performed without anaesthesia but this is now open to question. A penile ring block of lidocaine and bupivacaine may be used.

Action

1 Grasp the tip of the dorsal surface of the foreskin in the midline with a small artery forceps and gently pull it downwards until it is held on the stretch. If phimosis is particularly severe, use a second pair of artery forceps as a dilator to enlarge the opening. Using a silver probe in the infant, or artery forceps in the adult, gently free the foreskin from the glans so that it can be completely retracted, leaving no adhesions or inspissated smegma (Greek=soap) behind. Wash it with non-spiritous solution.

2 Gently pull the foreskin down over the glans and apply two straight artery forceps side by side in the midline on the dorsal surface of the foreskin. Divide it between these two (Fig. 47.1a). Continue the incision in the same direction with straight scissors about 3–6 mm short of the corona (Fig. 47.1b). From the apex of this incision, cut laterally until the incision reaches the lateral border of the glans (Fig. 47.1c). Now carry the incision towards the frenulum (Latin *frenum*=bridle), making sure that both surfaces of the foreskin are cut together. This ensures that the undersurface of the glans is not denuded of skin (Fig. 47.1d).

Alternative method

1 A more elegant alternative method is particularly useful for adults. Grasp the tip of the foreskin between two haemostats and gently stretch it over the glans. Make a circumferential incision in the penile skin at the level of the corona using a blade, taking care not to sever the veins that lie just below the skin. Divide the veins between haemostats and ligate them.

2 Make an incision through the dorsum of the foreskin to expose the glans penis followed by a second circumferential incision in the skin of the inside surface of the prepuce about the 0.5 cm from the corona. Free the foreskin by cutting the connective tissue that remains, until it is attached only by the frenulum. Place a small artery forceps across the frenulum, so catching the

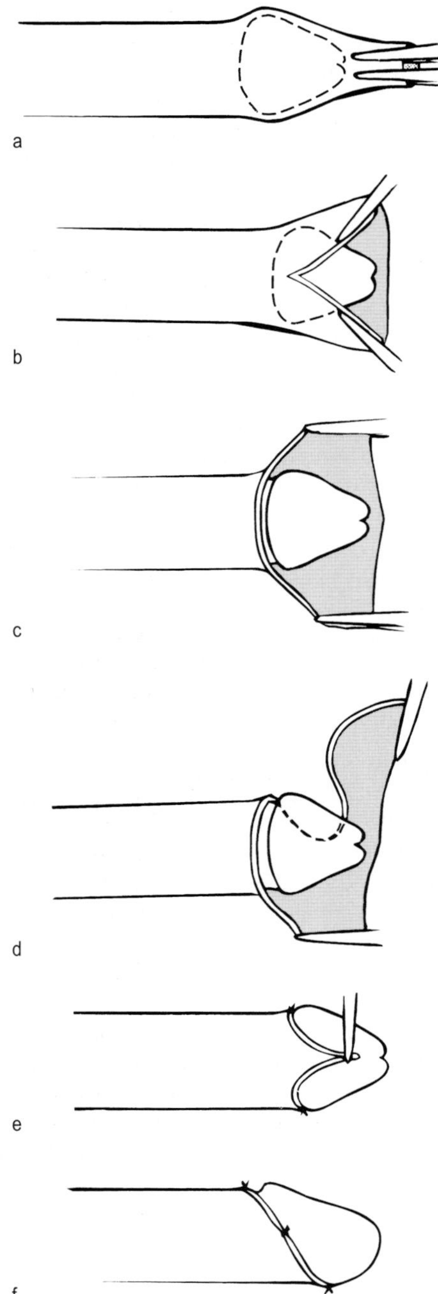

Fig. 47.1 Circumcision.

inverted-V extension of skin and frenulum together, and excise the foreskin (Fig. 47.1e).

3 Transfix the frenulum and apex of the shaft skin with a fine synthetic absorbable stitch and tie it firmly, releasing the artery forceps. Leave one end of the suture long to act as a stay suture. Search for, pick up and ligate with fine synthetic absorbable thread, all the bleeding vessels. There is usually an artery on each side of the shaft of the penis that tends to retract. Bring the two layers of the foreskin together with absorbable sutures. Leave a long end to the suture placed at the dorsal position so it can also act as a stay stitch. Appose, by gentle traction on the two stay sutures, the cut edges of the foreskin, ready for suturing. Avoid using too many sutures (Fig. 47.1f).

? DIFFICULTY

1. Do not pull downwards too forcefully on the foreskin once the initial two artery forceps have been applied, or you will remove too much skin.
2. Never use monopolar diathermy for circumcision in a young boy. If the penis is small, the high density of diathermy current at its base can lead to coagulation of the blood supply and necrosis of the penis. Bipolar diathermy is safer.
3. An adherent foreskin may be very difficult to separate from the glans. It may even require sharp dissection, particularly with longstanding phimosis in adults following repeated infections, or in balanitis xerotica obliterans.
4. Always make sure all bleeding is stopped. Infants cannot tolerate blood loss.

Aftercare

Dressings usually fall off and are unnecessary. A loose dressing is all that is needed.

In particular, avoid sewing dressings in place. Baby boys have been known to lose the glans penis through ischaemia caused by tight dressings or by constricting threads from a dressing.

Permit gentle bathing from the second postoperative day.

Warn the patient, or parents, that it will take several weeks for the penis to heal and achieve the final cosmetic result.

PARAPHIMOSIS

In paraphimosis (Greek *para* = beyond; beyond the glans), the retracted foreskin causes a constriction that interferes with venous and lymphatic return from the glans penis. The resulting oedema makes it even more difficult to reduce the paraphimosis. It is often possible to reduce it by gentle but prolonged squeezing of the swollen glans penis and manipulation of the foreskin. If this fails, operate. It is usual to use general anaesthesia but the penile ring block described above works well.

Hold the penis on the fingers of one hand, placing the thumb uppermost on the glans. Depress the glans downwards to expose the constricting band. In longstanding paraphimosis the resulting oedema makes it exceedingly difficult to identify this ring clearly. Transect the ring longitudinally with a small knife. This incision should be of sufficient length and depth to release the constriction and so enable the paraphimosis to be reduced. Leave the incision wide open, covered with loose dressings. Proceed to formal circumcision when all inflammation and oedema has settled.

MEATOTOMY

The indications for this operation are meatal (Latin *meare* = to go) stenosis or insufficient meatal size to allow free passage of endoscopic instruments. The operation most commonly performed in general departments is the standard meatotomy. Gently dilate the meatus until one blade of a straight artery forceps can be introduced into the orifice. Direct the forceps just to one side of the midline and introduce one blade until its tip lies in the fossa navicularis. Firmly clamp the forceps and leave it for 5 minutes, then remove it.

ADULT HYDROCELE

EXCISION OF HYDROCELE

This is suitable for very large or thick-walled hydroceles. Grasp the scrotum firmly with one hand and stretch the skin over the hydrocele. Choose an appropriate area between the vessels, which usually run transversely, to make a transverse skin incision. Carry the incision through all layers of the scrotum so you can deliver the entire scrotal contents and secure all bleeding points. Clean off all the coverings off the hydrocele sac with scissors. Incise the sac, drain the fluid and deliver the testicle.

Excise the sac only, keeping close to the testicle. Run a fine continuous haemostatic Monocryl or any other absorbable suture along the cut edge of the sac. Secure all small bleeding points with fine absorbable sutures and return the testicle to the scrotum. Grasp the dartos (Greek = skinned or flayed) muscle at each end of the incision with tissue forceps. Elevate them to bring the muscle into view and approximate them with a continuous absorbable suture. This gathers the muscle together and with it the skin, obviating the need for skin sutures.

Apply a firm Litesome or similar scrotal support, or use a 10-cm crepe bandage to wind around the scrotum to minimize any subsequent swelling.

If the sac is adherent, requiring scissors dissection to free it from the scrotum, there may be some oozing. Do not hesitate to insert a drain.

An alternative technique is the operation described by Mathieu Jaboulay (1860–1913) of Lyon. Instead of running a haemostatic suture along the cut edge of the sac, suture the edges together behind the epididymis.

LORD'S PROCEDURE

The procedure described by Peter Lord is particularly valuable when the sac is relatively thin-walled and has the advantage of requiring only a small incision in the scrotal skin and in the hydrocele sac itself, minimizing bleeding.

Incise the scrotum down to and including the hydrocele sac, securing all bleeding points in the incision. Widen it so you can just deliver the testis, everting the hydroceles sac behind it. Using interrupted sutures, pick up the edge of the sac and gather up the sac wall with a series of bites according to the sac size, finally taking a bite of the tunica. When all these sutures are in place, tie them, so bunching up and obliterating the hydrocele around the testis. Finally close the scrotal incision as described previously, with absorbable sutures and apply a scrotal support.

INFANTILE HYDROCELE

These hydroceles are hernias and should be treated as such. Do not attempt to excise the sac (see Ch. 43).

TORSION OF THE TESTICLE

KEY POINTS Diagnosis

- A swollen painful testis in a boy is a torsion until proved otherwise.
- Never delay operation: every minute counts. Never be tempted to leave the good side for another time; the child may leave the district and never return to hospital.

Carefully counsel the boy and his parents. Seek consent for exploration, orchidectomy if the testis is necrotic and fixation of the contralateral side. Counselling includes the information that the insertion of a testicular prosthesis can be considered in the future if the testis has to be removed.

Action

1 Incise the scrotum transversely as described for hydrocele operations. Continue the incision in depth until you can deliver the testicle and cord. Untwist the torsion and wrap the testicle in a warm pack. While you are waiting to see if the torted (Latin *torquere* = to twist) testis recovers, make a similar incision in the other side of the scrotum and deliver the non-twisted testicle, noting any abnormal anatomy that may be present.

2 With a fine nylon stitch, take a firm bite of the tunica of the testicle and anchor it to the side-wall of the scrotum. It is advisable to place three sutures for fixation taking care to avoid the vas, the epididymis and the blood supply to testis. Close the scrotal incision on the non-twisted side.

3 Remove the pack from the untwisted testicle and examine it carefully for viability. If it is obviously dead and remains black, remove it. Place a strong artery forceps across the cord and then remove the testicle and tie the cord with strong absorbable suture. If the untwisted testis appears potentially viable, return it to the scrotum, fixing it with fine nylon sutures as described for the other side.

ORCHIDECTOMY

SIMPLE ORCHIDECTOMY

The indications for simple orchidectomy are severe or recurrent attacks of acute epididymitis, chronic epididymitis including tuberculous epididymitis, severe testicular trauma when the testis is not salvageable, testicular infarction from a neglected torsion and in the management of advanced cancer of the prostate. Remember to discuss the possibility of inserting a testicular prosthesis.

Action

1 If the condition is inflammatory and involves the skin, then make the incision in the scrotum so as to excise the overlying attached infected skin. The incision therefore varies in shape and size according to the condition. Leave the involved skin attached to the underlying structures. Enter the scrotal sac away from the inflamed area. Deliver the testicle with the overlying attached area of skin. Do not hesitate to remove all the involved surrounding skin. The scrotal skin has amazing powers of regeneration. Apply gentle traction to the testicle and clean the cord structures to free 4–6 cm of cord.

2 Cross-clamp the cord at this level with two strong artery forceps, dividing it between them. Do not pull on the testicle or the divided upper end may retract from view. Tie the clamped upper end with strong absorbable suture, but do not release the forceps before applying a second tie. If the cord is very thick, tease it into two structures and cross-clamp each, to avoid creating a bulky tie. Use finger dissection and traction on the lower divided cord to remove the testicle.

3 Leave the scrotal wound unsutured to drain freely if there is infection. Otherwise insert a few interrupted absorbable sutures to approximate the skin edges. Apply loose dressings only.

TESTICULAR TRAUMA

Given the exposed position of the scrotum, this is mercifully uncommon and is largely confined to sporting injuries and assaults. The immediate pain may be excruciating, but in the excitement of a rugby match may be passed off as trivial and indeed may not manifest itself until some hours later. Later discovery may lead to the diagnosis of testicular torsion. Since exploration is mandatory in both circumstances this error is of no consequence. Explore the scrotum without fail when it is obvious that there is increasing size and pain. Otherwise simple support, rest and analgesics suffice. In the former circumstance there is a danger of increasing haemorrhage within the tunica vaginalis compressing and destroying the testicle; also, the pain of a disrupted testis can be so severe that exploration is necessary.

If the testis is completely disrupted, perform simple orchidectomy, although the testis can often be salvaged by simply evacuating the haematoma and loosely tacking the split and torn tunica albuginea together. Allow plenty of space for the blood to escape. Be willing to insert a small drain. Administer prophylactic antibiotics.

EXCISION OF EPIDIDYMAL CYSTS

Excise epididymal (Greek *epi* = upon + *didymos* = twin; upon the testes) cysts only when they become uncomfortably large. Removal of epididymal cysts is relatively contraindicated in young or unmarried males, as it may render that side sterile. The condition is multiple, so warn patients that recurrent cysts are likely.

Action

1. Incise the scrotum as described for excision of a hydrocele sac. Deliver the testicle along with its appendages, including the cysts. Remember that cysts are often multiple and commonly occur in the upper pole of the epididymis. Combine blunt and scissors dissection. Hold the testicle with one hand, or have an assistant hold it, while you clean off all the adventitial tissue surrounding the cyst.

2. With scissors, completely excise the cyst or else marsupialize it by cutting off the whole protruding surface. If there are very many cysts, excise that part of the epididymis bearing them. Oversew the raw area left following this, using fine absorbable sutures. Return the testicle to the scrotum and continue as described for hydroceles.

EXCISION OF VARICOCELE

Varicoceles, dilated veins of the spermatic cord, are common, particularly on the left side. Most of them do not require treatment. When you discover a varicocele, as a precaution order an ultrasound scan of the kidneys to exclude the presence of a mass interfering with venous drainage from the affected side. The evidence that varicoceles cause subfertility is questionable. Testicular pain is common and the coincidence of a varicocele does not mean that it is the cause of the pain. Varicoceles can cause a dragging scrotal discomfort but many men have continuing scrotal pain despite curative varicocele surgery. The testicular venous plexus rapidly regenerates and all types of treatment for varicocele have a high failure rate.

Action

Make an incision in the inguinal region as for a hernia. Expose the external oblique aponeurosis and open it in the line of its fibres into the external ring. Free the cord from the canal and deliver the testicle out of the scrotum. Dissect out, tie off with fine absorbable thread, and remove all the enlarged and tortuous veins that make up the pampiniform (Latin *pampinus* = tendril; resembling a tendril) plexus. Do this over the whole length of the cord. Do not be afraid to remove all the enlarged veins; leaving but a few prejudices the result. Make sure that all bleeding points are secure, then return the testicle to the scrotum. Close the external oblique aponeurosis with continuous 1 synthetic absorbable thread and close the skin. Fit a Litesome or similar scrotal support. In some specialist centres, laparoscopic ligation or percutaneous embolization are offered.

VASECTOMY FOR STERILIZATION

This operation results in more irritating, usually trivial, postoperative complaints leading to litigation in the courts, than any other urological procedure. Fully explain to the patient and his partner exactly what is entailed. Warn that, if a local anaesthetic is unsatisfactory, the procedure must be abandoned, to be performed later under a general anaesthetic, and that any operation on the scrotum is liable to cause pain, swelling and infection.

Sterilization is not immediate. The store of sperm must first be exhausted, which usually takes 2–3 months. To be certain, perform a seminal count at 3 months and 4 months; only when two consecutive completely negative counts are obtained a month apart is it safe to pronounce the patient sterile. If the counts are equivocal, be prepared to re-explore the procedure. Warn that re-canalization can rarely occur, in between 1 and 2 per 1000 vasectomies. It can occur years later and is not the result of surgical error or omission. If the partner shows signs of pregnancy, she should seek appropriate advice. Early re-canalization can be deduced from the equivocal postoperative sperm counts.

KEY POINT Consent form

- Make sure the detailed consent form covers all these points, that it is understood and signed.

Action

1 Grasp the upper part of the scrotum between the first two fingers and the thumb so as to be able to roll the scrotal skin between them. Identify the hard round structure of the vas and roll it away from the other structures of the cord (Fig. 47.2). Grip the vas between the middle finger, which invaginates the scrotum, and the thumb on the outside. Move the index finger nearer to the thumb. Now spread the index finger and thumb apart, so holding the vas firmly across the invaginating middle finger. This presents the vas in relief.

2 Make a 1-cm cut into the scrotal skin in the direction of the vas and extending down to it, cutting through the covering adventitia. Still firmly holding the vas, grasp it with tissue-holding forceps such as Alliss or, even better, with ring forceps especially designed to encircle the vas. It helps to make a longitudinal cut through the immediate coverings of the vas to reveal its glistening white muscular coat, before enclosing it with the forceps. Release the finger and thumb. The vas now protrudes from the incision, held by the forceps. Force an artery forceps under the vas to separate a length of it from its coverings and to be doubly sure that it cannot escape back into the scrotum.

3 Apply artery forceps about 3 cm apart on the vas and excise the segment between them. Tie each end with no. 2 Vicryl suture, burying the lower end deep in the scrotum. Incorporate the tied upper end into the subcutaneous tissues when closing each wound. This separates the two ends as widely as possible. Repeat the procedure on the other side. Preserve the excised segments for histological confirmation.

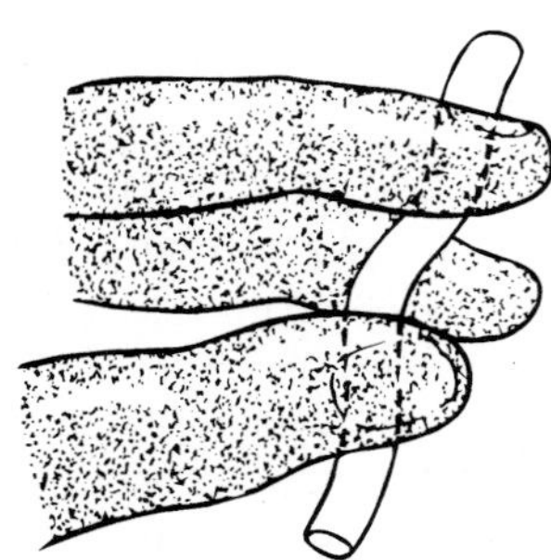

Fig. 47.2 Vasectomy: identifying the vas.

? DIFFICULTY

1. Do not attempt this operation under local anaesthesia unless the patient, and the scrotum, are relaxed.
2. If you use local anaesthesia, ensure that both the skin and the tissues immediately around the vas are infiltrated and that you have allowed sufficient time for the local anaesthetic to take effect.
3. If you lose the vas in the scrotum, try again. Never be tempted to grope blindly for structures in the scrotum.
4. If the operation is difficult, do not be content with simple division. Stop and try again on another occasion, after explaining the reason to the patient.

ORCHIDOPEXY

In adults, the testis is often atrophied, so consider whether orchidectomy is a better choice. The testis is often palpable in the inguinal canal or neck of the scrotum. In case of doubt, confirm its presence by ultrasound or CT (computed tomography) scanning. Maldescent of the testis (Greek *orkhis*) should be detected soon after birth but sometimes presents in childhood or later in life.

KEY POINTS Preserve spermatogenesis

- Always bring the testes down before the age of 2 years. After this time spermatogenesis decreases.
- Paediatric surgery is best performed by experts. The principles alone will be described.

Action

Make a small inguinal incision centred over the external ring. In young and fat boys, Scarpa's fascia may be thick and can be mistaken for the external oblique aponeurosis. Expose the external oblique over its medial third. In cases of ectopic testes, where the testis lies outside the external oblique, take care not to damage either the testicle or cord while exposing the external oblique.

If the testis lies in the superficial inguinal pouch, free it and the cord until the latter can be traced backwards into the external ring. The testis and cord should now be lying free, but there is insufficient cord length to bring the testicle down into the scrotum. Open the external oblique in the line of its fibres into the external ring. Free the cord from within the canal right up to the internal ring to add more length.

Gently insert your little finger under the cord and in through the internal ring, sweeping it gently from side to side. This frees the cord, vas and vessels from any posterior adhesions, again adding length. Look for an indirect hernial sac lying in front of the cord. If so, grasp it and gently pull it laterally. Hold the testis with one hand and apply gentle traction to the cord so that it is held taut. With fine non-toothed forceps, gently separate the vas and vascular pedicle from the adventitial bands that extend laterally to the hernial sac or retroperitoneum. Take care not to damage either the vas or vessels. This frees the maximum length of available cord.

Insert your forefinger into the scrotum, so widening the neck into it. This provides easy access to bring down the testis. Hold the scrotum stretched over the forefinger and make a small, 1-cm long, transverse cut in the scrotal skin over its most dependent part. Incise the skin only, leaving the dartos muscle intact. Now, with fine curved dissecting scissors, create a subcutaneous pouch between skin and dartos muscle for a distance of about 1 cm all round the incision. Thrust a fine artery forceps through the exposed dartos, out through the groin incision, and grasp the remains of the gubernaculums. Bring the testicle down through the scrotum and tease it out through the small hole in the dartos made by the forceps. Make sure the cord structures are not twisted. Place the testicle in the subcutaneous pouch and close the skin of the scrotum with fine synthetic absorbable thread. Using this technique of anchoring the testicle avoids any tension on the cord, which might endanger the vascular supply to the testicle. Close the inguinal incision.

? DIFFICULTY

1. For undescended testis, which may lie within the canal or just within the internal ring, use exactly the same technique. However, for these the cord length is often shorter, so take great care to obtain as much length as possible without either damaging the vessels or applying traction.
2. When there is not enough cord to bring the testicle into the scrotum, leave it as low as you can and try again when the child is older.
3. If the testicle is of very small size, with little cord length, and the contralateral one is normal, then remove it.
4. If you cannot find the testicle and cord structures at all, then close the wound and refer the case to a specialist.
5. If the condition is bilateral, explore both sides at the same operation. It is unkind to submit the child to two procedures.

PRIAPISM

Whatever the cause, commence treatment as soon as possible. If there is delay, the resulting sludging of the blood in the corpora and eventual fibrosis lead to impotence. Even with early treatment, impotence is common. Carry out the simplest procedure to obtain detumescence and then refer the patient to a specialist centre.

Either under local anaesthesia such as spinal or epidural, or preferably general anaesthesia, a wide-bore aspiration needle is inserted into the distal end of one corpus cavernosum and another into the proximal end of the opposite one, and the corpus is irrigated with 100–200 ml of physiological saline or heparin saline into the proximal needle until the efflux is reasonably clear. The corpora are then massaged to make them more flaccid. It may be necessary to repeat this process three or four times over the ensuring 48 hours before the corpora remain flaccid.

FURTHER READING

Blandy J 1986 Radical cure of hydrocoele. In: Blandy J Operative urology, 2nd edn. Blackwell Scientific, Oxford, pp 246–247

Blandy J, Fowler C 1996 Circumcision. In: Blandy J, Fowler C Urology, 2nd edn. Blackwell Scientific, Oxford, pp 445–447

Blandy J, Fowler C 1996 Orchidopexy. In: Blandy J, Fowler C Urology, 2nd edn. Blackwell Scientific, Oxford, pp 553–556

Blandy J, Fowler C 1996 Torsion of the testis. In: Blandy J, Fowler C Urology, 2nd edn. Blackwell Scientific, Oxford, pp 569–571

48

Gynaecological surgery

M. E. Setchell

CONTENTS

GENERAL CONSIDERATIONS

Diagnostic ultrasound and diagnostic and operative laparoscopy are used extensively in gynaecology (Greek *gynaikos* = woman). Nowhere is informed consent more important than in gynaecological surgery. Fully explain the probable operative procedure and its consequences, particularly if future fertility is likely to be affected. If the woman wishes, keep the partner informed as well.

Patients should stop taking the oral contraceptive pill 6 weeks before elective major gynaecological surgery. Pregnancy predisposes to thromboembolism, so give prophylactic heparin readily.

Menstruation is not a contraindication to gynaecological surgery, nor indeed to thorough examination.

Careless surgery in the female pelvis results in pelvic adhesions, which may drastically disturb a woman's fertility and affect the rest of her life and happiness.

Prepare

1 *Shave* pubic and vulval hair as little as possible to avoid the later discomfort when it regrows.

2 *Position the patient* for vaginal operations in the lithotomy position. Laparoscopy is best carried out with the patient in Lloyd-Davies stirrups, with steep head-down tilt. Perform abdominal operations with the patient supine and 5–10° of head-down tilt.

3 *Catheterize* the bladder before all abdominal procedures, laparoscopy included. Separate the labia and swab the urethral meatus with antiseptic solution. Without allowing the labia to close again, pass a silver or plastic catheter well into the bladder. Now let the labia approximate and press firmly and continuously suprapubically. When the urine flow ceases, gradually withdraw the catheter, taking care not to allow air to be sucked into the bladder.

MINOR GYNAECOLOGICAL OPERATIONS

DILATATION AND CURETTAGE

Diagnostic dilatation and curettage (D&C) is performed for heavy or prolonged vaginal bleeding; therapeutic dilatation and curettage is carried out for bleeding associated with retained products of conception. Any woman aged 13–50 years with heavy bleeding could have an incomplete or missed abortion; order a preoperative β-hCG (beta-subunit of human chorionic gonadotrophin) pregnancy test on blood or urine and a transvaginal ultrasound scan of the uterus before she is taken to theatre. Order a full blood count and 'group and save serum'. A preliminary hysteroscopy may be performed. If the D&C is for a miscarriage of greater than 10 weeks' gestation, ask the anaesthetist to give 5–10 units of synthetic oxytocin (Syntocinon) intravenously immediately beforehand. Through a Sims' or Auvard's speculum draw down the cervix, pass Hegar's uterine dilators and remove tissue with polyp forceps and curettage to send for histology.

BARTHOLIN'S CYST OR ABSCESS

An abscess is an acutely painful condition so deal with it as an emergency. The operation of marsupialization (Greek *marsyp(p)ion* = a pouch) is the procedure of choice since recurrence is very likely following simple incision and drainage.

LAPAROSCOPY

This is a very useful and important diagnostic procedure in the diagnosis of pelvic pain, both acute and chronic. It is particularly valuable in cases of suspected ectopic pregnancy (see Ch. 8).

OVARIAN OPERATIONS

This may be required for an ovarian cyst causing acute abdominal pain from rupture, torsion or haemorrhage. A preoperative abdominal or transvaginal ultrasound scan may suggest the diagnosis; colour Doppler scan demonstrates neovascularization, suggestive of malignancy. In no other gynaecological operation is fully informed consent more important, particularly when one or both ovaries may need to be removed once the abdomen is open and the clinical findings apparent. Order preoperative full blood count and take blood for tumour markers such as CA125 and carcinoembryonic antigen (CEA), even if results may be available only postoperatively.

If the tumour is likely to be benign use a transverse suprapubic incision, otherwise use a vertical incision. Distinguish a mature graafian follicle or a corpus luteum cyst from a neoplastic cyst. A luteal cyst may develop in early pregnancy; unnecessary removal can result in abortion. Do not risk sacrificing healthy ovaries – features of benign tumours are a smooth surface and the absence of ascites, peritoneal, omental or nodular metastases.

Ovarian cystectomy is the preferred treatment for benign ovarian cysts. Carry out salpingo-oophorectomy if there is evidence of malignancy, torsion, gangrene, or the tumour is very large and little normal ovarian tissue can be conserved.

If you suspect malignancy, explore the whole abdomen. If it is obviously malignant remove the uterus, ovaries and tubes, the omentum and as much metastatic tumour as possible. If it is simple, make an incision round the base of the cyst in the ovarian cortex and shell out the cyst intact (Fig. 48.1).

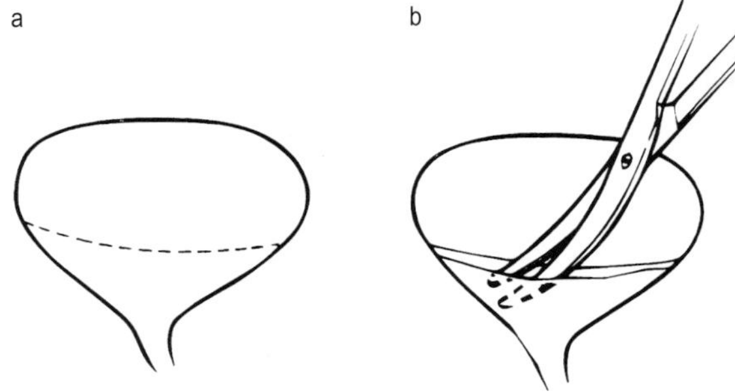

Fig. 48.1 Ovarian cystectomy (a) circumcision; (b) separation of cyst from ovary.

SURGERY OF ECTOPIC PREGNANCY

Classic ruptured ectopic (Greek *ek* = out of + *topos* = place) pregnancy presents as severe abdominal pain, guarding and rebound, and hypovolaemic shock. Tubal abortion or slowly leaking ectopic pregnancy demands ultrasound scanning, using a transvaginal probe, together with a rapid β-hCG assay to detect pregnancy. Laparoscopy is always required in the less acute forms of tubal abortion or slow leakage. In non-rupture, laparoscopic salpingotomy and aspiration of the pregnancy may be the treatment of choice if future pregnancy is desired. Very early ectopic pregnancies may be managed medically, with a single dose of methotrexate.

Once the diagnosis of ruptured ectopic has been made, take the patient to the operating theatre as soon as possible. Do not wait for blood to be cross-matched or hope that the patient's condition will improve. She will improve only when the fallopian tube is clamped.

Order a full blood count, group and save serum if not cross-matching, and secure intravenous access as soon as you suspect ectopic pregnancy. If the patient is shocked, take her to the operating theatre for immediate laparotomy. In less acute forms arrange for laparoscopy with a view to salpingotomy or salpingectomy.

Action

Make a generous incision, either midline or Pfannenstiel, provided you are used to this incision. As soon as the peritoneal cavity is open, aspirate blood with the sucker. Draw the uterus and appendages up into the wound. Identify the

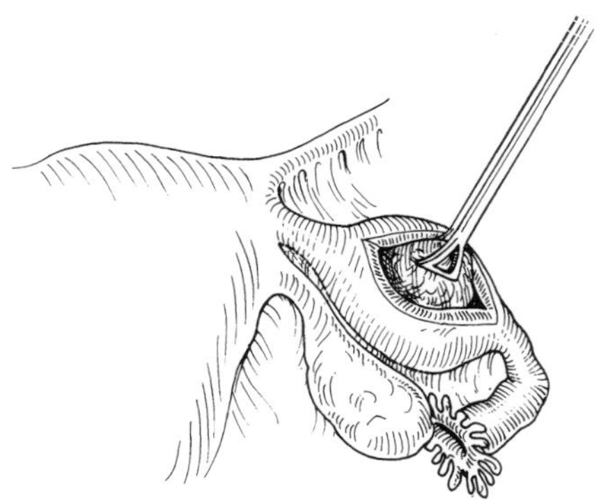

Fig. 48.2 Conservative management of an ectopic pregnancy. After removing the trophoblast through an incision in the free border of the salpinx, leave the tube to heal spontaneously.

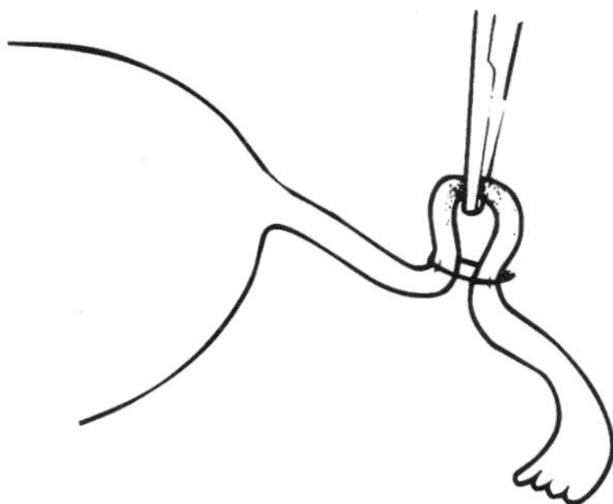

Fig. 48.3 Tubal ligation. Tightly encircle a loop of salpinx with an absorbable, synthetic ligature, then excise the isolated loop.

ruptured tube, clamp the mesosalpinx and the cornual end of the tube, then excise the damaged tube, ligate the pedicles but usually leave the ovary. Conserve the tube if the ectopic pregnancy is small, using a salpingotomy (Fig. 48.2). Inspect the contralateral tube and ovary but do not be tempted to tamper with it. Before closing the abdomen, aspirate and swab out as much blood as possible, and estimate the volume of blood loss. Washing the peritoneal cavity with Hartmann's solution may help to reduce adhesion formation.

TUBAL LIGATION

A sterilization procedure may be carried out in the course of a caesarean section operation or during the course of an abdominal operation.

Obtain prior consent from the patient. Avoid sterilizing a woman under the age of 30 years unless there is a good medical reason to perform it. Pick up a loop of fallopian tube with a Spencer Wells forceps 2–3 cm from the uterus. Tie an absorbable synthetic ligature tightly around the base of the loop and excise the end of the loop (Fig. 48.3). You may seal each end of the tube with the diathermy needle as an additional precaution.

HYSTERECTOMY

Hysterectomy may be for uterine disease or part of resection for ovarian, rectal or other cancer. If possible conserve at least one ovary in premenopausal women. Vaginal hysterectomy and radical (Wertheim) hysterectomy are also performed. Empty the bladder by catheterization and cleanse the vagina with an antiseptic. Bonney's blue or methylthioninium chloride (methylene blue) dye, making it more easily recognized at operation.

The uterus is removed through a Pfannenstiel or vertical incision after separating it from the broad ligament, ureters, bladder, and vagina, with or without the tubes and ovaries, after securing, doubly ligating and dividing the uterine vessels.

Close the vaginal vault or alternatively leave it open for drainage after running a haemostatic stitch round the edge.

MYOMECTOMY

This is the shelling out of fibromyomata from the uterus without performing hysterectomy. Now achieve haemostasis and close the serous surface of the uterus.

INCIDENTAL GYNAECOLOGICAL CONDITIONS

PELVIC INFLAMMATORY DISEASE

Suspected appendicitis may turn out to be acute salpingitis. The condition is almost always bilateral, although one tube may be more affected than the other. The tubes are oedematous and reddened, and pus is often seen dripping from the fimbrial end. Take a swab for bacteriological culture and close the abdomen. Start antibiotics at once, according to local antibiotic guidelines. This usually includes a cephalosporin and tetracycline to cover *Chlamydia trachomatis*, which is now the most common pathogen.

FIMBRIAL CYST AND PAROVARIAN CYST

Small cysts may be seen in relation to the distal end of the fallopian tube or broad ligament. They arise in remnants of the mesonephric (wolffian) duct and occasionally undergo torsion to produce acute abdominal pain. Remove them only if they have undergone torsion. Tie the pedicle before excision.

ENDOMETRIOSIS

This condition may involve the ovaries, forming chocolate cysts, or the pelvic peritoneum when it appears as small purple or dark-brown nodules. Rupture of a chocolate cyst produces acute abdominal pain. Occasionally it involves the intestine, when the appearance may mimic a carcinoma. In the large intestine it may produce subacute obstruction and can be extremely difficult to differentiate from carcinoma. Rarely, endometriomas may be seen in an abdominal scar.

CAESAREAN SECTION

The lower segment operation, performed under general or epidural anaesthesia, is almost universally employed nowadays.

Use a Pfannenstiel or vertical subumbilical midline incision. Pick up and incise the uterovesical peritoneal fold and incise the lower uterine segment, stretch it, incise the membranes, and deliver the fetus head first. Once the head is delivered, have the anaesthetist give an intravenous injection of synthetic oxytocin (Syntocinon) 10 units. Aspirate the infant's nose and throat. Have your assistant apply fundal pressure as you withdraw the baby. Clamp and divide the cord. Deliver the placenta and close the uterus using absorbable sutures before closing the abdomen.

PREGNANCY AND EMERGENCY SURGERY

The presence of a pregnancy may cause considerable confusion in the diagnosis of an acute abdomen and may make access more difficult at laparotomy. It should not, however, deter you from performing emergency abdominal operations when necessary.

Appendicitis

The appendix is pushed upwards and outwards during pregnancy, so that the physical signs of appendicitis may be considerably altered. Because the large pregnant uterus may prevent the normal walling-off of acute appendicitis, generalized peritonitis occurs more readily. Make a gridiron incision above and lateral to the normal site, or consider a right paramedian incision if there is doubt about diagnosis.

Cholecystitis

Acute cholecystitis and biliary colic are not uncommon in pregnancy, but the symptoms may be atypical, simulating hyperemesis or indigestion of pregnancy. If you make the diagnosis of gallbladder disease in pregnancy, prefer to wait until after delivery before carrying out cholecystectomy. If you need to perform the operation during pregnancy, prefer to do so in the middle trimester.

Red degeneration of a fibroid

Pregnancy and fibroids often coexist, and a fibroid growing rapidly during pregnancy may undergo red degeneration. This is an extremely painful condition; sometimes the pain is so severe that exploratory laparotomy is carried out. Once you diagnose fibroids do not attempt to remove them. Myomectomy in pregnancy risks catastrophic haemorrhage and loss of the fetus. The only exception to this rule is if a pedunculated fibroid has undergone torsion and is gangrenous.

Placental abruption

Placental abruption (Latin *ab* = from + *rumpere* = to break; sudden). Premature detachment of the placenta results in severe abdominal pain and uterine tenderness, which may or may not be accompanied by vaginal bleeding. It may cause profound shock and usually results in fetal death. Lesser degrees may cause diagnostic difficulty. Tenderness is localized over the uterus, and in the severe form the uterus acquires a characteristic woody/hard feel to it. Unless labour occurs spontaneously, induce it with prostaglandins and amniotomy – puncture of the fetal membranes.

Renal and ureteric calculi

Renal and ureteric calculi may occur during pregnancy. Manage them as in a non-pregnant patient, with analgesics and a high fluid intake, resorting to surgical management if this fails.

Pyelonephritis and urinary tract infection

Pyelonephritis and urinary tract infection are particularly common in pregnancy because of stasis produced by uterine pressure on the bladder, and progesterone-induced ureteric dilatation. The symptoms may not be typical, so include an MSU (midstream urine) specimen whenever you investigate an obscure abdominal pain in pregnancy. Avoid antibiotics that are known to have an adverse effect on the fetus.

Rectus sheath haematoma

Occasionally, a spontaneous haematoma occurs in the rectus sheath as a result of spontaneous haemorrhage from the inferior epigastric vessels in pregnancy. A tender mass appears in the abdominal wall. Treat the condition conservatively.

FURTHER READING

Hudson CN, Setchell ME 2004 Shaw's textbook of operative gynaecology, 6th edn. Elsevier, New Delhi

Setchell ME, Cass PL 1990 In: Williamson RCN, Cooper JM (eds) Emergency abdominal surgery. Churchill Livingstone, Edinburgh

Shaw RW, Soutter WP, Stanton SL 1997 Gynaecology, 2nd edn. Churchill Livingstone, Edinburgh

49

Ear, nose and throat

M. P. Stearns

CONTENTS

INTRODUCTION

You may need to decide if otolaryngological emergencies require immediate treatment or can be left for specialist care. You may be familiar with the techniques and so feel equipped to proceed if qualified aid is unavailable. As a junior doctor rotating through a number of attachments, when faced with an ear, nose or throat condition in the Accident and Emergency Department, you may be able to remove a foreign body from the nose or ear and control nasal bleeding, and initiate management of a fractured nose.

FOREIGN BODY IN THE EAR

The patient, usually a child, may complain of pain in the ear if the foreign object is irritating or has caused infection in the external ear canal. A live insect may cause noise in the ear. Most foreign bodies in the external auditory canal are found by chance.

Remove insects to relieve pain. Fill the ear with olive oil to asphyxiate it, or kill it with alcohol. Gently remove it by syringing the ear with water at body temperature.

Inanimate foreign bodies may yield to gentle syringing, but those that occlude, or nearly occlude, the meatus cannot be removed by syringing so they need to be extracted with an instrument. Commonly inserted small pieces of sponge rubber can be removed using crocodile forceps if they lie close to the external auditory meatus. Unless you are expert, do not attempt to remove solid foreign bodies, since you risk damaging the middle ear, including the ossicular chain. A general anaesthetic may be required.

If the child is cooperative, examine the ear in a good light, initially without, then with, an auroscope. When the child is relaxed and quiet, touch the foreign body with a fine probe to confirm its shape and texture. You may not need to insert an aural speculum to do this. Look for a graspable edge; if you can seize it with very fine Hartmann's crocodile forceps you may be able to remove it.

? DIFFICULTY

1. If the object is smooth and rounded, such as a bead, do not apply forceps; they cannot grasp the object, and risk pushing it deeper into the meatus, through the drum, ossicular chain, facial nerve and labyrinth.
2. The safest way to remove an occluding foreign body is under general anaesthesia, using an operating microscope. If this is not available, use illuminating loupes and the largest aural speculum the meatus will accept. Insinuate a stapedectomy hook beyond the object unless there is an obvious space above it, turn the hook to engage it, and ease it out by rolling or sliding. Alternatively, try the effect of using a small sucker.

3. *Golden rules*:
- Do nothing that could push the foreign body further into the ear canal.
- Pass hooks or probes anteroinferiorly, where the obliquity of the tympanic membrane allows you to insert the instrument more deeply without risk of injury.

REMOVAL OF NASAL FOREIGN BODY

Suspect a self-inserted foreign body in any young child with unilateral nasal discharge, which is usually foul smelling, obstruction or bleeding. The foreign body is commonly a screwed-up fragment of paper, vegetable matter, a plastic or metal bead, or plastic sponge.

As with aural foreign bodies, first gain the child's co-operation. You may succeed if the foreign body is graspable and if you have appropriate instruments, clear visibility, a headlight, and are skilful in using a nasal speculum. If any of these are lacking, it needs to be removed under general anaesthesia by a specialist with oral, not nasal, intubation.

If the object is graspable use fine forceps, otherwise use a small hook that can be passed above the foreign body, easing it downwards and forwards for delivery. Retain full visibility throughout.

MANIPULATION OF FRACTURED NOSE

Realignment of displaced nasal bones is not only a cosmetic operation because the septum may also be broken, and fractures often cause nasal obstruction. There may also be associated facial injuries such as a fractured maxilla or 'blow-out' fracture of the orbit. Do not fail to examine the patient for other facial injuries.

Try to manipulate nasal fractures within 2 weeks of the injury. The most suitable times to do so are either very early, before there has been much nasal swelling, or after about 5–10 days to allow much of the swelling around the fracture site to subside. If you try to manipulate the nasal bones while there is much swelling, it is difficult to see whether or not the nose is straight.

It may be possible to straighten the nose by digital pressure, easing the nasal skeleton back into the midline. You can often manipulate it without anaesthesia within the first hour or two after injury. Alternatively realign the nasal bones under local anaesthesia. You may feel a click as the fragments move into place. If you cannot reduce the fracture in these ways you need the aid of general anaesthesia.

▶ KEY POINTS General anaesthetic precautions

- You must either have the patient intubated or have the facility of using a laryngeal mask.
- Without these precautions sudden heavy bleeding into the airway puts the patient at great risk.

First, attempt manual reduction, pressing with your thumbs against the more prominent of the nasal bones. If this succeeds, over-reduce the fracture, and then mould the mobilized fragments into the desired symmetry. If this fails, insert one blade of a Walsham's forceps into the nostril and grasp one nasal bone. The rubber cuff on the other blade of Walsham's forceps should lie on the skin, protecting it from damage by the forceps. Rotate and displace the nasal bone laterally to disimpact the fractured nasal bone. Then grasp the other nasal bone with the other Walsham's forceps and rotate it laterally also. The nasal fragments are now mobile and can be centralized with digital moulding. Take great care to protect the skin from injury during manipulation with these instruments. If the septum is displaced, or the bridge-line is depressed, pass the blades of Asche's forceps into the nostrils, grasp the septum, and bring it into the midline, while lifting up the dorsum. If the reduced fracture is stable do not cover it with a splint. Grossly comminuted, unstable fractures require a plaster-of-Paris splint secured with adhesive strapping. Mould the splint and the underlying nose beneath, while the plaster sets. Leave the splint in place for 7 days.

FOREIGN BODIES IN THE THROAT

Fish bones lodge at any level, often in the tonsil or vallecula (diminutive of Latin *vallis* = valley). More substantial bones (e.g. from chicken, rabbit or chops) usually stick in the postcricoid region or upper oesophagus. Rarely, occluding foreign bodies such as sweets or a meat bolus can cause airway obstruction, leading to sudden death. Dentures, which are often broken, impact in the mid-oesophagus. A benign or malignant stricture may become occluded by a small bolus, such as a pea or piece of potato.

Inspect the throat carefully, using a headlight and tongue depressor. Look for the tip of a buried fish bone in the tonsil or base of tongue. Remove it with a fine pair of angled forceps, if necessary anaesthetizing the throat with a lidocaine topical spray.

If you cannot see the foreign body directly, use a laryngeal mirror, in the same manner as in indirect laryngoscopy, to examine the back of tongue and laryngopharynx. You can often retrieve a bone in these sites under indirect vision, using angled forceps. Have the patient grasp his own tongue with a gauze swab and draw it forward as far as possible. Hold the mirror in your non-dominant hand and the forceps in your dominant hand. You must grasp the foreign body in the forceps under vision or you risk causing serious damage.

If on examination with a mirror you see the foreign body deep in the pyriform fossa or postcricoid space, or if a radiograph demonstrates that it is in the hypopharynx or upper oesophagus, then you need to remove it by direct endoscopy under general anaesthesia. Use a laryngoscope or short oesophagoscope and suitable forceps to bring the foreign body into the lumen of the endoscope. Take care not to push a sharp object through the visceral wall. Try to rotate it so that its most traumatic aspect is disimpacted and either trails harmlessly or can be drawn within the endoscope as it is withdrawn.

? DIFFICULTY

1. Do not attempt to remove a denture bearing exposed sharp hooks from the oesophagus. Safe removal may be facilitated by passing a cutting forceps through the endoscope and cutting the denture into pieces.
2. In some cases the foreign body can be removed safely only by thoracotomy and oesophagotomy (see Ch. 36).

INCISION OF QUINSY (PERITONSILLAR ABSCESS)

Suspect the diagnosis of quinsy (acute suppurative tonsillitis) or peritonsillar abscess from a history of an extremely sore throat in a toxic patient. The patient has trismus (spasm of the jaw muscles) and dysphagia for solids and liquids, often with drooling because swallowing saliva is too painful. Although inspection may be difficult because of the trismus, a swelling of the soft palate may be seen in association with a contralateral tonsillitis.

Although incision of peritonsillar abscess is frequently described in textbooks, it is rarely performed because it usually responds to versatile systemic antibiotics. Treat early disease with high dosage given intravenously, and reviewed after 24–36 hours. Incise it only if the swelling is not subsiding or if there is a fluctuant peritonsillar abscess.

Action

1 Inject local anaesthetic into the palatal mucosa at the intersection of a horizontal line through the base of the uvula with a vertical line along the anterior pillar of the fauces. Preferably use a dental syringe and needle with 2% lidocaine and 1:80000 adrenaline. Allow at least 5 minutes for it to take effect.

2 Use a Bard–Parker handle with a no. 15 blade which can be wrapped in adhesive tape with the last 1 cm only exposed, preventing too deep penetration of the pharynx. Insert the knife blade backwards through the mucosa to a depth of 1 cm. When pus gushes out, widen the track with sinus forceps. As an alternative to incising the abscess, use a large-bore hypodermic needle. You can dispense with local anaesthesia. Take a swab for culture. Quite often, however, no pus is obtained, because the quinsy is not sufficiently mature.

▶ KEY POINT Caution

- Do not insert the blade more deeply than 1 cm, or you risk damaging the internal carotid artery.

INCISION OF RETROPHARYNGEAL ABSCESS

As a cause of acute illness with respiratory obstruction in infants and toddlers, this abscess tends to be to one side of the midline. In older patients the abscess may be truly prevertebral, strictly midline and, usually, tuberculous in nature, secondary to tuberculous osteomyelitis of a cervical vertebra, in which case treatment is not primarily surgical. If significant respiratory obstruction develops in spite of intravenous versatile antibiotic treatment in a young child or infant, you should incise a pyogenic abscess. Lateral retropharyngeal abscesses in particular are often associated with a foreign body. Consequently carry out a careful search for one when incising the abscess.

Action

Lateralized pyogenic abscess

Have the child anaesthetized by an experienced anaesthetist because, if the abscess is ruptured during intubation, the patient may inhale the pus. Have the patient held in a head-down position when being intubated and until the airway is protected by a cuffed endotracheal tube. When the tube is in place the abscess contents can be aspirated with a per-oral needle. Alternatively, it can be incised through a pharyngoscope or using a Boyle–David gag. Having incised the abscess send specimens of the abscess wall for histology and culture.

RELIEF OF UPPER AIRWAY OBSTRUCTION

Immediately relieve respiratory obstruction from major facial or laryngeal trauma, laryngopharyngeal tumours and impacted foreign bodies. Ensure that there is a clear airway if the patient is comatose. If necessary assist respiration with mouth-to-mouth breathing, Ambi bag, a laryngeal mask or endotracheal intubation. If necessary, ventilate the patient. An obstructed airway can frequently be expanded using positive pressure by mouth-to-mouth respiration or through a face-mask or oral tube, thus providing an adequate passage for air or oxygen.

Identify the cause of obstruction. Eliminate the cause if possible, or pass an endotracheal tube through or past it, or perform laryngotomy or tracheotomy to get below the obstruction. A totally obstructed patient can be partially relieved by inserting one or more large-bore hypodermic needles through the cricothyroid membrane.

LARYNGOTOMY

Lie the patient supine with extended neck. Make a horizontal stab incision between the cricoid and thyroid cartilages. Press the blade backwards until you feel the point enter the airway and air begins to hiss in and out through the wound with respiration (Fig. 49.1). With no loss of time, remove the knife and insert a small tube, curved downwards, inside the tracheal lumen. A correctly designed laryngotomy tube is flattened somewhat, so as to lie neatly between the cartilages, but if none is available use any type of tube – metal, rubber or plastic – even unsterile, if it maintains the airway. An improvised tube is difficult to keep in a correct position so control it manually until you can establish a stable airway. Unless the cause of acute asphyxia is quickly curable by removing an impacted foreign body or reducing angioneurotic oedema, perform an elective tracheostomy within 48 hours and close the laryngotomy incision.

EMERGENCY TRACHEOSTOMY

Always prefer laryngotomy to tracheotomy because it can be performed more quickly, with less haemorrhage. Rarely, if, for example, a subglottic lesion makes it impossible to perform laryngotomy and defies attempted incubation even through a rigid bronchoscope, you must perform emergency tracheostomy.

Lie the patient supine with extended neck by placing a sand bag or a 1-litre bag of fluid for intravenous infusion

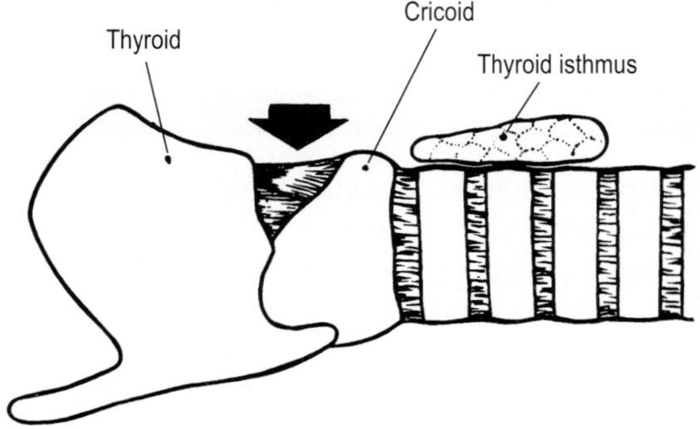

Fig. 49.1 Emergency laryngotomy: incision through cricothyroid membrane.

beneath the shoulders. Ensure the head is in a central position. Deliver oxygen by face-mask to give a few more minutes of operating time. If there is time, inject local anaesthetic such as 1% lidocaine with 1:100000 adrenaline (epinephrine).

Action

1 Cut vertically from the lower border of the thyroid cartilage in the midline, to the suprasternal notch. Deepen the incision and extend it between the strap muscles. Feel the first tracheal ring with the left index finger. Now divide the thyroid isthmus to expose the anterior tracheal wall. Control bleeding, which can be profuse, by pressure from an assistant. Decide quickly whether there is time to clamp major bleeding points before incising the trachea vertically through the second, third and fourth rings.

2 Insert a tracheal dilator to secure an airway. Introduce a tracheostomy tube. A cuffed tube prevents further aspiration of blood and allows ventilation, but is slightly more difficult to insert. Now control the worst of the bleeding. Use a tracheal suction catheter through the tube to clear blood that has already been aspirated into the trachea.

3 Subsequent decisions and procedures depend upon the cause of the obstruction and the patient's general condition. Monitor respiration and pulse during, and for several hours after, such a crisis. Institute assisted ventilation and/or cardiac resuscitation immediately postoperatively if necessary.

ELECTIVE TRACHEOSTOMY

This procedure is considerably easier to perform, in controlled conditions on an appropriately prepared and anaesthetized patient. Use either local or general anaesthesia. Ensure that you have available a correct-sized tracheostomy tube. If it has a cuff, test it for leaks. If you intend to ventilate the patient, use a plastic cuffed tube, not a metal one. Check the patency and security of connections from tube to anaesthetic equipment.

Action

1 Inject the surgical area with a solution of 1:200000 adrenaline (epinephrine) to help achieve haemostasis. Make a horizontal skin crease incision halfway between the cricoid cartilage and the suprasternal notch. Separate the pretracheal muscles vertically and divide the thyroid isthmus between artery clips. Seal the pretracheal vessels with diathermy just below the cricoid. Ligate the inferior thyroid veins, since diathermy is unreliable. Ligate or oversew the edges of the thyroid isthmus and expose the anterior tracheal wall. Having established haemostasis, make a 1–2-cm vertical incision, centred on the third or fourth tracheal ring (Fig. 49.2). Do not excise segments or cut flaps because there is a risk of subsequent stenosis. In addition, a tracheal flap may obstruct the passage of a tube.

▶ KEY POINTS Avoid extubation

- If a patient is accidentally extubated and the tube cannot be rapidly replaced, fatal respiratory obstruction can occur.
- Insert a strong stitch through the cut tracheal edge on each side and leave the ends long, protruding through the skin wound. These can be used to draw the trachea forwards and open the incision in it, to facilitate the reintroduction of a tube. This is particularly useful in paediatric tracheostomies.

2 Hold the tracheal incision open with a tracheal dilator. Ask the anaesthetist to remove the endotracheal tube to the subglottic level. Now insert, for example, a cuffed

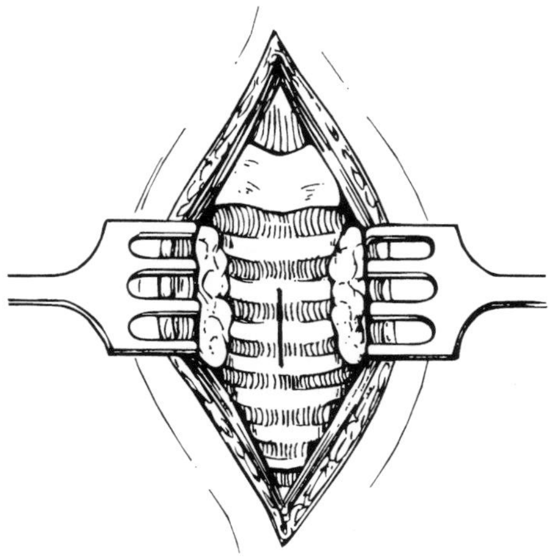

Fig. 49.2 Elective tracheostomy.

plastic tracheostomy tube. Inflate the cuff just sufficiently to prevent leakage around it when the anaesthetist inflates the patient's lungs. Overinflation of the cuff can lead to subsequent tracheal stenosis. The anaesthetist can now connect the tubing to the tracheostomy tube and withdraw the endotracheal tube. Have the endotracheal tube left until now, so that if there is any difficulty in inserting the tracheostomy tube, or, if the cuff bursts, the anaesthetist can continue to ventilate the patient through the endotracheal tube. When you have made certain there is no source of bleeding, close the skin loosely around the tube. Loose suturing allows drainage of any blood and also helps prevent air emphysema around the incision.

50

Oral and maxillofacial surgery

I. M. Laws

CONTENTS

GENERAL PRINCIPLES OF ORAL SURGERY

This chapter is limited to oral surgical procedures that as a trainee on rotation you are likely to assist with, some of which you may be invited to perform under supervision. The oral cavity is small, dark, sensitive and has a slippery surface. Patients may be nervous. They may tend to move their tongue or close their mouth at an inopportune moment. Consider giving intravenous sedation to anxious adults.

Ensure you have good illumination, arrange for adequate suction apparatus and make sure your assistant is efficient and can anticipate possible difficulties. If you operate under general anaesthesia, an endotracheal tube and a throat pack are required to prevent inhalation of blood and debris. Remember to remove the pack at the end of the operation.

Most minor procedures such as tooth extraction, biopsy, removal of salivary calculi and suturing of lacerations can be carried out using local analgesia. General anaesthesia is often preferable for children, patients with fluctuant abscesses and those allergic to local anaesthetic.

Hold the jaws apart with a prop or gag and stabilize the head in a rubber ring or horseshoe. Do not dislocate the jaw or scuff the lips, which tend to be dry following pre-operative anticholinergic drugs. Lightly coat the lips with petroleum jelly or keep them moist.

Prepare patients with bleeding disorders preoperatively. Achieve haemostasis by removing excess clot, suture tightly across a tooth socket and repair any lacerations. Apply pressure with a gauze pad for 10 minutes, timed by the clock. If necessary, lightly press resorbable haemostatic material, such as oxidized cellulose, into a bleeding socket. Sit the patient up at least 45° and if necessary give a sedative. Control secondary haemorrhage with pressure, treat infection with systemic and/or local antibiotics and prescribe 6% hydrogen peroxide mouthwashes.

For suturing, use a half-circle 22–24-mm needle with a reverse cutting edge and 000 sutures. Silk is easy to use, nylon is uncomfortable, both must be removed in 5–7 days. Polyglactin 910 remains intact in the mouth for 3–4 weeks and produces minimal reaction but the knots and ends are irritating. Insert the needle into the mucosa 3–5 mm from the edge, taking greater care on the more friable lingual edge. Use mattress sutures to give even tension and tie knots using the needle-holder rather than fingers.

Warn the patient that, until healing is complete, there may be constant discomfort because of the need to eat, swallow and speak.

If necessary prescribe analgesics, aspirin mixture to gargle, ice packs to reduce swelling, and recommend a soft diet. Following fixation of a fractured jaw make sure the patient does not inhale blood; have tools available to cut the wires if necessary. Give prophylactic antibiotics when operating on bone.

TOOTH EXTRACTION

Tooth removal is indicated when there is a large cavity in a painful tooth, a painful loose tooth resulting from periodontal infection, an alveolar abscess or a loose tooth following trauma that could be inhaled.

There are three basic types of extraction forceps and elevators to lever out broken roots. Obtain X-rays to reveal root patterns.

Action

1 As a rule have the patient seated, although the supine position is sometimes appropriate. Use local or general anaesthesia.

2 Stand in front of the patient for most extractions. Position the forceps blades on the buccal and lingual aspects of the tooth and push them under the gum as far as they will go along the root. Grip the tooth and move it to expand the socket. Deliver the tooth in the direction of the weakest wall generally the buccal. Avoid excessive force or you will fracture the jaw.

3 Squeeze the socket with your fingers to reduce the dead space and position a gauze pad for the patient to bite on until the clot has formed. Instruct the patient to avoid touching the clot for 24 hours, then bathe the wound frequently with warm saline until it heals. Inspect the socket if infection and pain develop a few days following extraction.

JAW INFECTIONS

DENTAL ABSCESS

Once pus has escaped from bone, its direction of spread is influenced by gravity and muscle attachments. Antibiotics given before there is significant fluctuation may suppress it. Order radiographs.

If there is no swelling, remove the tooth. Antibiotics are rarely required.

When fluctuation is present in the mouth, remove an accessible tooth and incise the swelling in the buccal sulcus or palate to release pus that has not emptied into the socket.

Pus around the muscles of mastication produces trismus and prevents easy access to posterior teeth. This usually presents as a submandibular abscess. Under endotracheal anaesthesia, incise the skin of the neck at the most dependent point of the swelling and parallel to the lower border of the mandible. Remove the diseased tooth when the acute phase is over.

CELLULITIS

Cellulitis involving the sublingual and submandibular spaces and the cervical fascial plane is named Ludwig's angina after the German surgeon who described it. It is usually caused by streptococcal infection, making breathing and swallowing difficult. Inspect an X-ray of the neck and mediastinum looking for gas bubbles. Administer parenteral penicillin, which will produce rapid improvement in early cases. Perform tracheostomy if dyspnoea threatens. If gas is present in the tissues, administer metronidazole.

OSTEOMYELITIS OF THE JAW

This rarely occurs in well-nourished populations. Most patients respond to long-term treatment with antibiotic therapy, but if the infection persists operation may be required at which the bone cortex is removed or drilled. For chronic disease the bone may need to be removed with subsequent bone grafting.

FACIAL FRACTURES

Facial injuries involve the nose, maxilla, zygoma and mandible. Fractures of the nose are dealt with in Chapter 49. Posterior and inferior displacement of the maxilla and blockage of the nose with blood clot causes respiratory distress. Bilateral fractures of the body of the mandible may result in lack of support for the tongue, which then falls back against the pharynx in a supine patient.

Exclude fractures of the skull and cervical fractures.

Emergency action

Respiratory obstruction from displacement of the maxilla will be relieved by pulling the maxilla forwards with a finger hooked around the back of the palate and following bilateral mandibular fractures by placing the patient in the recovery position.

Remove foreign bodies, such as broken teeth or dentures, from the mouth and pharynx. Plastic dentures are radiolucent and may not be apparent on a chest X-ray.

Unconscious patients with severe facial injuries generally require an elective tracheostomy.

Control persistent bleeding from the nose with posterior nasal packs.

Assess

Carefully look for deformity or loss of facial symmetry. Assess the number and position of teeth, and note any wear facets, in order to determine if the relationships have been altered. Identify and record the presence and site of skin lacerations.

Test for sensory loss to assess the possibility of nerve damage, including loss of smell, indicating possible olfactory nerve damage. Look for possible complications of fractures, such as diplopia and trismus. Carefully check for cerebrospinal fluid leakage from the nose or ear.

MANDIBLE

Plating is rigid and reduces the need for intermaxillary fixation and time off work. The technique is not difficult but intraoral access can make it complex. The plates are placed across the fracture line and where possible along the known stress lines in the jaw. Titanium is more malleable than steel but is less rigid. Neither needs to be removed unless it becomes infected or exposed. The plate, drill, screws and screwdriver must be made of the same metal to avoid electrolytic action. Alternatives are eyelet wiring, arch bars attached to the teeth, Gunning interdental splints or bandaging.

MAXILLA

A fractured maxilla is displaced posteriorly and inferiorly. Disimpaction involves moving the maxilla in the opposite directions after freeing it with disimpaction forceps. After disimpaction, fix the teeth in occlusion with a few wires round upper and lower teeth.

By applying pressure under the mandible, reduce the fracture between the maxilla and skull. Cranial fixation is then normally applied.

Reduction of the fracture may be difficult because of impaction of the bones and oedema. Access is easier after 3–4 days when the oedema has subsided. Inadequate reduction results in a concave profile that is difficult to correct.

Fixation may be from plating, a halo frame to which bones are fixed, and internal fixation with wires.

ZYGOMATIC COMPLEX (MALAR)

These are best treated within a week of injury, but allow excessive periorbital oedema to subside first. Through a small incision in the hairline skin and the temporalis fascia, insert a periosteal elevator (Fig. 50.1) to elevate the zygomatic arch.

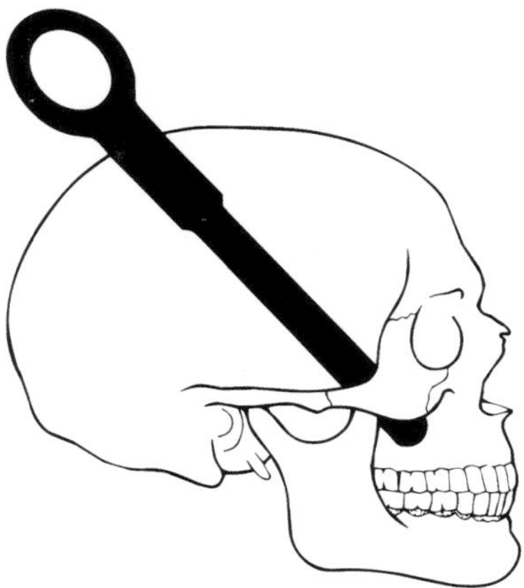

Fig. 50.1 Elevator under zygomatic arch.

FURTHER READING

Banks P, Brown A 2000 Fractures of the facial skeleton. Wright, Oxford

Ferraro JW 1997 Fundamentals of maxillofacial surgery. Springer, New York

Hawkesford J, Banks JG 1994 Maxillofacial and dental emergencies. Oxford University Press, Oxford

Langdon JD, Patel M 1998 Maxillofacial surgery. Chapman & Hall Medical, London

McGowan DA 1999 An atlas of minor oral surgery: principles and practice. Martin Dunitz, London

Miloro M 2004 Peterson's principles of oral and maxillofacial surgery, 2nd edn. Marcel Decker

Moore UJ 2000 Principles of oral and maxillofacial surgery, 5th edn. Blackwell Science, Oxford

51

Ophthalmology

J. D. Jagger, B. Mulholland

CONTENTS

INTRODUCTION

The procedures described here are semi-expert but do not require extraordinary technical skills. As a trainee you may encounter them during your rotations and have the valuable experience of assisting at some and even undertake some with the approval and supervision of your trainer. In an emergency make sure you work within your competence. Improve your appreciation of ophthalmic procedures by first revising the anatomy.

Many of the procedures described in this chapter can be carried out with small instruments available in a general surgical theatre. Ideally, however, a selection of special instruments will render these eye operations easier to perform:

- *Lid specula*: right and left, guarded, to keep the eyelashes away.
- *Forceps*: plain (Moorfields); 1-in-2 (Lister's); 1-in-2 fine (Jayle's or St Martin's); 2-in-3 fixation forceps; iris forceps (Barraquer's).
- *Scissors*: straight iris scissors; blunt-nosed straight and curved or spring conjunctival scissors; corneal scissors; De Wecker's iris scissors.
- *Knives*: disposable knife for entry into the anterior chamber (Alcon or Becton Dickinson) or diamond knife if available; Bard Parker handles with no. 11 and 15 blades.
- *Needle-holder*: coarse (Castroviejo); fine (Barraquer's).
- *Sutures*: black silk 3/0, 4/0, 6/0; 4/0, 6/0; synthetic absorbable such as Vicryl 4/0, 6/0, 8/0; nylon 9/0, 10/0; all these are available on atraumatic needles.
- *Muscle hooks*.
- *Iris repositors*.
- *Eyedrops and ointments*: antibiotics are chloramphenicol 0.5% and ofloxacin drops 0.3%, and fusidic acid (Fucithalmic) ointment 1% in gel; local anaesthetic drops are tetracaine (amethocaine) 1% and cocaine 4%, or proxymetacaine 0.5% (does not sting).

REMOVING AN EYE

The main indications for removal of an eye are irreparable injury with loss of sight, total or near total, severe pain in an already blind eye, or neoplasms such as a choroidal malignant melanoma that is too large for local irradiation.

There are two surgical approaches: Enucleation of the eyeball is removal from within Tenon's capsule – the sheet of connective tissue beneath the conjunctiva that covers both the eye and the insertion into it of the ocular muscles. Evisceration is removal of the contents after excising the cornea but the eyeball is not removed as the sclera is left in situ. It is often reserved for blind eyes with obvious gross intraocular infection but with no evidence of malignancy. Mobility of the prosthetic eye is better following evisceration than following enucleation.

ENUCLEATION

A general anaesthetic is usual but, in severely ill patients, local anaesthesia, including a retrobulbar injection of 1.5 ml of lidocaine 1% with adrenaline (epinephrine), may be adequate.

Sit at the head of the table and put in an eye speculum to separate the lids. Keep the lids about 20 mm apart by tightening the screw. Carry out a peritomy (incision of the conjunctiva around the rim of the cornea) by first opening the conjunctiva close to the edge of the cornea and encircling it. Undermine the conjunctiva backwards, allowing you to reach and open Tenon's capsule (the fibrous sheath enveloping the eyeball). Next expose the extraocular muscles through Tenon's capsule, and cut them.

Dislocate the globe forwards and divide the optic nerve. Attain haemostasis by packing the socket.

An orbital implant may be inserted, such as a ball, within Tenon's capsule. Finally, close the conjunctiva as a separate layer with 6/0 or 8/0 synthetic absorbable suture.

PROTECTING THE EYE: TARSORRHAPHY

Stitching the lids together may be done either centrally, which of course obscures vision, or laterally, where the protection given is due to the shortening and consequent narrowing of the palpebral fissure. Reserve central tarsorrhaphy for inability to close the lids (lagophthalmos) as this is a serious danger to the covering of the cornea, or for when ulceration is actually present. This type of tarsorrhaphy is indicated also when severe or protracted ulceration occurs for other reasons, for example in a numb cornea.

Strapping the lids, or supergluing the lashes together, may well suffice if the protective covering is required for a short period only.

In all cases, use local anaesthesia with tetracaine (amethocaine) 1% drops to the conjunctiva and 1% lidocaine with adrenaline (epinephrine) infiltration into the lid substance, both subcutaneously and subconjunctivally.

In tarsorrhaphy proper, prepare raw surfaces of the lid margins by simply dividing the lid into anterior and posterior layers through the 'grey line' (Fig. 51.1). Now insert horizontal mattress sutures of double-armed 4/0 black silk between the lids to draw them together. Put on antibiotic ointment and bandage the eye over paraffin gauze or non-adherent dressing and a pad only if bleeding has been excessive. Uncover the next day. Inspect again in a week and remove the sutures after 2 weeks.

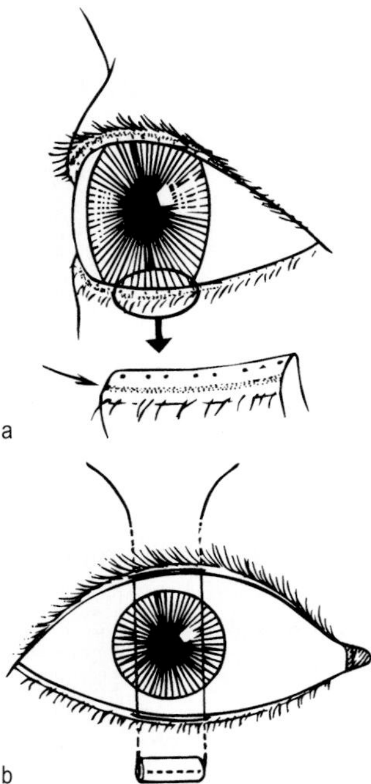

Fig. 51.1 Tarsorrhaphy: (a) division through the 'grey line'; (b) inserting the sutures.

EYELID INJURIES

Lacerations heal well, but there are important points to remember. If the lid margin is involved, try to appose the edges as accurately as possible. Use 6/0 Vicryl for the skin but try to insert a suture of 6/0 silk through the lid margin itself. Enter the needle on one side through the grey line 2–3 mm from the cut edge, emerging in the latter a similar distance down the cut and then in reverse through the other edge. After tying the suture, leave the ends 3 cm long and strap them down, then check that they do not abrade the cornea. Use the skin sutures to tie over the long ends of the lid margin sutures to keep them out of the eye.

If the lids are widely split, suture the tarsal plate before tackling the skin.

INJURIES OF THE GLOBE

LACERATIONS

- *Conjunctiva.* Leave small cuts (less than 5 mm) alone. Suture larger ones under local anaesthesia with interrupted 8/0 synthetic absorbable at 4-mm intervals, removing any prolapsed Tenon's capsule if excessive, or burying it.

- *Cornea and sclera*. Insert a speculum, and find and remove foreign bodies. Glass from windscreens is especially difficult. Put a drop of fluorescein in the eye; it may help to show small particles as well as corneal epithelial loss. Always X-ray a lacerated eyeball.

If obvious foreign bodies are present in the anterior chamber only, attempt to remove them with the finest small-bladed forceps under high magnification after re-forming the anterior chamber with Viscoelastic. Do this only during a procedure for a lacerated cornea. There is no substitute for Viscoelastic, so do not attempt to re-form the anterior chamber if none is available.

Insert sutures into clean lacerations of less than 5 mm only if aqueous humour is leaking. Place the stitches in, but not through, the tissue (Fig. 51.2). Enter and emerge about 1–1.5 mm from the wound edge. If the wound is irregular prefer to cover it with a conjunctival flap; cut the conjunctiva at the limbus, undermine it, and suture it in place with 9/0 or 10/0 nylon to cover the laceration.

BLUNT INJURIES

Evacuation of hyphaema

Hyphaema (Greek *hypo* = under + *haima* = blood; bleeding into the anterior chamber) is invariably treated conservatively initially, with bed rest and topical steroids to reduce the risk of further bleeding, such as dexamethasone (Maxidex) 0.1% four times a day. Cover the eye with a shield.

Ruptured globe

A totally disrupted eyeball may require enucleation, either immediately or within a few days of the injury, and the same applies to badly lacerated and collapsed eyes. Take the decision for enucleation, bearing in mind the possibility of the dreaded complication of sympathetic ophthalmia. Months, or even years later, the unaffected eye develops panuveitis with sight-threatening sequelae including glaucoma and cataract. Smaller posterior ruptures with some preservation of function may be diagnosed by the finding of a deep anterior chamber and chemosis from loss of the vitreous humour. An ophthalmic surgeon might explore the eye. You should manage the rupture conservatively.

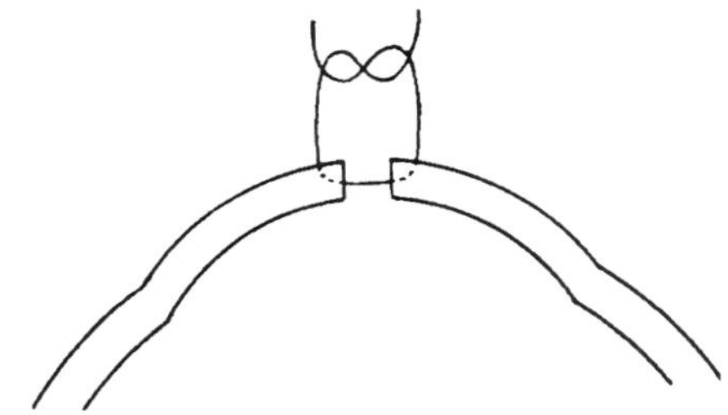

Fig. 51.2 Corneal and scleral sutures.

FOREIGN BODIES

INTRAOCULAR FOREIGN BODIES

These require specialist intervention if it is available. It is important that you recognize the possibility of the condition. A foreign body is easily missed when the entry wound is small and the initial disturbance minimal. If there is a history of something going into the eye, especially while hammering and chiselling, and you cannot detect a foreign body on superficial inspection, promptly order an X-ray of the orbit. Most small intraocular foreign bodies are sterile. Be willing to wait if this allows more favourable conditions for treatment. A large foreign body may cause a penetrating injury that requires to be dealt with in itself.

SUBTARSAL FOREIGN BODIES

Remove these by everting the upper eyelid after instilling proxymetacaine, tetracaine (amethocaine), oxybuprocaine or cocaine. Have a cotton-wool swab to hand before starting. Ask the patient to look down and keep doing so. Grasp the upper lid lashes with the thumb and forefinger of one hand and pull the lid down and forwards. With an orange stick, press the upper edge of the tarsal plate downwards (some 4 mm from the lid margin) and then lift the lashes so as to rotate the lid over the orange stick, which pushes the tarsal plate down and under the lid margin at the same time.

Once the eyelid is everted, keep hold of the lashes and press them against the eyebrow, instructing the patient meanwhile to keep looking down. Remove the orange stick and use your freed hand to remove the foreign body with the cotton-wool swab. Return the lid to its normal position by withdrawing both hands and asking the patient to look up.

CORNEAL FOREIGN BODIES

If you suspect the foreign body to be deep within the cornea, manipulation may push it into the anterior chamber. Unless you are expert, with available equipment, avoid tackling it. Superficial corneal foreign bodies can be removed after anaesthetizing the eye. Make sure you have a good light focused on the cornea, and magnification. Very superficial foreign bodies may be brushed off with a cotton-wool swab. Embedded foreign bodies require to be needled out. Insert a 19G disposable needle tangentially to the cornea to get behind the foreign body. Do not insert the needle directly at the foreign body but enter the cornea a little to the side. Lever the foreign body out. If any rust is left behind, attempt to pick it out, but do not persist too long. Rust that is slight and milk-chocolate in colour will disappear by itself. Remove as much dark rust as can be delivered easily. You may be able to remove more after a few days of softening up, inserting chloramphenicol ointment, three times a day.

Pad the eye after putting in an antibiotic ointment. Put in a mydriatic drug (a pupil dilator) according to the degree of required manipulation. If it was easy, no mydriatic is required; if it was moderately easy, homatropine 2% drops suffices; if it was very difficult, insert atropine 1% drops. Monitor the patient daily until it has healed and no longer stains with fluorescein.

BURNS

Chemical burns

Immediately concentrate on removing any matter mechanically and, in particular, copiously irrigate the eye using any harmless fluid you have at hand. Do not hunt for specific antidotes. If the cornea is affected, apply antibiotic/steroid ointments such as Maxitrol, containing dexamethasone 0.1%, neomycin sulphate 0.35%, hypromellose 0.5%, polymyxin B sulphate 6000 IU drops, or Sofradex containing dexamethasone 0.05%, framycetin sulphate 0.5% and gramicidin 0.005% drops, and atropine. Keep the conjunctival fornices patent to prevent symblepharon (Greek *syn* = together + *blepharon* = eyelid; adhesion of the eyelids to the eyeball), by twice-daily passing a glass rod between the lids and the eyeball after anaesthetizing the eyeball with oxybuprocaine 0.4% (Benoxinate) or tetracaine (amethocaine) hydrochloride 0.5% drops. Always admit patients with lime burns for observation as the effects may be delayed and you may need to institute half-hourly drops including vitamin C in high dosage. Also encourage the patient to eat citrus fruits, since vitamin C is an antioxidant and a cofactor in collagen synthesis.

Thermal burns

Treat those affecting the lids as skin burns elsewhere, but problems of ocular protection may arise. If there is loss of skin following a thermal burn, the ocular surface may also be severely damaged by the injury. If there is exposure of the cornea, apply lubricants such as hypromellose 1.0% and try to produce a moist chamber. In the longer term it will be necessary to reconstruct the lids using tissue from elsewhere, such as skin from behind the ear and hard palate grafts to recreate the tarsal plate.

INFECTIONS AROUND THE EYE

PYOGENIC INFECTIONS

These usually arise in the lids. A stye is an infection of a sebaceous gland of the lid. Meibomian cysts result from inflammation of glands on the under surface of the lids. Inflammation in the tear ducts – the lacrimal (Latin *lacrima* = tear) apparatus – is termed acute dacryocystitis (Greek *dacryon* = tear). Rarely, cellulitis within the orbit may point. Avoid incision wherever possible but, in the presence of a tense abscess causing pain, release it. A local anaesthetic may not be necessary for treating acute dacryocystitis if it is obviously pointing. Incise it from below the inner palpebral (Latin = eyelid) ligament/medial central tendon, downwards and outwards for 15 mm, parallel to the orbital margin. You do not need to drain it.

Infections of the eyeball itself may be localized, as for example a pyogenic corneal ulcer, or widely disseminated, as when a metastatic infection lodges in the choroid, spreading thence to the vitreous and all parts of the eye. A corneal ulcer may perforate and require a conjunctival flap to cover it and help it to heal. It may also be accompanied by pus in the anterior chamber (hypopyon); if this is unresponsive to intensive local and systemic chemotherapy, you may need to perform paracentesis to obtain a specimen for microscopy and culture. Application of superglue may provide emergency treatment of corneal perforation. Anaesthetize the eye first with tetracaine (amethocaine). Apply 2–3 drops of superglue to the perforation after drying the cornea with a sterile swab. Cover the eye with a bandage contact lens.

EVISCERATION

If the vital internal structures of the eye are destroyed by infection, with loss of vision, evisceration is indicated rather than enucleation, since mobility is better following evisceration. If you have any suspicion of an intraocular tumour, however, choose enucleation.

Insert a speculum to separate the eyelids. Cut off the cornea. Steady the eye by grasping the insertion of a rectus muscle with toothed forceps. Now cut through the periphery of the cornea circumferentially over a 5-mm length by progressively deepening a scalpel incision. Use the belly of a Bard Parker no. 15 blade or ophthalmic blade. Once you have entered the anterior chamber, cut right round the edge of the cornea with corneal scissors, if they are available; alternatively, use any narrow-bladed, blunt-nosed scissors.

Having topped the eye, scoop out all its contents – lens, iris and retina as well as the humours. It is important to do this thoroughly. A special scoop is available, but a large and not-too-sharp curette is adequate. End by wrapping gauze round it to wipe away all the remnants of the uvea (Latin *uva* = grape. Galen likened the choroid and iris as resembling a grape with the stalk torn out). Inspect the cavity to make sure that all that is left is sclera. Recent practice is to sever the optic nerve, split the posterior sclera and insert the implant behind the scleral remnant to reduce the risk of extrusion – a technique for the specialist. Finally, pack the socket with paraffin gauze, and apply a pad and bandage. Dress in 48 hours. No suture is required.

GLAUCOMA

Chronic open-angle glaucoma is difficult for a non-specialist to recognize. Acute glaucoma produces sudden pain, loss of vision, headache, nausea and vomiting. It may be preceded by episodes of seeing haloes in the evenings. The eye appears red, with a swollen conjunctiva and the pupil may be mid-dilated and unresponsive to light. The corneal reflex is often cloudy or glassy in appearance.

Treat acute angle-closure glaucoma with miotics (Greek *myein* = to blink, close; hence, causing pupillary closure), such as pilocarpine 4% 1 drop every hour, the beta-blocker timolol maleate 0.5% (Timoptol-LA) twice daily, dexamethasone 0.1% (Maxidex) four times a day. Since patients with chronic open-angle glaucoma are asymptomatic they may be managed with timolol maleate 5% or prostaglandin analogues such as latanoprost (Xalatan) 1 drop each day.

In primary acute closed-angle glaucoma the pressure can usually be lowered adequately, if temporarily, by acetazolamide (Diamox), 500 mg intravenously, miotic drops and osmotic agents.

NEOPLASMS

The most common important ocular neoplasms affect the lids and the uveal tract.

Small benign lesions of the lid

These can be removed by cautery or a variety of methods of excision under local anaesthetic or even lidocaine 2.5%, prilocaine 2.5% (EMLA) cream.

Larger benign and malignant lesions of the lid

Carefully decide upon the surgical approach after noting the size of the lesion and its position in relation to the lid margins. You need to remove at least 3 mm beyond the visible margin of the lesion of a malignant lesion, to allow for possible microscopic extension.

For larger lesions away from the lid margin, you may excise the lesion and arrange a local skin flap. Alternatively, insert a free graft of skin from the contralateral upper lid. As you distend the skin with the preoperative anaesthetic injection of 2% lidocaine with added adrenaline (epinephrine) to reduce bleeding, you can ensure that the graft is of adequate size, and also that you can close the donor site.

Major reconstructive surgery of the eyelids is beyond the scope of this section. Intraocular malignancies are again a matter for the specialist, but the general principle applies that, for lesions of any size (which to the non-specialist means any degree of obviousness), enucleation is indicated.

FURTHER READING

Collin JRO 1993 A manual of systematic eyelid surgery. Churchill Livingstone, Edinburgh

Leatherbarrow B 2002 Oculoplastic surgery. Martin Dunitz. London

Tyers AG, Collin JRO 1997 Colour atlas of ophthalmic plastic surgery. Butterworth-Heinemann, Oxford

Willshaw H 1993 Practical ophthalmic surgery. Churchill Livingstone, Edinburgh

Internet website

www.eyetext.net

Index

Note: Page numbers in *italics* refer to figures and tables.

B

C

D

G

H

I

M

N

O

P

Q

R

S

X

Z